HISTORY OF
THE SECOND WORLD WAR

UNITED KINGDOM MEDICAL SERIES

Editor-in-Chief:

SIR ARTHUR S. MACNALTY, K.C.B., M.A., M.D., F.R.C.P., F.R.C.S., F.S.A.

MEDICAL SERVICES IN WAR

THE PRINCIPAL MEDICAL LESSONS OF THE SECOND WORLD WAR

Based on the Official Medical Histories of the United Kingdom, Canada, Australia, New Zealand and India

EDITED BY

Sir ARTHUR SALUSBURY MacNALTY, K.C.B.

and

W. FRANKLIN MELLOR

Respice, Prospice

LONDON

HER MAJESTY'S STATIONERY OFFICE

1968

First published *1968*

© *Crown copyright 1968*

Printed and published by
HER MAJESTY'S STATIONERY OFFICE

To be purchased from
49 High Holborn, London W.C.1
423 Oxford Street, London W.1
13A Castle Street, Edinburgh 2
109 St. Mary Street, Cardiff CF1 1JW
Brazennose Street, Manchester 2
50 Fairfax Street, Bristol 1
258–259 Broad Street, Birmingham 1
7–11 Linenhall Street, Belfast BT2 8AY
or through any bookseller

Price £8 0s. 0d. net

EDITORIAL BOARD

EDITORIAL COMMITTEE

ACKNOWLEDGEMENTS

The Editors wish to express their thanks to the War Historians of the Royal Navy, Army and Royal Air Force Medical Services and to those of Canada, Australia, New Zealand and India for their contributions to this volume and for the valuable assistance they have given to its inception and progress.

They desire also to take this opportunity to place on record their appreciation of the research work carried out by Miss F. E. E. Harney, of the Ministry of Health, on this and previous volumes of the United Kingdom Official Medical History of the Second World War. In the task of finding, sorting and evaluating the 'bricks of History' and of ensuring their use to the best advantage, her collaboration has been invaluable.

FOREWORD

By The Right Hon. The Viscount Portal of Hungerford, K.G., G.C.B., O.M., D.S.O., M.C., *Marshal of the Royal Air Force.*

IN THIS volume of the *Official Medical History of the Second World War* the principal medical lessons of the war are set forth. The contributors to this endeavour are not restricted to the Editors of the nineteen volumes of the United Kingdom *History* which have been published since 1952. They include also the Editors of the various Commonwealth Medical Histories of the War, namely, those of Canada, Australia, New Zealand and India.

In no previous war—not even the First World War—were the whole resources of the nation more universally applied and brought to bear on achieving victory. For the Second World War was a strife of Nations as well as of armies. The aeroplane had abolished the island security of Great Britain against raiders and possible invasion. Hitler, imitating the attitude of Louis XIV who exclaimed when his Bourbon grandson became King of Spain, 'There are no more Pyrenees', declared, 'There are no more islands'. Hence in planning, the security of the civilian population had to be considered. The chapters in this volume show how this was done through nutrition (food rationing), evacuation of women and children from populous cities and towns, air-raid precautions, and the Emergency Medical Services, which provided for the care and treatment of the Fighting Services as well as for civilians. Hand-in-hand with such measures were the arrangements for rehabilitation, for calling up doctors for the Fighting Services and for maintaining the medical needs of civilians in hospitals and in their own homes.

In medical organisation great results were achieved. As important instances the Blood Transfusion Service which saved countless lives, the surgical units near the front line which dealt with wounded promptly and efficiently and the air evacuation of wounded and other casualties, may be cited. All these measures reduced wastage of man-power.

Medical research, both before and in the course of the war controlled many diseases, for example, malaria, cerebro-spinal fever and typhus, which had often proved fatal to combatants in previous wars. Active immunisation by toxoid injections against tetanus, a type of wound infection so deadly in the War of 1914–18, proved its value. Preventive inoculation by a vaccine and delousing with D.D.T. reduced the severity of louse-borne typhus fever and brought the serious epidemic in Naples in 1943–44 to a rapid end. The greatest practical advance was made in the control of malaria. In this volume the various methods in

ix

use are described. They kept the infection in check among the Allied troops, even in hyperendemic areas like Burma and Assam where, otherwise, the disease instead of force of arms might have been decisive. The value of the sulphonamides for various infective diseases was more accurately defined and new preparations of these drugs were introduced and studied.

In the later stages of the war co-operation with the United States of America in the production of penicillin assured its wider use and saved thousands of lives. It was followed by the discovery of other antibiotics which prove efficacious in a whole range of diseases due to bacterial infection, including tuberculosis.

In all these medical matters, administration as well as prevention and treatment, success was sometimes neither spectacular nor uniform, but on balance it was achieved and played a great part in the winning of the war.

The experience of the past is indispensable for future training and organisation. Hence all medical officers in the Armed and Civilian Medical Services should be acquainted with this book.

PORTAL OF HUNGERFORD

CONTENTS

xi

CONTENTS

INTRODUCTION

'He who neglects the lessons of history is condemned to
repeat them.' GEORGE SANTAYANA.

A SURGEON of the American Civil War wrote 'Any Government that fails to record the medical experiences of war commits a crime against the State and against those who may be called upon in future to aid in the defence of their country'.

Conversely, when such experiences have been set out and their lessons distilled for all to see, it becomes a crime to disregard them. To regard history—even recent history—as 'Bunk', as Henry Ford is alleged to have put it, is merely to close one's eyes to reality and one's mind to learning. It matters greatly that we remember something of what happened before and be armed against the necessity to relearn some of the old lessons the hard way all over again. This is particularly the case in war-time. Then the Medical Services of a nation become of paramount importance. Napoleon, although he approved of Baron Larrey's administration of the French Army Medical Services, ignored this consideration to his cost, especially in the Russian Campaign. In the Second World War their effectiveness greatly influenced the course of the struggle, particularly in the Far East, where the Allied Medical Services were manifestly superior to those of the adversary.

Today, in the Armed Services, health is prized above all else. It is a pre-requisite of military efficiency. In time of war no cost is reckoned too high if it can be preserved. When man-power is all-important every encouragement is given to those Services that can effect a reduction of wastage through preventable disease and the restoration of the wounded.

The manner in which these Services coped with their manifold problems is described in the Commonwealth Official Medical Histories. For the first time the Official Medical Historians collaborated closely in carrying out their respective tasks. A Liaison Committee, set up with the approval of the Commonwealth Governments in 1946, held meetings (to which the United States of America sent Observers) in Ottawa, Oxford, Canberra and New Delhi and provided a mechanism for a constant exchange of information and experience. Each national History has benefited thereby, both in accuracy and interpretation.

It is fitting, therefore, that this volume should include contributions from Canada, Australia, New Zealand and India. These countries saw the problems of war from their own standpoint and had to learn their own medical lessons. Some medical problems were common to all,

xiii

while others were peculiar to a particular country. The United Kingdom had, for example, many civilian as well as military medical problems to face and the lessons gained from the work of the Civilian and Colonial Medical Services and from that of the Medical Research Council take their place in this account. Each Historian realised the importance of putting on record the main lessons learnt and their joint experience and co-operation add to the comprehensive character of the volume.

Altogether, the Commonwealth Official Medical History volumes number 36. This volume is an epitome of and a guide to them. It offers handy reminders to those who find themselves concerned with the shaping of the present and future Medical Services and provides an opportunity for them to assimilate into their work the results of a vast and fruitful war-time experience.

If wars under new conditions and with new weapons should again menace the world many of the medical lessons of the Second World War will not be out of date. Some of them are fundamental and of permanent value.

The art of medicine, practised as it was by the Allied Medical Services during the war, with knowledge, ingenuity, courage and a high sense of responsibility, was no less important than the military victory. Both brought relief to the human spirit and a new lease of freedom.

W. FRANKLIN MELLOR

PART I

The United Kingdom

Detailed official accounts of the work of the United Kingdom Medical Services during the Second World War will be found in the following volumes.*

VOLUMES RELATING TO THE FIGHTING SERVICES

Royal Navy

The Royal Naval Medical Services . . . . .
Vol. I Administration . . . . } J. L. S. Coulter
Vol. II Operations . . . .

Army

The Army Medical Services
Vol. I Administration . . . . . .
Vol. II Administration . . . . . .

The Army Medical Services (Campaigns)
Vol. I Europe, Battle of Britain, Mediterranean, Middle East, Madagascar . . . } F. A. E. Crew
Vol. II Hong Kong, Malaya, Iceland, Faroes, Libya (1942–43), North West Africa . . .
Vol. III Sicily, Italy, Greece (1944–1945) . . .
Vol. IV North West Europe . . . . .
Vol. V Burma . . . .

Royal Air Force

The Royal Air Force Medical Services
Vol. I Administration . . . . . .
Vol. II Commands . . . . . . } S. C. Rexford-Welch
Vol. III Campaigns . . . . . .

VOLUMES RELATING TO THE CIVILIAN SERVICES

The Emergency Medical Services

Vol. I England and Wales . . . . .
Vol. II Scotland, Northern Ireland. Raids on Industrial } C. L. Dunn
Cities . . . .

The Civilian Health and Medical Services

Vol. I England and Wales . . . . . } Sir Arthur S.
Vol. II Scotland, Northern Ireland, the Colonies . MacNalty

Medical Research . . . . { F. H. K. Green and Sir Gordon Covell

Medical Statistics (Fighting and Civilian Services) not yet published.

CLINICAL VOLUMES

(Incorporating the experience of the Fighting and Civilian Services)

Medicine and Pathology . . . . . .
Surgery . . . . } Sir Zachary Cope

---

* Published by Her Majesty's Stationery Office, London.

The Royal Naval Medical Services

By Surgeon Captain C. H. Joynt, R.N.

CONTENTS

THE ROYAL NAVAL MEDICAL SERVICES

INTRODUCTION

IN A REVIEW of this length, it is not possible to give an account of all aspects of naval medical administration, and it is proposed to refer briefly only to a few major fields in which difficulties were experienced or deficiencies became apparent. Before doing so, it is perhaps necessary to outline cursorily the respective functions and responsibilities of the executive and the medical branch and their relationship to each other. In the Royal Navy, the executive is the responsible branch, and the medical and other branches act towards it, at all levels from Admiralty down to the individual ship or establishment, in the capacity of professional advisers. There is no medical chain of command as such, the senior medical officer of each ship or establishment being responsible directly to his commanding officer, and corresponding, on professional matters, with senior and other members of his branch through the command. The responsibility for accepting, modifying or rejecting professional advice rests with the command as, in consequence, does the contingent liability in the case of rejection of such advice. This system, which has been evolved over the centuries in response to long experience, arises in large part from the self-contained nature of the fighting ship and of the fleet or squadron at sea and, in general, works very well. It does, however, leave room for failure in certain circumstances, and matters of hygiene and preventive medicine did, sometimes, fail to receive the necessary priority and concern on the part of the executive in shore bases abroad.

By their nature, H.M. Ships are self-contained units in which health measures have been so carefully organised over the course of years that naval officers and ratings have come to accept them as a matter of course. Provided that the instructions concerning health and sanitation are observed, it should be impossible to obtain bad food or water. The seaman has for generations unwittingly observed the fundamental sanitary law of keeping his ingests separate from his egests by passing his excrement straight over the side of the ship into the sea, where it cannot possibly pollute food or flies. His ship has always been the sailor's home, accompanying him wherever he goes, affording him facilities for keeping himself and his clothes clean and allowing him changes of clothing which are an automatic safeguard against lice and typhus. So long as he remains in his ship he can isolate himself from the natives of primitive countries who are the chief reservoirs of many infectious diseases, and can avoid infection from insects which rarely travel far from shore across the water. The danger of this customary protection is, of course, that, in time, it comes to be taken for granted and may induce a sense of false security when circumstances change. This becomes most apparent when the sailor moves ashore. Several factors then come in. Firstly, precautions must be taken that are unaccustomed and may not appear to the executive to be very obviously necessary. The medical officer himself may not, because of lack of the necessary practical experience, be absolutely certain of what requires to be done and may, consequently, have difficulty in getting it across to the command. Unaccustomed to having to take an active interest in health matters, the command may not fully realise that the enforcing of hygienic measures to preserve the health, morale and fighting efficiency of their troops is as important as any other military duty. There may be a tendency to regard these as the doctor's concern, ignoring the circumstance that, as the doctor has no disciplinary powers and no resources of man-power beyond his own sick berth staff, who are normally fully occupied in work of a clinical nature, he is powerless to implement the necessary precautions without the active support of the executive. The importance of anti-malaria clothing, of the siting of sanitary arrangements, the provision of suitable facilities for ablution and a ceaseless campaign against flies, may not be realised and so not given the requisite priority. A state of affairs did come into being in some Commands, where such hygienic measures as were adopted were regarded as a purely medical responsibility and, worse still, it was implied that not only the responsibility but also the attendant liability was carried by the Medical Branch. It is not implied that this attitude was at all general, but that it existed is indicated by the issue of an Admiralty Fleet Order which, while primarily concerned with anti-malaria measures, indicated clearly that Their Lordships recognised it as the primary responsibility of the executive to ensure that the recommendations made by the Medical Branch for the prevention of preventable diseases were carried out. One of the operative paragraphs of this Order, which contained the gist of the matter, reads as follows:

'It is for medical officers, in consultation with medical officers of other units and Services in the same area, to advise on what anti-malaria measures are appropriate, but Their Lordships wish it clearly to be understood that they hold Flag and Commanding Officers responsible for ensuring that protective and preventive measures are undertaken and rigorously enforced. They desire that the provision of men for such duties as canalisation, oiling, digging trench latrines, where such measures are necessary, shall be regarded as of operational importance and shall have priority accordingly'. The last paragraph of this Order reads as follows: 'While malaria, owing to its supreme importance, has been specially selected in framing this Order, the same principles of discipline and responsibility apply equally to such preventable tropical diseases as dysentery, scrub-typhus and dengue. In fact, these principles should be implicit in all the measures taken to preserve the health of the Royal Navy. The medical officer can only advise as he has no executive authority over officers and ratings except when they are on the sick lists'. (Vol. I. *Admin.* p. 175.)

It ought to be stated here that there was never the slightest difficulty in convincing the executive of the necessity of such measures as were required for the treatment of the sick and wounded; difficulties, when they arose, were entirely concerned with preventive medicine and hygiene.

Another matter that occasionally caused difficulty was the necessity for secrecy and security about impending operations. The essential observation to be made here is that, if the full medical commitments of a ship (or, *a fortiori*, a fleet or squadron) were to be met in the course of an impending operation against the enemy, the medical department must be given sufficient information of the circumstances ahead, so far as they can be foreseen, to be able to make the necessary arrangements to meet them. This question arose on several occasions during the course of the Second World War. Some medical officers, including some holding appointments on the staffs of Flag Officers, complained that they were not fully acquainted with impending events. Other medical officers did not hold this view. There were, of course, occasions when security requirements granted Flag and Commanding Officers no discretion to reveal details of impending operations to members of their staffs and heads of departments. In cases where such discretion was allowed, it was doubtless exercised in different ways by different Flag and Commanding Officers, who would also be influenced in their decisions on a matter of such importance by their views on the character and discretion of the staff officer or head of department concerned. That this difficulty was not widespread is certain. That it did occur and occasionally gave rise to embarrassment is evident from the reports of several medical officers holding responsible appointments. It is obviously desirable that a medical officer should have sufficient notice to replenish or augment his supply of medical stores and to polish up final details of his organisation for action when the probability of its being called into action very shortly is apparent. That this notice was not always given is apparent from the following note in the action report of the medical officer of a cruiser which became heavily engaged during and subsequent to the landings in North Africa in 1942, who recorded that he had no knowledge of any impending operation or of the likelihood of enemy action until half an hour before the landings were carried out. He reports 'A brilliantly lighted port was visible in the distance, which I later discovered to be Algiers. At 0030 hrs. I was informed that we were part of a force for the invasion of North Africa. The beaches were actually

occupied half an hour later'. (Vol. II. *Ops.* p. 489.) The Senior Medical
Officer, Port Party 1500, who became responsible for the arrangements
for dealing with naval casualties at Arromanches states: 'It is fully
realised that in all intended naval and military operations, secrecy is
absolutely essential and vital, but this principle can be carried too far.
This is particularly so when officers, whose special departments are
expected to play a major part in the success of an enterprise, are not
fully informed of the object for which they have to plan. My own
experience of the Normandy landings was that I had to make repeated
requests before I could be fully informed of my responsibilities and
future commitments. By contrast, my Army opposite numbers, with
whom I was in daily consultation in combining our mutual medical
welfare, were always possessed of full information about what lay
ahead'. (Vol. II. *Ops.* p. 525.) This question of the difficulties caused
by considerations of security was not confined to the lower levels.
The Staff Medical Officer to the British Naval Commander at the time
of the North African landings remarks at some length on these matters,
and the Medical Department of the Navy (Admiralty) also had reason
for complaint. (Vol. II. *Ops.* p. 487.) It was not, in fact, until the
liberation of North Africa (Operation 'Torch') and the liberation of
Normandy (Operation 'Overlord') that the Department of the Medical
Director-General of the Navy was involved in the original medical
planning from the beginning. One important consequence of this
failure always to involve the medical department in forward planning
was the relative inexperience of the medical branch of the Navy
in Staff Operational Planning. This deficiency has been partly met,
or at all events lessened, by the inclusion of medical officers from time
to time in the Naval Staff Courses in post-war years.

NORTH RUSSIA (Vol. II. *Ops.* p. 417)

The provision, or lack of it, for the treatment in North Russia of
casualties and survivors of ships sunk during the severe and continued
battles fought by the Arctic Convoys in 1941 and 1942 came in for a
great deal of adverse criticism, some of it ill-informed but much,
unfortunately, justified. It is, therefore, worth while here to give a
brief outline of the nature of the problem, of the facilities available and
of some of the administrative difficulties, by no means all medical,
responsible for the admittedly unsatisfactory state of affairs which
prevailed. The places concerned were, firstly, the Kola Inlet area,
including Polyarnoe, nine miles north of Vaenga, Vaenga itself, and
Murmansk, eighteen miles further south, and secondly, Archangel. In
general, the convoys ended in the Kola Inlet between mid-December
and mid-July, and at Archangel during the remainder of the year when
the ice edge receded.

In the Kola Inlet area, apart from a small sick bay at Polyarnoe, staffed by one medical officer and a sick berth attendant, accommodating 20 beds in one room, with a second for use as a medical store and dispensary, reliance had to be placed on Russian hospitals for the treatment of casualties and survivors among Royal Naval personnel. At the start, late 1941 to early 1942, before enemy attacks on these convoys had really got into their stride, the reception of British patients in Russian hospitals in Murmansk was described as adequate and the local Russian authorities were very helpful. There were many conflicting reports on the conditions in these Russian hospitals, only one of which was a regular establishment, the others having been improvised in schools, etc. In general, it may be said that accommodation was very simple, there was much overcrowding, the sanitary arrangements were primitive and inadequate by British standards and, in view of the severity of the climate, the heating plants surprisingly insufficient. There was a great shortage of sulphonamides, plaster-of-Paris, narcotics and antiseptics, and a complete absence of inhalational and intravenous anaesthetics. On the other hand, the Russian nursing sisters were well-trained, competent and hard-working. There was, however, a great scarcity of them, most of the nursing being done by women of little experience. In general, the Russian medical officers were skilful and energetic, and they were always most helpful and co-operative. The Russian wards were desperately crowded and every available passage, hall and corridor was filled with beds or with patients still on stretchers, awaiting an empty bed. The Russians' difficulties were considerable. At one time the degree and effectiveness of enemy air attacks almost paralysed the life of Murmansk. There were periods of great activity on the North Russian front when casualties would arrive much faster than the hospitals could deal with them. As the attacks on the Arctic Convoys increased, the hospital accommodation of British casualties became progressively more difficult.

In contrast to the many favourable reports made on Russian hospitals in the area round the Kola Inlet, the corresponding reports on the medical and surgical facilities in the Archangel area seem to have been generally adverse. Archangel itself was not regarded as an agreeable place in which to arrive after running the gauntlet of the Arctic Circle convoy route. To the all-pervading smell of sewage, the consequence of the complete absence of any piped sewerage system (sewage lay in open cesspools in many places), was added in summer the annoyance of mosquitoes and other biting insects, while bed-bugs were a perpetual source of complaint. The local Russian hospitals did their best for British sick, but their beds were crowded and they suffered from severe lack of supplies. Absence of anaesthetics and occasional lack of skill were regarded as being responsible for much suffering among patients, especially where burns and fractures were combined. This combination of fractures and severe burns was a common feature in casualties from early Arctic Convoys, the result of air attack on ships, and was not experienced to anything like the same extent in land warfare, so that experience in dealing with it would necessarily be limited among the doctors and nursing staff of the Russian hospitals. In 1942, the British medical facilities at Archangel were limited to the nucleus of what had been a British Army Field Ambulance Unit for 18 beds, but from which the major in charge and his nursing orderlies had been withdrawn, leaving one Captain R.A.M.C., a sergeant dispenser, a corporal, a lance corporal and two orderlies, a cook and a carpenter. Their equipment consisted principally of consumables, most of which had already been expended. The unit maintained and manned two Medical Inspection Rooms at nearby ports and was responsible for a total of 90 R.N., Army and R.A.F. personnel scattered throughout the area.

If the strain on local resources at Archangel was already great in the early months of 1942, the demands which arose in mid-July of that year, with the arrival of the survivors of Convoy P.Q. 17, were incalculably more exacting, and it may be said that the local facilities were virtually overwhelmed. This convoy started out with 35 ships, of which only 11 completed the journey. It had been dispersed, and the surviving ships were stragglers, who made their way to Archangel largely independently and unescorted. During the first week in which these ships arrived, the total of survivors landed at Archangel reached 1,245, of whom 688 were British and Dutch and 557 American. They included 179 cases of immersion foot. None of these ships could send signals stating the number of cases to be accommodated and they staggered into port at indefinite times. Although many of these survivors were uninjured, 90 per cent. developed complaints of one sort or another. As they came in, improvised arrangements were made with the help of the Russians. For the hospital cases, such arrangements as were possible were made by the medical officer of the rescue ship *Zaafaran*, himself a survivor. This situation was dealt with and a base organisation set up, which, however, had to be run by any medical officer whose ship had been lost and who was awaiting return to the United Kingdom, so preventing the development of any continuity. In addition, transport was exceedingly difficult, with patients scattered in different hospitals over a wide area, and the greatest difficulty was experienced in getting the Russian authorities to allow visits to casualties and sick in ships in the anchorage. Efforts to provide hospital facilities under Naval medical control ashore at Murmansk and Archangel were made through the Admiralty and the Ministry of War Transport, and with the Russian Government through diplomatic channels, but, as will be shown later, without result by the time that Convoy P.Q. 18 was due to arrive in September, although it was known this convoy would be involved in strong enemy opposition and heavy casualties were anticipated. Fortunately, the medical officers of the escort of this convoy were able to arrange for survivors and casualties to be cared for afloat and to be nursed somehow on board until their arrival back in Scapa Flow. The year 1942 closed at Archangel without any change in the position which had provoked so much criticism among wounded and survivors there.

The reasons for the exiguous nature of Service medical arrangements in North Russia were complex and not a little due to the confused nature of the reports reaching the Admiralty from the local Naval authorities. A major part of the cause of this confusion was provided by the varying and alternating needs of the Kola Inlet and Archangel areas, according to which was acting as terminal port at the relevant time. To begin with, in the winter of 1941–42, in response to urgent appeals, the Admiralty sent two medical officers for duty ashore in North Russia. They were promptly sent back to the United Kingdom on the grounds that there was insufficient work ashore to occupy them. (Vol. II. *Ops.* p. 439.) In February 1942, the Admiralty was informed that the combined medical work at Archangel was insufficient to occupy the time of more than one Naval medical officer, and this report also commented favourably on the local hospital accommodation ashore. In May 1942, the Senior Naval Officer, North Russia, requested that either a hospital unit ashore or a hospital ship should be provided, but omitted to indicate where he required either to be. The Admiralty immediately prepared to send out 4 medical officers and 31 sick berth staff as a hospital unit and asked whether they were required for work at Archangel or in the Kola Inlet. On June 7, the S.N.O. indicated the need for the unit at Archangel, but four days later, signalled that the personnel for the unit were not necessary, and that the local Russian hospital resources were adequate for British requirements, provided that instruments and medicines could be supplemented. Meanwhile, the position ashore in the Kola Inlet remained uncertain so, on June 15, the Admiralty asked whether a hospital unit was required at Murmansk. The S.N.O. replied on the 16th, stating that such was not the case, but that one was required at Archangel! On June 19, a further signal was received from Archangel, asking for a medical officer ashore, but no medical stores or equipment. In view of this confusing series of contradictory communications, the Admiralty abandoned its plans and arrangements for a hospital unit in North Russia.

On July 30, the Commander-in-Chief, Home Fleet, expressed his great concern occasioned by the reports he was receiving as to conditions of casualties and survivors in North Russia, a concern that was fully shared by the Admiralty. On August 1, the Senior Naval Officer, North Russia, asked for a hospital unit to be sent to Polyarnoe, in the Kola Inlet. On August 17, medical stores and equipment and

4 medical officers, a dental officer, a warrant officer and sick berth staff were embarked in the U.S.S. *Tuscaloosa*, an American cruiser, to establish a Naval Auxiliary Hospital at Vaenga, in the Kola Inlet. The unit arrived on August 23. But immediately the divergent needs and alternating periods of activity between the Murmansk and Archangel administrations were revealed. The Senior Naval Officer, North Russia, decided to send two-thirds of the unit to Archangel at once, keeping the remainder for duty at Vaenga. The two-thirds arrived at Archangel but were never allowed to land, the result being that the unit returned to England forthwith, thus depleting the needs of Murmansk without any benefit to Archangel. Meanwhile, the remaining one-third of the unit which had remained behind in the Kola Inlet continued its preparations to set up a naval auxiliary hospital at Vaenga. On September 21, the Commander-in-Chief of the Soviet Northern Fleet received orders from Moscow that the arrangements for this hospital were suspended and that the unit was to be returned to England in Convoy Q.P. 15. Steps were taken to implement these instructions to withdraw, but on September 25, negotiations for the retention of this hospital were reopened at diplomatic level. These negotiations continued until October 2, when the Russian Government gave permission for 'a certain number of British medical collaborators' to work in Soviet hospitals, but refused permission for a separate British Service medical establishment to be set up on shore.

The Admiralty now decided to provision, staff and equip one of the Arctic Convoy Rescue ships as a small hospital ship, for permanent service as a base hospital at Kola Inlet. But barely had this project been raised when, on October 5, the Russian Goverment approved the establishment of a Royal Naval Auxiliary Hospital ashore at Vaenga Bay. This establishment opened towards the end of the year and, before it eventually closed, it received and treated altogether 735 patients. These figures included casualties sustained in some of the most severe actions of the Arctic convoy route, and the knowledge that a British hospital existed at Vaenga was a great stimulant to the morale of the Royal and Merchant Navy Fleet in Northern Waters. All attempts to make similar arrangements at Archangel were frustrated by Russian refusal to permit the opening of such an establishment in that area.

One further example of the difficulties experienced in North Russia is exemplified by the advance efforts made, independently of those just described, to provide for medical care of casualties and survivors from Convoy P.Q. 18 on their arrival in Archangel. As mentioned above, it was known that this convoy would meet with severe enemy opposition. With this contingency in view, a medical officer and 8 sick berth ratings, with stores and equipment, were sent to Archangel during August in H.M.Ss. *Blankney* and *Middleton*. On August 29, these personnel and stores were still embarked at Archangel and had not been permitted to land. On September 12, when the P.Q. 18 convoy battle was reaching its height and casualties were already known to be severe, the British ambassador in Moscow was refused permission, by the Russian Government, for the disembarkation of this hospital unit. On September 14, permission was given for the stores and equipment to be landed, but on September 14 the personnel had to be transferred to H.M.S. *Palomares* and returned to the United Kingdom.

The reasons for the tragic story of the attempts to make adequate provision for the care of casualties and survivors from the gruelling and cruel convoy battles on the Arctic Convoy route have been made sufficiently clear above. They may be summed up in the confusion occasioned by the intermittent and alternating nature of the requirements at the terminal ports, and active opposition on the part of the Russian Government authorities to the establishment of any non-Russian medical establishment ashore.

RESCUE OF SURVIVORS AT SEA
(Vol. II. *Ops.* pp. 449-463)

A parallel problem in connexion with the Arctic convoys was that of providing for the rescue of survivors from ships sunk during the heavy, prolonged attacks by aeroplanes, submarines and, occasionally, surface vessels, to which the merchant ships and the escorts were subjected for days on end, both going to and returning from Russia. The majority of losses were of merchant ships. The relatively small number of wounded to be treated among the large numbers of survivors was very noticeable, in contrast to the state of affairs observed when survivors were rescued in warmer climates. Among the reasons for this may be mentioned the following:

(i) A large number of deaths occurred instantaneously, probably due to the fact that a large number of ammunition ships blew up when hit, leaving few, if any, survivors.

(ii) Most ships sank very quickly, so that they had to be abandoned rapidly. It is no adverse reflection on the crews of these ships to say that this meant that, in some cases at least, the injured were not removed but were left on board.

(iii) Such injured and shocked casualties as did manage to escape did not survive many minutes in the very low temperature of the water. A number of ships reported that bodies, obviously badly injured, were seen floating in the sea.

In any case, as will be shown later, the nature of the weapons used, U-boats and torpedo-bombers predominating, meant that on the whole casualty rates were fairly low. Although wounds were relatively few in number, exposure proved a formidable problem, about 30 per cent. of all survivors needing strenuous medical attention for this reason. It is also of interest to note that the effects of exposure were severe despite the fact that rescue was always reasonably prompt. Three degrees of severity of effects of exposure were met with:

(i) Cold but dry. These cases usually came from lifeboats, and commonly responded quickly to warmth and hot drinks.

(ii) Wet, slightly shocked but conscious. This group included the majority of the survivors rescued. They had usually been in the sea for up to 20 minutes, and their condition seemed to depend largely upon the quantity of clothing they had been wearing at the time of abandoning ship. Treatment consisted in removing their wet clothing and wrapping them in blankets. When their shivering had ceased, they were usually fit to be given clothing and to join their companions. Navy rum was of great value in dealing with both these categories, but some experienced medical officers considered that it should not be given until clothing had been changed and recovery assured, because otherwise these men were inclined to lie about without making any effort to get dry and fixed up for clothing and accommodation, etc.

(iii) Grossly shocked, pupils widely dilated, limbs rigid, unconscious and stomach and lungs containing oil fuel. These men had usually been in the water for 30 minutes or more in varying degrees of undress. When brought on board, they were taken to a warm compartment, clothing was removed and they were wrapped in blankets. Artificial respiration was started at once and intra-muscular injections of camphor were considered to be of value. Mouth, nostrils and eyes were cleared of oil fuel. As soon as breathing became deeper and more regular, these patients were left until the pulse became palpable and the pupils began to contract. A prolonged bout of shivering now followed, after which consciousness would return. The patient was then moved to a warm billet and sleep induced. Warm drinks were of no value in these cases after return of consciousness, as they invariably resulted in the vomiting of blood-stained froth mixed with oil fuel. These men usually took 48 hours to recover, provided that no complications occurred meanwhile.

In order to deal with this problem of the rescue of survivors from ships sunk in the Arctic convoys, an extensive organisation was soon developed. All ships soon learned that an internal organisation was necessary. In general, survivors were received in an easily accessible, warm space, adjacent to the upper deck, where they could be quickly sorted into categories. In many ships, especially the smaller, no attempt was made to set aside sleeping accommodation for uninjured survivors, it being considered essential that the ship's company, upon whom depended the safety of the ship and survivors alike, should retain their own customary sleeping billets for such short periods as they could contrive to use them, while the uninjured survivors had to make use of such space as they could find elsewhere on board.

It soon became apparent, however, that further and special provision must be made for the rescue of survivors from the sea and for their subsequent care, which did not involve ships of the escort stopping to pick them up, exposing themselves to danger of attack while so occupied and denuding the convoy of cover and protection. As a result, the Rescue Ships were devised, and altogether twenty-one of them were in service during the war at various times. They were administered by the Ministry of War Transport in association with the Trade Division of the Admiralty. They performed much useful and gallant work in the saving of thousands of ship-wrecked personnel on convoy service. They were a mixture of Royal and Merchant Navies both in personnel and in administrative control, flew the Red Ensign and were in no sense 'Red Cross' ships, though their duties included that of acting as hospital ships for the convoy with which they sailed. They were 'hired' ships, of about 1,000 to 2,000 tons, most of them capable of 10 to 13 knots, were coalburners having a range, without re-fuelling when specially bunkered, of 3,000 to 5,000 miles, specially equipped for rescuing survivors from wrecked and blitzed ships in convoy. Their crews averaged about 70, made up of master, officers and crew, all Merchant Navy, one Naval medical officer with two sick berth attendants, and a mixed gunnery crew of Royal Navy and Army gunners. They had bed accommodation for 100–150 survivors and mattresses for as many more. Each had a well-equipped sick bay and also carried complete sets of clothing for 200 survivors. The British Sailors' Society, Women's Voluntary Services and many Naval welfare societies kept them well stocked with comforts and amenities. Rescue nets were fitted along the sides and it was found that nets on booms that could be swung out at right-angles near the bows were very desirable to prevent men being swept out and away by the bow wave. There were two cranes forward in the well deck, from which could be swung out large baskets, each capable of lifting two men at a time. There were also large numbers of life-belts, heaving lines and ropes, which could be thrown to men in the sea. Much difficulty was often experienced in getting on board men who were covered in oil fuel. It was necessary for somebody to climb down the rescue nets with heaving lines which they tried to pass round the chest of the survivor. Even then, the line was liable to slip and allow the man to fall back into the sea. A not uncommon feature, observed in other waters as well as in the Arctic, was that many survivors who had managed to get themselves to the point of being helped from the sea, collapsed when safety was within reach, and required to be handled in the same manner as those who had been helpless while still in the water.

The commonest injuries treated were compound fractures of the limbs, head injuries and burns and scalds. Plasma transfusions were given when necessary.

TRANSPORT OF SICK AND WOUNDED
(Vol. I. *Admin.* p. 119)

The provision of hospital ships raised a serious problem throughout the war, one that was immeasurably increased when it became necessary to make provision for them to accompany the British Pacific Fleet as part of the Fleet Train, where great endurance, reasonable speed, oil fuel and reliability were essential to enable them to keep within reach of the Fleet. The finding of suitable ships was very difficult and they were a source of constant complaint, on the part of Flag Officers handicapped by their shortcomings, and of the medical staffs who sailed in them. The principal defects might be summed up as excessive age, insufficient speed, poor accommodation for staff and difficulty in providing accommodation for tuberculous patients. There were serious difficulties in dealing with Asian patients, because of unsuitable heads, lack of galleys for separate cooking to meet the ritual requirements of Muslims and Hindoos and lack of rice. Their power boats were a constant problem, and as lifeboats were unsuitable. A further difficulty was often that, when suitable boats were supplied, crews could not be found out of the small ship's company characteristic of the Merchant Navy.

At first sight, it might appear that hospital ships might be used in common for service with the Army or with the Navy as occasion or need arose. This, however, was rarely the case, because the requirements of the two Services and consequently the internal arrangements needed, were different. In general, the Army required hospital ships for the evacuation of patients from shore hospitals to base hospitals further from the scene of operations. The Navy, on the other hand, used its hospital ships themselves as base hospitals, equipped for and capable of carrying out all the functions of such and able to keep up with the Fleet Train and remain with it for such time as was necessary. Exchange service was always unsatisfactory, as the Naval hospital ship was found to have insufficient accommodation and was too slow for use as a carrier, while the Army hospital ship was inadequately equipped and the accommodation too overcrowded for use as a base hospital. The details of the problems associated with the provision of hospital ships is given at length in the naval volumes of the Medical History of the Second World War, and are too long to be included here.

For the transport and evacuation of casualties from the beaches in combined operations, use was made of specially equipped tank landing ships (L.S.T.) and motor fishing vessels (M.F.V.). (Vol. I. *Admin.* p. 93, Vol. II. *Ops.* p. 509.) The use of L.S.T., specially fitted to carry casualties for limited distances, was adopted during the war for medical transport afloat and proved most valuable. In the assault phases, when only limited numbers of hospital carriers could be made available and as hospital ships could not be used until a port had been captured, these L.S.T. were practically the only vessels used for evacuating casualties in the early stages. So far as the British assault area in Normandy was concerned, 70 L.S.T. out of the total employed in the operation were specially fitted with stretcher racks on each side of the tank deck, and a dressing station was arranged at the after end of the hold. The latter consisted of a small enclosure aft, curtained off by a canvas screen, fitted with special lighting over an operating table, hot and cold water supplies, and a small basin and sink with suitable drainage sump. Accommodation was available for 300 to 350 stretcher cases on the tank deck, while a further 160 walking cases could be carried on the troop decks on the port and starboard sides of the main deck. Special medical staffs were embarked in each of these 70 medically fitted L.S.T., 40 being manned by R.N. medical personnel. Some 18,000 casualties were evacuated from Normandy to the United Kingdom in these vessels until hospital ships could be satisfactorily employed. It may be necessary to add, at this interval since the war, that the rigging of the dressing station and the stretcher supports was carried out after the disembarkation of the tanks and while awaiting the arrival of the casualties during the time that the L.S.T. was dried-out on the beach. Special reception hards were constructed at Gosport, Stokes Bay, Southampton, etc., for the disembarkation of casualties on arrival in the United Kingdom.

Motor Fishing Vessels, fitted to carry eight to ten cot cases and some twelve to twenty walking cases, were supplied through the Director of Small Vessels Pool at the Admiralty, whenever the Medical Director-General was satisfied that such vessels were a necessary requirement. These M.F.Vs. performed invaluable duties for medical transport afloat as they were good, seaworthy craft, capable of going alongside ships lying at anchor outside ports and harbours, and were employed in transporting invalids from one port to another by coastal routeing, as was necessary in Iceland. They were used extensively in other parts of the world, and some 50 medically fitted M.F.Vs. were in service at various times during the war.

Stretchers were the subject of criticism from time to time. Those used were the Army type, constructed of wood and canvas; a rather similar, but lighter, stretcher made of steel tubing and wire netting 'not collapsible', and the Neil-Robertson stretcher, made of bamboo and canvas, into which a patient could be strapped to allow of his being passed through narrow hatches and along alleyways. Each had its drawbacks. It was found that the Army type was very heavy and rapidly exhausted bearers when used for loading L.S.T. across wide stretches of beach at low tide. It was also unsuitable for transferring patients between ships with their decks at different levels and over the sides of ships to a jetty alongside. The steel stretcher was lighter than the Army pattern, but was similarly unsuitable for use in narrow hatches, alleyways, etc. The Neil-Robertson stretcher, while generally admirable for the purposes for which it was designed, also suffered from defects. It was too short for many patients, and it caused a great deal of pain to badly burned patients—a criticism which was repeated some years after the war, when a very large number of severely burned casualties had to be landed in Malta after an explosion of aviation spirit in an aircraft carrier. Many medical officers were of the opinion that the Stokes litter, as used in the United States Navy for all purposes, should be introduced. This consists of a light, shallow wire basket, into which an unconscious patient may be strapped if necessary, which fulfils the functions of both the Army pattern and the Neil-Robertson stretcher. A Stokes litter, obtained from U.S. Naval sources, was a prized possession in many ships.

THE MEDICAL CARE OF NAVAL COMMUNITIES ASHORE

During the Second World War a large proportion of the Royal Navy found itself serving ashore, at home and abroad, in training camps, port parties, Naval Air Stations and many other establishments. At home, in general, the provision of medical facilities and the implementation of the necessary sanitary and public health precautions involved no serious problems. Abroad, the problem was often more complex and some aspects of this have been dealt with above. It might, however, be added here that two other factors were of importance. The first of these, in malarious areas, was the lack at the beginning of the war of a suitable uniform for wear after sunset to protect the wearer from the bites of mosquitoes. 'Tropical rig', universally worn at sea and ashore in warm climates, became stabilised shortly after the outbreak of the war (it had been in use for some years before that) and consisted of short-sleeved, open-necked shirt, shorts, woollen stockings and leather shoes or boots. As time went on, this became modified by the abandonment of the helmet as an item of uniform and the substitution of sandals for boots or shoes and stockings. Eventually, too, shirts came to be abandoned while working about the ship or establishment, and the sailor's costume, when not engaged on formal duties, came to consist of shorts, sandals and cap. The difficulty of finding a suitable rig for evening wear in malarious areas was solved by the introduction of Action/ Working rig, primarily for wear in action by persons not requiring full anti-flash gear, as described later. It was, unfortunately, often difficult to ensure that this rig was always worn, as the sailor, in hot climates, preferred to continue in the state of near undress in which he had passed the day, and it was often difficult to persuade officers of the watch, chief and petty officers, of the necessity to take disciplinary measures against ratings who failed to wear their action/working dress after dark. The problem of a suitable evening rig for officers in similar conditions was never really adequately solved, the shirts worn after dark by them being almost universally short-sleeved, although they did wear long trousers. The alternative of the tight-collared No. 10 white tunic was almost intolerable under tropical conditions, besides raising very difficult problems of laundry. (Vol. I. *Admin.* p. 196.)

Another problem, largely due to shortage of medical man-power, was the difficulty of affording courses in tropical hygiene, and the practical application of the methods laid down in various handbooks, to medical officers appointed to shore stations abroad. A certain number of medical officers were so fortunate as to attend the Army's course at Mytchett, and this was of the greatest value, but these were in a minority. Parallel with this problem went another, not confined to tropical stations. This was the lack, often inevitable, of information concerning the conditions with which they would have to contend and of the availability of other sources of medical aid and hospital facilities, which they would meet after getting ashore. For instance, in the Norwegian Campaign in 1940, it was found that, on one or two occasions, provision was made for the setting up of specifically naval sick bay accommodation for the early treatment of casualties in places where local facilities were adequate, while at other places, where there were none, no separate naval arrangements had been planned. (Vol. II. *Ops.* p. 299.) It is appreciated that the Norwegian Campaign was planned and laid on as a matter of great urgency and that consequently such uneven provision of scarce facilities was unavoidable. It would have been valuable, however, had 'Intelligence' known that a severe epidemic of typhus was being experienced in North Africa at the time of the landings there. The Army long ago learned its bitter lesson in Walcheren, the Crimea and South Africa, but the Navy had, from long immunity to shore diseases, failed to learn, to anything like the same extent, the relative importance of weapons and disease in the production of casualties in time of war.

TENTED HOSPITALS

The provision of hospital facilities for special, entirely or predomi-
nently Naval or Royal Marine operations ashore overseas, raised a
difficult problem. It is not proposed to deal with this at any great length
because, as a result of the lessons learned during the Second World War,
the organisation for dealing with combined operations has been materially changed and much more use would be made in future operations
of Army methods and organisations. The first example of this difficulty
was provided by the Mobile Naval Base Defence Organisation
(M.N.B.D.O.), a requirement that had been foreseen before the war,
the primary object of which was the capture and defence of a port or
base from which future operations could be supported. (Vol. II. *Ops.*
pp. 120–149.) Each M.N.B.D.O. consisted of an underwater unit,
including booms, indicator loops and a controlled minefield with the
necessary personnel; an A.A. brigade with associated searchlights; a
coastal defence brigade; a communications company, and a landing,
transport, maintenance, workshop and administrative unit, with ancillary
supply and accounting, meteorological and comprehensive medical
services. The M.N.B.D.O. was manned and organised entirely by the
Royal Marines and, as the Army were not involved, there were no
Army medical facilities available, at least in the early stages, and all
medical provision had to be made by the Royal Navy. The medical
organisation devised for each M.N.B.D.O. (two M.N.B.D.Os. were
eventually formed), included the supply and staffing of two tented
hospitals, complete with tentage and all stores, besides provision for
the setting-up of outlying sick bays to deal with detached units.

The Naval medical branch had no experience in the erecting of tents
and the management of such an establishment, and considerable difficulties were encountered in training and eventually mastered by each of
the four tented hospitals in turn. Much difficulty was experienced in
the transport and reassembly of medical stores, which inevitably were
spread over a number of different ships and, in some cases, became
widely separated, even arriving in different and widely separated ports.

The history of each of these units after proceeding overseas varied,
and is too long and complex to be satisfactorily outlined here. Suffice it
to say that one of them acted as a Casualty Clearing Station in Crete
before being evacuated with loss of all stores and transport. Another
never seems to have operated as a tented hospital at all, becoming
completely split up into various sick bays dealing with scattered units.
Another joined the Royal Marines during the invasion of Sicily and also
eventually dispersed, and the fourth was set up, after various adventures
in North Africa, as a hospital in the Maldive Islands during the early
stages of the preparation, by the Royal Marines, of a base at Addu Atoll.
This last hospital, incidentally, had to deal with a widespread epidemic

of scrub typhus, which completely overwhelmed its resources and necessitated the despatch of a hospital ship to provide necessary hospital and laboratory cover before the epidemic was brought under control by appropriate preventive measures.

An essential difficulty encountered by the tented hospitals, apart from those due to novelty and inexperience, which were overcome by experience, was that they were isolated units not fitting into any larger organisation or command. The requirement, in the event, was found to be of very brief duration, for except in the Maldives, in each case in which a M.N.B.D.O. went into action, it did so in company with Army units, or was followed up by them very shortly, so that the separate provision of tented hospital accommodation rapidly became unnecessary, and the position of the Naval unit became anomalous.

MOBILE LANDING CRAFT ADVANCED BASES (M.O.L.C.A.BS.)
(Vol. II. *Ops.* pp. 150–167)

A not dissimilar provision was made, towards the end of the war, in the shape of M.O.L.C.A.Bs., which were large Naval units, designed for the establishment and support of landing craft bases overseas during the reoccupation of enemy occupied territory. Again, each M.O.L.C.A.B. included two tented hospitals, making provision for 100 beds each. As a result of experience with the M.N.B.D.Os., planning and equipment were greatly improved. Two M.O.L.C.A.Bs. were eventually formed, and it is proposed to refer to these in only the briefest outline. Each was commissioned as a ship, H.M.S. *Landswell* and H.M.S. *Landlock*.

The officers and men of the Royal Navy and Royal Marines required for M.O.L.C.A.B.1—H.M.S. *Landswell*—assembled at Hayling Island in November and December 1943. The total complement numbered 43 officers and 525 men. The medical staff included 8 medical officers and 35 sick berth ratings. There were also 2 dental officers and 2 sick berth ratings (D), and the complement included a trained anti-malaria section of one officer (Royal Marines) and fourteen men. The sick berth staff included specialist ratings, qualified as operating-room assistant, laboratory technician, radiographer and physiotherapist. During the time that the equipment and stores were being assembled and loaded it was possible to arrange for certain medical officers and the Royal Marine Officer appointed for anti-malaria duties to attend the London School of Tropical Medicine. All medical officers attended a course in tropical medicine at the Royal Army Medical College at Millbank, and also received training at the Army School of Hygiene at Mytchett. Unfortunately, it proved impossible for any of the sick berth staff to be so trained.

The personnel, stores and equipment of M.O.L.C.A.B.1, including the medical section, were embarked in five L.S.T. at Southampton and sailed at the end of January 1944, passing through the Mediterranean and the Red Sea to Willingdon Island, Cochin, where a period of acclimatisation and training had been planned. They were accommodated in a camp which had been constructed by the Engineers of the Indian Army for the Royal Indian Navy. At the time of arrival of M.O.L.C.A.B.1, this camp was not really ready for occupation, and the personnel learned a valuable lesson in the implementation of the hygienic and other measures necessary for the preservation of health in a tropical climate. As the future planned occupation of the unit required that its stores and equipment should be kept intact, a sick bay was set up in one of the huts at the camp, stores being drawn as required from a neighbouring Naval establishment, and hospital facilities provided by the Combined Military Hospital, Ernakulam. Owing to changes in the plan of campaign, the operation for which M.O.L.C.A.B.1 was intended did not materialise, and a prolonged stay had to be made at Cochin. During this time, it was possible to arrange for further courses for medical officers at the Royal Naval School of Tropical Medicine at Colombo and the specialist medical officers were able to work in the Civil Hospital at Ernakulam, while the anti-malaria unit performed valuable work in mosquito control in connexion with an epidemic of filariasis then prevalent among the native civilian population. Indeed, this waiting period, although very trying from many points of view, afforded much valuable experience to all concerned.

M.O.L.C.A.B.1 was eventually moved to Singapore at the end of August 1945, after the surrender of the Japanese, had led to the modification of the operation which had been planned for about this time. At Singapore, the unit took over the former Boom Defence Base at Loyang at the north-east end of the island, and became involved in the reoccupation of the Naval Base. The medical party became responsible for the care of prisoners-of-war and the civilian population, so that they never, in fact, operated as planned, viz. as two tented hospitals, accommodation being found in the buildings at Loyang and the base. The personnel, as will be realised, found an enormous amount of work to be done, and the anti-malaria party were fully occupied in restoring the anti-mosquito organisation, which had been completely neglected by the Japanese. The history of M.O.L.C.A.B.2, which left England in April 1944, was very similar to that of M.O.L.C.A.B.1 and it, too, ended up on Singapore Island, where it took over the reorganisation of medical arrangements in the southern part of the island.

Although these two units never performed the function for which they were designed, and instead became involved in post-war local relief and reconstruction of areas formerly occupied by the enemy, it would be

impossible to exaggerate the valuable part they played in the rehabilitation of this part of Malaya.

MEDICAL ESTABLISHMENTS ABROAD—
INTER-SERVICE CO-OPERATION

At this point, some reference should be made to inter-Service co-operation, which was extensive throughout the war and increased from year
to year. In many places abroad, large demands were made on the Army
for medical stores by Naval establishments and sick bays far from Naval
medical depots, and these demands were always met at once and, so far
as stocks permitted, in full. In the absence of Naval hospital and specialist
facilities, those of the Army and R.A.F. were always freely available,
and this acceptance of patients belonging to another Service was, of
course, reciprocal, and merely extended normal practice in the years
between the wars.

A novel, and more complicated form of co-operation was provided by
the setting-up of the Naval Wing, planned from the start, in the 64th
General Hospital in Alexandria in 1940. The Naval Wing was housed
in the same group of buildings and was under the control, so far as the
purely Naval side of administration was concerned, of a Naval medical
officer, overall command being exercised by the Army Officer Commanding. Medical and nursing staff performed duties in both Army and
Naval sections as required, a large proportion of the nursing duties
being carried out by Naval sick berth attendants, while administrative
duties were carried out mainly by Army personnel. (Vol. I. *Admin.*
p. 390.)

Similar arrangements were later made in Malta, where the Naval
hospital on a hill overlooking the Grand Harbour had to be largely
vacated, only first-aid and emergency facilities being maintained, while
the greater part of the medical and nursing staff were transferred to the
Army hospital at Imtarfa, situated in the central part of the island, and
away from the Grand Harbour, the main target of enemy air attacks.
(Vol. I. *Admin.* p. 397.) Again, at Trincomalee in 1945, the 54th British
General Hospital became the Combined Services Hospital, in this
instance under overall Naval control, the Navy providing all specialist
services and staffing the European wards, while the Army provided the
nursing staff for the Asian wards. (Vol. I. *Admin.* p. 417.)

Although these arrangements worked well and amicably in all
instances, there were inevitable difficulties of an administrative and
disciplinary nature because of different methods, regulations and
routines characteristic of the two Services, but these were always dealt
with satisfactorily and harmonious relations were maintained. Certain
problems did, however, remain. One of these was the disposal of

patients admitted to a hospital managed by a Service other than their own. In the Army, it was normal practice to evacuate casualties and sick to the rear shortly after admission, in order to keep beds available for emergencies. In many instances, patients from ships, discharged to an Army hospital suffering from conditions from which early recovery could be anticipated, were evacuated from the theatre, even to the United Kingdom, leaving the ship without, perhaps, an important officer or a key rating for many months until a relief could be sent out from the United Kingdom. Another problem, more important because of the larger scale, was occasioned by the alternating requirements of the two Services. This situation arose, for instance, in Alexandria in March 1944, when the Military authorities informed the Naval authorities that, because of political pressure to return to the Egyptian Government the buildings occupied by the 64th General Hospital, it was proposed to close this establishment and to transfer its staff and equipment to Amirya. This would have been so far from Alexandria as to render its use impracticable by the Navy, and it became necessary to make arrangements for the opening of a purely Naval hospital. After some difficulty, a suitable building was found, but the assembling of stores and equipment proved very difficult. The R.N. Auxiliary Hospital, Alexandria eventually opened for the reception of patients in September 1944, and cared for over 5,000 patients, including out-patients, before it was closed in November 1945. (Vol. I. *Admin.* p. 394.) A rather similar situation also arose in Cochin, South India, in 1943 and 1944, when constantly changing arrangements were planned for the development of a combined Services hospital, plans undergoing considerable modification as Army requirements diminished with the changing strategic situation in the Eastern Theatre, while Naval requirements continued to increase, being largely connected with the development of landing-craft bases in connexion with the reoccupation of Burma and Malaya. (Vol. I. *Admin.* p. 429.) This brief outline will, perhaps, serve to indicate that there was widespread co-operation and co-ordination between the medical services throughout the war, but that it was not always easy to achieve and was not without its difficulties and problems. The superficial assertion that since sailors, soldiers and airmen all suffer from the same complaints and require the same treatment they should be treated in the same hospitals by members of one, combined Service, ignores all the multiplicity of procedural, administrative and logistical problems involved in implementing this very obvious premise. The staffing of a hospital by medical and nursing personnel of one combined medical service would present few difficulties; the logistical problem—the provision and perhaps the building and support and defence of the hospital—which must inevitably be by one of the user Services, would remain and might even be increased.

HABITABILITY

Among the more important factors involved in the maintenance of the health and well-being of ships' companies during long periods spent on board, whether in harbours in which there were often few facilities for sport and recreation, or on long voyages in the cold of the Arctic or the heat of the Tropics, may be included clothing, diet and all those items which contribute to habitability. (Vol. I. *Admin.* p. 184.) During the nineteen thirties, ventilation standards had been laid down, calling for the supply of 2,000 cu.ft. of fresh air per man per hour, not to fall below 1,500 cu.ft., representing a complete change of air every five minutes, and the maintenance, in cold climates, of a temperature on the messdecks and in working compartments of between 60°F. and 65°F. Efforts to achieve these standards were handicapped by many factors, some inherent in the structure of ships of war, including the absolute necessity for versatility, the essence of which is that a ship should be capable of efficient service in any part of the world and in any extreme of climate at short notice. For example, during the war, one ship, on one occasion, went from Algiers to Murmansk in three weeks in January, from a mean temperature of 70°F. to one varying between 18°F. and minus 30°F. Habitability problems, always severe in ships of war because of minute watertight subdivisions and the virtual absence of means of natural ventilation, were greatly increased by war-time conditions, including voyages of great length, long periods closed-up at Action and Cruising Stations, blackout, and a vast increase in 'wild heat', generated by constant running of main engines and the maintenance of the reserve of energy needed to allow of the availability of full power at short notice. The largest single factor, however, was the rapidly increasing complexity of ships and their weapons and equipment, including radar, with associated need for increased stowage space, encroaching on the already exiguous living-space available for the personnel on the mess-decks, and requiring large numbers of extra hands to man them. In some cases, complements rose by nearly 60 per cent.

In hot climates, especially in older ships designed primarily for service in the North Atlantic, these factors combined to produce excessively hot, humid conditions on the messdecks and in store-rooms, W.T. compartments and other confined working spaces, while in some compartments, particularly in engine-rooms, conditions might, on occasion, become quite intolerable. In H.M.S. *Barham* at Dakar, the dry-bulb temperature on the messdecks ranged between 100°F. and 110°F. while in the forward Medical Distributing Station it reached 140°F. when the ship was closed-up at Action Stations. Only nine cases of heat exhaustion were reported. In H.M.S. *Resolution*, on the same occasion, 64 cases of heat exhaustion occurred, one of whom died. Included were 12 per cent. of the engine-room complement, who had been exposed in the dynamo- and boiler-rooms to temperatures varying between 126°F. and 136°F. Long-continued and constant exposure to less severe conditions than these led to increased incidence of skin diseases, headache, lassitude, inability to concentrate and serious loss of efficiency.

In cold climates, one of the most trying factors was the liability to sudden and rapid variations of temperature, primarily due to changes of wind intensity and direction. There might be a rise or fall of 20°F. in as many minutes as a result of a change of course. There was usually a film of ice on the insides of bulkheads in living and working spaces. As a result of a sudden rise in temperature this would melt so that the decks became covered by, and everything sodden with, water, which subsequently froze when the temperature again fell, perhaps as suddenly. This occurred even in engine- and boiler-rooms, where stalactites of ice formed, hanging down from the air supply lines. In bad convoys, fighting their way mile by mile, large numbers of the crew were at action stations, out in the open, for days on end. Such measures as were taken early on were aimed, not at improved habitability, but at preventing the freezing-up of gun mechanisms, technical machinery and navigational instruments, upon which the safety of the ship depended. Later, steps were taken to improve matters by the introduction of an elaborate heating system, a process known as Arcticising. Steam-pipes were laid through living and working spaces and even to certain situations on the upper deck. To begin with, these measures were not entirely satisfactory, as internal temperatures tended to rise too high, so that everything became covered in slush and it was so hot that a man with a few moments to spare for rest must first strip off his clothes to tolerate the heat; otherwise, he became soaked in sweat, and started to freeze when he went outside again. With growing experience, these defects were greatly reduced, and it became possible to maintain fairly reasonable conditions between decks. As time went on, too, men learned, usually by bitter experience, the basic precautions necessary in the Arctic. They acquired the habit of remaining constipated, they went about making faces at each other so as to feel whether or not they were getting frost-bitten cheeks, lips or nose, and they learned not to touch bare metal with the hands, or tin mugs with the lips, for fear of freezing to them. Apart from frost-bite, these conditions produced no physical ailment specifically attributable to the climate alone. Numerous common ailments were aggravated by the cold. Pediculosis was very prevalent in some ships, related to the wearing of clothing for prolonged periods. Foot troubles, such as sore feet, eczema and exacerbations of epidermophytosis, were aggravated by wearing sea-boot stockings for many days or even weeks without taking them off. It was hard for both officers and men to keep themselves clean. Reference to the mental effects of these conditions is made later.

As the adverse effects upon efficiency of these conditions, alike in cold and hot climates, became more and more apparent, the Habitability Sub-Committee of the Royal Naval Personnel Research Committee, itself a sub-committee of the Medical Research Council, was set up and, in 1943, conducted an enquiry by constructors, ventilation engineers, physiologists, psychologists and selected executive and medical officers, into living conditions in ships and establishments in all parts of the world. Much was found that could be done by the ship's own efforts, and improved morale resulted in ships visited when it was realised that an interest was being taken. The most important discovery, however, was the lack of useful data and records and it was soon apparent that conclusions from research in factories were not applicable in men-of-war because of a greater production of 'wild heat', combined with a high density of population. Among the results of the investigation was the setting-up of arrangements to collect the necessary definite data to prove that increasing weapons and machinery produced no benefit if the living conditions became so bad that the morale and physical conditions of the ship's company deteriorated. A research unit was established to conduct experiments and collect data and, as a result, it was decided to set as a provisional standard, in hot climates, an Effective Temperature not above 80°F. as desirable and an upper limit of 86°F. beyond which efficiency was likely to be impaired. At the same time, a set of instruments was devised to measure the effective temperature, calculated by tables, from the temperature of the air, the humidity and the degree of air movement. The instruments included a whirling hygrometer, silvered Kata thermometers, 130°–125°F. and 150°–145°F., a globe thermometer, stop-watch, vacuum flask and support for the globe thermometer, together with a book of instructions on the use of the instruments.

CLOTHING (Vol. I. *Admin.* p. 194)

At the outbreak of the war in 1939, provision of cold-weather clothing had remained unchanged since 1918. When extremely cold conditions were met with, much depended on local improvisation. Naval stores could provide long, thick underpants and vests, a limited number of pairs of seaboots for wear by upper deck personnel and a number of duffel coats, which men going off watch exchanged with those coming on. These supplies increased as time went on. At the same time, large supplies of 'Woollies'—Balaclava helmets, thick jerseys, sea-boot stockings, mufflers, etc.—were supplied to ships by numerous voluntary organisations and were very welcome. As a result of experience in the Arctic convoys, it became apparent that greater provision must be made and, in association with the British Industries Research Association, the 'Anarak' suit was developed, and remained the chief form of naval Arctic clothing for the rest of the war. The problem as regards the Navy was not the same as that of the Arctic explorer who was engaged in strenuous exercise in the open pulling a sledge or following a dog-team. What was required was something which a man could wear sitting still in the open for long periods, with temperatures often many degrees below freezing point.

As has been indicated above, official recognition was given to the costume that had been worn on occasion on hot stations for some years before the war, *viz.* shorts and shirts. Sandals instead of shoes were introduced, partly because of coolness but also, and largely, because of the consequent reduced incidence of foot infections when leather shoes and woollen stockings were discarded. The sun helmet was abolished, and the discarding of shirts at work was approved. This costume brought other risks in its train, *viz* the liability to extensive burns of personnel exposed to flash. In order to combat this, anti-flash gear was developed for wear by personnel working on the upper deck in action, and Action/working dress—dark-blue long trousers and light-blue, long-sleeved shirt—for wear by others. The effectiveness of these measures was strikingly shown at the sinking of the *Prince of Wales* and the *Repulse* off the Malayan coast at the end of 1941. In the *Prince of Wales* where anti-flash gear was not being worn on account of the heat, there were many cases of very extensive burns due to flash and fractured steam-pipes. In the *Repulse*, where all men working on the upper deck wore anti-flash gear, long-sleeved shirts and long trousers tucked into the tops of boots, and many of those not so protected wore boiler suits, burns were confined to the face and hands and occurred mainly in engine-room personnel.

No change had taken place in flying clothing since 1929. An overall, a Sidcot suit or an Irvine suit was worn over Naval uniform. The first move was made, in association with the R.A.F., to meet the requirements of pilots ditched in aeroplanes launched from catapults from C.A.M. ships accompanying Atlantic convoys. When these C.A.M. ships were discontinued, on their replacement by carriers, further consideration was given to the question of suitable flying clothing, and the Naval Immersion Suit was devised and introduced into the Service in 1943. This suit was very popular and increased the expectation of life after crashing into the sea from about ten minutes in very cold climates to over an hour.

It is worthy of mention that it was found, by bitter personal experience, that certain proprietary inflatable waistcoats showed a tendency to slip upwards and over the head, especially if there were much oil fuel on the surface of the sea, because the buttons came out of the button-holes.

This was represented to the makers, with a view to the substitution of some more suitable form of fastening for the buttons. A warning was also issued to the Fleet, drawing attention to this danger.

DIET (Vol. I. *Admin.* p. 240)

In general, the provision of food was satisfactory throughout the war, apart from the inevitable shortages of particular items at different times, shared by all members of the Services and the civilian population at home. As regards quantity, the heavy manual work of the days of sail and of hand-fired boilers no longer takes place, almost all heavy work being done by machinery, and caloric requirements were actually less than those of the Army. Many medical officers were of the opinion that ship's companies ate too much and got too little physical exercise. The Admiralty planned to provide adequate quantities, but made no attempt to plan different dietaries for different climatic conditions, leaving this to individual ships. Attempts to vary dietaries often came up against the innate conservatism of the Naval rating in the matter of food— the same menu was demanded in the Tropics and the Arctic.

VITAMINS

Scurvy was a disease of the times of long sea voyages before the art of preserving food was understood and had ceased to occur at sea long before the discovery of the vitamins, which became news between the wars. As a result of advertising and commercial propaganda, many people, including some senior executive officers and some doctors, felt during the war that there must be a shortage of vitamins in the diet if these were not being issued in synthetic form. The Medical Director-General of the Navy issued information on the subject through Admiralty Fleet Orders, but 'scurvy scares' continued to arise from time to time. All were scientifically investigated and it was invariably found that the sponginess of the gums, which had given rise to the alarm, was the result of Vincent's disease. No case of scurvy occurred in any of H.M. Ships during the war.

It was at one time thought that Vitamin A played a large part in the acuity of night vision. It was demonstrated, however, that the amount of this vitamin in a normal Service diet was more than enough to prevent deterioration of night vision in which many other factors played a part, that individual night vision varied greatly quite apart from any question of diet and, finally, that Vitamin A in excess of ordinary requirements brought about no increase in visual acuity in the dark.

The question of the addition of synthetic vitamins was raised again and again by the executive, including, on occasion, flag officers infected by vitamin publicity campaigns, especially in the U.S.A., and sometimes it was difficult to convince them that such additions were not necessary.

In general, however, it was rightly accepted that with a little care in the provision of vegetables and jams, ships could depend on obtaining everything that was required for a complete and adequate dietary. The introduction of dehydrated vegetables did much to simplify this provision, although in the early days they often left something to be desired in the matter of palatability. Early in the war the Admiralty took care to inform commanding officers that they were to accept responsibility for the important matter of cooking to preserve palatability and vitamin content of victuals and that 'They must constantly guard against the possibility of good rations and their essential content being reduced in nutritional value by bad cooking, with the inevitable result that fighting efficiency would be impaired'.

ACTION MESSING

This was a requirement that arose during the Second World War because of air attacks which might last for hours and even days on end, so that it was necessary to make provision for meals that could be delivered to and consumed by the sailor at his place of duty during lulls in action. No general directive was issued, individual ships making their own arrangements. These varied with the size, type and age of the ship, the size of the ship's company, climatic conditions and the type of operation on which she was engaged. This provision was primarily the responsibility of the Supply Officer, but the Medical Officer was often consulted. In Northern Climates, action messing involved the constant supply of hot soups, tea or cocoa, with such items as meat pies, etc., which could be eaten by hand. Some shelter was needed and it was important to remember that china or plastic mugs or cups were to be preferred to metal utensils, which were liable to freeze to fingers or lips. In the Tropics, the greater requirement was ample supplies of fluids, and it was found that, in general, prolonged action in hot climates inhibited a man's appetite, and he tended not to feel hungry. Attention was paid to the needs for water and salt and recommendations were made to all ships in the light of results of investigations made by the U.S.N. Medical Authorities in 1943.

Action messing produced very serious problems, particularly in the Arctic, when men had to be fed at their guns, sometimes for days on end, during such lulls as occurred. The extinguishing of galley fires when action was imminent, for instance, meant that hot drinks had to be provided by means of steam heating. The cooks did wonderful work. While, during short lulls, other ratings might have a chance to snatch a few minutes sleep or rest, the cooks, who had been on duty in magazines, etc., had to start to do some cooking. The Medical Officer of one ship engaged on Arctic convoys remarked in his report 'In our case, the cooking was done by a handful of chaps relieved from their action stations, who never could have got a rest of any kind, and who did absolute miracles'. Incidentally, when survivors from other ships had been picked up from the sea, supply ratings might find themselves similarly occupied in issuing clothing and bedding to large numbers of men who had lost all their own.

MEDICAL ORGANISATION OF H.M. SHIPS IN ACTION

At the outbreak of the war in 1939, the medical organisation of a ship in action was virtually the same as that laid down throughout the First World War, and was based on the assumption that the most important incident likely to occur was a Fleet action with ships of the enemy, the major weapon being the gun. (Vol. II. *Ops.* p. 5.) The potential strength of enemy aircraft was not generally recognised and the magnetic mine had yet to be encountered. The Medical Staff were to be placed in a protected space—in an armoured ship below the armoured deck—and were to remain there during the heat of the action, care being taken that they were not exposed to danger of suffocation, etc., by being left there too long. The object was to ensure that the medical staff would be available to attend to the wounded after the battle was over and only first aid was to be carried out, during action, by parties specially trained and detailed for this purpose. Wounded men were to be moved only to sheltered positions near where they had been wounded, so as to be out of the way of others and form no obstruction to the efficient fighting of the ship. No effort was to be made to take them to dressing stations until such time as the command, during a lull, gave the necessary instructions and the medical parties were called out of their refuges. Two Medical Distributing Stations were set up, so far as possible at opposite ends of the ship, so that one or other might be used should the other have been damaged. First-aid bags were distributed before action to first-aid parties. It was recommended that if there were large numbers of wounded they should be treated in suitably screened areas of the upper deck and that, should further action appear to be imminent, they should be removed to a protected position, beneath armour if possible. It was further ordered that 10 per cent. of the ship's company should be trained in first aid. There was only one Medical Officer in each Destroyer Flotilla, the Coxswain, who received a special course of training being responsible for the care of sick and wounded in other destroyers.

It was recognised, prior to the outbreak of hostilities, that these arrangements were probably insufficient and inappropriate to modern conditions but, in the absence of actual experience, the nature of what would be required was not obvious. Experience was quickly obtained as numerous incidents afloat began, including the sinking of the aircraft carrier *Courageous*, of the old battleship *Royal Oak*, the mining of the

Adventure, *Nelson* and *Belfast*, the Battle of the River Plate, etc. The
earliest change effected was the appointment of a Medical Officer to
each destroyer, at first in the Western Approaches, and later throughout
the Fleet. This was done in part for the benefit of morale, which was
found to be improved with the assurance that somebody would be
available to treat the wounded should casualties occur. This was, of
course, the reason which first led to the appointment of surgeons to
the ships of the mediaeval navies in the 13th century.

Before going on to outline the changes that took place in the nature of
weapons used, in the consequent nature of the injuries sustained, in the
general characteristics of Naval actions and to describe the new medical
organisation devised to meet these changes, it would be well to refer
briefly to the defects shown in the old organisation when exposed to
modern conditions. (Vol. II. *Ops.* Chaps. 3 and 4.) It was found that
all medical personnel, placed together behind armour, had in one or two
cases all been killed or wounded, so defeating the principal object of
so placing them, *viz.* to ensure as far as possible that they would be
available at the end of the action. Again, spaces nominated as Medical
Distributing Stations had been found in some cases to be difficult of
access through man-holes in hatch covers, tortuous passages, watertight doors, etc., through which wounded on stretchers could not
conveniently be carried. Sometimes the M.D.S. could not be approached
at all when watertight integrity, essential to the preservation of the ship,
must be preserved. Further, the old organisation was far too rigid and
it soon became apparent that the medical officer, if there were but one,
or the S.M.O., if there were more, must be free to move about, so far as
conditions permitted, to positions where his presence was required.
Not the least of the differences was caused by the prolonged nature of
air attacks, which sometimes lasted all day or, with but little interval
during daylight, for several days on end.

As reports began to come in, it was apparent that, not only had the
nature of naval action itself altered, but also that the nature of the
casualties sustained had changed greatly. In general, it could be stated
that shell-fire, as in the Battle of the River Plate and in a number of
subsequent actions, produced mainly lacerated wounds of soft parts,
with few fractures and few burns. For instance, in H.M.S. *Ajax* at
the River Plate, there were 13 killed and 22 wounded, all by shell
splinters. There were no fractures and only one case was complicated
by burns. Similarly, on another occasion, in H.M.S. *Berwick*, 7 were
killed and 9 wounded, 6 being splinter lacerations, one of the chest.
There were three fractures, but two of these were fingers jammed,
not the result of shell-fire, and one was struck by a door blown away by
blast. In 13 incidents, up to the end of 1940, there were 42 dead and 113
wounded, of which only 10 were fractures and 11 burns. In Armed

Merchant Cruisers, the picture was different. Burns were more frequent because of wooden decks and the presence of ready-use ammunition in exposed positions near the guns. In a gun action in the *Alcantara*, nine men were accidentally injured by dropping projectiles on themselves. It should be added that these accidents were contributed to by the necessarily imperfect arrangements for loading and transport of ammunition in merchant ships converted to carrying guns without the provision of turrets.

The assessment of injuries caused by torpedoes was difficult as the majority of ships hit were sunk, while those that survived suffered relatively little damage. In the larger ships that survived, it was found that the casualties varied with the compartment hit and the number of men in the vicinity. The *Ark Royal* and the *Calypso* were both sunk by torpedo fire without sustaining any casualty directly attributable to the torpedo. It became apparent as the war progressed that, provided the ship survived, the limited number of casualties caused by the actual explosion of the torpedo was recorded too frequently to be regarded as merely fortuitous, and certain general conclusions could be reached. Fractures predominated, and appeared to be due to men being thrown down (in contrast, as will be shown, to injuries caused by the magnetic mine). There was a conspicuous absence of such severe injuries as dislocated knees and fractured spines. There was no definite ratio between numbers killed and wounded, such as came to be expected in mine or bomb explosions and there were few lacerations and no high incidence of burns. H.M.S. *Liverpool* produced an apparent exception to this last conclusion, when there was a large number of burns. Investigation showed, however, that these resulted from the explosion of the ship's petrol tanks some twelve minutes after the hit by the torpedo was sustained. This incident also showed the inadequacy of tropical dress—shorts and shirts—as a protection against burns.

Shells and torpedoes had been used in the First World War and their effects were already known, although probably not well remembered. The effects of air attack had not been experienced at the beginning of the Second World War, and, of course, so far as some members of the Naval Medical Service were concerned, the advent of the magnetic mine was quite unexpected. Some time elapsed before the pattern of the injuries likely to be caused by these new weapons had been worked out in the light of analysis of reports. It ought, perhaps, to be explained at this stage that the magnetic mine differed radically in its effect from the mines used in the First World War, in that, while the latter exploded in close contact with the hull of the ship, and their effects were analagous with those resulting from a torpedo explosion, the magnetic mine exploded sufficiently far below the ship's bottom to allow of the development of a tremendous water-hammer effect, producing very severe,

though often localised, damage to the ship's structure and lifting the
ship bodily in the water. The casualties sustained varied little from ship
to ship, provided that it was not sunk outright. When a ship was struck,
the effects were sometimes remarkably local and in most ships the
casualties were confined to the immediate vicinity of the explosion.
Casualties were of the kind associated with a fall from a height—the
effect of the ship having been lifted violently. Injuries commonly
affected the lower extremities, and simple fractures of the leg and thigh
were common, while dislocations and torn collateral ligaments of the knee
and ankle joints were often recorded. More rarely, the pelvis was fractured.
Compression fractures of the lower dorsal vertebrae were fairly common
in some ships, and there were also cases of fracture of the skull and
the maxilla. Burns and scalds were relatively uncommon and there
were few references to the effects of blast.

The development of air attack produced conditions and considerations
that had not been previously experienced. Surprise and the frequently
prolonged nature of the attacks were features peculiar to the weapon.
Instances of continuous attacks upon the ship by waves of bombers
for perhaps ten hours or more at a time produced special problems
in maintaining the nervous and physical endurance of personnel.
An unexpected feature was a state of dazed apathy and inertia induced
in physically uninjured persons by a successful bombing attack. There
might be a complete lack of initiative, leading on more than one occasion
to large numbers remaining motionless in a compartment from which
they could easily have escaped had somebody started to move, and
this occurred after a near miss as well as after a direct hit. A specific
job of work was the best preventative, assisted by the attainment of
good morale by training, exhortation and other similar methods.

The physical injuries resulting from air attack varied according to
whether the ship sustained a direct hit or a near miss. In the case of the
near miss, although men might be thrown into the air or sustain fractures
of limbs, spine or skull, the great majority of casualties were due to
splinter wounds. In one ship, of 13 killed and 32 wounded by a near miss,
all were cases of splinter wounds and all occurred on the upper deck.
Splinters tended to follow a curved, upward path and wounds were
almost invariably above the hips, the lower limbs being protected by
the ship's side and decks—an argument in favour of keeping well inboard
during attack. It was shown that the incidence of these wounds could
be materially reduced by the enforcement of the order to 'Lie flat
with your head inboard during raids if not required for duty'. The
splinters varied in size, but many were little larger than a large pea.
The track of the wounds was usually from below upward and, although
the wound of entry might be minute, it was no indication of the extent
of the resulting internal damage. Splinter wounds of the abdomen and

chest were excruciatingly painful, but wounds of the limbs showed numbing for an hour or so. Head wounds were common, with penetration of the skull and brain damage resulting even from tiny fragments. Scalp wounds might occur even when upper-deck personnel were wearing steel helmets, splinters passing directly or by ricochet upwards through the headband. On the whole, eye injuries were remarkably rare. Although wounds by bomb splinters were most likely to affect upper-deck personnel, persons between decks were not safe from harm when near misses occurred. Splinters could pass through the side plating of a destroyer. Altogether, near misses were greatly dreaded, because they could cause more widespread damage to a particular part of a ship than a direct hit would have done elsewhere.

The injuries caused by direct hits were more varied and serious. A certain number of fractures of limbs or of ribs occurred from men being thrown against hatches and bulkheads and some fractures of spine or skull from the decks rising. These effects were relatively few and far less devastating than those sustained in the immediate vicinity of the explosion. It was found that, wherever a bomb exploded between decks, the majority of men within 20 ft. were killed instantly, their bodies being dismembered, eviscerated and even totally disintegrated. In the case of survivors at a distance of over 20 ft., wounds were usually caused by flying fragments of the ship itself rather than by bomb splinters. The total mortality from all causes in direct hits was usually 50 per cent. of those in the space hit or in the direct path of the blast through an open door. Practically every survivor, whatever the nature of his other injuries, would be suffering from burns, the extent depending upon the amount of skin surface exposed. These burns were the most characteristic effect of a direct hit. In one ship with 71 casualties, there were 32 dead and all the rest were burned. Flash usually scorched all exposed skin and even travelled up the legs of the trousers unless they had been tucked into the tops of the boots. Apart from the flash of the explosion there were other sources of fire in the ship itself and cordite was likely to ignite, with the added danger of irritating and toxic nitrous fumes. Less serious effects included rupture of the tympanic membrane. All members of the ship's company were issued with rubber ear plugs, but these were often uncomfortable, needed to be cut down to fit the meatus and it is doubtful if they gave more protection than plugs of cotton wool, though they were doubtless of psychological value.

Gas gangrene was an extremely rare complication and, when it did occur, was usually confined to thigh wounds. Its incidence was too rare to justify the undertaking of major surgery unless the ship was likely to be at sea for more than another thirty hours. In any case, conditions on board rendered major surgery excessively hazardous and difficult, and the problems of nursing and after-care were such as to discourage the undertaking of such operations save in exceptional cases of great urgency. It was generally accepted that major surgical procedures in a man-of-war can be justified only to save life or to relieve severe pain and, even in the latter event, other less drastic measures were to be preferred.

Machine-gun attack from the air was not, in general, a cause of many casualties, except in the case of survivors in the water. In one transport, however, off Dunkirk, seven soldiers were killed and 100, as well as seven of the ship's company, wounded. The conditions were quite exceptional, in that the upper decks of ships engaged in evacuating troops from Dunkirk were crowded with soldiers. While dealing with the nature of injuries caused by various forms of attack, it ought to be mentioned, although records did not become available until towards the later stages of the war in the Pacific, that the 'Kamikaze' or 'Suicide plane' attack resulted in splinter wounds and, especially, numerous and extensive burns caused by the explosion of the petrol tanks of the attacking plane.

Depth charges exploding under water after the abandonment and sinking of a ship produced very characteristic injuries among survivors in the water. H.M.S. *Tweed* was struck by a torpedo at 1615 hrs. on a fine, calm afternoon in the Atlantic in January, and at once started to settle by the stern, sinking within three minutes. No boats and only one Carley float got away; very few men went down with the ship. While survivors in the water were swimming away from the ship, and the bow was still sticking out above the sea, a depth charge exploded, probably at 250 ft. This was responsible directly or indirectly for all the casualties, as everyone was in the water. Nobody could have been more than 100 yards from the centre of the explosion. The force was considerable and felt as though something had squeezed the chest and abdomen tightly and suddenly. The majority of men immediately began to cough up bright blood and became incontinent of urine and faeces. Some must have been killed instantly while others obviously began to drown. Fifty-three survivors were picked up just before sunset. One was dead and two others died a few hours later. All the survivors had cramping abdominal pains, diarrhoea, melaena and some haemoptysis. It was noted that fat or well-covered men were much less affected than thin ones, while those wearing lifebelts or swimming on their backs seem to have suffered less from the effects of underwater blast. Similar injuries were sustained in many other cases exposed to underwater blast as a result of the explosion of depth charges. In those who came to autopsy, it was observed that no outward sign of injury was apparent, but dissection revealed extensive blast injuries of the lungs and multiple perforations of intestines. In one case complete rupture of the recto-sigmoid junction was recorded. A perhaps unexpected added hazard affecting survivors in the sea was illustrated in the case of the sinking of the *Dunedin* in the South Atlantic in November as a result of torpedo attack. The ship sank rapidly after being hit by two torpedoes, and only 140 men appear to have abandoned ship out of a ship's company of 470. In three days, 73 died of exposure and the bites of small fish, about 1 ft. long, which were in the company of many sharks. Of 71 picked up by the American S.S. *Mishmaha*, four died soon after rescue and 43 were landed later and sent to hospital in Trinidad. The most serious cases were observed to be suffering from multiple punched-out ulcers, caused by fish-bites.

The many changes in medical organisation for action that were necessitated by the changes in the nature of attacks and of weapons and their effects, as outlined above, gradually became apparent, and a number of these changes were implemented during 1940 and 1941 by local arrangements or individual enterprise. In April 1942 a comprehensive Fleet Order was promulgated, which recognised officially that modern circumstances of action afloat called for modern medical measures. This Order stated that before 1941 the organisation for action in H.M. Ships had been centralised in the medical distributing stations. War experience had now proved the necessity for a much greater degree of decentralisation and for more posts where emergency treatment could be carried out. It was recognised that considerable latitude must be allowed in its application, having regard to the great variations in the size and construction of H.M. Ships. But, while the arrangements recommended were primarily intended for larger ships, it was considered desirable that in smaller types the principles should be followed as far as possible.

The following posts for medical use were recommended in all H.M. Ships wherever possible:

(a) *A Main Distributing Station.* It was recommended that this position be sited either forward or aft, as convenient, in a compartment of the ship under protection. Where possible, it was to be allocated as such in the ship's plans, and appropriated and fitted out solely for medical purposes.

(b) *An Auxiliary Distributing Station.* This position should be sited towards the end of the ship remote from the main D.S., in a compartment under protection and of considerable size. Suggested positions were a messdeck, laundry, store room, any space which, although primarily allocated for other purposes, could quickly be converted for use as a medical distributing station. With this end in view, it was important that any permanent fittings provided should interfere as little as possible with the primary use of the compartment.

As regards these distributing stations, an important change of policy was based on the great harm experience had shown might be done to wounded men by carrying them through a series of narrow passages and man-holes to the treatment centres. It was now considered of primary importance that the distributing stations should not only offer adequate room for treatment, but also should be so sited as to afford access for stretcher cases.

(c) *First-Aid Posts.* A number of First-Aid Posts were recommended to be sited principally on the upper decks near to action stations. The types of compartment suggested for consideration were crew spaces, bathrooms, recreation spaces, captain's quarters, gun-room, sick bay, wide lobbies and posts in the 'island' on the flight deck of aircraft carriers. In selecting compartments for use as First-Aid Posts, the following main requirements were to be observed:

Working space; protection from the weather, explosive blast, and shell and bomb splinters; accessibility from fighting and working parts of the ship; easy passage of stretchers; the minimum of interference with the working and fighting of the ship; proximity to hot and cold water supply; adequate light and ventilation; adequate telephone communication; stowage space for first-aid equipment.

The recommendations recognised that the number of these stations could not be defined with accuracy, but must depend upon the local arrangements in each ship. A broad principle was laid down which aimed at every man-of-war being divided into areas, each area having its own first-aid post as a casualty reception centre. It was also recognised that the number of such first-aid posts which could be established in any particular ship would be affected by the number of personnel available to man them in action. In general, it was considered desirable that each first-aid post should be occupied by a sick berth rating or a specially qualified first-aid worker, together with a less skilled assistant. If possible, a medical officer was to be in charge of each of the two distributing stations but, should only one medical officer be carried, he would be in charge of the main station and the senior sick berth rating of the auxiliary. In addition, a minimum of two competent first-aid assistants was to be allocated to each distributing station, and the ship's master-at-arms was to be allocated to the main distribution station for the important function of recording the designation and particulars of casualties as they occurred.

By means of this reorganisation it became possible to split up trained medical personnel so that they were available in different parts of the ship, so eliminating the possibility of a large proportion being rendered casualties by any one incident. It was also considered important that the employment of medical personnel should be fluid and elastic. With this in view, it was considered vital that the senior medical officer should on no account be required to immobilise himself at any one point, but should be free to move about as necessary to supervise and adjust his organisation to meet changes in the situation which were bound to arise during the actual course of the action. In order to support the new policy of greater decentralisation, steps were taken to ensure that a far greater number of personnel in every ship should be qualified in first-aid than had been considered necessary in the past, and it was now stated that the 10 per cent. so trained, formerly required by regulations, should be regarded as an absolute minimum, and that as far as possible all officers and men should receive instruction in first-aid. Furthermore, it was provided that certain selected persons should be given more advanced instruction, including the technique of hypodermic injections. Concurrently with this provision, further instructions were issued which concerned the issue of omnopon in the form of tubunic ampoules.

The new Order gave lists of suggested fittings, items of equipment, dressings, etc., that should be available in each distributing station and first-aid post, but it is not proposed to enumerate these here.

This Order outlined the broad principles which should be observed in implementing an efficient modern medical organisation for action afloat. It was considered that, during the course of the action, casualties occurring in the immediate vicinity of the first-aid posts could be dealt with readily, while casualties occurring in situations beyond easy reach would be moved to the nearest cover and receive simple first-aid treatment from the nearest qualified person. Should opportunity offer, sorties would be made from the first-aid posts in order to render more skilled assistance to the more serious cases, which would, from time to time, be moved to the nearest first-aid post where they would be treated and retained until the end of the action. It is important to note that no attempt was to be made to transport a casualty to any position but a first-aid post during the course of the action and this point was emphasised in the Fleet Order; no attempt was to be made to take any case to a distant distributing station during the course of an action, except on the instructions of a medical officer. The reasons for this prohibition were two-fold, *viz.* to obviate the increased harm that might be done to the injured man by moving him further than was advisable before his condition had been assessed by a medical officer, and in order to prevent hazard to the watertight integrity of the ship through the unauthorised opening of watertight hatches and doors, upon which the safety of the ship might depend.

The mention of the issue of tubunic ampoules of omnopon raises the question of the use of morphia in the treatment of shocked casualties. By the end of the war, a number of experienced naval medical officers had expressed some criticism of the routine administration of morphia to casualties in action afloat. The opinion (which was not, of course, confined to naval medical officers) was that the sole criterion should be the existence of pain, and that morphia should not be used in cases of shock where there was no pain. The feeling was that a wounded man who had received morphia might subsequently lose the will to make an effort to save himself should his ship start to sink. Also, a school of thought arose which considered that morphia was always likely to increase shock in the case of casualties suffering from exposure at sea. This was particularly so in the case of wounds and shock accompanied by exposure in Arctic waters. This opinion was later incorporated in a Fleet Order.

BURIAL OF THE DEAD

A problem of great, and immediate, if not primarily medical, importance, was the disposal of the bodies of those killed in action. (Vol. II. *Ops.* p. 85.) Four possible courses presented themselves, *viz.*

(*a*) Immediate disposal during the course of the action;

(*b*) A funeral at sea before returning to harbour after action;

(*c*) A funeral at sea from another ship after returning to harbour, and

(*d*) Burial ashore.

The third and fourth courses involved much labour and such funerals placed a great strain on the ship's company, especially during the period of mental reaction and rehabilitation after a severe naval engagement.

Large numbers of corpses to be landed, perhaps placed in store, and transferred to another ship for burial, placed very great strains on a possibly small base with limited staff and facilities. Transport, accommodation and materials for suitable wrapping or encasement were all additional problems and, of course, there was the strain on the ship's company of the ship carrying out the disposal. As regards the first course, in at least one ship there was nothing demoralising or lacking in reverence in the action of a seaman who himself 'Buried' 15 members of his gun's crew during a short lull in a heavy action.

In general, it became evident during the war that every effort should be made to clear a damaged ship of her dead while still far out at sea. There might be bodies that were quite inaccessible, but every effort should be made to get at them. In hot climates, of course, immediate committal was essential. Attention to small details could greatly reduce the strain on a ship's company during committal—adequate and secure covering of bodies, adequate weighting, slits in the covering to prevent the formation of air pockets. Should a religious service not be possible at the time, a ceremonial memorial service should be held ashore later if at all possible. Immediate committal benefited by making use of the brief period of exaltation that followed action before reaction set in.

MORALE (Vol. II. *Ops.* p. 94)

The Royal Navy accepted as a basic factor that the newly recruited sailor is not, by nature, a hero and that it was necessary to make him into a fighter by training him to such a degree that he was able to overcome instincts of self-preservation and to carry out his task to the limits of his mental and physical capacity. To this end, reliance was placed on methods based on the power of suggestion and consisting of rigorous training and discipline, of leadership and confidence in officers, of an overwhelming pride in the individual ship and its achievements, and in the traditions of the Service, such as saluting the quarterdeck, the ceremony of colours and so on. The object of training was to create in him such a personal pride that failure to do his duty would become unthinkable. It was realised that, from the time a man first joined the Navy, he might well be in a state of emotional disturbance, because of worry over domestic affairs at home, the strangeness of his new surroundings and anxiety about the future. Later on, this anxious state might well be exacerbated by the presence of constant danger at sea. Probably the most potent of these factors was worry about domestic affairs at home, and great care was always taken over ensuring the quick delivery of mails. Although letters from home did much to support morale at sea, there were also times when they could cast him down. One medical officer recorded in his Journal that 'The vast majority of men who reported to me with minor physical and mental complaints did so immediately after receiving a worrying letter from home'. War-time training directed itself towards the idea that 'I am a British sailor. The British sailor has always been the best seaman and the finest fighter, and the hero of the people. Therefore I am a hero'. The principle was that nothing in the course of a man's instruction or surroundings must be allowed to arouse counter-suggestions to this conception of himself. Everything was done to reinforce this conception by insisting on smartness of dress, erect carriage, rigid discipline and personal pride in self, ship and the Navy. It was considered, rightly, that the exigencies of war were no excuse for relaxing Naval traditions, even as regards minor customs of the Service, which the newly-entered officer or man might regard as irksome or even as a waste of time and energy. It was found that the exigencies of war called for an even more meticulous observation of Naval traditions as this went far towards identifying the modern sailor with the sailor heroes of the past. Officers were taught that to praise a recruit under training was all important in order to justify his confidence in his own ability and that, where a reprimand was necessary, it was essential to couch it in terms that would leave a man's pride and self-respect intact, for a man without pride could not be expected to fight well.

Having once established a man's morale, the next difficult task was to sustain this morale through long periods of tedious and monotonous routine afloat, and this brought other factors into play. As in the case of the soldier and airman, so in the sailor, the commonest source of conflict in his mind was usually bound up with the fear of failure and the possibility of personal cowardice. Many medical officers recorded evidence which suggested that all emotion must have an outlet either in activity or in free discussion, and that should this outlet be denied, the results tended to display themselves as a continuous sense of anxious unrest caused by the conflict of three impulses. These were the natural urge to run away, the disciplined need to fight and the profound underlying fear of being thought a coward. From 1941 onwards, it became customary in many ships to give explanatory lectures on the reaction of the mind to fear, and there is no doubt that the experienced medical officer could do much in this way to diminish individual liability of some men to 'nervous breakdown'. These explanatory lectures adopted the approach that fear must inspire some reaction, the most primitive form being the reaction of flight. Officers responsible for training were taught that this primitive reaction could always be replaced by other action provided that training was thorough. The importance of meticulous and detailed instruction was urged, so that every man in the ship would know his exact job under all circumstances. The men themselves came to understand that the essence of the control of fear was to abolish uncertainty. Panic was never likely to occur without uncertainty as to what to do or where to go, and such uncertainty could be prevented by training. Concurrently, the Navy was always able to rely upon the power of example of its officers. This feature of leadership has been described in some quarters as depending on hero worship. Be this as it may, there is little doubt that the power of example remained throughout the war the most important and fundamental element in the mind of the naval rating. Although its psychological mechanism would be difficult to explain, and even more difficult to prove, there is probably much to be said for the view that each man tended to identify himself with his leader, and within broad limits would be likely to imitate him. The great sea captains of the past owed much of their success to this power of example and during the Second World War the behaviour of the officers of a man-of-war was again the keystone of the whole structure of the morale of her ship's company.

It came to be recognised that mood is the mirror of morale, and that the most dangerous mood is one of boredom, depression and 'bloody-mindedness'. To combat this, the Navy was always careful to see that a man should feel that his personal welfare was being considered as much as possible under the prevailing conditions of service. The organisation of incoming and outgoing mails was regarded as of the greatest importance, and leave and recreation were studied as much as possible. Encouragement, reassurance, praise and example were redoubled when men were tired, while the feeling of hate, too, could be instilled with value should the opportunity or need arise. A further important measure which was encouraged in all men-of-war was that, when a ship was in action, a special officer was detailed to stand at a microphone and broadcast what was going on so that men between decks and engineers and stokers in the bowels of the ship should not be left in ignorance of the details and progress of the action. The Second World War once again showed that a man-of-war is the finest background possible to foster morale by virtue of two qualities. One is the affectionate, sentimental pride felt alike by officers and men for their ship, and the other the sober fact that, in a naval action, the safest activity is steady devotion to duty rather than flight.

It has to be recognised that individual tolerance of conditions of active service afloat and threshold of fear vary, and that, while the individual threshold can be increased by rigorous training and good leadership, prolonged mental strain and physical hardship endured through months and even years of active service could not fail to reduce the threshold. It was well to realise that, no matter how high an individual's morale might appear to be, if pushed too far too long, there must come a time when his threshold would be reached and passed, with the result that the individual might suddenly collapse. This sequence of events was always more liable to happen in the case of the senior executive officer, who carried on his shoulders the ultimate burden of the ship's welfare and efficiency. Moreover, this officer's high sense of duty caused him to control and hide his personal feelings as part of his code for setting a good example to his subordinates. He tended to regard signs of strain in himself as a personal weakness which he would struggle to overcome, thereby further burdening himself and establishing the foundations of a vicious circle both mentally and physically. In this struggle to preserve his own high sense of duty, it would be only natural that he would demand the same of others, and would be quick to regard the normal by-products of mental and physical strain among his subordinates as weaknesses for which they themselves were personally responsible. In the early stages of the war there is no doubt that many commanding officers were permitted to remain too long in sea commands, and this was particularly so in the case of the many overworked destroyers and smaller units of the Fleet. Later, sea commissions were sensibly shortened and twelve to eighteen months of active service afloat at one stretch came to be regarded as the average period during which a commanding officer could be expected to give of his best. To some extent, this principle also came to be observed in the case of all officers and men as the war progressed.

It was of paramount importance that the medical officer should be so well acquainted with his fellow-officers and with the rest of the ship's company, especially senior ratings in key positions, as to be able to recognise early signs of failure of tolerance, in order that action might be initiated to arrange necessary rest. Sometimes the evidence of impending collapse might be so slender that great experience on the part of the medical officer was necessary before he could take action, and even then the medical officer himself might be tempted to delay in making the report which it was his duty to make, on account of his personal friendship with the officer concerned, and on account of the reluctance to initiate that personal resentment which might so frequently result. By 1943, the Navy had firmly established a clinical entity honourably labelled 'Fatigue'. This was applied to many officers and men who had fought hard and successfully, and replaced what would formerly have been a diagnosis of 'Anxiety State', thereby avoiding an implied slight on the man's character and adverse effect upon his Service career. Above all, it enabled a tired man to be rested, and used to fight again later.

At the same time, it was necessary that steps should be taken in the reverse direction to ensure that abuse did not arise. (Vol. II. *Ops.* p. 103.) It was vital that the number of men found medically unfit for sea service should be limited to those whose medical state justified this classification. It was unfortunately true that there were a number of men whose only real ailment was an unwillingness to serve at sea. To draw attention to these, an explanatory Fleet Order was published, laying down the course of action to be taken in regard to cases suspected of malingering. Many medical officers serving in the Navy at that time had had little Service experience, and their natural inclination was always to make the presumed well-being of their patient their only consideration. Medical Officers were reminded, however, that experience showed that there were other factors which had frequently to be taken into account, and that these other factors involved both the interests of the Navy and fairness to other ratings. It often happened that a patient who was determined to avoid sea service, sometimes with truly stated, and sometimes with untruly stated symptoms, got himself discharged to hospital or depot for investigation. Such a man, should his symptoms be false, would be found by the naval hospital fit, and would subsequently be drafted to sea. On arriving in his new ship, the man would re-state his symptoms, adding the information that he had already been in hospital for the same trouble. He might then well be discharged once again to hospital or depot for further investigation. He had now established for himself a 'hospital history', which eventually made it almost impossible to get him to, or to keep him at, sea.

The Fleet Order fully appreciated the difficulties confronting medical officers when dealing with such men, who 'knew the ropes', and the natural desire of heads of departments in a ship in which such men were employed to get rid of a 'passenger', *via* the medical route if possible. The serious effect on morale of better men and the cumulative effect of large numbers becoming unfit for sea service were, however, pointed out, and instructions issued for the procedure to be adopted in order that suspected malingerers might be adequately and fairly dealt with. Closer co-operation between medical officers on the one hand, and the executive officers, heads of departments and divisional officers on the other, was urged. An insight into the man's character was to be afforded to the medical officer by the officers under whom the man was employed, and the existing Fleet Order, under which an executive officer was to render a report on all neuro-psychiatric cases was now extended to include all cases suspected of malingering. Should the medical officer decide, after full discussion with the executive officer concerned, to send the case to hospital or depot for investigation, a full statement, including the executive report, was to accompany the man. In the case of a man suspected of substantial malingering, this suspicion was to be recorded on his medical history sheet, as well as the result of any investigations and a record of any disciplinary action already taken. Suspected malingerers, on discharge from hospital, were to be made the subjects of special reports in detail, and of thorough investigation by naval depots. Hospital specialists were to be consulted as necessary and, should disciplinary action be applicable, this was to be taken by the depot authorities before the man was redrafted to sea.

ARCTIC CONVOYS (Vol. II. *Ops.* p. 464.)

The especially arduous conditions experienced in the course of the Arctic Convoy battles brought out a number of interesting and valuable features concerning morale. Study of available records allows those persons who displayed a loss or lowering of morale to be divided into two classes, *viz*, survivors of ships which were lost, and those whose ships had not been lost.

As regards the former group, in general the morale of survivors was considered to be low. This appeared to be due, not so much to lack of personal courage as to a combination of a number of the factors which are outlined below:

(i) Having been resuscitated on board the rescuing ship, most survivors were then unoccupied, which was bad for their morale, especially during subsequent action.

(ii) Most of the officers and men concerned were professional seamen of the Royal or Merchant Navy. They were now travelling as passengers in the ship which had rescued them and they found this status irksome and, being themselves unoccupied and currently disorientated, they were not slow to shower adverse criticism on the qualities of seamanship displayed by their hosts.

(iii) Many survivors were 'lifeboat and raft conscious' for a considerable period after the rescue. They were apprehensive during subsequent enemy action and found it difficult to remain below decks. After rescue, in a crowded ship at sea, it was more than obvious that there was inadequate boat and raft accommodation for the large numbers on board should the rescuing ship herself become a casualty.

When possible, British Royal and Merchant Navy survivors were absorbed into the organisation of the rescuing ship, with marked improvement in their morale. In the case of survivors of other nations, this was not always possible. In the latter case, it was often noticed that the lower deck survivors assumed that their officers no longer had authority over them, and the morale of both officers and men suffered in consequence.

Once landed in North Russia, every factor that might have helped to restore morale was lacking. Their homes, corporate ship life, discipline, occupation, even their uniforms and to some extent their identities, had disappeared. Accommodation available to them was crowded, inadequate, uncomfortable and lacking in many of the simplest amenities, being usually in requisitioned and improvised buildings. The result was seen in large numbers of men loitering in the streets of Archangel and Murmansk, hanging about gloomy hospitals, with shaved heads and dressed in a miscellaneous assortment of garments, which themselves went far to remove the supports of crumbling self-respect. Boredom, vodka and hope deferred were usually added to their initial trials until they could be accommodated in homeward-bound ships which had to run the gauntlet of further severe enemy attack before safety was reached in the United Kingdom.

Among personnel in the other group, morale was found to be extremely high during the course of operations. But the constant strain of action left its mark on many and manifested itself in various forms after the experience was over. The outstanding effect was fatigue, so that every action—to climb a ladder, even to brush the hair—became a major problem of energy. (Vol. II. *Ops.* p. 426.) From one ship, nine officers were invalided at the end of one year in commission. 'There was nothing wrong with the morale of these officers, all of whom had fought magnificently and did so again'. These effects tended to worsen with repeated voyages. One medical officer said, in his Journal, 'I am finding the apprehension much worse, even though things are quieter than on my other trips. But I have never felt so tired. Our men seemed to get hyper-emotional and disorientated on this convoy and I must admit that a lot of it is a mental blur to me. I found it common enough for a responsible officer or rating to sit alone with me and weep a little and dry his eyes and go back to his job. At one time, I can't remember which day, I saw a seaman aiming at an aircraft, and he broke down and sobbed because his hands were too cold and clammy to work his gun'. This was a particularly bad convoy. There was, after a ship had been on many successive convoys, a reaction to the prolonged and repeated stress and strain, shown by an increase in the numbers attending the sick bay and, collectively, by the development of apathy and listlessness which had previously been quite foreign to the nature of the ship's company. Individual reactions fell roughly into three classes:

  (i) The man who came up and said outright that he was afraid and could stand no more. These often responded to suggestion and sedatives.

  (ii) The man who veiled his mental state by assuming a physical malady. Some of these, too, responded to suggestion and sedatives.

  (iii) The man who sought a means of escape in alcoholic intoxication. (Vol. II. *Ops.* p. 466.)

Many medical officers considered that no one, except those who actively desired to stay, should remain in a ship for longer than 18 months.

In many cases, reaction did not manifest itself until later, by which time the environment associated with unpleasant experiences had become the ship itself, from which there was no escape. A period of rest ashore, or even transfer to another ship, would mean a change of environment, which would bring forth a new mental and psychological adjustment.

Another medical officer remarked 'In my opinion, the greatest danger of the Arctic in time of war afloat is the mental effect of the climate. I have no doubt at all that fear against the Arctic background is a far more difficult thing to control than fear in other theatres of war. My own mental attitude had always differed in the Mediterranean and the Tropics, where I knew that the water was warm and most of the surrounding lands would at least be populated, even if you were taken prisoner-of-war. But here, in the Arctic, there was just nothing. The noise was dementing and behind it all was the awe-inspiring beauty of the Arctic with its cruel cold, its dreadful loneliness and what seemed to be the utter hopelessness of survival should the worst happen'.

H.M.S. STANDARD

In conclusion, some reference should be made to the commissioning of H.M.S. *Standard*, a rehabilitation centre established in Northumberland in January 1942, to form a labour unit in which men, whose conduct had been unreliable but who had no medical complaints justifying invaliding, could be employed in work of naval importance while remaining under naval discipline. (Vol. I. *Admin.* p. 151.) The selection of trainees was an executive decision, arrived at with the assistance of the medical authorities. When a man's conduct was such that he was considered unreliable and useless in general service, but physically fit and amenable to training, he was placed in category C/Q and sent to H.M.S. *Standard* for training to become fit for full or restricted service in the Navy. This system allowed both the Executive and the Medical Authorities the opportunity to remove from general service, without actual discharge from the Navy, those troublesome individuals who were constitutionally unfitted for life at sea in time of war. The particular group of men whose needs were served were to some extent both culpable and abnormal, but they were neither pure psychiatrics nor pure delinquents who could be dealt with either in hospital or in detention quarters. As many of the men concerned might have a history of repeated desertion, it was necessary to choose a site which would render such an offence difficult. It was also necessary to provide an environment free from the distraction of cinemas, public houses and camp followers and the disturbances of air raids. This was achieved by the discovery and adaptation of a former Ministry of Labour Training Centre for the unemployed, in the heart of the Cheviots.

The view of the Admiralty was that the establishment should be a place where hard manual work might be substituted for the hazards and hardships of active service afloat, the primary object being to instil self-discipline, and to show the individual that privileges are the reward for correct conduct and steady industry, and not his prerogative. This having been achieved, the intended procedure was to place the man in due course in a situation where the environmental circumstances would not prevent his giving reliable service. The camp was under Executive control and represented a combined operation between the Executive and the Medical Authorities, and was never regarded either as a hospital or as a penal establishment. Discipline was strict, isolation was extreme. Leave was restricted and was not granted at all until after a probationary period of one month's good conduct. After four Saturday afternoons ashore without untoward incident, each man became entitled to a week-end leave at home, and a further week-end each month subsequently. Men who had responded well were granted seven days' leave before drafting to a ship or shore service abroad.

In addition to general measures, special treatment by way of personal influence formed a most important element in the system of rehabilitation. There was here probably more personal and individual attention than anywhere else in the Navy, made possible by the comparatively large number of officers staffing the establishment in relation to the usual strength of the trainees, normally limited to 100. Each trainee was interviewed frequently by the commanding officer, schoolmaster, chaplain, medical officer and psychiatrist, and these various officers each exerted an influence from his own particular aspect, and they were ready to pool their knowledge for the benefit of others. In this way, a common policy could be reached. The final phase of treatment aimed at an assessment by the commanding officer from the executive aspect, after obtaining a clear impression from the psychiatrist. As time went on, methods were gradually altered. The aggressive type of trainee required an outlet for his impulses, which was provided by physical training, games and manual work in the open air. The timid and heavy-hearted were encouraged to exert themselves both mentally and physically in an effort to improve their morale. Behind the daily work and exercise, there was a constant round of naval routine, in which hoisting of colours, divisions, church, rounds and the rum issue, all played their part in keeping the trainee in touch with the Service to which it was hoped he would return as a useful member.

After three months in H.M.S. *Standard*, the suitability of the trainee for draft came up for discussion. Between three-and-a-half and four months proved to be the usual length of stay. Four months after taking up a draft, a report was made to H.M.S. *Standard* by the medical officer of the ex-trainee's present ship or establishment. This drafting of the trainee was the most important function of H.M.S. *Standard*, and the response of the individual to training enabled a definite decision to be made in many problem cases. Certain trainees were recommended for discharge as useless, while others merited purely medical disposal. In the bulk of cases it was possible to suggest the best type of future employment in the Service—service in a depot ship, boom defence vessels, small coastal craft or shore bases at home or abroad, but over a third were considered fit for general service, and, of course, each man sent to restricted service released a fit man for general service, an important consideration in time of war.

H.M.S. *Standard* was closed in July 1945, having received 842 trainees, of whom 680 were returned to useful Service employment, including 271 to general service.

The Army Medical Services

By Professor F. A. E. Crew, D.Sc., M.D., LL.D., F.R.C.P. Ed., F.R.S.

CONTENTS

(95349)

DIAGRAMS

ABBREVIATIONS

A. . . .	. The Adjutant-General's Branch
A.A. . . .	. Anti-Aircraft
A.A.I. . .	. Allied Armies in Italy
A.B. . . .	. Army Book
A.C.C. . .	. Ambulance Car Company, R.A.S.C.
A. & D. . .	. Admission and Discharge (book)
A.D. Corps. .	. The Army Dental Corps
A.D.G. . .	. Assistant Director-General
A.D.H. . .	. Assistant Director of Hygiene
A.D.M.S. .	. Assistant Director of Medical Services
A.D.S. . .	. Advanced Dressing Station (of a field ambulance)
A.F. . . .	. Army Form
A.G. . . .	. Adjutant-General
A.L.F.S.E.A. .	. Allied Land Forces South East Asia
A.M.D. . .	. The Army Medical Directorate
A.S.C. . .	. Advanced Surgical Centre
A.T.S. . .	. The Auxiliary Territorial Service (now W.R.A.C.)
B.A.O.R. . .	. The British Army of the Rhine
B.E.F. . .	. The British Expeditionary Force, France, 1939
B.D.S. . .	. Beach Dressing Station
B.G.H. . .	. British General Hospital
B.L.A. . .	. British Liberation Army
B.T.E. . .	. British Troops in Egypt
B.T.G. . .	. British Troops in Greece
B.T.U. . .	. Base Transfusion Unit
C.A.E.S. . .	. Casualty Air Evacuation Squadron (R.A.F.)
C.A.M.S. . .	. Commander Army Medical Services
C.C.P. . .	. Casualty Collecting Post
C.C.S. . .	. Casualty Clearing Station
C.D.P. . .	. Casualty Disembarkation Point
C.E.P. . .	. Casualty Embarkation Point
C. in C. . .	. Commander-in-Chief
C.M.W.C. .	. The Central Medical War Committee
C.O.S.S.A.C. .	. Chief of Staff to the Supreme Allied Commander
C.R.A.S.C. .	. Commander Royal Army Service Corps
C.R.S. . .	. Camp Reception Station
D.A.A.G. . .	. Deputy Assistant Adjutant-General
D.A.D.A.P. .	. Deputy Assistant Director of Army Psychiatry
D.A.D.H. . .	. Deputy Assistant Director of Hygiene

D.A.D.M.S.	. .	Deputy Assistant Director of Medical Services
D.B.P.	. .	Di-butyl phthalate
D.C.I.G.S.	. .	Deputy Chief of the Imperial General Staff
D.D.G.A.M.S.	. .	Deputy Director-General of Army Medical Services
D.D.M.S. .	. .	Deputy Director of Medical Services
D.D.S.T. .	. .	Deputy Director Supplies and Transport
D.D.T.	. .	Dichloro-diphenyl-trichlorethane
D.G.A.M.S.	. .	The Director-General Army Medical Services
D.M.P.	. .	Di-methyl phthalate
D.M.R.	. .	Director(ate) of Medical Research
D.M.S.	. .	Director of Medical Services
D.U.K.W. .	. .	A $2\frac{1}{2}$-ton amphibious vehicle
D.Z. .	. .	Dropping Zone
E.M.S.	. .	The Emergency Medical Services of the Ministry of Health and of the Department of Health for Scotland
Fd.Amb.	. .	Field Ambulance
F.D.C.	. .	Field Dental Centre
F.D.S.	. .	Field Dressing Station
F.S.T.	. .	Field Surgical Team
F.S.U.	. .	Field Surgical Unit
F.T.T.	. .	Field Transfusion Team
F.T.U.	. .	Field Transfusion Unit
G. .	. .	General Staff Branch
G.D.O.	. .	General Duty Medical Officer or General Duty Orderly
Gen.Hosp. .	. .	General Hospital
G.H.Q.	. .	General Headquarters
G.S. .	. .	General Service
G.1098	. .	Mobilisation Equipment Scale
H.A.A.	. .	Heavy Anti-Aircraft
H.Q. .	. .	Headquarters
I.A.M.C.	. .	The Indian Army Medical Corps
I.M.S.	. .	The Indian Medical Service
I.1248	. .	Medical Mobilisation Equipment Scale
L.C.I.	. .	Landing Craft, Infantry
L/Cpl.	. .	Lance-Corporal
L.C.T.	. .	Landing Craft, Tank
L. of C.	. .	Line or Lines of Communication
L.S.I.	. .	Landing Ship, Infantry

L.S.T.	. . .	Landing Ship, Tank
L.V.T.	. . .	Landing Vehicle, Tracked
L.V.W.	. . .	Landing Vehicle, Wheeled
M.A.C.	. . .	Motor Ambulance Convoy; Motor Ambulance Company, R.A.S.C.
m/c.	. . .	Motor Cycle
M.D.T.	. . .	Mobile Dental Team
M.D.S.	. . .	Main Dressing Station (of a field ambulance)
M.E.H.D.H.Q.	. .	Medical Embarkation and Hospital Distribution Headquarters
M.F.S.U.	. .	Maxillo-facial Surgical Unit
M.F.T.U.	. .	Medical Forward Treatment Unit or Malaria Forward Treatment Unit
M.N.S.U.	. .	Mobile Neurosurgical Unit
M.O.	. .	Medical Officer
M.O.U.	. .	Mobile Ophthalmic Unit
M.R.C.	. .	The Medical Research Council
M.S.	. . .	Military Secretary
N.C.O.	. .	Non-commissioned Officer
N.O.	. . .	Nursing Orderly
O.2E.	. .	Officer-in-charge 2nd Echelon, G.H.Q.
O.C.	. .	Officer Commanding
O. i/c.	. .	Officer in charge
Operation 'Neptune'	.	The assault landing on the Normandy shore, 1944
O.R.	. . .	Other Rank
P.	. . .	Provost Branch
P.A.C.	. .	Prophylactic Ablution Centre
Para.	. . .	Parachute
P.o.W.	. .	Prisoner(s)-of-War
Pte	. . .	Private
Q.	. . .	Quartermaster General's Branch
Q.A.I.M.N.S.	.	Queen Alexandra's Imperial Military Nursing Service (now as below)
Q.A.R.A.N.C.	.	Queen Alexandra's Royal Army Nursing Corps
R.A.	. . .	The Royal Regiment of Artillery
R.A.D.C.	. .	The Royal Army Dental Corps
R.A.F.	. .	The Royal Air Force
R.A.F.M.S.	.	The Royal Air Force Medical Services
R.A.M.C.	. .	The Royal Army Medical Corps
R.A.M. College	.	The Royal Army Medical College
R.A.P.	. .	Regimental Aid Post

R.A.S.C. . . . The Royal Army Service Corps (now The Royal
                Corps of Transport)
R.E. . . . . The Corps of Royal Engineers
R.H.U. . . . Reinforcement Holding Unit
R.M.O. . . . Regimental Medical Officer
R.M.P. . . . Regimental Medical Post (A.A.)
R.N. . . . . The Royal Navy
R.T. . . . . Radio Telephony

S.A.C.S.E.A. . . Supreme Allied Commander South East Asia
S.B. . . . . Stretcher-bearer
S.D. . . . . Staff Duties
S.H.A.E.F. . . Supreme Headquarters Allied Expeditionary Force
S.M.O. . . . Senior Medical Officer
S.R.N. . . . State Registered Nurse
S. & T. . . . Supply and Transport

U.K. . . . . The United Kingdom
U.S. or U.S.A. . . The United States of America

V.A.D. . . . Voluntary Aid Detachment (B.R.C.S.)
V.D. . . . . Venereal Disease
V.D.T.C. . . . Venereal Diseases Treatment Centre
V.D.T.T. . . . Venereal Diseases Treatment Team

W.H.O. . . . The World Health Organisation
W.R.A.C. . . . The Women's Royal Army Corps (formerly A.T.S.)
W.W.C.P. . . . Walking Wounded Collecting Post

INTRODUCTION

DURING the war years, 1939–45, the British Army Medical Services discharged their manifold functions in a wide variety of physical, climatic and demographic settings and in an equally wide diversity of tactical situations. Much of great and immediate value was gleaned from the experience gained and was incorporated into policy and practice while the war was still being fought. Each senior administrative medical officer during and at the end of a campaign recorded his opinions as to the ways in which improvements in the organisation and functioning of these Services might be achieved and these opinions merit very careful study.

Campaigns.

The planning for each of these campaigns was advantaged by the lessons that had been learnt in the earlier ones and it can be stated without fear of contradiction that by the time Operation 'Overlord' was launched in 1944 the Army Medical Services, taking full advantage of the advances in medical knowledge and skill that had occurred, had developed an organisation and a series of procedures that enabled them to attain a truly remarkable degree of efficiency. The power to repair the damage

(95349)

C*

that resulted from enemy missile, accidental injury and disease, possessed by these Services surpassed that of the vast majority of the agencies causing disability and death.

The introduction of the atomic bomb, which brought the war to an abrupt and startling end, though it in no way affected the organisation and functioning of the Army Medical Services during its course, created a completely new situation for which these Services were in no way prepared. The power of the weapon to maim and kill suddenly came to exceed by far that of the Army Medical Services to repair and prevent. These Services, like all the other components of the Armed Forces of the Crown, were to be called upon in the post-war years to attune themselves to entirely new concepts of strategy and tactics and to prepare themselves for participation in two kinds of warfare, one in which, for a variety of reasons, only pre-atomic-bomb weapons or modifications of these (the so-called conventional weapons) would be employed and the other in which the nations possessing the lineal descendants of the bomb that obliterated Hiroshima would be involved and in which these weapons would be used.

It is difficult in these circumstances to estimate the extent to which and the length of time during which the lessons learnt during 1939–45 will continue to be of value. In so far as general principles are concerned they will continue to have their applications in all forms of warfare, irrespective of the kind of weapons that are used. But in respect of detail, it is reasonable to assume that they will be of value only in that kind of warfare in which the conventional weapons are employed. The billowing cloud of the exploding atomic bomb heralded the passage of mankind from one era into another, the two being as distinct as were the stone and bronze ages of man's early history.

Military medicine, in its endeavours to ensure that for the wounded and the sick the very best medical care shall be provided, has become sub-divided into so many specialties that no one man can possibly be sufficiently acquainted with all of them and with the war-time developments in each of them as to be able to decide which of these developments were of an enduring kind. Nor can one man, reviewing the opinions of the senior administrative medical officers presented in the different volumes of this History, hope to identify all those which have influenced post-war policy and practice. The views and considered opinions of such as had served in the Army Medical Directorate during the war years either as consultants or administrative officers were therefore sought and those who had served as senior administrative medical officers in the different campaigns were invited to look once more at the reports they had written. These are the men who during the war years either initiated or else witnessed and guided such developments as occurred and who are now best equipped to assess their value.

This is particularly so in the case of the man who for the greater part of the war years so successfully headed the Army Medical Services as D.G.A.M.S., Lieutenant-General Sir Alexander Hood, G.B.E., K.C.B. For the most part the opinions of these consultants and senior administrative medical officers have been interwoven into the texture of this account without special acknowledgement. But, where it seemed more appropriate, these opinions are included as quotations and their authorship is indicated by the initials of the persons concerned.

This account deals with the administrative and organisational aspects of the 'clinical services', surgery, medicine, pathology; their professional aspects are dealt with elsewhere in this volume. In so far as psychiatry is concerned the administrative and organisational developments that took place were so comprehensively covered by Dr. Ahrenfeldt in his response to a request for his views, that it was decided that his account should appear under his own name. Dr. Ahrenfeldt held the position of D.A.D.A.P. in the Army Medical Directorate shortly after the end of the war and wrote an excellent book on *Psychiatry in the British Army in the Second World War*. In this he had done for this specialty that which is to be attempted here for all the others.

It seemed reasonable to assume that the lessons that had been learnt and which seemed to possess a relatively permanent value would quickly become incorporated into the administrative and instructional procedures of the R.A.M.C. in the immediate post-war years. A comparison was made, therefore, between things as they were in the years immediately before and after the war, making use of the 1935 *R.A.M.C. Training Manual*, and Lieutenant-Colonel T. B. Nicholls' *Organisation, Strategy and Tactics of the Army Medical Services in War*, 1937, which was based upon this manual, and the 1950 *R.A.M.C. Training Pamphlet* No. 2. It was assumed that by 1950 all that had been learnt and that was regarded as being of value would have been incorporated into policy and practice. It was assumed also that this was far too soon for the repercussions of the dropping of the bomb on Hiroshima to have exerted any profound effect upon the affairs of the Army Medical Services.

List of those whose opinions are quoted, together with a statement of their wartime appointments:

A.H.   Lieutenant-General Sir Alexander Hood, G.B.E., K.C.B. D.D.M.S. B.E.F. (France and Belgium 1939–40); D.D.M.S. Scottish Command; D.G.A.M.S. 1941–48.

A.P.   Brigadier Sir Arthur Porritt, Bt. G.C.M.G., K.C.V.O., C.B.E. Consulting Surgeon Second Army (N.W. Europe).

E.A.S.   Major-General E. A. Sutton, c.b., c.b.e., m.c. O.C. 9 B.G.H.;
            D.D.M.S. Alexandria Area (L. of C. Western Desert, Greece,
            Crete); D.M.S. East Africa Force; D.D.M.S. C.O.S.S.A.C.;
            Deputy Chief Surgeon S.H.A.E.F.; D.M.S., A.A.I.

E.P.   Major-General Sir Edward Phillips, k.b.e., c.b., d.s.o., m.c.
            A.D.M.S. Ind. 10 Div. (Iraq and Iran); D.D.M.S. XIII
            Corps; D.D.M.S. XXX Corps; D.D.M.S. Eighth Army
            (Western Desert, Sicily, Italy); D.D.M.S. Second Army;
            D.M.S. B.L.A. and B.A.O.R. (N.W. Europe).

E.W.W.   Brigadier E. W. Wade, d.s.o., o.b.e. A.D.H. Scottish Command;
            A.D.M.S. 52 Div.; D.D.M.S. III Corps; D.D.M.S. First
            Army (N. Africa); Inspector of Medical Services, War Office.

G.E.M.   Major-General G. E. MacAlevey, c.b.e., d.s.o., m.c. A.D.M.S.
            Ind. 17 Div.; D.D.M.S. Fourteenth Army (Burma).

H.O.   Major-General Sir Heneage Ogilvie, k.b.e. Consulting Surgeon
            East Africa and Middle East.

I.A.   Lieutenant-Colonel Ian Aird (later Professor of Surgery in the
            London Post-graduate Medical School). Commanded one of
            the earliest mobile surgical units in the Western Desert.

J.C.D.   Major-General J. C. Dowse, c.b., c.b.e., m.c. O.C. 11 B.G.H.;
            A.D.M.S. 44 Div.; Inspector of Medical Services, War Office;
            D.D.M.S. A.F.H.Q. (N. Africa); D.M.S. Eighth Army (Italy);
            D.M.S. Cairo; D.D.G.A.M.S. War Office.

J.C.W.   Colonel J. C. Watts, o.b.e., m.c. Surgical Specialist 2/5 C.C.S.
            (Western Desert Force); 8 B.G.H., Alexandria; 9 B.G.H.,
            Cairo; 2 C.C.S., Haifa and Damascus; 16 B.G.H. Jerusalem;
            O.C. Reserve F.S.T., Eighth Army, Tripoli, Zuara and Sfax;
            Surgical Specialist 59 B.G.H., Salerno and Castelamare; O.C.
            F.S.U. 78 Div. and Polish Carpathian Div.; Surgical Specialist
            195 A/L Fd. Amb. 6 Airborne Div.; D.A.D.M.S. 6 Airborne
            Div. (N.W. Europe); O.C. 225 Para. Fd. Amb. (Far East).

J.H.J.C.   Colonel J. H. J. Crosse, o.b.e. A.D.M.S. First Army; A.D.M.S.
            (Ops.) A.F.H.Q.; A.D.G., A.M.D.8.

J.M.M.   Major-General J. M. Macfie, c.b., c.b.e., m.c. D.A.D.M.S.
            B.T.E.; A.D.M.S. G.H.Q. Middle East; D.D.G.A.M.S.
            (Admin.) War Office.

J.R.R.   Brigadier J. R. Rees. Consulting Psychiatrist to the Army.

N.C.   Lieutenant-General Sir Neil Cantlie, k.c.b., k.b.e., m.c. O.C. 12
            C.C.S.; O.C. 28 B.G.H.; A.D.M.S. 46 Div.; D.D.M.S. V
            Corps (N. Africa and Italy); D.D.M.S. Eastern Command,
            India. (Succeeded Sir Alexander Hood as D.G.A.M.S.)

R.D.C.   Major-General R. D. Cameron, c.b., c.b.e., m.c. Medical Adviser to the Ministry of Supply; A.D.M.S. 43 Div.; A.D.M.S. 42 Armd. Div.; A.D.M.S. 3 Div. (Operation 'Neptune'); D.D.M.S XXX Corps (N.W. Europe); Inspector of Medical Services, War Office.

S.D-E.   Brigadier Sir Stewart Duke-Elder, g.c.v.o., f.r.s. Consulting Ophthalmic Surgeon to the Army.

T.O.T.   Lieutenant-General Sir Treffrey Thompson, k.c.s.i., c.b., c.b.e· D.D.M.S. Army in Burma; D.D.M.S. Eastern Army; D.M.S. 11 Army Group; D.M.S. A.L.F.S.E.A.; D.M.S. G.H.Q.(I.). Member of Medical Advisory Division at H.Q. S.A.C.S.E.A.

W.E.T.   Major-General W. E. Tyndall, c.b., c.b.e., m.c. A.D.M.S. Base Sub-area Norway; A.D.M.S. 11 Armoured Division; D.M.S. G.H.Q. Home Forces; D.D.G.A.M.S.(Ops.), War Office; D.M.S., A.L.F.S.E.A.

THE ARMY MEDICAL SERVICES

The Enlargement of the Concept of the Nature of Health

I T WAS during the war years that in several countries and especially in the United Kingdom the movement that was to expand the content and scope of Preventive Medicine so greatly gained impetus. The concepts relating to the nature and causes of disease are invariably associated with the prevailing notions concerning the nature of man. When man is regarded as a multicellular organism composed of a number of mutually interdependent parts, each of which makes its own special contribution to the smooth functioning of the whole community of parts, the individual, disease is looked upon as the consequence of the failure of one or more of these component parts to function normally. The failure of a part leads to a disharmony within the community and thus to disease. When man is thought of as a member of an ecological system, sharing his world with a multitude of other forms of living things, some of them having habits related to individuation and to reproduction that render them pathogenic to man, then disease is regarded as the consequence of the development of disharmony, of the disruption of an equilibrium, within the ecological system in which mutual tolerance and peaceful co-existence become replaced by conflict. Disharmony between the individual and the content of his external physical world, living and non-living, is the cause of disease. The great edifice of modern scientific medicine rests firmly on the foundations of these two concepts. Man is regarded as a biological being living in an external physical world. The whole organisation of the profession of medicine is a reflection of these concepts. There is the medicine of the part, cardiology, ophthalmology, etc. and of the region, chest surgery, etc. and there is the medicine of the ecological system, helminthology, malariology, etc., etc.

With the growth of the social sciences man came increasingly to be looked upon as a social being living in a social milieu and being affected by the attitudes and actions of other members of the group and by social institutions, aims and values. It came to be recognised that disharmony between the individual and the conditions and circumstances that obtained within the community was the cause of much ill-health and so the search for causation became extended from the physical to the social environment of individuals and groups.

This development had its repercussions in the Adjutant-General's

Branch during the war years. A Directorate of Personnel Selection was created to play its important part in the task of ensuring that as far as possible the mental and physical attributes of the individual soldier should be matched with the nature of the rôle he was to be called upon to play. To the Army Medical Directorate a Directorate of Psychiatry was added and consultants in psychology, psychiatry and physical medicine appointed. The PULHEMS system of medical and occupational classification was adopted by the Directorate of Hygiene. (*Admin*. I. p. 357.)

These happenings were in part evoked by similar though more ambitious developments that had been taking place in the medical services of the Canadian Armed Forces. The suggestion had been made that the Royal Canadian Army Medical Services should be greatly enlarged and transformed into the Royal Canadian Army Health Service, the word health in this context being given a meaning far more extensive than it can claim in orthodox medical circles. It was proposed to combine into one service medicine, personal and social psychology, social science, personnel selection and those specialties designated as being auxiliary or ancillary to medicine. In this way it was to be proclaimed that health and welfare were not to be dissociated and that health was the concern of many professional groups other than the medical.

The scheme was not adopted. It would have been difficult to effect such drastic changes in time of war and with the coming of peace there were many other reconstructional developments that claimed a higher priority and greater urgency. However, since the ideas from which these proposals stemmed were essentially sound, it is not improbable that with the passing of time some such enlargement as was then suggested will occur.

In the British Army these developments specially affected the Directorate of Hygiene which added to itself specialists in nutrition and physical medicine. (*Admin*. II. p. 26.) The great expansion of the interests and responsibilities of this directorate is outlined in the narrative of the campaign in Libya. (*Campaigns* II. p. 395.) There the statement is made that the Army Hygiene Service 'now accepts responsibility for studying all influences likely to enhance or undermine the vigour, fitness, well-being and efficiency of the soldier. Man-management is now included in the province of modern military medical services'.

It was in order to indicate the nature and magnitude of the changes that had occurred that the term hygiene was dropped and health inserted in its place in the titles of the Directorate of Army Health and of the Army Health Service.

'The demonstration which the British and Canadian Armies gave, and to a lesser extent the U.S. Army at a later date, certainly influenced

W.H.O. and other international bodies in stressing the essential need for inter-professional work and thought in dealing with matters of health as opposed to dealing with sickness and disability. Whether health is thought of as physical, mental or social, it must always involve a considerable team of people of different disciplines and outlook.' (J.R.R.)

The Need for Co-ordination between the Medical Services of the Royal Navy, the Army and the Royal Air Force

'During the war years there was inevitably an overall shortage of medically qualified persons to serve the civil population and the Armed Forces. The three Directors-General were obliged to compete in their demands before the Medical Man-power Committee. In the field of research it was difficult to avoid unnecessary duplication. In the various theatres of war the senior administrative medical officers of the three medical services acted more or less independently in matters of medical policy, e.g. numbers, sizes and locations of hospitals, needs and methods of evacuation, sanitation, priorities of supplies, of personnel, transport and equipment. On one occasion it was found necessary to ask a civilian arbitrator to decide upon the site of a hospital to serve all three services since the services themselves could not agree. The most economical and most efficient use of the resources available was rendered impossible by this division of the medical services into three. In every theatre there should be one head of all the medical services. Complete integration of the medical services of the Royal Navy, the Army and the Royal Air Force undoubtedly would be the best solution; it is bound to happen eventually for the reason that it would most certainly yield a far more efficient and economical service.' (A.H.)

'In a war of any magnitude Britain will always be stretched to the full to find the necessary man-power, particularly specialised man-power such as medical. The resources available will be limited and will have to be used in the most economical and efficient manner. With the development of combined operations and of combined joint command, the time has surely come when the medical provision for the three Fighting Services (and also for the civil population in time of war) should be amalgamated.' (T.O.T.)

This question of the complete fusion of the three medical services is one that has been investigated by a number of committees. The Mond-Weir Committee, 1922, was the first to study the possibility and desirability of the integration of these services. It recommended that there should be no amalgamation but that a Joint Committee on Medical Services should be appointed and charged with the task of achieving greater efficiency and economy through co-ordination. Then, in 1946, immediately after the end of the War of 1939–45, an interdepartmental committee was formed to study the possible advantages of drawing together certain of the administrative services, including the medical services, and of forming a combined organisation to provide common services. In the *Statement on Defence*, 1948 it is stated that 'further examination has not led His Majesty's Government to the conclusion that such a complete amalgamation would be in the real interests of economy and efficiency, either in existing circumstances or in those which are likely to obtain for many years to come. The Government consider, however, that a greater measure of co-ordination between these services is desirable.' A new Co-ordinating Committee was brought into being to replace the Joint Committee. Next came the Waverley Committee, 1953, appointed by the Minister of Defence to review the arrangements for providing medical and dental services for the Armed Forces at home and abroad, in peace and war and to make recommendations. This committee reported in 1955. It was in favour of integration at the hospital level but was of the opinion that this was not desirable in so far as forward medical units were concerned. Like the Mond-Weir Committee it decided that the objects which might be achieved by amalgamation could better be attained by co-ordination.

In 1958 a Select Committee was appointed by the Government to examine the estimates with a view to effecting economies. One of its sub-committees concerned itself with Services' estimates in so far as these related to the medical services. Much time and thought were given to the consideration of the possibility of integrating the three Services and ultimately (*Fourth Report from the Select Committee on Estimates, Medical Services of the Armed Forces*, 1959. *H.M.S.O.*) the committee recommended that the Services should adopt integration of both the medical and dental services as a long-term objective. The Ministers' comments upon this proposal were published in the *Sixth Special Report from the Select Committee on Estimates, Session* 1959–60. *H.M.S.O.* They stated that previous enquiries into the possibility of integration of the medical services had unanimously rejected it and that nearly all the evidence given to the Select Committee from all sources had been either against it or had not supported it. It was their view that there were grounds for believing that it would adversely affect recruiting; that there would be no economy and that a rise in cost was by no means inconceivable. Integration, they held would tend to blur the responsibilities of commanders for the care of their troops and might ultimately confuse ministerial responsibility. That being so it would be wrong to take the risk of changing over to a system which might well prove less effective in meeting the needs of the three Services, which, in the Ministers' view, must be regarded as the overriding criterion.

The Select Committee had recommended that the structure and

operation of the Canadian Forces Medical Services should be closely studied as a guide and that the Canadian progress towards integration should be followed in the United Kingdom. To this the Ministers replied that they would watch the Canadian scheme with interest and any good results would be made use of, but they pointed out that the scheme was as yet in its infancy. (The Indian Armed Forces adopted a similar scheme of integration for their medical services.)

The Ministers reported that, after further consideration, they rejected the idea of integration. They proposed to establish a small panel of civilian professional advisers who could be available for consultation and for the consideration of professional problems. They did not suggest that co-ordination was incapable of being carried further but suggested that if this is carried too far the dangers of over-centralisation, of slow reaction to change and of divided responsibility are likely to arise. They maintained that in respect of such co-ordination the point had already been reached where the dividends from eliminating duplication were becoming small.

At the end of this report the Select Committee on Estimates expressed its dissatisfaction with the Ministers' reaction to its recommendations and urged that the issues should be debated in the House of Commons.

In the evidence given by the representatives of the medical services much emphasis was placed upon the differing specialised medical needs of the three. But when this evidence is carefully examined it is found that the argument that such different needs made integration quite impossible is far from convincing. Of course aviation medicine, for example, is of prime importance to the R.A.F. and it is to be expected that the R.A.F. medical services will continue to be much occupied in the further development of this branch of occupational medicine. But aviation medicine is also of importance to the Royal Navy and to the Army for the R.A.F. has no monopoly of aviators and aircraft. Surely in the modern world aviation medicine has to be looked upon as a specialised branch of medicine of which all practitioners of medicine must know the elements and in which specialisation is to be encouraged.

The resistance of these representatives to any suggestion that a single hospital system could adequately serve the Navy, the Army and the Air Force could have surprised no one who remembered the difficulties of documentation, discipline and disposal that arose when, for example, a soldier was admitted to an E.M.S., R.N. or R.A.F. hospital during the war years. But such difficulties are not insurmountable.

Very little attention was paid by the committee to the hygiene, pathology and dental services. The nursing service was not considered at all. It would be very difficult indeed to maintain that the needs of the Navy, the Army and the Air Force are so different in respect of these that integration is unthinkable.

The argument that integration would have a very adverse effect upon the recruitment of medical officers was forcefully presented but was necessarily rooted in opinion and impression unsupported by any factual information.

It is not to be expected that the fusion of the three medical services will ever be easily achieved for many imponderables are involved, e.g. the loyalty of men to organisations with proud traditions and the satisfaction of really belonging to the Royal Navy or to the Royal Air Force or to the Army, as the case may be, and of being an heir to its glory. It is not to be expected that many members of these three Services would ever find it possible to suggest that his own should lose its identity. Nevertheless, the considered opinion of Sir Alexander Hood, who enjoyed unique opportunities for studying the matter and whose ability to reach sound conclusions through the exercise of cold reason is undisputed, is one that cannot easily be disregarded. It seems most likely that it will turn out to be a prophecy.

'During the war years the Emergency Medical Services of the Ministry of Health for England and Wales, the Department of Health for Scotland and the Ministry of Home Affairs in Northern Ireland actively co-operated with the medical services of the Armed Forces and accepted responsibility for the care of very large numbers of wounded, injured and sick from home commands and from overseas theatres of war. This sharing of responsibilities between military and civil medical services resulted in a number and variety of troublesome difficulties. (*Admin.* I. p. 194.) It is for consideration whether in the future any form of emergency medical service should not form part of one unified medical service.' (A.H.)

'The E.M.S. rendered very great service to the Army. To begin with there were difficulties arising out of the lack of understanding on the part of the members of the E.M.S. of the Army's needs and methods. But when once this deficiency had been remedied the medical officers of the E.M.S. were as helpful as they would have been as members of the R.A.M.C.' (J.R.R.)

It is to be noted that the vast majority of those who held commissions in the medical services of the Armed Forces during the war years were, on first appointment, just as unacquainted with the specific requirements of the military environment as were the medical officers of the E.M.S. They were 'civilians in uniform' who had taken with them into the strange new life ideas and attitudes that had been developed in, and that were appropriate to, civilian practice. It was not at all easy for many of them to accept and to act upon the view that the prime purpose that lay behind their professional activities was that of cutting down to the irreducible minimum man-power wastage due to injury or to sickness, to return to the line at the earliest possible moment the sick and the injured, cured and restored. The interests of the Army tend to override those of the individual. It is in this connexion that the military and the civilian points of view can diverge and even clash.

The question as to whether it would have been better had the E.M.S. been merged along with the medical services of the Armed Forces into one unified service is an important and very difficult one. In a war such as that of 1939–45 there was inevitably a very considerable wastage from the Armed Forces, very large numbers being found unfit for further military service and therefore being returned to civil life. The needs of these, in respect of rehabilitation preparatory to such return, are very different from the needs of those who, recovering from sickness or injury, are to resume their military activities. The latter must be dealt with in a military atmosphere, the former need a civilian-orientated atmosphere. A unified service, unified on a military basis presumably, could not deal adequately with rehabilitation for both military and civil life, could not provide both kinds of atmosphere. There was need, it would seem, for a civilian medical service to deal with this problem of rehabilitation for civil life.

Factors Affecting the Quality of the Functioning of the Army Medical Services

'The 1939–45 War was the first major conflict since the Crimea in which it was not found necessary to appoint a Commission of Enquiry to deal with some breakdown or failure on the part of the Army Medical Services. An examination of the reports of these Commissions reveals that two main causes operated to yield such breakdown (1) failure on the part of the General Staff to appreciate the nature and magnitude of the problems with which these Services were confronted and (2) failure on the part of the Army Medical Services to present their requirements for the performance of the tasks to be undertaken by them in a sufficiently convincing manner. The various components of the Army knew far too little of each other's organisation and special functions. Intelligent co-operation, based upon mutual understanding, was therefore difficult, if not impossible. In the 1939–45 War this state of affairs no longer existed.

'During the decade 1920–30 there developed a widespread acceptance of the view that for the attainment of efficiency it was imperative that between all arms and services within the Army there must be close co-operation based upon an understanding of each other's affairs. Following upon this, the system evolved whereby officers of all branches attended courses of instruction at the Army School of Hygiene while officers of the R.A.M.C. attended courses at all army schools of instruction, including the Staff College and the Senior Officers' School where they functioned both as students and instructors. It came to be the rule that medical problems were included in all training exercises from company training to army manoeuvres. Questions involving medical matters were also included in the promotion examination papers for branches other than the medical.

'In this way all officers, medical and others, came to cultivate the same system of ideas, to speak the same language, and were thus able to apply their own specialist knowledge to the solution of problems common to all. That which the medical officers learnt at the non-medical army schools of instruction was passed on to their colleagues during R.A.M.C. training. That which the non-medical officers learnt from their contacts with medicals in these schools enabled them to develop a clear conception of the special tasks that were undertaken by the Army Medical Services, of the importance of these in the establishment and maintenance of military efficiency and in the conservation of man-power, and of the requirements of the medical services in the field.

'It is safe to say that in the future, as in the past, the quality of the contribution that the Army Medical Services make to any given military enterprise will be determined by the extent to which the various components of the army, including its medical services, understand each other's problems, potentialities and needs.' (A.H.)

'By the time the war had ended it is safe to say that the A.M.S. had achieved a state of efficiency unequalled in the past and unlikely to be bettered in the future. The reasons for this were, in my opinion:

1. The experience gained by the older age-groups when serving in the A.M.S. in the 1914–18 War. They were "blooded" as youngsters and they came to constitute the solid core of the senior administrative medical officers in the 1939–45 War.

2. The greater understanding by, and therefore the closer co-operation with, army and corps commanders who really did seem in 1939–45 to appreciate the worth of the A.M.S. in the conservation of man-power and in the maintenance of morale. The Crimean and Boer Wars, the slaughter of Passchendaele and the Somme, the scandal of Mesopotamia and the tragedy of the porters in East Africa, grim and tragic as these were at the time, taught lessons that were learnt and not forgotten.

3. The unfailing support given at all times to the man on the spot by the Army Medical Directorate.

4. The intelligent construction of a multiplicity of new medical units on an as required and often *ad hoc* basis by Ds.M.S. and D.Ds.M.S. in the different theatres, ably advised by their consultants.

5. The vastly expanded powers of the Army Hygiene Service in the fields of health-promotion and disease prevention.

'Could the great captains of the past have been able to return as spectators of the conflict, what would have astonished them would not have been the new weapons and the new strategies but the fact that hundreds of thousands of troops could live for years under war conditions in many different parts of the world and yet not be decimated by the great epidemic diseases.' (E.A.S.)

This last sentence merits elaboration. Up to the beginning of the present century wars were invariably associated with, and were followed by, great epidemics of such diseases as plague, cholera, typhoid, typhus and dysentery. Larrey, the great military surgeon of Napoleonic times, had good reason to record that 'the greatest enemies of the soldier are not the bullets of the enemy but cold weather, poor food and disease'. Napoleon's indirect attack upon Britain through the Middle East in 1798 was largely wrecked by trachoma in Egypt and by bubonic plague in Syria. Haiti remained an independent Negro republic for the reason that yellow fever intervened when Napoleon sent an army of 30,000 men to the island in 1801–02. When some 23,000 of these had been stricken down by this disease the French withdrew and left the island to its Negro population, which enjoyed the great advantage of an acquired immunity. In the Crimean War of 1854–56 the number of battle casualties was quite insignificant when compared with the number of those who died from disease. In the Boer War at the turn of the century some 8,000 were killed in action while some 14,000 succumbed to disease. In the expeditionary force as a whole one man in every six went down with typhoid fever and of those who did 8,022 died.

Throughout history, right up to the end of the 19th century, wars invariably brought great danger and even disaster to the peoples of the countries in which they were fought. The pestilences that attended and followed in the wake of the Thirty Years War in the first half of the seventeenth century, for example, turned much of North-west and Central Europe into a veritable desert; three-quarters of the population died, the depopulated cities fell into decay and agriculture languished through lack of labour.

It was in the Russo-Japanese War of 1904/5 that for the first time in history the old alliance between the sword of the soldier and the sickle of the Grim Reaper was broken. Of the total Japanese dead only 2·1 per cent. died from disease. Behind this truly remarkable achievement lay a grand record of peace-time discovery in the medical field and of the war-time application and exploitation of the fruits of such discovery in the military sphere. Vaccination and inoculation became the means whereby men could be equipped with new biological qualities that would enable them to flourish in strange ecological systems. By them the individual was provided with a shield of immunity that protected him against the assaults of pathogenic micro-organisms. The records of the last half-century reveal how very successful this protection has been. Armies have moved amid populations in which the great epidemic diseases were rife. When it has been found necessary to banish such diseases from the civil population of an area, this has been done, as in the case of typhus in Naples. In the wake of an army epidemics no longer sweep through a country.

Throughout man's history his mastery over his physical environment has at all times been greatly impeded by malaria. From the greater part of North-west Europe this disease has been banished but in most other parts of the world, wherever the appropriate species of the mosquito are found, it is exceedingly prevalent. The wars of Imperial Britain, including that of 1939–45, took her armies into highly malarious regions and upon them this disease levied a very heavy toll. It is not surprising, therefore, to learn that Field Marshal Lord Wavell found it necessary to state that 'In the theatres where future operations are likely to take place, we may well find that disease, and especially malaria, is a more dangerous factor than enemy resistance . . . We must prepare to meet malaria by training as strict and earnest as against enemy troops; we must be practised in the use of weapons against it—the mosquito net, long sleeves and trousers, the flit-gun—as we are with the rifle. We must study the habits of the mosquito as we do the tactics of the Japanese'.

In Burma, as elsewhere, two campaigns were being fought synchronously, the intra-specific war against the human antagonist and the inter-specific war against the malaria parasite. To have been beaten in the latter would have meant defeat in the former. One important reason why the Allies were able to defeat the Japanese was that they were able to hold the malaria parasite in check, while the Japanese were not. Of the many new weapons with which the Allied armies were equipped none excelled in military value those gifts of the chemist, mepacrine and dichloro-diphenyl-trichlorethane. No contribution to the winning of the war was of greater value than the demonstration that with the aid of mepacrine malaria could be 'suppressed' for considerable periods of time and that with the aid of D.D.T. the insect vectors of disease could be banished from the physical environment of an army. 'The demonstration that great forces operating in highly malarious areas could be kept practically free from malarial symptoms was, I think, an outstanding feature of the Burma campaign'. (G.E.M.) (*Campaigns* V. p. 640.)

THE RESPONSIBILITY FOR DISEASE-PREVENTION

Although it has long been understood that the battalion, company and platoon commanders, and their equivalents in units other than infantry, are actively interested in the health and welfare of the men under their command and that the regimental medical officer is the source of information and advice concerning the methods to be adopted by the individual and the unit for the achievement and maintenance of a high standard of healthiness, it was only during the War of 1939–45 that it was made perfectly clear that it was indeed the responsibility of the unit officers to give effect to this advice.

'The importance of Preventive Medicine to an army cannot be exaggerated. It is not enough to have a highly trained and professionally skilful medical service if the fighting man himself is not taught the rules of self-protection against disease. Instruction must be given to all ranks from the Commander-in-Chief to the most recently joined recruit. All commanders must be made aware of their responsibilities in respect of health promotion and disease prevention. It is the duty of the medical services to offer the necessary instruction and the commander's to see that the rules are kept.' (J.C.D.)

In Fourteenth Army's 'A' Branch a non-medical officer was appointed to supervise and generally control those activities which had for their purpose the reduction of the incidence of malaria. The fitness of a commander to command was judged by the extent to which anti-malaria measures were exercised in his formation or unit.

'Good doctors are no use without good discipline. More than half the battle against disease is fought, not by the doctors, but by the regimental officers. It is they who see that the daily dose of mepacrine is taken, that shorts are never worn, that shirts are put on and sleeves turned down before sunset, that minor abrasions are treated before, not after, they go septic, that bodily cleanliness is enforced. When mepacrine was first introduced and turned men a jaundiced yellow, there was the usual whispering campaign among troops that greets every new remedy —the drug would render men impotent—so, often the little tablet was not swallowed. An individual medical test in almost all cases will show whether it has been taken or not, but there are a few exceptions and it is difficult to prove for court-martial purposes. I, therefore, had surprise checks of whole units, every man being examined. If the overall result was less than ninety-five per cent positive I sacked the commanding officer. I only had to sack three; by then the rest had got my meaning'. (Field Marshal Sir William Slim. *Defeat into Victory* p. 180.)

'The use of suppressive drugs was by far the most valuable anti-malaria measure; but to ensure that these suppressive drugs were actually taken by the troops was a very difficult matter indeed.

'To sack an able and gallant commanding officer because the anti-malaria discipline in his unit was bad was exceedingly distasteful to all concerned but it was certainly a measure of the real appreciation by higher command of the nature of medical problems and of the value of medical recommendations.' (G.E.M.)

'In Burma scrub typhus, with its very high mortality-rate, caused great anxiety among the troops. For protection against the mite D.B.P. (Di-butyl-phthalate) was widely used but, as its application was a tedious affair, it was necessary, as in the case of suppressive drugs for malaria, to make it a unit responsibility'. (W.E.T.)

The lesson learnt in Burma made it certain that after the war Fourteenth Army's example would be followed. The appointment of a special staff officer (D.A.A.G. Health Discipline) to the staff of each division in a malarious area, to ensure the strict enforcement of anti-malaria discipline, was sanctioned.

Planned Recruitment and Planned Release

In the War of 1939–45 the recruitment of medically qualified persons for service with the Armed Forces of the Crown was the responsibility of the Central Emergency Committee of the British Medical Association which on the outbreak of war became the Central Medical War Committee and which placed its executive powers in the hands of a Committee of Reference. This committee was representative of all sections of the medical profession and of the various government departments intimately concerned with the question of recruiting medical personnel. A register of all practitioners of medicine willing to undertake military service had been compiled before the outbreak of war. In June 1940 the practice of medicine was removed from the schedule of reserved occupations and doctors thereupon became liable for compulsory military service. The War Office, the Admiralty and the Air Ministry informed the C.M.W.C. of their requirements in respect of medical officers and this committee then decided the quota of practitioners to be found by each of the districts into which the country had been divided. Local medical war committees then chose the practitioners they considered to be the most suitable for service in the Armed Forces. The names of these were submitted to the C.M.W.C. and the final allocation between the three Services, the Admiralty, the War Office and the Air Ministry, lay with this committee. The War Office then communicated with the practitioners allotted to the Army Medical Services, offering them commissions in the R.A.M.C. and requesting them to attend at a specified place for medical examination and interview. If a man declined the commission he became liable for calling-up for service in the same way as non-medical citizens. (*Admin.* I. p. 158.)

This planned system of recruitment was equitable and would have been entirely satisfactory had there been enough medically qualified persons in the community to satisfy the needs of the three Services and of the civilian population. As early as November 1940 the C.M.W.C. asked the Minister of Health to arrange for an immediate enquiry into the supply of medical men for the Armed Forces whose demands it was unable to satisfy. The Robinson Committee (*Admin*. I. p. 160), the Shakespeare Committee (*Admin*. I. p. 163) and the Cranborne Inquiries (*Admin*. I. p. 175) all wrestled with this problem without success and none of the Services obtained all the medically qualified personnel they maintained they needed. This was a problem with which D.G.A.M.S. had to live throughout the war years.

At the time of the end of the war in Europe the strength of the Army (British and Indian and Colonial and Women's Services) was 5,699,000. The strength of the Medical Services (R.A.M.C. and I.A.M.C.) was 16,903 officers. The ratio of medical officers to troops was 2·98 per 1,000. (*Admin*. I. p. 197.)

The release of medical officers at the end of the war was likewise planned. The C.M.W.C. had formulated a plan which was based upon the principle of priority for age and length of service but this differed from the scheme that had been devised for the Armed Forces as a whole and it was therefore unacceptable.

Those serving in the Armed Forces were divided into three categories, class A, those rendered surplus to requirements and available for release, on grounds of personal entitlement, in groups determined by a combination of age and length of service; class B, those released in the national interest to satisfy civil needs; and class C, compassionate release on account of exigencies of a private and domestic nature. As regards the medical, dental, nursing and certain other professions, it was specially provided that release would be effected only on individual sanction by the War Office.

This scheme, applied to medical personnel, it was pointed out, must inevitably encounter a number of serious difficulties. The end of the war in Europe would bring little reduction in the medical commitment for with the transfer of troops to the Far East there would arise the need for increases in the medical services since there was no E.M.S. in India. It was estimated that not less than 1,000 medical officers, including 500 specialists, would be required as reinforcements. Considerable numbers of the medical officers then in the United Kingdom were ineligible for service in the Far East on account of age or low medical category or for the reason that they had already completed a long tour of service overseas. In class A of the demobilisation scheme was a disproportionate number of specialists who necessarily belonged to the higher age-groups. It was suggested that there should be an exchange between the doctors in uniform and those serving in the E.M.S. But this and other suggestions could not be accepted for a variety of reasons and the protracted discussion that brought satisfaction to no-one was brought to an end by the decision of the Prime Minister in May 1945 that 1,600 doctors should be returned to civilian life forthwith from the Forces. (*Admin.* I. p. 235.) The Army's share, 1,100, involved the demobilisation of Groups 1–11 and it was planned to complete this by the end of August 1945. But within these eleven age and length of service groups there were no less than 467 specialists.

These could not all be released without replacement in view of the demand for 700 specialists of various kinds for India and South East Asia. At the beginning of August the demobilisation of 12–16 began. In these groups there were some 700 medical officers. A real crisis seemed imminent when the news that Japan had surrendered changed the whole situation and the release programme was able to proceed. But it was not until early in 1947 that the restrictions placed upon the demobilisation of medical officers could be relaxed and that a ratio of 2·5 medical officers per 1,000 total strength of the army could be regarded as satisfactory.

Developments within the Army Medical Directorate

The significant differences between the pre-war and early post-war organisation of A.M.D. were:

1. The addition of A.M.D. 7, the Clinical Staff branch of the directorate. During the war years A.M.D. 7 had been the Directorate of Pathology and the consultant group, greatly enlarged, had been moved from the R.A.M. College to A.M.D. there to cluster around D.G.A.M.S. After the end of the war the consultants returned to the College to be borne upon its strength but served as part-time directors of their particular services, e.g. surgery, medicine, pathology and psychiatry. A.M.D. 7 accommodated them in A.M.D.

   'The move of the consultants from the R.A.M. College to A.M.D. was absolutely essential. It made it possible for the consultants to make the right contacts and to render the greatest possible service.' (J.R.R.)

2. The inclusion of psychiatry in the clinical group and the appointment of an Army Psychiatry Advisory Committee. During the war years there had been a Directorate of Army Psychiatry, A.M.D. 11. At the end of the war this directorate was dropped and the consultant in psychiatry was borne on the strength of the R.A.M. College.

3. The change of name of A.M.D. 5 from the Directorate of Hygiene to the Directorate of Army Health which included a special statistical section and a pool of officers for employment in research projects. This section and the pool were integral parts of the

war-time Directorate of Medical Research (*Admin*. II. p. 498.), but when at the end of the war this directorate was discontinued, these parts of it were taken over by A.M.D. 5.

4. The redistribution of responsibilities of A.M.D. 1, 2 and 3, resulting in a much clearer and more precise definition of their respective functions. A.M.D. 1 became the 'A', 'P' and 'M.S.' section of the Army Medical Directorate; A.M.D. 2, along with A.M.D. 1, the 'G' section with a special sub-section, A.M.D. 2 (a), concerned with training, planning and the preparation of the Army Medical Services for war while A.M.D. 3 became the 'Q' section of the directorate.

During the war years it had been found necessary to create a special branch of the directorate, A.M.D. 8, to deal with the matters handled by A.M.D. 2 (a) after the war's end.

5. The appointment of an Inspector of Medical Services. In 1941 this appointment, which had been allowed to lapse, was revived (*Admin*. I. p. 123) as an inspectorate of training.

'During the reorganisation that followed the return of the B.E.F. from France and Belgium in 1940, it came to be recognised that drastic changes were necessary if the Army was to hold its own in a novel kind of warfare in which mobility was the essential feature. The Inspector of Medical Services of earlier days used to concern himself with the professional aspects of the work of the R.A.M.C. officer and with the functioning of military hospitals. D.G.A.M.S., recognising that the supervision of the purely professional work of the Corps could safely be left to the consultants and that there was an urgent need for the supervision of field training, introduced new terms of reference for the Inspector who was placed in charge of all field units.' (J.C.D.)

THE NEED FOR A D.D.G.A.M.S.(ADMIN.) AND A
D.D.G.A.M.S.(OPS.) IN WAR-TIME

'During a war it is essential that D.G.A.M.S. should acquaint himself with the conditions in every theatre of war. He must not be tied to the War Office but must personally visit each theatre there to examine the major problems of a medical kind and to discuss them with those on the spot. If he is to enjoy this freedom he must have two deputies, one for day-to-day administration and one for operational planning.' (A.H.)

LIAISON BETWEEN THE MEDICAL AND OTHER
BRANCHES OF THE STAFF IN LONDON IN WAR-TIME

During the war years dispersal of headquarters was inevitable for a variety of reasons. The adverse effects of such dispersal can be avoided only by adequate means of intercommunication. When A.M.D. was situated in 39, Hyde Park Gate, far removed from all other components of the War Office, one small motor car was made available for the transport of the dozens of members of the Directorate who were required to attend in person conferences and the like at the War Office main block, the Air Ministry, the Ministry of Health, the Medical Research Council's many committees in the London School of Hygiene, Civil Affairs committees in Northumberland Avenue, etc. etc. The alternative means of transport was the omnibus. Perforce this had to be used by most members of the staff of A.M.D. on most occasions with much loss of time and no little anxiety when 'Top Secret' documents were being carried. (The consultants as a group used their own private cars.)

'When Operation "Overlord" was being planned there had to be frequent discussions between the medical directorates of the Navy, Army and Air Force and between A.M.D. and S.H.A.E.F. and the medical branches of the Canadian and U.S. Headquarters. Because of the most unsatisfactory transport facilities it was at all times difficult to maintain a satisfactory liaison.

'The medical services fall within the A.G's. Branch of the War Office. In operational planning the medical tactical plan is submitted through "A" channels. It was found, time and time again, that D.D.G.A.M.S. (Ops.) had to deal direct with the "G" and "S.D." branches for the reason that time did not permit the medical tactical plan to be passed *via* "A". Such non-observance of the rules could lead to difficulty.' (W.E.T.)

MEDICAL EMBARKATION AND HOSPITAL
DISTRIBUTION HEADQUARTERS

In October 1939 this organisation, quite separate from A.M.D., was brought into being to deal with the reception of casualties arriving from overseas theatres and for their distribution among the hospitals in the United Kingdom. It was modelled upon a similar organisation with similar functions that was set up during the War of 1914–18. It consisted of a D.D.M.S. with a staff of 12. It had outposts at Southampton, Newhaven and Liverpool. At each of these places was an A.D.M.S. and his staff. At Southampton No. 3 Company R.A.M.C. functioned as a depot for the supply of personnel to hospital ships and ambulance trains. When Southampton could no longer be used as a port of disembarkation this company moved to Liverpool. When any other port was used a party from this company was sent there for temporary duty.

By 1942 it had become evident that between this headquarters, many of the branches of A.M.D. and the Ministry of Health there was much unnecessary duplication and a committee of investigation recommended that M.E.H.D.H.Q. should be abolished and its functions distributed within A.M.D. (*Admin.* I. p. 424.) It was decided, however, to create a new branch (A.M.D. 12) to take over these functions. At the same time the Liverpool medical embarkation staff was reorganised. It became the Medical Embarkation Pool (United Kingdom and Northern Ireland) and placed in charge of an A.D.M.S. (Embarkation). The pool of medical personnel for duty in troop transports, previously forming part of No. 11 Depot R.A.M.C., was transferred to Liverpool and attached to No. 3 Company R.A.M.C.

A.M.D. 12 was a war-time creation to meet war-time needs; with the coming of peace this branch was closed down.

The Army Nursing Service

In 1942 the term 'Nursing officer' for Q.A.I.M.N.S. and T.A.N.S. personnel was first introduced and effect was given to the decision that the Q.A.I.M.N.S. should be included as part of the Armed Forces of the Crown. The Matron-in-Chief's rank became equal to that of a brigadier; that of a chief principal matron equal to that of a colonel; of a principal matron, a lieutenant-colonel; of a matron, a major; of senior sisters of ten years' service, assistant matrons and sisters-in-charge, a captain; and that of a sister equal to that of a lieutenant. (*Admin.* II. p. 15.)

After the end of the war working parties were appointed to consider future developments within the Army Nursing Service and out of their deliberations came the decision to change the name from Q.A.I.M.N.S. to Q.A.R.A.N.C., Queen Alexandra's Royal Army Nursing Corps. (*Admin.* II. p. 24.) This had complete military status, the nursing officer becoming subject to the full provisions of the Army Act in common with all other officers of the Army. Officers were appointed to commissions in the Corps in the undermentioned ranks:

Senior Controller   equal in rank to a brigadier
Controller   ,,   ,,   ,,   ,,   ,, colonel
Chief Commander   ,,   ,,   ,,   ,,   ,, lieutenant-colonel
Senior Commander   ,,   ,,   ,,   ,,   ,, major
Junior Commander   ,,   ,,   ,,   ,,   ,, captain
Subaltern   ,,   ,,   ,,   ,,   ,, lieutenant.

In 1950 the rank titles were changed again to become the same as those for male officers in the Army.

THE EMPLOYMENT OF NURSING OFFICERS
IN FRONT OF THE C.C.S.

Concerning this matter there was much debate during the war years and it seemed that two conflicting schools of thought concerning it were developing, one presenting the view that they should not be so employed, the other that they should. In fact there was no conflict of opinion, the disputants' differing opinions were reflections of different circumstances.

'This depends upon the operations being undertaken and the conditions in the field. In the winter of 1942–43 in First Army in North Africa nursing officers were not allowed in C.C.Ss. This was a mistake, in my opinion, because conditions were static and not unsuitable. Indeed nursing officers could have been sent forward for detached duty with F.S.Us. with great advantage, for these units at this time were accommodated in buildings which made the retention of wounded for quite long periods possible and provided ample scope for skilled nursing.' (N.C.)

'The reason why nurses were not employed in the winter of 1942–43 in the C.C.Ss. in North Africa was that the British troops were very thin on the ground and could only be reinforced by fortnightly convoys from the U.K., whereas the enemy was flying in reinforcements daily from Sicily and Italy and could have launched an attack at any moment. It was decided that the presence of women in the C.C.S. at this particular time could have seriously affected their mobility'. (E.W.W.)

'I would always use nursing officers as far forward as possible, even though the enemy could be expected to behave as did the Japanese in the Second World War and even knowing how they might be treated if captured. They are quite capable of roughing it and in medical units holding casualties their presence makes all the difference; this was certainly so when the patients were suffering from scrub typhus.' (T.O.T.)

'In the winter of 1942–43 in Algeria conditions were static in the area of First Army. No sudden or extensive advance or retreat was to be expected. The forward surgical units were usually accommodated in buildings and nursing officers could certainly have been attached to them. But the question is whether or not there would have been any real advantage in so employing them.

'A nurse can provide no skill in nursing or in theatre work that a good nursing orderly cannot. She can give comfort and a feeling of security to a soldier broken in body and in spirit that no man can give. But the chief thing that such a man needs is removal from the scene, noise and memory of combat and the right thing is not to bring the nurse to him but to remove him at once to a place where nurses are the normal attendants of the sick.

'In Abyssinia and in the Western Desert during the same period the most valued quality of the forward surgical units was their ability to move suddenly, quickly and for considerable distances and to evacuate serious cases as soon as possible and as far as possible. In the circumstances that then obtained a nurse would have been better than an orderly only in exceptional cases when casualties could not be evacuated. The special needs of the nursing officer in transport, accommodation and feeding would have interfered with that free mobility on which the usefulness of forward surgery depends.

'In these theatres the nursing officer could have been employed in front of the C.C.S. as soon as conditions became stable, in the Western Desert after Sousse had been taken and in Abyssinia after the fall of Addis Ababa.' (H.O.)

'A C.C.S. is the furthest forward point at which major surgery should be performed, except in very exceptional circumstances. The rôle of the field ambulance is now the same as it was when the unit was first invented—the rapid collection and evacuation of casualties. Serious casualties can be evacuated considerable distances before operation (particularly if evacuation by air is possible) whereas after operation patients have to remain *in situ* for several days.

'Os.C. general hospitals and C.C.Ss. should not allow themselves to be persuaded into using hotels and schools as hospital accommodation just because an excellent operating theatre can be formed in them. The disadvantages of these buildings are that there are far too few lavatories, bathrooms and kitchens and that these deficiences cannot at all easily be made good. It is far better under most circumstances to select a site in a field, well away from possible bombing targets and rely upon the Geneva Convention by laying out huge Red Crosses on the ground.' (E.W.W.)

'I am quite convinced, in the campaign in North-West Europe, that the employment of nursing officers in forward areas was a good policy, provided they were well chosen. I am sure that the old dictum "that where major surgery is done there should be nurses" is a good one both from a technical and a morale point of view.' (A.P.)

'I would never allow nursing sisters forward of the C.C.S. level. If a casualty is of such a nature as to require the skilled attention of a trained female nurse, the sooner he is in a base hospital the better for him and all concerned'. (E.A.S.)

The aim of the senior administrative medical officer in the field is to make such arrangements as will ensure that the casualty and the surgeon-nurse team shall be brought together as quickly as possible, in circumstances that are as propitious as possible for the fruitful exercise of the surgical and nursing arts. Surgery and nursing are not to be dissociated but must be considered as a combination. Both are attended by the best results when practised in quiet, peaceful surroundings well back from the clamour of battle. When speedy, safe and, if possible, comfortable evacuation is at all feasible, despatch of the casualty to the rear to the C.C.S. level is the rule. But the coming of the F.S.U. introduced a complication. This was a specialist surgical unit that could function in front of the C.C.S. when circumstances permitted, being attached to some parent unit, F.D.S. or M.D.S. of a field ambulance, which was capable of holding the immobiles among its patients. The question now became not whether or not Q.A.I.M.N.S. personnel should be employed in front of the C.C.S. but whether or not major surgery should be undertaken there since certain forms of it yield a proportion of immobiles that require skilled nursing.

In every theatre there were occasions when casualties could not be evacuated to the rear. In the Anzio beachhead, for example, there was no rear. In Italy during periods of severe wintry weather it was impossible to get casualties back. In all campaigns there are relatively quiet periods when surgical and nursing facilities can be sent forward with advantage.

In the opinion of some the presence of females in areas in which they were exposed to the possibility of being wounded or killed by enemy missile was the cause of much anxiety and also of not a little difficulty for the reason that appropriate accommodation for them could not be provided. This chivalrous attitude is praiseworthy but it disregards the doctrine that the one to be considered above all others is the casualty, not the doctor and not the nurse, both of whom are dedicated to his service. The members of the Army Nursing Service would be the first to claim equality with those of the R.A.M.C. in respect of taking risks for the sake of the wounded and the sick. This claim is completely justified by the record of the Q.A.I.M.N.S. during the war. (*Campaigns* V. p. 638.)

Bearing directly upon this question of the employment of nursing officers in the forward areas is another, the question as to whether or not male nurses with the S.R.N. qualifications should be admitted to the R.A.M.C. as non-medical officers or to the Q.A.R.A.N.C. as nursing officers, equal in every way to the female nursing officer.

The numbers of men with this qualification are steadily increasing and male nurses are gaining their places in the higher ranks of the nursing profession. They will certainly seek admission to the Q.A.R.A.N.C. or to the R.A.M.C. and to find a satisfactory reason for rejecting them will not be at all easy. As for their entrance into the R.A.M.C. as non-medical officers it is perhaps sufficient to state that this nursing qualification in no way especially equips them for employment in the fields of administration, sanitation or quartermastering.

To add male nursing officers to the existing male nursing orderly/ female nursing officer organisation would in no way advantage the patient. They could be employed in the forward areas but it certainly will remain the rule that whenever possible the wounded will be evacuated rearwards at least to the level of the C.C.S. so that there is no point in legislating for the very exceptional and in any case such evacuation is desirable from the point of view of the casualty. Though male and female nurses can be completely equal in respect of professional knowledge and skill they still remain distinct for one is male and the other female. This difference would seem to be of considerable importance in so far as nursing is concerned, for the casualty, because of his illness or injury, is a child-like dependent creature, often frightened and insecure, who sees in the female nurse a mother-figure, tender and compassionate. In the patient/nurse relationship this ingredient would seem to advantage the patient greatly.

The Army Hygiene Service

Of the very many developments that occurred in the field of hygiene the following can claim an unusual importance.

In the Directorate itself among the war-time posts created was that of a staff-captain concerned with military intelligence. (*Admin*. II. p. 26.) He established profitable contact with the Directorate of Military Intelligence.

Although every directorate and branch of A.M.D. was indirectly advantaged by this liaison, this officer was primarily concerned with the interests of his own directorate. D.D.G.A.M.S. (Ops.) and the planning branch A.M.D. 8, for example, certainly needed the information which this officer gleaned even more than did A.M.D. 5. It is imperative that in time of war information of the 'military intelligence' as well as of the 'medical intelligence' kind shall flow into A.M.D. It remains to be decided whether the creation of this post was the best possible method of securing information of this kind and of disseminating it within the Army Medical Directorate.

In the interests of medical man-power economy the field sanitary section was formed to take the place of the field hygiene section in corps and L. of C. areas. Its commanding officer was a non-medical officer. (*Admin*. II. p. 31.)

The field entomological unit was formed to undertake field trials of new insecticides. (*Admin*. II. 34.)

Because in the army of 1939–45 there were so very many different national and ethnic groups no less than 198 different ration scales had to be designed to satisfy their various needs. Each of these scales had to be in harmony not only with the peculiar dietetic habits of the consumers but also with local climatic conditions. (*Admin*. II. p. 69.) The development of operational ration packs constituted one of the major advances during the war years. (*Admin*. II. p. 69.)

Crash helmets became an issue for D.Rs. and parachute troops. (*Admin.* II. p. 94.)

One of the major casualties of the war was the solar topee. (*Admin.* II. p. 91.)

Traditionally, the combat head covering of the soldier was designed to intimidate the enemy and to protect the wearer against his weapons. With the passing of time the first of these purposes was disregarded. The steel helmet and its forerunners have all been designed to protect the head of the wearer against the weapons of the time, club, mace, axe, sword, bullet, mortar or shell fragment.

The headgear worn by the soldier at other times has usually been a part of a smart uniform that has been designed to magnify the martial qualities of the wearer. In certain instances it has been meant to provide protection against the elements. In the Tropics, until very recently, exposure of the head and neck to the rays of the sun was regarded as highly dangerous by many peoples and special attention was given to their protection. This notion can be traced back beyond the days of imperial Rome and ancient Greece. The blame for the damage that was supposed to be caused was ascribed to various factors, for example, to an imbalance between the cerebro-spinal and the sympathetic nervous systems, to the sun's rays striking through the orbit or to the ultra-violet rays (the actinic theory).

In Mesopotamia, during the First World War, the British troops suffered severely from what was then called sunstroke, in spite of the wearing of pith helmets, a variety of solar topee (or topi) and broad spine pads. Nursing sisters, working in tents with double roofs of thick canvas, were required to wear their helmets during the daylight hours in the hot weather. Sir Victor Horsley, the consulting surgeon, who scoffed at these practices, was said to have died of 'heatstroke' at Asmara and this event was regarded by some as complete proof that his opinion concerning this particular matter was utterly mistaken.*

Yet in 1913 Castellani and Chambers had cast grave doubts upon the suggestion that the sun's rays were directly responsible for the disease and had maintained that so long as the temperature of the body was maintained within normal limits, exposure of the head to the sun's rays was without effect. Slowly it came to be noted that 'heatstroke' could strike a man down just as easily in the dark boiler-room of a steamer as it could in the scorching desert and that the sun's rays were important only in so far as they increased the heat-load.

---

* The belief that Sir Victor Horsley died of 'heatstroke' is open to doubt. Dr. Anthony Feiling, who attended him at Asmara in 1916, informs me that he diagnosed Sir Victor's death as due to an attack of Paratyphoid A, which was raging in epidemic form at the time; this diagnosis was not proved bacteriologically owing to lack of facilities at the time.—A.S.M.

It was about halfway through the Second World War that the wearing of pith helmets between 0900 and 1700 hrs. ceased to be compulsory in the hot weather in India. In the early days of the campaign in the Middle East the topee was to be encountered in the Western Desert but man was ceasing to be a hat-wearing animal and soon Australians, British and New Zealanders were living unharmed in the burning desert either bare-headed or wearing the lightest of headgear. In Burma's steaming jungles and arid plain the slouch-hat was worn by all save General Wingate who had managed to equip himself with a pith helmet of a Boer War vintage.

There were many cases of 'heatstroke' in Tenth Army and among troops employed on railway duties in the region of the Persian Gulf, a well known danger spot. There were two main categories of cases, the newly arrived and as yet unacclimatised and those on transports in which on account of operational necessity medical recommendations concerning overcrowding had to be over-ridden. Much effort was spent by the Directorate to ensure that salt tablets and abundant drinking water were provided. Mobile heatstroke centres were devised to accompany convoys. It was concluded that of all the prophylactic measures, acclimatisation was the most valuable. (*Admin*. II. p. 179.)

Advances in knowledge concerning the effects of heat, humidity and atmospheric movement upon the temperature of the human body and upon the functioning of the sweat-glands and concerning the body's needs in respect of water and mineral salts, many of them made during the war years, gave strong support to the growing inclination to discard the pith helmet and the topee. (*Med. and Path.* p. 278.)

By the end of the war the topee had become nothing more than a status symbol. It owes the name solar topee to the pith of the sola plant *Aeschynomena paludosa*, an Indian rush, and by a process of association it came to be thought of as a solar topee (L. *solaris* from *sol* the sun). In a standard work on *Health in Hot Countries*, published in 1904, it is stated that 'No material appears to be so effective in intercepting the peculiar vibrations which cause sunstroke, wherever they may be, as the pith of the Indian rush.' It is of interest to note that no such head covering was developed in those parts of South America where the climatic conditions are very similar to those found in the East. It seems that the topee gave illusory protection against a non-existent disease.

Important developments occurred in the production of impregnated clothing; veils, gauntlets and socks impregnated with D.M.P. (Di-methyl-phthalate) to protect against the mosquito; socks and trouser-leg bottoms impregnated with D.B.P. (Di-butyl-phthalate), for protection against the *Trombiculid* mite. (*Admin*. II. p. 90.) To protect the troops in the campaign in North-West Europe against the hazard of typhus they were issued with some 750,000 shirts impregnated with the louse-killing D.D.T. (Dichloro-diphenyl-trichlorethane). (*Campaigns* IV. p. 81.)

The large-scale use of D.D.T., first synthesised in 1874, and of gammexane for insecticidal purposes constituted the most outstanding development during the war years in the field of preventive medicine. (*Admin.* II. p. 121.) They were successfully used against the mosquito, the fly, the louse, the bed-bug, the sandfly and the flea.

Considerable difficulty was caused by the urgent need for economy in the use of soap and soap powders which were strictly rationed. (*Admin.* II. p. 135.)

The financial penalties in connexion with V.D. were abolished. (*Admin.* II. p. 241.)

Towards the end of 1944 it was decided to establish a central syphilis register at the War Office with branches in overseas commands to ensure and check the adequacy of individual treatment. The scheme worked well. (*Admin.* II. p. 237.) With the man's consent (in writing) the medical officer of health of the county or county borough in which the man proposed to go after release from the army was notified in a letter marked 'strictly confidential' that the man was about to be discharged. The man himself was in possession of a form on which particulars of his medical history were given. (*Admin.* II. p. 240.)

The procedure for dealing with repatriated prisoners-of-war on their return to the United Kingdom included arrangements for their reception, cleansing, if necessary, medical examination with a view to determining their nutritional state, sorting out those who required immediate hospitalisation and increased dietary for those despatched on recuperative leave. (*Admin.* II. p. 270.) The directorate prepared a most useful pamphlet, *Hints on Diet during Recuperative Leave for Liberated Prisoners-of-War.* (*Admin.* II. p. 273.)

The Army Dental Service

Of the many differences between the 1935 *R.A.M.C. Training Manual* and the 1950 *R.A.M.C. Training Pamphlet No. 2*, none is more striking or more meaningful than that which relates to the Army Dental Service. In the Manual the Army Dental Corps is not even mentioned although it had been in existence since 1921. It was not until 1935, however, that the Dental Directorate (A.M.D. 6) was created as a branch of the Army Medical Directorate, the head of it being given the title of Director of the Army Dental Service. In the 1950 Pamphlet a whole, if brief, chapter is devoted to the organisation and functions of the Army Dental Service in the field. Moreover, the Corps is referred to as the Royal Army Dental Corps, a title that the high quality of the work it had performed during the war years and the widespread recognition of the value of this work had earned for it. The volume of this work was immense for the dental condition of very large proportions of the intakes was deplorable and when these were made dentally fit they required a great deal of maintenance. It says much for the Army Dental Service that at all times the discharge rate on account of dental disease was remarkably low.

Within this service there were two developments of lasting importance —the elevation of the status of the dental officer within the Army Medical Services and the creation of mobile dental units that, by taking dental care into the forward areas, could prevent much loss of man-power caused by the despatch of men requiring dental treatment to the rear.

The Army Dental Service had grown from very small beginnings under the shelter of the Army Medical Services to reach, during the war years, a stage of development when it understandably sought a measure of administrative detachment from its overwhelmingly large parent body. The purely professional interests of the doctor and the dentist became increasingly merged but in the administrative field the Army Dental Corps claimed and was given a large measure of autonomy. The Dental Directorate functioned with a quiet, smooth efficiency.

As the Corps expanded with the growth of the Army there was much up-grading of the posts held by dental officers in the Army Medical Directorate and in H.Qs. of commands at home and overseas. In 1940 a consulting dental surgeon joined the consultants group in A.M.D.

When in 1941 a war establishment for the maxillo-facial surgical team was introduced, specialist status for the dental officer attached to such teams was sought. It was agreed that he should be classified as a specialist maxillo-facial dental surgeon, be given the rank of major and receive additional pay. In this way the dental officer achieved equality with the medical officer. Then came the creation of the post of dental surgeon specialist, one to each command at home and overseas, who, in his own field, was the equivalent of the medical or surgical specialist and functioned in a consultative as well as in an executive capacity. Approval for the granting of such specialist status and additional pay was given early in 1943. (*Admin*. II. p. 313.)

In addition to these specialist appointments open to officers of the A.D. Corps there were also the following: specialist dental surgeon and graded dental surgeon on the staffs of 1,200 and 600-bed hospitals and graded maxillo-facial dental surgeon with the M.F.S.U.

In the pre-war list of field medical units no dental unit of any kind is included. In the post-war list the following appear: the field dental centre, the field dental laboratory and the mobile dental team.

The Field Dental Centre

	Officers	O.Rs. R.A.D.C.	Weight of Equipment	Transport
Class A	1	1	$\frac{1}{4}$-ton	
B	2	2	$\frac{2}{5}$-ton	
C	3	3	$\frac{3}{5}$-ton	
D	4	4	$\frac{3}{4}$-ton	

The Field Dental Laboratory 1   11 $2\frac{3}{4}$-ton 1 m/c.
                                       1 truck 15 cwt. G.S.

These units were creations of the early years of the campaign in the Middle East. F.D.Cs. were distributed in the L. of C. and base areas to match the distribution of troops. Since they were not self-supporting they had to be attached to some parent unit for maintenance and administration. A field dental laboratory was established to serve several F.D.Cs. and like them was attached to some medical parent unit.

Having proved their worth they were carried over into the post-war period.

The Mobile Dental Team

1 officer and 3 O.Rs. (clerk-orderly, dental mechanic and 1 driver R.A.S.C.)
1 lorry 3-ton
Combined weight of G.1098 and I.1248 equipment—$1\frac{3}{4}$ tons
Function. To provide specialist dental treatment in the forward areas.

This unit was first introduced in the Middle East (*Admin*. II. p. 335). It proved to be so useful that several were raised for the invasion of North Africa and many more for the invasion of the Continent of Europe. The allotment came to be 1 per armoured division, 2 per infantry division, 3 per corps plus an increment of 1 for each division in the corps. The M.D.Ts. with divisions and corps were classified as army troops and the incremental teams as G.H.Q. troops. When employed with air-portable formations the teams were given a jeep and trailer in place of the lorry. M.D.Ts. were not self-accounting and were therefore attached to some parent unit for maintenance and administration. They were capable of undertaking comprehensive dental treatment including denture work.

The Army Transfusion Service

The immense value of the contributions made by this service, like that of those made by the other 'clinical' services, is revealed upon almost every page of the medical sections of the campaign narratives and in those sections of this volume that deal with the subjects of medicine, surgery and pathology. Here it is sufficient to record that specialist status was not awarded to the transfusion officer until after the cessation of hostilities in Europe (*Admin.* II. p. 389.), although transfusion itself was regarded as a specialty, a consultant in resuscitation and transfusion having been appointed in 1941. The transfusion orderly became a tradesman. (*Admin.* I. p. 319.)

Medical Provision for the Auxiliary Territorial Service

The creation of the A.T.S. and its great expansion during the war years presented the Army Medical Services with many novel problems of considerable magnitude and complexity.

THE FORMATION OF A.M.D. 9

When in late 1940, the A.T.S. Council was formed, it came to include a woman doctor who was given the rank of lieutenant-colonel and the title of Woman Medical Adviser and attached somewhat loosely to A.M.D. 1. As the A.T.S. expanded and her responsibilities enlarged, a new branch of A.M.D., A.M.D. 9, was formed to deal with all the problems of the medical administration of the A.T.S. and the W.M.A. became an A.D.G. functioning as a co-ordinator, interpreting the needs of the A.T.S. to A.M.D. and keeping D.A.T.S. informed of the medical aspects of the problems with which the A.T.S. Directorate was dealing. (*Admin.* I. p. 123.)

It so happened that the personal and professional qualifications of both of the officers who held the post of A.D.G. were such as equipped them admirably for the difficult rôle they were called upon to play. Because each in her turn attracted the respect of her colleagues in the two directorates concerned, the interests she represented claimed their earnest attention. As a result of the experience gained it was possible to reach the following firm conclusions: 'In war-time at any rate, a medical officer of standing is absolutely necessary to watch all aspects of the medical provision for women. There is every advantage in putting a woman doctor in this position and the best place for her is in whatever co-ordinating branch there is in the Army Medical Directorate, with free access to D.A.T.S. and her staff.' (*Admin.* II. p. 423.)

THE APPOINTMENT OF WOMEN SPECIALISTS

In December 1940 women were appointed to specialist posts in medicine, surgery and gynaecology and later to similar posts in a number of other specialties including psychiatry, orthopaedic surgery, radiology and pathology. In June 1941 a woman medical officer was attached to the medical branch of each of four home commands, with the rank of major, to advise the D.D.M.S. on all matters relating to the

A.T.S. In certain of these commands this officer was used for general medical staff duties. Later in the same year these officers became D.A.Ds.M.S.(W.) and in 1942 these posts were extended to cover all home commands. By 1944 the purely A.T.S. work of these officers had begun to shrink but it was decided that they should be retained and absorbed into the general staff and so the W. was dropped from their title. A few women became A.Ds.H., one became D.A.D.M.S. in a base sub-area in B.A.O.R. and another D.A.D.M.S. at Rhine Army H.Q. (*Admin.* II. p. 424.)

CRITICISM CONCERNING MEDICAL ATTENTION

The Army Medical Services during the war years quickly learnt that a great deal of public attention was continually focused upon the A.T.S. Complaints, mostly unjustified, that these young women were not getting proper medical attention were not uncommon. During a mild but widespread epidemic of influenza and of German measles it was far from easy to find adequate accommodation for the very large numbers of the sick and there was much unhelpful criticism of the camp reception station and hospital accommodation that was provided for the A.T.S. It was learnt that it was a far simpler matter to provide improvised accommodation for the sick among the men than it was to do so for the sick among the women and that the champions of the latter were numerous, vehement and vociferous. Most of the A.T.S. personnel who required hospitalisation were accommodated in E.M.S. hospitals.

PROBLEMS OF PREGNANCY

It was agreed that the Army was no place for a pregnant woman. In the case of the married woman there was a widespread opinion among laity that continued service with the A.T.S. would probably lead to miscarriage. It was important therefore that the state of pregnancy should be recognised at the earliest possible stage. In the absence of the biological tests for pregnancy—the Ascheim-Zondek or the Hogben— it was not until the twelfth week that the medical officer could be quite sure. It was most unfortunate therefore that the use of these tests had to be restricted to special cases. The stocks of one of the largest breeders of mice in England were destroyed by enemy action, there was a chronic shortage of animal feeding stuffs and *Xenopus laevis*, the claw-toed frog of South Africa, could be imported only with the greatest difficulty.

When A.T.S. personnel were included in overseas drafts it became possible for a girl, six to eight weeks pregnant, to be included. By the time she reached her destination, in the Middle East, for example, her pregnancy could be so far advanced that she could not be returned to the United Kingdom. Since normal pregnancy constitutes neither sickness nor injury she could not travel in a hospital ship as a protected person and a troopship was certainly not suitable for her conveyance. Air transport was regarded as being quite unsuitable in war-time because of the danger of anoxaemia to the foetus. It was learnt that it was most desirable that all A.T.S. proceeding overseas should be examined for pregnancy by some test that would detect the condition in its earliest stages. There are real difficulties attached to any such scheme, some legal and others practical. The consent of the woman had to be obtained and so the non-volunteer could escape the draft. The biological tests that were in use during the war years will doubtless be replaced by others that will not require test animals.

In the married woman discharge occurred around the fourteenth week of pregnancy; in the unmarried around the twentieth. No way of detecting pregnancy in a really determined woman who wished to conceal her condition was discovered.

Eight to 15 per cent. of the women in the A.T.S. were married and these contributed from 66–75 per cent. of the pregnancies. The married pregnancy-rate rose steadily as the war progressed, being about a quarter of the married strength in 1942, about a third in 1943 and nearly a half in 1944. The unmarried pregnancy-rate was about $1\frac{1}{2}$–$1\frac{3}{4}$ per cent. of the unmarried strength in 1941, 1942 and 1943 and then rose to $2\frac{1}{2}$ per cent. and stayed there until the end of the war. This rise, the reason for which was not to be discovered, occurred in the other Women's Services and also in the civil population. All the evidence that was available strongly suggested that the unmarried pregnancy-rate in the Women's Services was significantly lower than that of the civil population.

GENERAL SICKNESS RATES

There was an exceedingly high rate of minor sickness and a remarkably low rate of major sickness among A.T.S. personnel, relative to the men. The admission-rate to camp reception stations was consistently double and the hospital admission-rate approximately two-thirds that of the men. The C.R.S. admission-rate is a reflection of the attitude that existed in the A.T.S.; the woman was encouraged to report sick and was put to bed for complaints that the soldier was encouraged either to ignore, or at least to treat lightly. The hospital admission-rate of male and female differed partly because the average age of the A.T.S. was lower than that of the Army generally.

Discharges on account of pregnancy were four times as numerous as were discharges on medical grounds. Discharge on medical grounds was much more common among married as compared with unmarried personnel. About 50 per cent. of the discharges on medical grounds were for psychiatric reasons (about 30 per cent. for males). It is reasonable to think that the term psychiatric in this connexion covered many conditions other than those included in the standard textbook of the subject.

The Physical Development Centre

A physical development centre had been established at Aldershot in 1936 for the development of the sub-standard peace-time recruit. This venture proved to be a marked success, preserving for the Army a large number of recruits who would otherwise have been rejected. As a result of the remedial treatment they received they reached a satisfactory physical standard.

Three such centres were opened during the war years, at Kingston-on-Thames, Skegness and Hereford. They were equally successful. Of the first 4,059 soldiers admitted to one of them, 81 per cent. were raised in medical category at the end of the course and of these, 85 per cent., or 69 per cent. of the total admitted, were placed in category A.1. It was in connexion with these centres that the specialists in physical medicine were able to make their most dramatic contributions to the war effort. (*Admin.* I. p. 376.) The A.T.S. Reconditioning Centre was a combination of convalescent depot and physical development centre designed especially for members of the Auxiliary Territorial Service. In 1946 the name was changed to A.T.S. Convalescent Establishment. Two such units were formed, one near Cobham in Surrey in 1943 and the other near Brussels in 1944. Like the centres for the male, these units received such as needed toning up, exercise and general re-orientation—the weedy, the undernourished, the pallid, the convalescent —but they were remarkable for the number of girls with severe foot defects and postural anomalies who were admitted and who profited greatly from the skill of the specialist in physical medicine. (*Admin.* II. p. 431.)

The Directorate of Medical Research

The Medical Research Council, dealing directly with the Army Council, assumed responsibility for the initiation and conduct of scientific investigations on behalf of the Army. (*Admin.* II. p. 499.)

The Army Council had a scientific adviser, a professional academic physicist. It became necessary, therefore, for the Director-General of the Army Medical Services to do two things, to add to his staff a professional academic scientist to act as liaison officer between the Army Medical Directorate as a whole and the Medical Research Council and make certain that it was understood by all that he, the D.G.A.M.S. was the adviser of the Army Council in the medical and biological sciences. To the post of liaison officer a Territorial officer serving in the R.A.M.C. was appointed and he was accepted by the D.C.I.G.S. as the representative of D.G.A.M.S. in his capacity as scientific adviser to the Army

Council in the medical and biological sciences. The officer concerned was qualified to act in this capacity for in civil life he was a university professor of genetics, possessed a medical degree and was a Fellow of the Royal Society.

It was when the M.R.C. began to send teams of investigators overseas, there to examine some problem of importance to the expeditionary force, that this post of liaison officer became transmuted into that of director of medical research. It could not possibly be satisfactory, for example, to have teams of scientists in mufti wandering about army, corps and divisional areas examining casualties among tank crews or cases of infective jaundice. It was manifestly much more convenient and satisfactory for the members of such a team to be in uniform and to be representatives of a branch within the Army Medical Directorate. So, the Directorate of Medical Research formed a research pool which could carry the scientists nominated by the M.R.C. and could arrange for their employment by the medical branch of the H.Q. of the expeditionary force concerned. This scheme proved to be most satisfactory.

It is to be noted that the sub-committees of the Military Personnel Research Committee came to interest themselves in problems that could not possibly be regarded as being medical in their nature, physiological, psychological certainly but not medical since they related to a man's efficiency as a soldier and not to his health and welfare as a human being. Certain of the research teams of this directorate of medical research were called upon to investigate such problems and so the question presented itself—can a man wearing the uniform of the R.A.M.C. and claiming to be a protected person properly engage in activities that are in no way concerned with health and disease but with a man's fighting efficiency or with the offensive value of a weapon? An answer to this question was sought and it was ruled that the Directorate of Medical Research must restrict its activities to investigations which were, beyond all question, medical in nature. This ruling did not affect the activities of the sub-committees of the M.P.R.C.

So, half of the pool and half of the staff of the Directorate of Medical Research was transferred to the Scientific Adviser to the Army Council whose territory was enlarged to include all physiological and psychological problems, other than the purely medical, that were of concern to the Army. This solution was not completely satisfactory for the reason that the physiologists and many of the psychologists who were transferred had medical degrees and were in the R.A.M.C., being therefore protected persons. (*Admin.* II. p. 506.)

As a result of this diminution in the scope of the Directorate of Medical Research it was reorganised and, as its main activity, began to use statistical methods for the provision to the different branches and directorates of A.M.D. of information concerning the health of the troops in the different theatres of war. This was a service of considerable value and satisfied an urgent need.

Undoubtedly the Director-General acted wisely when he created the post of liaison officer between A.M.D. and the M.R.C. When the whole of the nation is mobilised for war it becomes divided into two parts, those in uniform and those not so garbed and between these two categories there inevitably develops a degree of mutual repulsion. Furthermore, it is by no means exceptional for civilians in high places to regard the military mind as being somewhat limited and difficulties in intercommunication between the civilian and the soldier often develop. It was the responsibility of the liaison officer to remove these difficulties. It is by no means certain that his holding army rank and wearing uniform advantaged him in the performance of this task. It is to be noted that the scientific adviser to the Army Council and the scientific advisers who were associated with Combined Operations H.Q. and later with S.A.C.S.E.A., remained civilians. There can be no doubt, however, that when the liaison officer, in his capacity as director of medical research, visited overseas theatres to prepare the way for the research teams, his army rank and his uniform were of considerable help. The wearing of a borrowed uniform by a civilian scientific adviser on a visit to an overseas theatre and the display of rank badges to which he is not entitled could lead to very serious difficulty.

A member of the R.A.M.C. is a protected person and enjoys certain privileges for the reason that his activities are concerned with the care of the sick and the wounded. If such a person becomes involved for example in the designing of body armour or of an armoured vehicle, both intended to protect a man from harm, can he claim the protection of the Geneva Convention and should he remain in the R.A.M.C? The considered opinion of higher Army authority in 1939-45 was that he could not and should not.

'The question of the extent to which a medical officer may participate in activities not strictly medical and yet ethically remain entitled to protection under the Geneva Convention is an interesting and debatable one.

'It would seem that the brightest future of medicine lies in the preventive field and if this applies in peace it logically should do so in war.

'The quality of clothing, the constituents of food, the provision of safety belts in motor vehicles and planes, the actual details of construction of vehicles—all these are examples of matters which, from the preventive point of view, may affect vitally the physical condition of the medical officer's patients. It is perfectly ethical for him to vaccinate a soldier to prevent him dying of smallpox; surely it is just as ethical to advise on the construction of floor boards in an armoured car with the intention of preventing fatal accidents from mine explosions.

'A medical officer doing research into the various types of crash helmet or protective clothing is working towards the saving of life just as much as if he is transfusing or operating upon a patient. His aim is the preservation of life just as much as were the activities of the *armed* medical officers in the Burma campaign.

'It would seem, therefore, that both logically and ethically medical officers carrying out such para-medical preventive assignments should be given protection under Geneva Convention regulations.' (A.P.)

A review of the researches undertaken by the various investigational mechanisms of the Army during the war years reveals that in the early years of a protracted global war the major problems of the Army are those that arise from the necessity of producing in ever expanding quantity, machines and equipment of ever increasing ingenuity, precision and lethality. In the later years the most pressing problems are those which relate to the numbers and quality of men, to their health, their efficiency and their morale. To begin with the Armed Forces lean very heavily upon the physical sciences for the production of weapons and equipment. Later, they were forced by the shortage of man-power, to turn to the biological and social sciences for the provision of their most urgent requirement, men capable of making the fullest possible use of the tools which the physical sciences, in application, had so abundantly supplied.

Though it is desirable, even essential, that the problems that embarrass an army should be investigated whenever and wherever they present themselves, it is to be noted that the solution of a problem does not necessarily mean that the army is thereby immediately advantaged. It was found during the war years that in many an instance by the time a solution had been reached the problem had lost its importance. It took about a year for a recommendation based upon the outcome of an investigation to be translated into routine practice. Time, much time, is required to define the problem, to formulate precisely the questions that are to be asked, to devise the methods whereby an exact answer can be secured, to design and test methods for the application of the information gained under active service conditions, to frame and to submit the recommendations to the proper authority and for these recommendations to be translated into action. (*Medical Research* p. 28. *Admin.* II. p. 512.)

The Employment of Scientists

During the war years a considerable number of professional scientists were included in the research pool of the Directorate of Medical

Research—biologists, physiologists, psychologists, malariologists, statisticians, physicists, chemists, etc., etc. A lesson that was re-learnt was that a scientist, a well educated and well trained person, could tackle a wide range of problems successfully after a relatively short acquaintance with them even though they did not pertain to his own particular branch of science. It became clear that what mattered was not the man's initial knowledge of a subject but his ability to grasp the essential facts and to apply to their analysis the mode of thought that is common to all forms of scientific activity. An educated person well versed in one particular field of science can quickly make himself competent in another if the urge to do so is sufficiently strong. Indeed it can be profitable to introduce a physicist into a biological field or a biologist into that of the physical sciences for the reason that the new-comer will not be entangled in the orthodoxy of the science.

Special Leave for Private Medical Treatment

In peace-time the Army had very clear-cut rules concerning medical treatment outside its own medical resources. Other ranks were entitled to free treatment and were not permitted to seek and obtain it at their own expense from civilian practitioners. Officers were not entitled to free medical care and could make their own arrangements so long as they bore the cost. They were eligible for free treatment within the Army, however, when this was available.

During the war years the Army came to include very large numbers of non-Regular soldiers and many of these, when sick, wished to consult their own peace-time doctors. So also did many of the young women of the A.T.S. Permission to do so was withheld but by the middle of 1942 it had become obvious to all that many soldiers and auxiliaries were, in fact, making their own arrangements. The matter was referred to the Army Council and after a great deal of attention had been given to it, the announcement was made that special leave for private medical treatment could be given, subject to certain safeguards, the more important of these being that:

(i) The treatment must be necessary and approved and must be given by a registered medical practitioner.

(ii) Skin, psychiatric and venereal diseases were excepted.

(iii) The soldier or auxiliary undertook not to hold the Army responsible for the cost of the treatment or for any risk or injury incurred thereby.

(iv) A medical report had to be forwarded weekly to the soldier's or auxiliary's commanding officer who transmitted it to the senior administrative medical officer of the area or district.

(v) The Army reserved the right to have the patient examined by a military medical officer or to remove the patient to a military or E.M.S. hospital at any time, should there be reason to consider his or her progress to be unsatisfactory.

These arrangements referred to soldiers and auxiliaries serving in the United Kingdom. The scheme regularised a practice that had become fairly common and one that could not easily be checked. From the Army's point of view it was unsatisfactory for the reason that the A.M.S. could not exert any kind of control over the treatment given. It occasionally led to difficulties when the patient displayed stubborn reluctance to return to duty. (*Admin*. II. p. 425.)

The same option was permitted, for the same reasons, in the Royal Navy and the Royal Air Force. In the U.S. and Canadian Expeditionary Forces neither officers nor other ranks were permitted to have any medical treatment outside their own medical services. But here the situation was different for the American and Canadian troops were serving outside their own countries.

The Appointment of Consultants

Before the war there were two full-time consultant posts within the establishment of the A.M.S., those of consulting physician and consulting surgeon to the Army. These appointments were combined with those of the professorships of tropical medicine and of surgery in the R.A.M. College. The occupants of these posts were closely concerned with A.M.D. both as advisers and as the administrative heads of the Army medical and surgical services. It was intended that both of them would form part of the medical branch of the G.H.Q. of an expeditionary force, should war break out. (*Admin*. I. p. 136.)

In order to obtain consultants for an expanding army, subsequent to mobilisation, and for other expeditionary forces, the D.G.A.M.S. approached the Royal College of Physicians of London and the Royal College of Surgeons of England in September 1938, asking them to select and nominate a number of civilians with appropriate qualifications for appointment as consultants within the A.M.S. Those selected would be given emergency commissions in the R.A.M.C., being gazetted as lieutenants and immediately promoted to the rank of colonel. This was the beginning of an arrangement that served the Army well. Similar arrangements were later made with the Royal Colleges of Edinburgh.

As was to be expected, it was not long before the question of the rank, status and pay of these consultants began to command the attention of the War Office, the C.M.W.C., the Army Council, the two Royal Colleges and the Army Medical Advisory Board. After a long-continued argument the medical bodies among the above-mentioned group of interested parties overwhelmed the opposition and in May 1943 three temporarily commissioned consultants, two in the United Kingdom and one in the Middle East, were promoted to the rank of major-general. (*Admin.* I. p. 143.) The rest became brigadiers. This was a matter that should have been settled before the outbreak of war; the disputation occupied the attention and consumed the energies of many at a time when far more important matters demanded the most careful study.

At the beginning of the war there was not a single stenographer in A.M.D., only copy typists. Certain of the consultants found it necessary to employ medical secretaries of their own since there was no establishment for anybody at that level.

It is of interest to note that during the war, officers, other than medical, were commissioned only after they had shown themselves to possess certain qualities that were held to be desirable in one placed in charge of others. The only qualifications demanded of a medical officer, G.D.O. or consultant, were a medical degree and a certain level of physical fitness. It was accepted that to a very large extent military and civil medicine had a very great deal in common and that in the Army the practitioner of medicine functioned primarily as a doctor. It was hoped that he might come to be a good soldier while serving. A specialist was required to have more professional knowledge and skill than a G.D.O. and a consultant to have more than a specialist. It can be said of the consultants that the great majority among them quickly adjusted themselves to the novel environment in which they found themselves and to the strange responsibilities they were called upon to shoulder.

One of the responsibilities of the senior administrative medical officer in a theatre of war is that of making the fullest possible use of the consultant group with which he has been provided. He and his consultants and medical advisers have to cultivate a common system of ideas and to share a common aim. It is for them to make recommendations of a medical kind, stemming from a sufficient knowledge of medicine and of the conditions and circumstances in which the action that is recommended has to be unleashed. It is for him, if he thinks fit, to translate recommendation into policy and action. For this particular task of using a consultant group to the best advantage the Regular medical officer can have no peace-time training. In war he can suddenly find himself associated with a group of men of high repute professionally, much better qualified than himself and with little or no knowledge of the Army. He has to be able to understand the significance of what each of them has to say about his own specialty and he has to help each of them to become a component member of the Army and of a team of which he himself is the head. This can never be an easy task.

The consultants to the Army, as distinct from those appointed to specific commands, were actually part of the establishment of the R.A.M. College, but had their offices and clerical staffs in the Army

Medical Directorate during the war years. This arrangement was in every way satisfactory for it brought them into close contact with the branches with which they were continually dealing and also made them immediately available to D.G.A.M.S.

The Graded Specialist and the Trainee

Following the outbreak of war and with the rapid enlargement of the Army it quickly became apparent that the number of experienced specialists available for recruitment was insufficient to meet the requirements of the Army Medical Services. The Central Medical War Committee was therefore notified that in the circumstances a proportion of younger and less experienced men would be acceptable for appointments in the various specialties. These would be posted to general hospitals with an authorised establishment for more than one specialist in a particular branch of medicine and would work as assistants under the guidance and supervision of more experienced officers of full specialist status. They were designated as graded specialists, drew specialist pay, but held rank as G.D.Os. Officers already serving in the R.A.M.C. holding the appropriate qualifications and being recommended were also eligible for employment as graded surgeons, graded physicians and the like. (*Admin*. I. p. 148.)

In 1942 the qualifications of an officer applying for recognition as a graded specialist were exactly defined. (*Admin*. I. pp. 151, 153.) This scheme, admirable as it was, failed to produce all the specialists that were needed and it became necessary to devise another whereby the G.D.O. could receive training within the Army Medical Services and graduate as a graded specialist. D.Ds.M.S. commands were required to discover young G.D.Os. of promise and to recommend them for training in one of the specialties. The directors and consultants in A.M.D. examined those recommended and such as passed the test of interview were posted as G.D.Os. to vacancies in the establishments of hospitals where they could receive instruction. Aspirant pathologists were posted to command laboratories. (*Admin*. I. pp. 150, 153.)

Rather more than a quarter of the total medical officers serving in the Army Medical Services were employed as specialists, graded specialists and trainee specialists. The trainee scheme was very successful indeed and did much to maintain the morale of the A.M.S. at a high pitch. There were no graded specialists in hygiene but officers with suitable qualifications were given courses of training before posting as D.A.Ds.H. or as officers commanding field hygiene sections. (*Admin*. I. p. 152.)

Women Medical Officers

Though a considerable number of medically qualified women served with the R.A.M.C. during the war years they never belonged to the

Corps. They were not commissioned in the R.A.M.C. but in the Women's Forces and their rank was a relative rank. (*Admin.* I. p. 206.)

From 1937 onwards throughout the war years the Medical Women's Federation had been demanding that women doctors should be employed in the medical services of the Armed Forces on terms of parity with men. This agitation had commanded the full support of the British Medical Association and was the cause of much disputation.

At the beginning of the war the Armed Forces were far from ready to cope with the situation that was soon to be created by the large scale recruitment of women and the great expansion of the women's services. Before the passing of the Defence (Women's Forces) Act in 1941 it is certainly true that medical women serving with the R.A.M.C. were in a most unenviable position. The category within the Army to which they belonged was very indeterminate and their duties and responsibilities were ill-defined. They had no actual rank or title and even the details of the uniform they were supposed to wear remained unprescribed. The Act made all things clear; they were to be commissioned in the Women's Forces, but it failed to satisfy the Medical Women's Federation and the British Medical Association for the inequality in respect of status between male and female still remained.

Equality in all respects between the sexes was a well-established and accepted principle in the civil medical world, but to apply this to the Army at this particular time was bound to be a very difficult matter. Before the passing of the Defence (Women's Forces) Act, no female could be an officer in His Majesty's Forces within the meaning of the Army Act in its existing form and special legislation was needed before the granting of commissions to women could be authorised. At that time women were enrolled and not enlisted in the women's services. None of the professional and technical corps admitted women to their commissioned ranks; the women officers serving with them and participating in their professional or technical activities held commissions in the women's services. To make an exception in the case of the medical women serving with the R.A.M.C. would have been exceedingly difficult. Within the A.M.S. it was generally accepted that although women were capable of filling very many of the appointments within the medical services of an expeditionary force they could not possibly be posted to such units as a field ambulance which functioned well within the range of the enemy's guns. Furthermore, the R.A.M.C. officer had duties that were purely military, he had to exercise command and maintain discipline among soldiers in their capacity as fighting men. Save in the atmosphere of the hospital, soldiers were unaccustomed to receive orders from a woman officer. A woman holding a commission in the R.A.M.C. would be burdened with responsibilities that she would find difficult to discharge and would be placed in a position, *vis à vis* the soldier as soldier, that would be embarrassing to her and to others. A commission in the Women's Forces did not carry with it the need to exercise command or disciplinary powers outside the scope of purely professional duties.

No agreement between the champions of the rights of women and the Army authorities was ever reached, but the controversy died down in 1942 and the subjects of the status of women in the Army, the exact nature of the commissions they should hold and the terms and conditions of service that should be offered to them were put into cold storage until the war ended.

The Non-Medical Officer, R.A.M.C.

Before the war, excluding quartermasters, all officers of the R.A.M.C. were required to hold degrees registrable with the General Medical Council. At the end of the war there were 642 officers who lacked such qualifications and who were serving as bearer officers with a field ambulance, administrative officers in a general hospital, C.C.S. or F.D.S., or officer commanding a field hygiene section. (*Admin.* I. p. 214.)

'During the war a non-medical officer was at the head of A.M.D.3, the branch of the Army Medical Directorate that was concerned with medical equipment. Several others held Grade 2 and Grade 3 staff appointments in this directorate and in the medical branches of H.Qs. commands and armies. A non-medical officer, in the rank of colonel, succeeded shortly after the end of the war to the important appointment of O.i/c R.A.M.C. Records.' (J.M.M.)

This development had been forced upon the Corps by the severe overall shortage of medically qualified men in the country as a whole. The Hartgill Committee had considered this impending shortage and had recommended that non-medical officers should be employed as officer-in-charge of a bearer section of a field ambulance.

It was found that though the possession of a medical degree was an advantage it was not an essential qualification for such as occupied the positions listed above. The field hygiene section could be commanded as competently by a man holding a diploma in sanitary science as by one with a medical degree and a diploma in public health.

The post-war field hygiene section was commanded by a non-medical officer.

R.A.M.C. Trades

In peace-time every O.R. R.A.M.C. is a tradesman and is trained in the medical units of the Corps. With the outbreak of war the peace-time procedure governing the classification of tradesmen and their advancement in their trades fell into abeyance and in its stead the prescribed arrangements for the general training and classification of tradesmen under war conditions came into force. These, subsequently amended as found expedient, were devised to ensure more intensive training and more rapid advancement of tradesmen to meet the requirements of individual trades and also to give a wider scope for the acceptance of civil qualifications in substitution for training within the Corps after joining the Army. (*Admin.* I. p. 319.) The number of R.A.M.C. trades and their variety were subject to modification from time to time, some being suspended and others being introduced as the situation changed. Among the war-time recruits to the Corps were very many who could never have hoped to qualify as tradesmen; they would never have been admitted in peace-time. These had to be employed in general duties outside the scope of any particular trade.

R.A.M.C. Trades included the following:

Trained nurse	Clerk	Dispenser
Operating room assistant	Storeman (technical)	Mental nursing orderly
Laboratory assistant	Chiropodist	Transfusion orderly
Optician	Hospital cook	Clerk orderly (clinical)
Nursing orderly	Masseur	Sanitary assistant
Special treatment orderly	Radiographer	

A.T.S. personnel served as clerks, storewomen, G.D.Os., cooks (hospital and ordinary), telephonists, masseuses, radiographers and almoners, having entered the A.T.S. in the ordinary way and being employed in their own professions or civilian occupations by special War Office authority. There was a special A.T.S. trade, medical orderly. The duties of such were to look after the M.I. Room and to help the M.O. at sick parade. (*Admin.* II. p. 435.)

The Voluntary Organisations

No account dealing with the work of the A.M.S. during the War of 1939–45 would be complete if in it no mention was made of the very great assistance these Services received from such bodies as the Venerable Order of St. John of Jerusalem, the British Red Cross Society and the St. Andrew's Ambulance Brigade. This assistance took a variety of forms. There were the convalescent and auxiliary hospitals (*Admin.* I. p. 408), the Military Hospitals Reserve (*Admin.* I. p. 19), the welfare officers attached to military hospitals (*Admin.* II. p. 22), the comforts and food parcels for the P.o.W. (*Admin.* II. p. 261), the ambulance car companies that were heavily engaged in the distribution of patients in home commands and also of casualties returning to the United Kingdom from overseas (*Campaigns* IV. p. 68) and the Voluntary Aid Detachments. (*Admin.* I. p. 21.) It is impossible to praise these voluntary organisations too highly for the work they did and for the way in which they did it. The A.M.S. and the nation as a whole are deeply indebted to them.

As was to be expected the inter-relationships of V.A.D. and A.T.S. and of Q.A.I.M.N.S. and V.A.D. had to be regularised. It was suggested by the Army Council that the V.A.D. organisation should be merged into the A.T.S. This was fiercely opposed and the matter was referred to the Elliot Committee in 1943 which recommended that the V.A.Ds. should retain their separate identity under their existing name. (*Admin.* II. p. 21).

The Need for the Training of the R.A.M.C. Officer in Administration and Staff Duties

'In wars such as that of 1939–45 the great majority of the officers of the Army Medical Services must necessarily consist of non-Regulars. Inevitably the small core of Regular officers must come to occupy positions primarily concerned with administration and planning. It is essential, therefore, that the Regular R.A.M.C. officer shall be trained for this destiny from the earliest days of his service. His responsibility in time of war is necessarily heavy for it is for him to make the best possible use of the great wealth of professional talent that is placed at the disposal of the Army when the whole of the medical profession is mobilised. He must be well trained in administration and at the same time well versed in the practice of modern medicine; he must be a good soldier as well as a good doctor.' (A.H.).

Field Training

'The maintenance of a high morale in a fighting force depends to a large extent upon the efficiency of its medical services. To be efficient the medical services must display a number of qualities that are essential to the carrying out of their numerous and varied tasks.

1. The professional standards of the members of the medical services must be high.

2. The medical services in the field must have the most up-to-date equipment and be well exercised in its employment. In respect of mobility the medical units must be able to match the formations they serve.

3. The transport facilities for the carriage of casualties must be highly efficient, well manned and up to date.

'On the outbreak of war the professional standards of the Regular Officers were of a high order. But the personnel of the A.M.S. were not ready for active service in the field for in peace-time there had been no systematic training for field medical units, indeed, such units did not exist in peace-time save in a modified form in the Territorial Army.' (J.C.D.).

During the war years attempts were made to remedy this state of affairs. (*Admin.* I. p. 318). A 'battle' course of instruction was offered by 167 Field Ambulance and the Inspector of Medical Services was placed in charge of all field units. This 'battle' school had a lineal descendant in the post-war years in the Field Training School, R.A.M.C. (1949–53). This became the Field Training Centre (1953–62) and this in turn became the Field Training Wing of the R.A.M.C. Depot and Training Establishment.

The Senior Administrative Medical Officer of a Formation as Commander Army Medical Services

In the reports of D.Ds.M.S. and A.Ds.M.S. in the field the opinion was frequently expressed that the dual functions of the D.D.M.S. and A.D.M.S. should be overtly recognised. To make it perfectly clear to all concerned that those holding these positions were actually in command of troops and were engaged in the tactical handling of units, it was suggested that they should be given the title of C.A.M.S. in the same way and for the same reasons that the senior S. & T. officer in a formation was C.R.A.S.C. (*Campaigns* III. p. 577.)

Though no action was taken, the recommendation itself is surely reasonable. In Burma, it is to be noted, the field medical units were armed. (*Campaigns* V. p. 337.)

The Medical Advisory Division, S.A.C.S.E.A.

Within the Services it is firmly maintained that because their tasks, weapons, organisations, problems and the elements in which they function are so very different it is essential that the Royal Navy, the Army and the Royal Air Force should each retain its own identity. Each has its own medical services and during the war years each of them, and combined operations also, had its own scientific advisers and teams of investigators and its own contacts with the Medical Research Council and its many committees. In every overseas theatre there was to be encountered a more or less strong desire to manage its own affairs and a more or less strong reluctance to endure any kind of interference from without. As a general rule the attitude of the medical branch of an expeditionary force H.Q. was a faithful reflection of that of the commander.

This attitude can readily be understood for it was displayed by men heavily burdened with responsibility who knew the local conditions and who were eager to get on with the job. There can be no doubt, however, that this desire for autonomy and this separation of the medical services did tend to hamper the rapid acquisition of knowledge concerning the nature of the problems of a medical and biological kind that harassed the forces in the field and the rapid dissemination of the fruits of scientific investigation.

S.A.C.S.E.A. in Kandy, Ceylon, was very remote from London. It was required to deal also with New Delhi. It was a highly complex and composite organisation with U.S. and British Naval, Army and Air Force elements. The Supreme Commander found it desirable to bring into being a medical advisory division consisting of four senior administrative medical officers—one representative from each of the medical services of the Royal Navy, the Army, the Royal Air Force and of the United States Forces. The group was called a division for the reason that this G.H.Q. was modelled upon the naval pattern. It is to be noted that it was found necessary to appoint one of the members of this division as its chairman or director, for though the group of advisers may be a large and composite one, there can only be a single channel along which its communications with the commander flow. (*Campaigns* V. p. 416.)

Certain trends are to be noted. In the *Third Report from the Estimates Committee, Session* 1962–63 the view is once again presented that 'it can be argued that in the military circumstances which apply today this (*the existence of three separate headquarter organisations of the Navy, Army and Air Force*) is not the most efficient method of conducting national defence'. Though this view is not that of the heads of the three Services it is one that is gaining ground. So also is the notion that the three medical services should become merged. The war-time development of the 'task force', compounded out of Naval, Army and Air Force elements, has been carried over into the post-war period and in a number of overseas commands there is to be found the equivalent of the war-time supreme commander.

If this process of integration proceeds it is most unlikely that the medical advisory mechanism at the headquarters of the commander will be fashioned on the model of this medical advisory division. It is much more likely that the integration of the three medical services will become more and more complete and that one man will occupy the post of senior administrative medical officer and that he will be assisted by an appropriate number and variety of administrative medical officers, consultants and advisers in the different specialist fields of medicine and in the sciences on which medicine rests.

Medical Intelligence

During the course of a long-continued war when a large proportion of the medical man-power of the country consists of civilians in uniform far removed from their practices it becomes desirable, even necessary, to devise some means whereby these men may be kept informed of recent developments in the kind of medicine with which they are familiar, the medicine of general practice and the medicine of the hospital sphere. In the absence of such information they are inclined to become anxious about the future and dissatisfied with the present.

During the War of 1939–45 the Directorate of Pathology was made responsible for the production of a bulletin containing brief accounts of recent developments in the medical field. This appeared at frequent intervals, was prepared by the editor of the *Lancet* (then disguised as a major, R.A.M.C.), and was distributed to all officers of the Army Medical Services. It did much to maintain the morale of the A.M.S. at a high level particularly among those whose misfortune it was to be functioning in localities where 'nothing ever happened'.

The A.M.S. produced nothing like the medical intelligence reports of the U.S. medical services. These were very impressive indeed, giving full and detailed accounts of the medical features of the countries into which the Allied armies were about to enter. With such information before him, the senior administrative medical officer's task of preparing a medical appreciation was greatly facilitated.

The British Army had, for centuries, been serving and fighting in very many different eastern countries and had accumulated a vast store of information of this kind. In 1939–45 the A.M.S. and I.M.S. included men who knew the countries of the Middle and Far East as well as others knew their England or Scotland or Wales. A publication such as that produced by the Americans was not so necessary in A.M.S. circles; it would have been very helpful, nevertheless, for in it the information was systematised and presented in a most convincing manner.

The Organisation of the Army Medical Services in the Field

When the lists of the field medical units that relate to the pre-war and the early post-war years are compared the magnitude of the effects of the impact of the war upon the Army Medical Services is most clearly revealed.

Pre-war	Early Post-war
1. Regimental Medical Establishments	1. Regimental Medical Establishments
2. Field Ambulance	2. Field Ambulance
3. Casualty Clearing Station	3. Casualty Clearing Station
4. Field Hygiene Section	4. Field Hygiene Section
5. Ambulance Train	5. Ambulance Train
6. General Hospital	6. General Hospital
7. Convalescent Depot	7. Convalescent *Training* Depot

Pre-war	Early Post-war
8. Hospital Ship	8. Hospital Ship
9. Advanced Depot of Medical Stores	9. Advanced Depot of Medical Stores
10. Base Depot of Medical Stores	10. Base Depot of Medical Stores
11. Mobile Hygiene Laboratory	11. Mobile Hygiene Laboratory
12. Mobile Bacteriological Laboratory	12. Mobile Bacteriological Laboratory
13. Motor Ambulance Convoy	13. Motor Ambulance Company, R.A.S.C. (Combination of 13 and 14. Pre-war units.)
14. Ambulance Car Company, R.A.S.C.	

15. Base Malaria Field Laboratory (in malarious areas)
16. Base Transfusion Unit
17. Beach Medical Unit (only in opposed landings)
18. Burns Team
19. Central Pathological Laboratory
20. Chest Surgery Team
21. Field Dressing Station
22. Field Hygiene Company
23. Field Medical Company
24. Field Surgical Team
25. Field Transfusion Team
26. Malaria Control Company (only in malarious areas)
27. Maxillo-facial Surgical Team
28. Medical Forward Treatment Unit (only in tropical or sub-tropical countries)
29. Mobile Ear, Nose and Throat Team
30. Mobile Malaria Field Laboratory (only in malarious areas)
31. Mobile Neuro-surgical Team
32. Mobile Ophthalmic Team
33. Special Treatment Team

No less than 19 new medical units were born of the experience gained during the war. These had been created to satisfy the needs of the time and place and had proved to be so valuable that they had been incorporated into the post-war organisation of the Army Medical Services in the field. All of the 14 units that had existed before the war were still to be found in the early post-war list but almost every one of them had been subjected to more or less drastic modification.

1. REGIMENTAL MEDICAL ESTABLISHMENTS

	Pre-war	**Post-war**
R.A.M.C.	1 M.O.	1 M.O. and 1–6 N.C.Os.
Regimental	1 L/Cpl. (orderly)	1 N.C.O.
	1 Pte. (batman)	

The R.A.M.C. element had become considerably increased.

2. THE FIELD AMBULANCE

Pre-war Two types, infantry and cavalry.

The Infantry Field Ambulance

3 per infantry division and 1 per corps.
13 officers and 225 O.Rs.
42 vehicles including 8 six-wheeled motor ambulances and 3 trailers.
Weight of combined G.1098 and I.1248 equipment—21 tons.
Capacity: 150 patients but not limited to this number.
Organisation: H.Q. and two companies. The H.Q. formed the M.D.S. and each of the companies could form an A.D.S.

The A.D.S.

One or at the most two per divisional front. The centre from which the field ambulance S.B. squads worked to clear the R.A.Ps. and in which the casualties were collected, given first aid and then evacuated by the ambulances of the unit to the M.D.S. The A.D.S. could provide sheltered accommodation for about 50 casualties. When the carry between R.A.P. and A.D.S. was long or more than usually difficult, a number of Bearer Relay Posts was set up between them. When large numbers of casualties were expected, in order to prevent the A.D.S. becoming bogged down, a W.W.C.P. was sometimes established by a company of one of the divisional field ambulances or of the corps field ambulance on the route between A.D.S. and M.D.S. and nearer the former. The W.W.C.P. set up reception, recording, dressing and evacuation sections. Evacuation was by lorry and the like, provided by 'Q', direct to the C.C.S.

The M.D.S.

One per divisional front. Its organisation indicates its functions. It had receiving, recording, resuscitation, dressing, gas and evacuation sections. In the receiving section the casualties were sorted into those fit for immediate further evacuation to the C.C.S. and those who needed to be retained for a while to receive urgent medical care. Evacuation from M.D.S. to C.C.S. was by M.A.C.

When circumstances permitted, casualties were evacuated from the

A.D.S. direct to the C.C.S. by the ambulance cars of the field ambulance and no M.D.S. was then opened. When this happened the field ambulance attached a number of clerks to the C.C.S. to record the admissions from the division which the field ambulance was serving.

The Rest Station

When circumstances permitted, in order to retain the minor sick in the divisional area and to lighten the load of the C.C.S. it was customary to open a divisional rest station, using one of the divisional field ambulances or the corps field ambulance. Here simple medical treatment was provided.

The Cavalry Field Ambulance

2 per cavalry division.

10 officers and 167 O.Rs.

42 vehicles including 12 six-wheeled ambulance cars and 2 trailers.

Weight of G.1098 and I.1248—4 tons 10 cwt.

Organisation: H.Q. and 4 sections. The H.Q. formed the M.D.S. and each of the sections could provide a small A.D.S., much less elaborate than that of the infantry type of field ambulance but much more mobile and self-sufficient.

Tank battalions had their own regimental medical establishments. The clearance of their R.A.Ps. was incorporated into the general arrangements for the collection of the wounded and their evacuation made by the formation to which the tank battalion was attached. For the armoured brigade, especially when this was acting in an independent rôle, the cavalry field ambulance was regarded as the most suitable medical unit to satisfy its needs.

Post-war

1 standard type.

3 per infantry division and airborne division, 2 per armoured division, 1 per independent infantry brigade group, 1 per independent armoured brigade, 1 per army.

13 officers and 221 O.Rs.

54 vehicles including 16 ambulances and 6 trailers.

Weight of combined G.1098 and I.1248—when serving with infantry or armoured formations and units $11\frac{1}{2}$ tons, with airborne $9\frac{1}{2}$ tons.

Organisation: H.Q., H.Q. section and 1 company divisible into 3 sections.

The H.Q. formed the A.D.S., the H.Q. section assisted the A.D.S. and was used for leap-frogging movements and for augmenting and relieving the sections of the company. Company H.Q. administered and controlled the activities of the 3 sections, each of which could form a

C.C.P., the equivalent of the old A.D.S. Whenever possible evacuation from R.A.P. to C.C.P. was by jeep ambulance.

The A.D.S.

This was the equivalent of the old M.D.S. but in it the sorting of the casualties had become far more systematised (*Admin.* I. p. 472.). There were three categories of casualties, Priority 1, those requiring resuscitation and/or urgent surgical intervention. Priority 2, those requiring early surgery and possibly resuscitation, and Priority 3, all others. Priorities 1 and 2 were quickly evacuated by M.A.C. to the C.C.S. receiving at the time or to the A.S.C. if this had been established. Priority 3 cases, except those who could reasonably be expected to return to their units within a few days and who were evacuated to the F.D.S. were likewise sent by M.A.C. to the C.C.S.

'The grading of stretcher cases into the three categories, as practised in 1939–45, was not without its dangers. Its success depended very largely indeed upon the commonsense of the medical officer who carried out the grading. There were occasions when the forward units were grossly overcrowded with patients awaiting operation when, had these been evacuated to the rear in the normal manner, they would have had their operations sooner and under better conditions.' (E.W.W.)

The transformation of the chain R.A.P.—A.D.S.—M.D.S. into R.A.P.—C.C.P.—A.D.S. was the direct outcome of the experience gained during the earlier years of the war. It was strongly recommended by the Hartgill Committee (*Admin.* I. p. 466.). The creation of the F.D.S. had made the M.D.S. superfluous. The field ambulance of the early post-war years was better equipped, far more flexible, mobile, and efficient than its predecessor. During the war years the cavalry field ambulance had become the light field ambulance. The standard type field ambulance could satisfy all the needs of an armoured formation and with its modified equipment was well suited for service with airborne formations.

3. THE CASUALTY CLEARING STATION

Pre-war

1 per division. Army troops (or with a small force G.H.Q. troops.)

12 officers and 86 O.Rs., plus 2 more when X-ray plant was installed.

2 lorries for drawing rations and stores. 10 three-ton lorries were needed to move the light section of the unit, 22 to move the whole unit; these were supplied by 'Q'.

Capacity: 200 patients, 50 in beds the rest on stretchers.

Organisation: A heavy and a light section. Receiving (and sorting), resuscitation, gas, pre-operation, theatre, dressing, evacuation, dental and X-ray sections, office.

The C.C.S. was the pivot of the whole evacuation system, being the first point down the line where proper surgical facilities existed and where skilled nursing could be offered. (Note: No Q.A.I.M.N.S. on the establishment.) It was usual to group several C.C.Ss. and to open them in succession. The C.C.S. usually had to deal with casualties occurring in the rear areas, collecting them with the help of the M.A.C.

The C.C.S. could furnish 3 surgical teams out of its own resources. As many as 5 additional surgical teams from the general hospitals could be attached to a C.C.S. during battle.

An Advanced Operating Centre could be formed by a C.C.S. in front of its own position in order to cut down the time interval between the receipt of a wound and the intervention of a skilled surgeon.

At the outbreak of the War of 1939–45 there was only one C.C.S. in being, 2/5 C.C.S. formed for the Palestine emergency and sent to the Western Desert a week before war was declared. It had one surgeon on its establishment and only one theatre. It was intended to reinforce this unit with unequipped surgical teams from general hospitals. Its surgical potential was very low. During 1940–41 this C.C.S. was reinforced by a surgical team from 8 B.G.H. and as its own surgeon was in process of being replaced there happened to be three surgeons available for a time. Its light section, with two of these surgeons, went forward to Mersa Matruh and set up an operating centre at the M.D.S. of 2/1 Fd. Amb. When the Italians retreated, the unit, acquiring a variety of vehicles and a quantity of surgical equipment, was able to move forward with its host, the field ambulance. It was from this *ad hoc* arrangement that the mobile surgical unit, consisting of a surgeon, an anaesthetist, 2 O.R.As., 2 N.Os. and a staff car and one lorry with driver, was evolved. Among the medical arrangements for the battle of Sidi Barrani, December 1940, was the improvisation of a mobile C.C.S., built out of the light sections of 2 (Ind.) and 2/5 C.C.Ss. and a number of surgical teams. Though this unit lacked beds, Q.A.I.M.N.S. personnel, special dietaries and the like, it did possess the essential property of mobility since one of its components had its own transport. (*Campaigns* I. pp. 205, 234.) Later the mobile C.C.S. with its 10 additional lorries was invented; its light section could be transported in the unit's own transport and the whole of the unit could be moved in three lifts. It could keep pace with the advancing formations and could open in the divisional area. The Hartgill Committee recommended that sufficient transport should be given to a C.C.S. to enable the unit to be moved in one lift by the transport of two such units.

As Eighth Army moved westwards to join up with First Army in Tunisia, the system of forming a forward surgical centre, in which a number of C.C.Ss. with added surgical units was congregated, developed to give rise later to the corps medical centre.

Post-War

3 per corps and 1 per army. Army troops.

16 officers, 131 O.Rs. and 22 Q.A.R.A.N.C.

9 vehicles including 1 four-stretcher ambulance and 3 trailers.

Weight of combined G.1098 and I.1248—39 tons.

30 three-ton lorries were needed to move the unit; these were provided by 'Q'.

Capacity: 200 patients, 120 in beds and the rest on stretchers.

Organisation: Medical and surgical sections. Each C.C.S. had two surgeons and two theatre staffs on its establishment and by attaching six surgical teams from general hospitals for use as F.S.Ts., each working a 12-hour shift, the total surgical output of the unit was approximately 100 cases in 24 hours. Eight such teams, working in four theatres was the maximum that could be conveniently used.

The C.C.S. had pre- and post-operative wards, resuscitation ward, X-ray, reception, evacuation and theatre sections.

Evacuation from the C.C.S. was by M.A.C. ambulance train or by air.

The post-war C.C.S. was a larger unit than its predecessor and carried Q.A.R.A.N.C. on its establishment. It had more transport but was still an immobile unit. The creation of the F.S.T. greatly multiplied its surgical potential while the adoption of the plan to form an Advanced Surgical Centre by attaching F.S.Ts. and F.S.Us. to a field ambulance had made the provision of an advanced operating centre by the C.C.S. unnecessary.

4. THE FIELD HYGIENE SECTION

The early post-war unit had far better transport and was therefore much more mobile than its predecessor. The cavalry type—the light field hygiene section of the war years—had disappeared. (Hartgill Committee. *Admin*. I. p. 470.) The allotment had changed from 1 per division, infantry and cavalry, plus such as were required for non-divisional troops, L. of C. and bases, to 1 per corps and 1 per base area and sub-area.

When the organisation of the medical services in the field was reviewed at the end of the war, the divisional field hygiene section was abolished and replaced by a D.A.D.H. and 8 hygiene assistants for inspectorial duties. At corps level there was an A.D.A.H. and a field hygiene section commanded by a non-medical officer. At army H.Q. there was an A.D.A.H. and a field hygiene company.

5. THE AMBULANCE TRAIN

The post-war ambulance train was smaller than its predecessor (accommodation for 250 patients instead of 360) and had a smaller staff

(2 M.Os., 2 Q.A.R.A.N.C. and 34 O.Rs. as compared with 3 M.Os., 3 Q.A.I.M.N.S. and 45 O.Rs.).

6. THE GENERAL HOSPITAL

Pre-war

Allotted to a force on the basis of the number of beds required, usual figure 10 per cent. of the force.

Two types, 1,200 and 600 bed, both of these increasing by multiples of 100 beds.

1,200-Bed (including 200 beds for officers).
  35 officers, 80 Q.A.I.M.N.S. and 229 O.Rs. With each additional 100 beds 1 officer, 4 Q.A.I.M.N.S. and 9 O.Rs.
  Organisation: Medical and surgical divisions. The staff included a surgical team that could be used to reinforce the surgical potential of a C.C.S.; it consisted of a surgeon, anaesthetist, theatre sister and 1 O.R.A.

600-Bed (including 60 beds for officers).
  23 officers, 50 Q.A.I.M.N.S. and 144 O.R.s (no detachable surgical team). With each additional 100 beds 2 officers, 5 Q.A.I.M.N.S. and 11 O.Rs. Weight of combined G.1098 and I.1248—1,200-bed, 223 tons 16 cwt; 600-bed, 134 tons 14 cwt.

Transport	1,200-bed	600-bed
Bicycles	3	3
Carriers, stretcher	20	12
Carts, hand	3	3
Carts, water tank	3	3
Disinfectors, Thresh	2	1

Post-war

Allotted according to the number of beds required. Staff and equipment were adjusted on a sliding scale from 50 beds, increasing by 50 beds to 300 and thereafter by 100 beds to 1,200 beds. The commonest requirement was expected to be for 1,200- and 600-bed units. When mobility was a major consideration the 200-bed would be favoured. The 300-bed and over were divided into H.Q., medical and surgical divisions. The larger sizes could be divided into heavy and light sections (each of these being a multiple of 50 beds). This arrangement made the movement of the hospital a simple matter since a section of 50 beds was fairly self-contained.

Staff, Transport and Weight of Equipment:

Tons		Offrs.	Q.A.R. A.N.C.	O.Rs.	Cars Utility G.S.	Trucks 15-cwt.	Trucks Water 15-cwt.	Lorries 3-ton	Trailers
50-bed	14	4	5	36	—	—	1	—	—
200 „	51	14	22	114	1	—	1	—	1
600 „	134	23	50	217	1	1	2	2	3
1,200 „	271	34	80	343	1	1	2	2	3

The change from bicycle and hand-cart to utility car and lorry was but a reflection of the completeness with which the internal combustion engine had affected the habits of the industrialised world. Transport vehicles were plentiful and so the hospital could be organised to take advantage of their existence. The invention of the basic section of 50 beds, readily transportable, and the adoption of the block or brick system of packaging stores constituted a very great advance.

During the war years the immobility of the indivisible large hospital had frequently and seriously affected the medical services' ability to provide adequate bed-cover when the advance was rapid or the withdrawal hurried, as in Libya 1940–43, France and Belgium 1940 and N.W. Europe 1944–45. Not only was the large general hospital, functioning on the L. of C., exceedingly difficult to move quickly, it was also difficult to find a suitable site for it. In Libya (*Campaigns* I. p. 269, II. p. 263) it was found necessary to improvise a mobile military hospital.

'During the course of the campaign in N. Africa it was quickly realised that the distance between corps C.C.Ss. and Army general hospitals was likely to become too greatly extended. So, during the winter of 1942–43, the 200 and 600-bed Army general hospitals were reorganised, in respect of tentage, equipment and personnel, into 50-bed blocks, so as to make the units more mobile. Thereafter these units were frequently moved forward by such blocks'. (E.W.W.)

The post-war general hospital was much more useful than its predecessor; one of any given size (so long as this was a multiple of 50 beds) could be provided to match the site and the existing need and it could be moved with relative ease by self-contained sections of 50 beds.

7. THE CONVALESCENT DEPOT. THE CONVALESCENT TRAINING DEPOT

Pre-war

No definite allotment, possibly 4–5 per cent. of the ration strength. Accommodation for 2,000 convalescents.

A.M.S. Staff: 4 officers and 5 O.Rs. (R.A.M.C. and A.D. Corps).

Non-medical Staff: 9 officers and 105 O.Rs.

Post-war

1 per army. For women on an as required basis.

A.M.S. Staff as above.

Organisation: H.Q. and 4 companies each of 250 men. An officers' wing (100) could be added. Women: H.Q. and 2 platoons each of 75 (including 10 per cent. officers).

The unit had changed its name to define more exactly its function. The post-war unit was half the size of its predecessor but had the same A.M.S. staff. The rapid development of physical medicine had greatly increased the efficiency of the unit. The development during the war years of the A.T.S. Reconditioning Centre (*Admin.* II. p. 431) and its record led to the provision during the post-war years of a Convalescent Training Depot for the W.R.A.C.

8. THE HOSPITAL SHIP

Hospital carriers, hospital ships and ambulance transports remained very much the same in respect of the A.M.S. elements of their establishments.

9. THE ADVANCED DEPOT OF MEDICAL STORES

Pre-war

1 per corps. Usually sited at railhead.

Q.M. and 8 O.Rs., including one attached driver R.A.S.C.

1 30-cwt van

Weight of ordnance and medical stores—26 tons 15 cwt.

Post-war

1 per corps, 1 per army.

1 officer and 16 O.Rs.

1 truck 15-cwt G.S., 1 truck—water 15-cwt, 3 three-ton lorries.

Weight of stores—35 tons.

Organisation: The staff was divided into a main store, holding section and a small mobile element consisting of 2 drivers and 2 lorries.

The post-war depot, much larger than its predecessor, was so organised and equipped that it could discharge its function of replenishing forward medical units far more efficiently and speedily. The mobile element was a war-time development that claimed its place in the post-war organisation. (*Campaigns* IV. p. 314.)

10. THE BASE DEPOT OF MEDICAL STORES

Pre-war

1 in each base.

2 officers and 20 O.Rs.

No transport of its own.

Weight of stores—113 tons $13\frac{1}{2}$ cwt.

Post-war

1 per 150,000 of the force.

3 officers and 52 O.Rs.

1 truck 15-cwt G.S. and 1 three-ton lorry

Weight of stores—205 tons.

Organisation: H.Q. and traffic, supply, repair and regimental sections. In selected base depots there was also a returned store and repair section which included a R.E.M.E. sub-section. This undertook major repairs of equipment and provided mobile teams which visited medical units to maintain their equipment. When several base depots were established in a theatre one of them was designated as the central base depot and given an increased staff to be responsible for the receipt of all imported stores and for their distribution among the other base depots.

A Port Detachment R.A.M.C. was attached to a convenient unit in the port area to assist in the identification and despatch of imported medical equipment to the central base depot.

The post-war depot's staff was double that of the pre-war unit and was organised into a number of specialised sections. The system of block supply, evolved during the war years, had been carried over into the post-war organisation. These developments made the post-war unit far more efficient.

11. THE MOBILE HYGIENE LABORATORY

Remained essentially unchanged.

12. THE MOBILE BACTERIOLOGICAL LABORATORY

Remained essentially unchanged.

13 and 14. THE MOTOR AMBULANCE CONVOY. THE AMBULANCE CAR COMPANY, R.A.S.C. (Pre-war.)
THE MOTOR AMBULANCE COMPANY, R.A.S.C. (Post-war.)

The pre-war M.A.C. was a medical unit, commanded by a major R.A.M.C. and was organised into H.Q. with a Medical Wing of 2 officers and 7 O.Rs., R.A.M.C. and a Transport Wing (3 officers and 58 O.Rs. R.A.S.C.) and 3 sections each with a Medical Wing (7 O.Rs. R.A.M.C.) and a Transport Wing (1 officer and 42 O.Rs. R.A.S.C.).

Its first line transport consisted of:	*H.Q.*	*Section*	*Totals*
Motor cycle, solo	5	2	11
Motor cycle with sidecar	1	1	4
Motor cars	2	—	2
Motor ambulances	—	25	75
Lorries 3-ton, 6-wheeled	7	—	7
Trailers, kitchen, water-tank	2	—	2

Second line transport:

Lorries 30-cwt., 4-wheeled

An Ambulance Car Company R.A.S.C. was included in the order of battle of the B.E.F. in France and Belgium, 1939–40. It consisted of H.Q. and a Workshop section together with 3 sections each of 25 motor ambulances. For later campaigns the unit was reorganised and came to consist of 4 sections of motor ambulances and 1 section of troop-carrying vehicles (T.C.Vs.).

At the end of the war when the organisation of the field units was reviewed a War Office Standardisation Conference recommended that the rôles of the M.A.C. and the A.C.C. could be undertaken by one standard unit to be known as the Motor Ambulance Company R.A.S.C. (*The Second World War* 1939–45. *Supplies and Transport*. Vol. I. Chap. 3 and Vol. II. pp. 308, 324 and 344.) (*Also* the Hartgill Committee *Admin*. I. p. 470.)

The Motor Ambulance Company R.A.S.C.

   1 per corps, 1 per army, with additional companies for the L. of C. and base areas as required. Commanded by an officer of the R.A.S.C. and administered by D.D.S.T. Under the operational control of the administrative medical officer of the formation to which the M.A.C. was attached.

   Organisation: H.Q. and Workshop platoons, 2 relief driver increments, 3 ambulance car platoons each of 30 cars and 1 platoon of T.C.Vs. Each platoon consisted of 5 sections each of 6 vehicles. To M.A.Cs. allotted to corps a medical platoon of 34 orderlies R.A.M.C. was added.

This change was eminently reasonable. It meant the saving of 2 medical officers per M.A.C. Experience had shown that no adverse effects were associated with evacuation in the A.C.C. as compared with the old M.A.C. so long as care was taken to ensure that only those fit to be moved were loaded into the ambulances and that an orderly R.A.M.C. accompanied such as needed close attention *en route*. The R.A.S.C. provided for the transport and maintained it; the R.A.M.C. shouldered the responsibility for the care of those transported, an uncomplicated relationship.

When necessary a control post could be established at some convenient point along the route of evacuation and an ambulance car relay post placed at some suitable point so that when a loaded ambulance car from the forward area passed through, it could be replaced by an empty one sent forward.

'In the R.A.S.C. it is the custom for vehicles to move in convoys. In casualty evacuation it is usually preferable to have ambulances move independently as soon as each of them is loaded. In the early days of the campaign in N. Africa it took a little while to break down this "convoy complex".' (E.W.W.)

The Ambulance Control Post, Capua and Cassino

This was an innovation that merits careful examination. It was the distributing centre for all Eighth Army casualties during the Cassino battles. In its long lane of tents ambulances from all sectors of the front unloaded and, with a minimum of delay, patients found themselves in other ambulance cars bound for British, Canadian, New Zealand, Indian or other hospitals. The distributing officers maintained a list of the bed-state of all the hospitals in the hospital centres. The loaded ambulances moved off singly. The odd case that needed emergency treatment was retained at the control post, but the vast majority, their dressings having been examined, passed quickly on their way to the medical centres at Caserta or Naples. The post had a holding capacity of 250 and facilities for life-saving surgery as well as for staging, sleeping and feeding the ambulance car crews. (*Campaigns* III. p. 262.)

UNITS BORN OF THE EXPERIENCES OF 1939–45

15. THE BASE MALARIA FIELD LABORATORY

1 per force in malarious theatres.

5 Officers and 16 O.Rs.

2 jeeps, 2 trucks 15-cwt G.S. and 2 trailers 10-cwt.

A mobile unit that was attached to a parent medical unit at the base or on the L. of C. for maintenance and administration.

Functions: The O.C. acted as adviser in malariology to the D.M.S. when there was no consulting malariologist with the force. To conduct malaria surveys, to prepare malaria maps, to carry out research in the field of malariology and to impart instruction in anti-malaria measures.

As the 'camp' diseases, typhoid, typhus and dysentery, passed under control through the application of scientific knowledge concerning their causes and mode of spread, malaria came to occupy their place as an instrument of death and disability impeding and disrupting military enterprises in tropical and sub-tropical regions. In the campaigns in the Middle East, in Sicily and in Italy and especially in that in Burma, this disease was the cause of constant anxiety. The search for the means of bringing it under control began soon after the outbreak of hostilities and as the years passed new medicaments, new insecticides and new repellents and methods of using them, endowed the medical services with the power so to reduce the incidence of this disease that it ceased to have any great military importance. (*Med. Res.* pp. 155, 164. *Med. and Path.* Chap. 7.) For the fullest exploitation of this new knowledge and new techniques new units were required. The base malaria field laboratory and the mobile malaria field laboratory were the direct lineal descendants of units of the same name that were created during the war years. (*Admin.* II. p. 33.) The acquisition and the exercise of the power greatly to reduce the incidence of malaria was, without doubt, one of the major triumphs of the war years.

16. THE BASE TRANSFUSION UNIT

1 per theatre. The standard unit was based upon the estimated requirements of a force of two corps. For each additional corps or army additional personnel were authorised for the unit.

4 officers and 69 O.Rs. plus a pool of transfusion officers.

2 motor cycles, 2 cars utility, 3 trucks 15-cwt, 11 lorries 3-ton, including refrigerator lorries.

Combined weight of G.1098 and I.1248—13 tons.

Organisation: H.Q., 1 blood-collecting section and 1 forward distributing section to each army. The O.C. acted as adviser in resuscitation and transfusion to the D.M.S. When dried plasma could not be supplied from the United Kingdom a plasma-processing section was added to the unit. When whole blood could be supplied from sources outside the theatre the blood-collecting section was withheld. Forward distribution of transfusion materials was effected by maintaining an advanced blood bank of 2 refrigerator vehicles in each corps. (*Admin.* II. p. 385. *Campaigns* V. p. 650.)

17. THE BEACH MEDICAL UNIT

3 M.Os., 3 non-medical officers and 69 O.Rs. Pioneers or infantrymen of the beach group were attached to the medical unit to act as S.Bs.

5 jeeps, 2 two-stretcher motor ambulances, 1 truck 15 cwt G.S., 1 amphibian and 5 trailers 10-cwt.

Functions: To take care of casualties occurring on the beach both among beach-group personnel and assault formations so as not to immobilise the field medical units of the latter; to form a C.E.P. for the documentation and despatch of casualties to vessels at sea, pending the opening of a port. (*See* also p. 152.)

Assault landings were fairly common operations during the war and by the time of the invasion of Sicily the beach brick or beach group had taken shape. It was an organisation specially designed for the administration of the affairs of a landing beach during the assault stage of the enterprise until the arrival, about D-day + 6, of the personnel of a sub-area who then took over from the brick. This brick or group consisted of some 2,000 officers and men and included a brick battalion and an A.A. battery together with representatives of the different services, including the medical. The brick, landing on the heels of the assaulting troops, made arrangements for the siting of dumps, dressing stations, C.E.Ps. and the like and facilitated in all possible ways the onward passage of troops, equipment and stores.

The Middle East establishment of the medical element of the brick was:

S.M.O., clerk and D.R. with a motor cycle.
2 M.Os. and 40 O.Rs. R.A.M.C.
2 hygiene N.C.Os.
3 drivers R.A.S.C.
There was in addition the brick battalion's M.O. and 21 regimental
  S.Bs. and the A.A. battery's M.O. and 5 regimental O.R.s.
2 four-wheel-drive ambulance cars.
The equipment of a light field ambulance much augmented in respect
  of G.1098 stores, drugs and tentage.

The N. African establishment for the medical element was one field ambulance less one company. (*Campaigns* III. p. 6.)

With the passing of time and as experience was gained the establishment of the medical element of the beach group underwent changes. For Operation 'Neptune', the initial landing on the Normandy beaches in 1944, two F.D.Ss., two F.S.Us. and 2 hygiene N.C.Os. were allotted to each of the six beach groups. (*Campaigns* IV. p. 42.)

18. THE BURNS TEAM

3 officers, 2 Q.A.R.A.N.C. and 4 O.Rs.
Weight of equipment—4 tons.

An immobile unit that had to be attached to some parent medical unit, e.g. a general hospital, for maintenance and administration.

In a highly mechanised army inflammable fuels are everywhere present and their use and especially their misuse lead to countless accidental burns. To the treatment of burns, very unsatisfactory at the beginning of the war, much thought and time were given (*Med. Res.* pp. 74–78), and it became very much of a specialist occupation. Out of this experience the Burns Team was derived.

19. THE CENTRAL PATHOLOGICAL LABORATORY

1 officer and 10 O.Rs.
Weight of G.1098 and I.1248—$1\frac{1}{2}$ tons.

An immobile unit that had to be attached to some parent medical unit, e.g. a general hospital, for maintenance and administration.

The urgent need for a laboratory in which major pathological investigations could be undertaken was clearly recognised during the war years and towards the end such a unit was brought into being. The post-war laboratory is a direct descendant of this.

20. THE CHEST SURGERY TEAM

4 officers, 4 Q.A.R.A.N.C. and 8 O.Rs.
Weight of G.1098 and I.1248—$\frac{1}{2}$ ton.

In the sphere of military medicine, as in that of civil medicine, thoracic surgery developed as a specialty. Two small thoracic surgical units were formed for service in the Middle East (*Campaigns* I. p. 298.) and a chest surgery team was included in the medical order of battle for N.W. Europe. (*Campaigns* IV. pp. 111, 649.) It was but reasonable that such a team should be included in the post-war organisation.

21. THE FIELD DRESSING STATION

1 per infantry and armoured division and 1 per airborne division when employed in a ground rôle, 2 per corps as corps troops and 1 per army as army troops plus 1 for each corps in the army.

7 officers and 115 O.Rs.

25 vehicles including 4 four-stretcher ambulances.

Weight of G.1098 and I.1248—5 tons.

Organisation: H.Q. and 2 sections maintained by H.Q. but capable of acting apart therefrom.

Accommodation: 100 patients, 40 in beds and 60 on stretchers.

Functions: To maintain the fighting strength of a formation by holding all minor sick and injured and all mild exhaustion cases within the formation's area. Usually the holding period was seven days. In exceptional circumstances, the divisional F.D.S. could be employed in the divisional evacuation plan. The corps F.D.S. discharged its function in one of several ways, (i) by treating corps troops in the same way as the divisional F.D.S. dealt with divisonal troops, holding them in the corps area, (ii) by acting as a filter for a C.C.S., the reception section of the F.D.S. diverting minor cases to the F.D.S. and the more severe to C.C.S., (iii) by acting as a centre for the treatment of some special type of case, e.g. exhaustion, gas or V.D., (iv) by acting as a parent unit for an advanced surgical centre and (v) by acting as a reception unit on an airfield to accommodate casualties awaiting evacuation by air.

The F.D.S. was one of the new medical units designed by the Hartgill Committee. (*Admin.* I. p. 467. *Campaigns* II. p. 262.) It was intended to discharge two quite different and distinct functions. In a divisional area, where it was suggested these units should be provided on the scale of 1 per armoured and 2 per infantry division, it was to serve primarily as a resuscitation centre for casualties suffering from severe shock (exhaustion) though it could also be used as an A.D.S. to serve divisional troops. In the corps area where the suggested allotment was one per corps plus an additional one for each division in the corps, the F.D.Ss. were to be employed chiefly to form advanced surgical centres by combination with one or more of the newly designed F.S.Us. The corps F.D.S. could also serve as a rest station or as a centre for dealing with a special type of casualty, e.g. gas.

E*

During the war years the F.D.S. attracted the commendation of all who were concerned with its utilisation and there was never any doubt that it would find a lasting place in the organisation of the A.M.S. in the field. It proved to be a most useful multi-purpose unit and was a most effective means of preventing unnecessary loss of man-power through the evacuation from the forward areas of the minor sick and injured. It satisfied the need for a mobile holding unit.

22. THE FIELD HYGIENE COMPANY

1 per army. Army troops.

10 officers and 213 O.Rs.

8 motor cycles, 29 jeeps, 8 trucks 15-cwt G.S., 1 truck water 15-cwt, 4 lorries 3-ton, 29 trailers 10-cwt.

Weight of combined G.1098 and I.1248—24 tons.

Organisation: The O.C. was a specialist in Army Health. H.Q., an instructional wing and six platoons, each of these being much the same as the standard hygiene section. Two of the platoons included workshop personnel. The instructional wing was designed to train up to 200 students (officers or O.Rs. of every arm and service other than the medical) at any one time. Two of the platoons were available for attachment to independent divisions in special situations. The other four platoons were for employment in supervising sanitation in the army area.

The field hygiene company with its authorised establishment and with its own transport would not encounter the difficulties which must necessarily be associated with any attempt on active service to create a novel unit out of such bits and pieces as happen to be available. It was learnt during the war years that it was essential that the individual soldier should make his own personal contribution to the safeguarding of his own health and that to this end it was necessary that he should receive instruction in the elements of preventive medicine.

During the war years, because so large a proportion of the army consisted of categories other than Regular soldiers with relatively long service, those who had attended courses of instruction at the Army School of Hygiene were few and far between. It was found necessary in the Middle East and in North Africa to form a school for the instruction of all and sundry in the simple rules and techniques of health-promotion and of disease-prevention. (*Campaigns* II. p. 399. *Admin.* II. pp. 43, 48.) Many and various difficulties were encountered in obtaining suitable establishments and equipment. These two hygiene schools did excellent work and demonstrated beyond all doubt that some such instructional machinery was an essential part of an overseas force of any considerable size, especially when this was operating in an area in which strenuous efforts had to be made to protect the troops from epidemic disease.

23. THE FIELD MEDICAL COMPANY

1 per army and on an as required basis for L. of C. and base areas.

12 officers and 50 O.Rs. plus a pool of officers for duty as officers in medical charge of troops of units without M.Os. of their own.

2 motor cycles, 9 cars utility, 2 two-stretcher motor ambulances, 1 truck 15-cwt. G.S., 4 lorries 3-ton.

Organisation: The unit was so equipped as to be able to form a number of reception stations (5–100 beds) up to a maximum of 350 beds.

Functions: To provide medical cover for troops in L. of C. and base areas belonging to units without M.Os. of their own.

In every theatre during the war years the need for some unit designed to provide medical cover for the many units and parties in the rearward areas with no M.O. of their own was keenly felt. The use of field ambulance or C.C.S. personnel for this purpose was found to be most unsatisfactory and wasteful. This unit should prove to be among the most useful of post-war creations.

24. THE FIELD SURGICAL TEAM

2 per infantry and armoured division, 6 per airborne division.

Surgeon, anaesthetist, 6 orderlies and 2 drivers.

1 jeep, 1 lorry 3-ton and 1 trailer 1-ton.

Weight of G.1098 and I.1248—4 tons.

Organisation. A completely mobile specialist unit which was attached to some parent medical unit for maintenance and administration.

Function: To provide or to reinforce the surgical potential of the medical unit to which it was attached, usually a C.C.S. but on occasion a F.D.S. with which it formed an A.S.C.

In an airborne operation 2 F.S.Ts. were attached to each airborne field ambulance to provide surgical facilities until such time as the ground forces established contact with the airborne when the F.S.Ts. were usually withdrawn. When the F.S.T. was so employed its equipment was modified to suit the rôle it was to play.

It was the custom before the war and also during its earliest years to reinforce the surgeons of the forward C.C.Ss. with surgical teams provided out of the staffs of the 1,200-bed general hospitals. But such teams, useful as they were, were not mobile and had no transportable equipment. Their employment in the Middle East quickly disclosed their deficiencies. (*Campaigns* II. p. 262.) It was not surprising, therefore, that the Hartgill Committee recommended that in place of these teams and of others hastily compounded out of such surgeons and anaesthetists as happened to be available, a unit with an establishment, with equipment and with transport of its own, should be created. This field surgical unit was designed and equipped to undertake 100 major surgical operations without replenishment of stores and to be able in association with the corps F.D.S. to form an advanced surgical centre. (*Admin.* I. p. 467.)

The F.S.Us. proved to be of the greatest usefulness; they were freely employed to augment the surgical potential in the forward areas and in very difficult circumstances were able to provide skilled surgical intervention far in front of the C.C.S. After the end of the war the F.S.U. became the F.S.T.

'In the Western Desert the F.S.U. satisfied the needs of forward surgery in mobile warfare as no other unit had done before and as no other unit could do under those conditions. The line of battle in the open desert might move as much as twenty or even fifty miles in a day in either direction and facilities for necessary surgery had to be provided wherever men were being wounded.

'F.S.Us. formed an entirely fluid surgical potential that could be modified according to the needs of the time. The simplest grouping was one F.S.U. attached to a section of a light field ambulance. Further elaborations were the grouping of several F.S.Us. to which were added F.T.Us. in a less mobile site with several field ambulances or sections of C.C.Ss. Such an A.S.C. was established at Burg el Arab in the early stages of the battle of Alamein.

'The unsupported F.S.U. was essential for the saving of life when the main problem was major haemorrhage, but in little else. Nursing was difficult and further transportation precarious. The real contribution of the single F.S.U. depended upon the ability of the surgeon commanding it to think in terms of the need of the wounded man. Apart from a few urgent cases the majority of wounded men, after a rapid assessment, were better sent further down the line to better equipped and staffed units where they could be retained.

'A tendency that was difficult to combat was that of the administrative medical officers to attach single F.S.Us. as a morale booster to a mobile force where they could do no useful surgery. Forward surgery must be good and a point is reached when "the further forward the worse it is".'

(H.O.)

In the Italian campaign the F.S.Us. and F.T.Us. were heavily involved in the Cassino battles which raised such difficult problems for the medical services. The time taken to get a casualty back to the A.D.S. in this terrain was abnormally prolonged; he had to be carried down steep, treacherous paths for two miles or more through a series of stretcher-bearer relay posts stationed every 200 yards or so along the track, under fire for most of the way and in rain or snow. At the end of this hand-carry in the valley the F.S.Us. and F.T.Us., under canvas extensions to specially equipped lorries, waited to offer full surgical facilities.

25. THE FIELD TRANSFUSION TEAM

3 per corps and 2 per Army. Army troops.

1 officer (a specialist in transfusion), 2 transfusion orderlies.

1 driver.

1 three-ton lorry

Weight of G.1098 and I.1248—2½ tons.

D.D.M.S. Army distributed the F.T.Ts. to medical units in corps or army, one team usually being attached to each C.C.S., passing under the control of the senior administrative medical officer of the formation which the C.C.S. was serving. Sometimes attached to an A.S.C. The unit to which the F.T.T. was attached maintained and administered it. The usual proportion of F.T.Ts. to F.S.Ts. was 1 : 2 but the F.T.T. could be reinforced by the attachment of a second transfusion officer from the pool at the B.T.U.

Function: To provide a mobile and expert transfusion service in forward areas.

The original design of the Army Transfusion Service was drawn up by the Royal College of Surgeons of England soon after the Munich crisis in 1938. A key staff for the Army Blood Supply Depot and for an overseas Transfusion and Surgical Research Laboratory was ear-marked. (*Admin.* II. p. 373.) This laboratory left for France on October 5, 1939 and thereafter was supplied with transfusion materials by the Army Blood Supply Depot, which had opened in Bristol. After Dunkirk the laboratory was disbanded and in its place the B.T.U. appeared. The Hartgill Committee recommended that the field transfusion unit should be created. This was very much the same as the post-war F.T.T. The war-time F.T.Us. proved their worth in all the theatres and it was always certain that they would find a place in the post-war organisation.

26. THE MALARIA CONTROL COMPANY

1 per army in malarious regions.

12 officers and 156 O.Rs.

11 jeeps, 15 trucks 15-cwt G.S., 9 lorries 3-ton and 11 trailers 10-cwt.

Combined weight of G.1098 and I.1248—14 tons.

Organisation: H.Q. and 1 section for each corps.

Function: To control civil labour for undertaking anti-malaria measures.

During the war years the arrangements for the control of locally enlisted civilian labour for employment on anti-malaria schemes were haphazard and unsatisfactory. Since the work done was so important a contribution to the prevention of malaria among the troops—the transformation of Dimapur from a place where no one could hope to avoid this disease into something approaching a health resort is an instance of this—it is not surprising that in the post-war organisation of the A.M.S. in the field a place had to be found for this unit adequately staffed and equipped for the undertaking of its difficult tasks.

27. THE MAXILLO-FACIAL SURGICAL TEAM

1 per army, additional teams being provided for G.H.Q. troops on an as required basis.

7 officers, 8 Q.A.R.A.N.C. and 16 O.Rs. (The officers included surgical and dental specialists).

2 jeeps, 2 lorries 3-ton and 2 trailers 10-cwt.

Combined weight of G.1098 and I.1248—3 tons.

Function: To provide specialist treatment for maxillo-facial injuries.

Organisation: The team was divisible into two smaller teams each capable of working independently. The unit was attached to some parent unit for maintenance and administration.

During the war years the first of the Maxillo-facial Surgical Units, as they were then called, was formed in the United Kingdom in 1940, the second in Alexandria in 1941. (*Campaigns* I. p. 297.) They soon proved their worth and it was quite certain that they would be represented in the post-war organisation.

28. THE MEDICAL FORWARD TREATMENT UNIT

1 per corps, as army troops in tropical or sub-tropical areas or elsewhere if required.

19 officers, 13 Q.A.R.A.N.C. and 187 O.Rs.

5 trucks 15-cwt. G.S. and 1 trailer 1-ton.

Combined weight of G.1098 and I.1248—122$\frac{1}{4}$ tons.

Organisation: H.Q. and 4 sections, one or more of which might be detached. Capable of treating 1,000 minor cases. 100 beds and 900 stretchers.

Function: A general hospital on a light scale equipped to deal with sick (rather than with the wounded) likely to be fit to return to their units within a limited period. The M.F.T.U. was used to save transportation of sick to the rear and was usually sited in the corps maintenance area. The beds of the M.F.T.U. counted against the total allotment of hospital beds to the force.

This unit originated as the Malaria Forward Treatment Unit, designed in Burma for the treatment of malaria patients in the forward areas at a time when this disease was the main cause of wastage. By holding and treating such patients men were not lost to the divisions to which they belonged. They proved their worth abundantly and when malaria ceased to be the major medical problem these units were used for the holding and treatment of men with other forms of sickness.

In the campaign in Burma, especially, it was almost certain that any man who was evacuated beyond the corps area would be lost to his division for the reasons that the L. of C. was so very long and the base was so very far away. It was imperative that every effort should be made to hold in the forward areas such men as could be treated satisfactorily in such units as the F.D.S. and the M.F.T.U. (*Campaigns* V. p. 124.)

29. THE MOBILE EAR, NOSE AND THROAT TEAM

1 per corps as army troops.

1 officer and 5 O.Rs.

1 three-ton lorry.

Combined weight of G.1098 and I.1248—$\frac{1}{2}$ ton.

Function: To provide specialist treatment for E.N.T. cases in the forward areas. The unit was mobile and carried its own equipment but was dependent upon some parent medical unit for maintenance and administration.

In so far as the British Army Medical Services are concerned this unit was a post-war creation. During the war years there had been E.N.T. specialists on the strength of the general hospitals but no mobile teams which could take their specialist knowledge and skill into the forward areas. The creation of this unit completed the coverage of the whole range of the specialties. It was another example of the system of taking medical care into the forward areas there to deal with such as could be treated satisfactorily away from the large general hospital instead of arranging for such as required specialist examination and treatment to be sent back to the general hospital level.

30. THE MOBILE MALARIA FIELD LABORATORY

1 per army, 1 per independent force in malarious regions.

4 officers and 17 O.Rs. The officers: a specialist in Army Health, 2 malariologists and 1 entomologist; the O.Rs. included laboratory assistants and drivers.

1 car utility, 3 trucks 15-cwt G.S., 1 lorry 3-ton.

Combined weight of G.1098 and I.1248—$1\frac{1}{2}$ tons.

Function: To provide facilities for investigation and control of malaria problems in the field. Attached to a parent medical unit for maintenance and administration.

This unit was a war-time creation of the Army Hygiene Service. It proved its worth time and time again and inevitably it claimed its place in the post-war organisation. (*Admin.* II. pp. 32, 33.)

31. THE MOBILE NEURO-SURGICAL TEAM

> 1 per army, additional teams being provided for G.H.Q. troops on an as required basis.
>
> 6 officers, 6 Q.A.R.A.N.C. and 11 O.Rs.
>
> 2 jeeps, 2 lorries 3-ton.
>
> Combined weight of G.1098 and I.1248—16 tons.
>
> Function: To provide specialist treatment for neuro-surgical cases. The team was divisible into two smaller teams each of them capable of working independently. The unit was attached to a parent medical unit for maintenance and administration.

The first of the mobile neuro-surgical units as they were then called served in France and Belgium in 1939–40 and was captured at Dunkirk. It was reformed for the campaign in Libya at the Military Hospital for Head Injuries, Oxford and came to consist of a neuro-surgeon, a neurologist, an anaesthetist, 2 Q.A.I.M.N.S., 4 G.D.Os., 4 orderlies and 2 drivers R.A.S.C. It had to depend upon some host unit for beds, X-ray and pathology services and for nursing. The post-war M.N.S.T. grew out of the war-time M.N.S.U. and was an improved form of this.

32. THE MOBILE OPHTHALMIC TEAM

> 1 per corps. Army troops.
>
> 1 officer and 6 O.Rs.
>
> 2 lorries 3-ton.
>
> Combined weight of G.1098 and I.1248—$1\frac{1}{4}$ tons.
>
> Functions: to treat eye injuries and to prescribe or replenish spectacles in the forward areas. The team was dependent upon a parent medical unit for maintenance and administration.

A mobile ophthalmic unit was formed in the Middle East upon a 1914–18 model, being developed from the specialist surgical resources of Eighth Army and came to consist of an ophthalmologist, an optician, theatre orderlies and drivers R.A.S.C. It was a unit capable of undertaking any major ophthalmic operation but its main function was to treat and retain in the forward areas cases of refractive errors and minor ophthalmic lesions. It carried a supply of optical material to satisfy local spectacle needs. In certain circumstances an ophthalmically-trained Q.A.I.M.N.S. sister and a trainee-anaesthetist-refractionist were added to the unit. The allotment of these units ultimately came to be one per corps.

'In First Army in N. Africa an ophthalmologist with sufficient equipment to treat eye injuries and to carry out refractions, and accompanied by a sergeant optician who had outfits of spectacle frames and lenses, was provided with a 3-ton lorry from Army M.A.C. He spent his time travelling round divisional units and in so doing saved very many man-hours which would otherwise have been expended by men travelling rearwards to the C.C.S.' (E.W.W.)

'The main function of the A.M.S. is the conservation of man-power. The M.O.U. contributed greatly to this. In the population as a whole and in any representative sample of it there are very many individuals of sufficiently high physical and mental calibre capable of becoming effective soldiers who are handicapped only by an error of refraction. When problems of man-power necessitate the service of such as cannot reach and maintain their efficiency without optical aid, provision must be made to correct their refractive errors. In the rough and tumble of active service spectacles are commonly broken or lost and must be rapidly replaced. The M.O.U. working in the forward areas, could do this.

'The M.O.U. in the forward areas undoubtedly reduced the number of excised eyes considerably. The F.S.U. was not equipped with specialised personnel and material to deal with ocular wounds. A trivial wound, such as a corneal abrasion, can lead to the development of infection and to the loss of an eye unless treated promptly and effectively at an early stage. The M.O.U. changed the prognosis of eye injuries.' (S.D-E)

THE SPECIALIST TRINITY

The co-existence of the M.N.S.U., M.F.S.U. and M.O.U. in the Middle East inevitably encouraged the development of what came to be known as 'the specialist trinity', a close association and co-operation of the three units to form a centre for the treatment of wounds of the head. (*Campaigns* III. p. 183.)

The value of the specialist surgical units, maxillo-facial, ophthalmic and neurosurgical, was abundantly demonstrated during the Cassino battles. In most conditions most wounds are of the limbs. The reasons for this are the design of the human body and the conditioned reflexes of the experienced soldier. But when the battleground consists of the rocky slopes of mountain-sides and deep intervening valleys, an unusually high proportion of head wounds is to be expected. A shell or mortar bomb bursting on rock sends its fragments, and also slivers of rock, hurtling in all directions. On a mountain side the only protection is the sangar and this is quite inadequate. In the valleys in the Cassino area 'schu' mines had been sown in their thousands. Though these had wooden casings they had small metal hinges and a few metal parts in their firing mechanism. When trodden on they exploded and the metal parts were flung upwards and commonly lodged in the face of the victim, often in his eye. So great was the number of such wounds that 92 B.G.H. had largely to be set aside for ophthalmic cases and 65

B.G.H. for facial and neurosurgical cases, being reinforced by specialists in these fields.

'The grouping of the M.F.S.U., M.N.S.U. and M.O.U. after the passing of Tripoli at the foremost C.C.S. led to greatly improved work on head injuries.' (H.O.)

'In the Middle East certain of the specialist surgical units displayed a tendency to operate for insufficient reasons. One of them, in spite of protests, took a man off combatant duties for several weeks in order to re-graft a forehead burn sustained in childhood, because it was said to be giving him a feeling of inferiority. Another refused to take a number of surgeons from C.C.Ss. for a course of instruction in the primary treatment of head wounds in patients who could not be evacuated to a special centre. The results of this attitude were unfortunate.' (H.O.)

33. THE SPECIAL TREATMENT TEAM

1 per corps. Army troops.

2 officers and 7 O.Rs.

1 car utility, 1 lorry 3-ton.

Combined weight of G.1098 and I.1248—$\frac{3}{4}$ ton.

Function. To provide specialist treatment for cases of venereal diseases in the forward areas.

The team was attached to a parent medical unit for maintenance and administration.

During the war years the availability and potency of the sulphona-mides and of penicillin made it possible to hold cases of venereal disease in the forward areas and to treat them there. In Italy the New Zealand Army Medical Services had their V.D.T.C. as did also the Indian Medical Service while the Canadians had their V.D.T.T. In the British Army both a venereal disease treatment centre and a venereal disease treatment team had been formed in the Middle East. The centre, author-ised in 1941, had 100–200 beds and was attached to some selected general hospital. The team, a much smaller unit, functioned in the forward areas, as could also a section of the V.D.T.C. The records show that these units did excellent work. (*Campaigns* III. p. 533. V. p. 124.) But no such units were included in the medical order of battle of Second Army for the invasion of the Continent of Europe. In this there were 20 P.A.Cs. (in which treatment was not attempted) and four general hospitals with a total of 3,900 beds set aside for V.D. cases. This arrangement meant that treatment was not undertaken in the forward areas.

In the post-war organisation of the A.M.S. in the field the V.D.T.T., in the form of the special treatment team, appeared.

The Corps Medical Centre

It had long been recognised that subject to the requirements of the tactical situation, greater efficiency resulted from the concentration of the field medical units in which treatment was offered, than from their dispersal. General hospitals and C.C.Ss. were commonly grouped to form a medical area at base and on the L. of C. During the War of 1939–45 this practice became further developed as new medical units were created and as evacuation by air became the method of choice. In Burma, for example, the corps medical area of the campaign in N.W. Europe became the corps medical centre. This arrangement greatly simplified the evacuation procedure from the divisions since all their casualties were sent to one place, a matter of the greatest importance when evacuation is by air. It also greatly eased the functioning of the grouped units since casualties on arrival at the centre could be sorted out and distributed by one reception mechanism; by controlling the flow of casualties into each of the C.C.Ss. and F.D.Ss. in turn, the casualty distribution officer could ensure that none of them was overwhelmed by the numbers of casualties seeking admission.

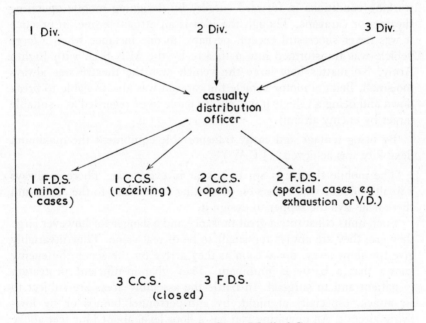

FIG. 1. Layout of a Corps Medical Centre

'It would have been impossible for transport aircraft to touch down at half a dozen different units to collect casualties. For one thing the construction of runways for transport aircraft at such units would have involved enormous and unnecessary labour, and for another, the number of transport aircraft was very limited and only just sufficient to maintain the army. Only by running to a very strict time-table could this maintenance be achieved. To have dissipated these resources by routeing transport aircraft to individual C.C.Ss. or M.F.T.Us. would have so slowed up their turn-round as to have invited disaster. The grouping of medical units was thus an absolute necessity.' (G.E.M.)

In Burma towards the end of the campaign the grouping of the divisional, corps, and Army medical units to form divisional, corps and Army medical centres became the rule.

The arrangement proved to be so satisfactory that it was inevitable that after the end of the war with further developments in systems of air evacuation the corps medical centre would be retained. (*Campaigns* IV. p. 289. V. Divisional, pp. 377, 407, 446. Corps, pp. 170, 364, 377, 380, 403, 405, 407, 414, 449, 525, 560. Army, pp. 525, 560.)

The Mobile Operating Theatre

In the Middle East at least nine attempts were made to improve the working conditions in forward surgery by designing mobile operating theatres or caravans. Though the idea is an attractive one, in practice it was never successful except, perhaps, in one instance when a large vehicle was transformed into a theatre by the M.N.S.U. with Eighth Army. No matter how large the vehicle was the theatre was always too small. Being a motor vehicle the caravan was always liable to break down and being a vehicle it was always liable to be regarded as a suitable target by enemy aircraft.

'By using tentage and easily transportable equipment the maximum flexibility was achieved.' (J.C.W.)

'The mobile theatre is apt to appear in every war. There is always a wealthy donor who insists on presenting such a unit to the Army and there is always the sapper to design it.

'Such units constitute a great nuisance and a danger for however large they are, they are always too small to be of real value. They invariably give the show away, for as soon as they arrive on the scene the enemy knows that a battle is imminent. They give insufficient protection to patient and to surgeon. In battle the assembly areas are subject to air attack, especially at night, by anti-personnel bombs or by low-flying aircraft. An operating van has a floor level about four feet above ground level and both patient and surgeon feel exposed. A tented F.S.U. can be protected quite quickly to a height of three feet by digging-in.' (H.O.)

'The vast distances of the Western Desert and the promise of a rapidly moving war demanded mobile, self-contained units, capable of opening and closely rapidly, and of moving quickly, efficiently and without breakdown over open desert. Such units had to be suitable for grouping and regrouping in a changing pattern, and for working in field ambulances or casualty clearing stations according to the fluidity of the tactical situation and the elastic variation of the evacuation line. Experience finally decided the contest for supremacy between the theatre caravan which was comfortable in operation, relatively sandproof and easy to open but expensive and lost temporarily or permanently if a chassis defect developed and the tented theatre which was slower to open and less sandproof but movable with its equipment from one truck to another in case of breakdown.' (I.A.)

The provision of the small motorised independent surgical unit, the F.S.U., was the final outcome of these developments.

Inter-Communication within the Corps

'In 1935 a cavalry field ambulance was mobilised in Egypt and a training camp for personnel in the use of a field ambulance in the desert was established. A variety of field exercises were carried out and at the end of the training a report was submitted to Army H.Q. in which it was stated that it was necessary for the A.D.M.S. of a division and his field ambulances operating in the desert to be on the divisional wireless net. This suggestion was disregarded.' (A.H.)

'It is essential that all forward medical units should have wireless facilities to enable them to keep in touch with each other and with their brigades.' (J.C.D.)

'It was conclusively demonstrated that in mobile warfare the medical services could not keep pace with a rapid advance, whether it be an armoured or an infantry pursuit, unless they had their own wireless net to provide a speedy means of inter-communication. Without a separate medical wireless net orders could not get through to medical units sufficiently quickly for them to keep pace with a rapid advance and as a result the medical units tended to lag behind the fighting formations. This inevitably resulted in a thinning out of the medical resources in the forward areas so that there was a serious risk of initial delay in the evacuation and treatment of casualties incurred during the contact battle as the pursuit closed.' (D.D.M.S. Second Army. *Campaigns* IV. p. 642.)

As new systems of inter-communication were developed it was inevitable that sooner or later they would be made available to the medical services in the field. When considerable and enlarging distances separate the different forward field medical units from each other and from the H.Q. of the formation with which they are serving and especially when the battle is fluid and the movement of formations rapid, no system other than R.T. could possibly prove to be satisfactory. The developments that occurred during the war years ensured that after the war R.T. sets would be part of the modern equipment of the Army Medical Services in the field.

In 1950, D.D.M.S. corps was allotted R.T. sets for inter-communication with corps medical units and with A.Ds.M.S. divisions.

Air-Transportability

'An early instance of the movement of a large and complete medical unit by air was that which occurred in N. Africa. In 1942 there was a large U.S.A.A.F. formation at Biskra, on the edge of the Sahara, which had no immediate medical cover. It happened that at that time there was a 200-bed hospital in First Army reserve. This was placed at the disposal of the American formation and the U.S.A.A.F. transported the unit, personnel and all equipment, save the disinfestor, by air, a performance that in those days was an astonishing feat.' (E.W.W.)

The idea of transporting whole units by air for immediate functioning on arrival at their destination underwent a speedy development during the war years. An outstanding example of this is provided by the two air-transportable brigades (9th of Indian 5th Division and 99th of Indian 17th Division) in the race for Rangoon at the end of the campaign in Burma. (*Campaigns* V. p. 530.) Such a development inevitably affected medical units and it is to be expected that in the post-war years these will be so modified in respect of loads, that they will become air-transportable when occasion demands.

The Medical Services of an Armoured Division

Since during the war years there was very considerable development of the armoured fighting vehicle and of the tactical use thereof, it was inevitable that there would be corresponding developments in the tactical use of the field medical units attached to an armoured formation. The cavalry field ambulance, which became the light field ambulance, was dropped and the standard unit took its place.

The number of casualties to be expected in an armoured division employed in its normal rôle was found to be less than that in an infantry division but the mobility of the former greatly exceeded that of the latter, an armoured division moving as much as 50 miles in a day.

The A.D.M.S. kept control of the A.D.Ss. of his two field ambulances and placed the field ambulance companies under the control of brigade. He took care to ensure that at all times there was a dressing station open on the divisional centre line. To this all casualties were evacuated from the C.C.Ps. The O.C. of the field ambulance acted as S.M.O. brigade and kept in close touch with brigade H.Q. during operations.

His task was that of clearing casualties, with the field ambulance company section, from the brigade front to the A.D.S. on the divisional centre line that was open. The A.D.M.S. leap-frogged the two A.D.Ss. up the divisional centre line and controlled their opening and closing until the conclusion of the operation.

In an advance the order of march of the two field ambulances was as follows:

(i) Sections of the companies of the field ambulances moved in support of the regiments or battalions.

(ii) Company headquarters of the field ambulances moved with brigade H.Qs.

(iii) The leading field ambulance, less its company moving on the divisional centre line, under command of brigade for movement, prepared itself to open an A.D.S. as and when required.

(iv) The second field ambulance, less its company under command of brigade, under the command of the A.D.M.S. moved with divisional H.Q.

Medical Services for Airborne Formations

It was only in November 1941 that the first airborne divisional headquarters was formed, that of 1st Airborne Division of two parachute brigades, an air-landing brigade group and a depot. Its H.Q. included the ordinary divisional medical staff officers while each of the parachute brigades had its parachute field ambulance and the air-landing brigade its air-landing field ambulance. The first of these, 181 Air-landing Fd. Amb., came into being in January 1942 and was responsible for much of the pioneering work associated with the development of the medical services for airborne formations. In the following April, 16 Para. Fd. Amb. was formed out of a number of R.A.M.C. volunteers of all ranks. In June 17 Para. Fd. Amb. was raised but it was never recruited to strength and was replaced by converting 127 Para. Fd. Amb., a standard infantry-type field ambulance, to a parachute rôle, the volunteer members of 17 Para. Fd. Amb. being included. New equipment had to be designed, new loading tables for personnel and equipment were evolved and a complete battle drill produced. Before the end of 1942, two more field ambulances, 133 and 224, were transformed into the parachute type. In June 1943 when 6th Airborne Division was formed, it became necessary to supply more airborne field ambulances and so 195 became an air-landing unit and 225 a parachute unit. In December 1943 H.Q. Airborne Troops, later to be designated as 1 Airborne Corps, was formed with a D.D.M.S. included in its staff. (*Admin.* I. pp. 505–514.)

The medical services of airborne formations were, therefore, war-time creations. Because of the development of the aeroplane it became inevitable that such airborne formations and their medical services would be carried over into the post-war organisation of the Army. In this there was no air-landing field ambulance but only a parachute field ambulance which had exactly the same establishment as the standard field ambulance serving with an infantry or with an armoured division, differing from this only in respect of the weight of its combined G.1098 and I.1248 stores, $9\frac{1}{2}$ tons instead of $11\frac{1}{2}$. In an airborne operation the field ambulance was divided into an air party and a sea or land tail. All the essential equipment was broken down into manloads, special packs being provided in the A.F.G.1098 and key personnel were widely distributed throughout the different aircraft. The air party comprised the bulk of the unit and the two attached surgical teams. Most of the personnel of the party dropped by parachute but a few, including the R.A.S.C. drivers, proceeded by glider along with the light vehicles and the heavy equipment. The sea or land tail consisted of all the remainder of the transport and of the medical and ordnance equipment. When the tail joined up with the air party the unit could function fully in a ground rôle.

The air party element was divided into sections placed under command of each of the parachute battalions and the rest which flew in with the brigade H.Q. H.Q. of the field ambulance opened an A.D.S. when instructed to do so by the brigade commander. This was usually sited within the perimeter of one of the battalions but near to brigade H.Q. The officer commanding the field ambulance functioned as S.M.O. brigade group and assumed responsibility for the medical administrative arrangements on all the D.Zs. in the brigade area. There could be no evacuation until the arrival of the ground troops.

Medical Services for the Anti-Aircraft Formations

It was as part of the system of the defence of Great Britain against air attack that the first anti-aircraft division was formed in 1936 by the transformation of an existing Territorial division. Its medical services at this time consisted solely of the regimental medical establishments. In December of the same year a second A.A. division was formed by the same process and to it an A.D.M.S. was appointed. In 1938 the number of these divisions had grown to five with 22 groups altogether and an A.A. corps was formed. Early in 1939 this corps became A.A. Command and to this formation a D.D.M.S. was appointed. Two more divisions were formed. (*Admin.* I. p. 32.)

These formations of the Territorial Army were intended to undertake very unusual tasks and for this reason developed an unusual structure. For the most part their component troops were to be distributed in small pockets widely separated from each other and often on sites far removed from towns and hospitals and general practitioners of medicine. The areas allotted to the divisions did not coincide with the commands and districts of the Army and operationally the functioning of the A.A. regiments R.A. and of the searchlight battalions R.E., of which these divisions were composed, was quite unrelated to that of the formations in the different commands and districts.

Medical Services for these A.A. formations were gradually evolved. (*Admin.* I. p. 35.) Each A.A. regiment R.A. had 2 R.M.Os.; each searchlight battalion R.E., 3. Each M.O. had a 1-ton van capable of carrying two stretcher cases. Each division had a divisional medical company R.A.M.C., T.A. and to each of the groups a section of this company was attached. Two motor ambulances were attached to each of the regiments R.A. and battalions R.E. Each regiment had 2 regimental medical posts each with 3 beds and each battalion had 3 of these R.M.Ps. each with 5 beds. The staff of the 3-bed R.M.P. was 1 M.O., 1 corporal and 3 N.Os. There was a D.D.M.S. corps and an A.D.M.S. and D.A.D.M.S. in each division. All who required hospitalisation were evacuated to the nearest military or civil hospital.

A.T.S. personnel had been serving with regimental and divisional headquarters of the Territorial Army units from the beginning. In 1941 it was decided to form mixed H.A.A. batteries and this meant that young women would be working side by side with men as combatants and in very rigorous conditions in isolated localities. A number of interesting repercussions occurred. It was found necessary to give the women the full male ration. The young women, though living on the tops of hills in all weathers in the depth of winter, disliked the woollen stockings and the long woollen pants with which they were issued. The inevitable rumour that the radar equipment used in gun-laying could be the cause of sterility, cropped up from time to time and had to be killed. In 1943, as the man-power shortage worsened, A.T.S. searchlight units were formed and functioned very efficiently. (*Admin.* II. p. 460.)

A.A. Command and its medical services were creations of the period of the Second World War. They served their purpose and with the ending of the war they disappeared.

Casualties

THE CALCULATION OF THEIR NUMBERS

Non-battle

In 1935 the daily admission-rate to medical units on account of sickness and injury was calculated at 3 per 1,000. In 1950 this estimate had become 1·5 per 1,000 of the force in a temperate zone and in the absence of any epidemic. In the Tropics, owing to the greater prevalence of diseases such as malaria, it was reckoned that the daily admission-rate could easily become 3 per 1,000—still far lower than it had been in the same regions in 1935.

This very considerable lowering of the daily admission-rate on account of sickness and injury is a trustworthy indication of the progress that had been made in the intervening years in the field of health-promotion and of disease-prevention. To this improvement there must, of necessity, be a limit, for from no considerable group of individuals will sickness and injury ever be completely absent, but this limit has not yet been reached. As mechanisation progressively proceeds it is to be expected that injuries will become more common.

Battle

Prior to the War of 1914–18 the estimate of the Austrian General Cron was in common use. He assumed that only three-fifths of the total force would be at risk and that of these 10 per cent. would become casualties, i.e. 6 per cent. of the total force. During that war, however, it became very obvious that no formula could be expected to provide an accurate forecast. In the Medical History of that war the average casualty-rate in a series of selected battles is given as 9·5 per cent.—Somme 17·1, Arras 7·8, Messines 5·7, Ypres 7·5. Nicholls, in his *Army Medical Services in War* 1937, gives a table of approximate casualties in a large series of battles of the War of 1914–18 and finds that the average figure is 9·62 per cent. of the force at risk.

In the 1950 pamphlet the following estimates are given:

Formation	Daily Average for All Days in Action	Severe Battle Day
Brigade	2·5 per cent.	12–15 per cent.
Division	1·0 ,, ,,	5–6 ,, ,,
Corps	0·5 ,, ,,	2–3 ,, ,,

It is obvious that the number of casualties in any engagement is determined by the operation of many factors, the most important of these being the relative strengths and the relative fire-power of the forces involved and the nature of the operation, whether of an offensive or a defensive kind.

THE RATIO OF KILLED TO WOUNDED

1935   1 : 5   1950   1 : 3·5

As the precision and the lethality of weapons increase the proportion of the killed among the casualties enlarges.

THE RECOVERY-RATE OF THE WOUNDED

Nicholls gives the following figures for the War of 1914–18:

Disposal	Approximate Percentage		
R.T.U. (Front Line) from forward medical units	7 }	64 }	82
R.T.U. (Front Line) from hospital and con. depot	57 }		
R.T.U. on L. of C., garrison or sedentary occupation	18		
Died	7		
Invalided	8		
Disposal otherwise but not stated	3		
	100		

In the War of 1939–45, 92 per cent. of the wounded recovered and approximately 14 per cent. of them were invalided.

As the power to control infection and to counteract the effects of haemorrhage enlarges, as surgical techniques improve and as evacuation becomes more speedy and comfortable, the recovery-rate rises and the size of bed-cover needed becomes lessened.

THE RECOVERY-RATE OF THE SICK AND INJURED

Nicholls gives the following figures for the War of 1914–18:

Disposal	Approximate Percentage		
R.T.U. (Front Line) from forward medical units	21 }	84 }	93
R.T.U. (Front Line) from hospital and con. depot	63 }		
R.T.U. on L. of C., garrison or sedentary occupation	9		
Died	1		
Invalided	4		
Disposal otherwise but not stated	2		
	100		

In the War of 1939–45, 50 per cent. of the sick and injured were retained in divisional or corps areas and were fit to return to duty within a week. Of the remainder 80 per cent. were fit to return to duty within one month.

CALCULATION OF TRANSPORT FOR THE EVACUATION
OF THE WOUNDED

1935

Front line to A.D.S. 25 per cent. will require lying-down transport
         75 ,, ,, will make their own way back

A.D.S. to M.D.S. 30 per cent. will require lying-down transport
         70 ,, ,, ,,   ,, sitting transport

W.W.C.P.—rearwards 5 per cent. of those reaching the W.W.C.P. will
              require lying-down transport
         95 ,, ,, will require sitting transport

M.D.S. to C.C.S. 50 per cent. will require lying-down transport
         50 ,, ,, ,,   ,, sitting transport

C.C.S. to Gen. Hosp. 50 per cent. will require lying-down transport
         50 ,, ,, ,,   ,, sitting transport

1950

Front line to C.C.P. 40 per cent. will require lying-down transport
              (stretcher, jeep amb., amb. car)
         60 ,, ,, will make their own way back

C.C.P.—rearwards 40 per cent. will require lying-down transport
         60 ,, ,, ,,   ,, sitting transport

HOSPITAL BED-COVER

1914–18

   France and Flanders 4 per cent. of the strength of the force
   Egypt and Palestine 10 ,, ,, ,, ,,   ,, ,, ,, ,,
   Macedonia   14 ,, ,, ,, ,,   ,, ,, ,, ,,
   East Africa   25 ,, ,, ,, ,,   ,, ,, ,, ,,

plus beds equal to 8 per cent. of the strength of the force in France
and Flanders set aside in the United Kingdom for casualties from that
theatre.

1939–45

   N.W. Europe 4 per cent. of the strength of the force
   N. Africa   6 ,, ,, ,, ,,   ,, ,, ,, ,,
   Middle East   8 ,, ,, ,, ,,   ,, ,, ,, ,,
   Far East   10 ,, ,, ,, ,,   ,, ,, ,, ,,

plus beds equal to 3 per cent. of the strength of the force in N.W.
Europe set aside in military and E.M.S. hospitals in the United Kingdom
for casualties from that theatre. Owing to the extensive use of air-
evacuation from this theatre to the United Kingdom the number of
beds actually required in N.W. Europe never exceeded 3 per cent.

The very considerable reduction in the number of beds provided is a
reflection of the advances made in preventive medicine leading to a

reduction in the incidence of 'camp' diseases, of changes in strategy leading to a reduction in the number of casualties and of the advances made in the field of curative medicine which led to a reduction in the 'duration-of-stay' in hospitals.

N.W. Europe	*Mean Monthly Admission-rate per 1,000 Strength*	
	1914–18	*1939–45*
Non-battle casualties	53·9	23·7
Battle casualties	30·4	14·5

The sulpha drugs and penicillin were heavily involved in the reduction of the duration-of-stay in 1939–45.

Non-battle casualties

About one-third of the total admissions to medical units on account of sickness or injury (1·5 per 1,000 per day in temperate climates) are retained in the forward areas and do not reach the general hospitals so that the total hospital bed-cover can safely be reduced to 1 per 1,000. The average duration-of-stay in hospital of the non-battle casualty is approximately 20 days.

Battle Casualties

During the War of 1939–45 the average daily admission to general hospitals did not exceed 0·6 per 1,000 of the total force. (In the campaign in N.W. Europe the rate for British troops was 0·48). The average duration-of-stay was taken to be 50 days.

The total requirement of hospital bed-cover becomes:

Non-battle casualties 1 × 20 = 20 per thousand of the force or 2 per cent.

Battle casualties 0·6 × 50 = 30 per thousand or 3 per cent.

A total of 5 per cent. plus 20 per cent. of this, or 1 per cent., for a dispersion factor. A grand total of 6 per cent. The dispersion factor allows for that proportion of the authorised beds which are packed for shipment or for move within the theatre, for the beds that are not available for general use, being reserved for special purposes and for the seasonal fluctuations in the incidence of disease.

The figure of 6 per cent. is the minimum total requirement of hospital beds. In a non-temperate climate or in a pandemic it would be increased by a further 2 per cent.

HOLDING POLICY

It is this that largely determines the relative proportions of the bed-cover to be provided in an overseas theatre and in the United Kingdom respectively. It is decided by the War Office with the agreement of the overseas force commander and is expressed in terms of days. Factors influencing this decision are the distance of the overseas theatre from the United Kingdom, the operational conditions in the overseas theatre and the availability of ships and aircraft for casualty evacuation.

In the Middle East it was found that as a general rule it was far more economical to provide sufficient hospital beds to allow the holding of the sick and wounded up to 120 days or even longer. In N.W. Europe, on the other hand, during the assault phase only such cases as were unfit to be moved were retained and as the campaign developed the holding policy was extended to 7, 30 and ultimately to 42 days.

DOCUMENTATION

Before the war army medical statistics were based upon two army forms, A.F. I.1220, a personal record of each case treated in hospital and A.F. A.31, a consolidated monthly return from hospitals showing bed-state, admissions and numbers remaining, by diagnosis.

In the field the first point along the evacuation chain at which a permanent record was usually made was the M.D.S. or W.W.C.P. if the latter was opened. Whenever circumstances permitted a manuscript record was maintained at the A.D.S., this being a duplicate of the nominal roll of casualties that was sent to the M.D.S. It was usual for extra clerks to be sent to assist any medical unit or part thereof that was being hard pressed. Nominal rolls of casualties from each formation were maintained. The field medical card A.F. W.3118 (and its envelope A.F. W.3118A) which had been filled in and fixed to the clothing of the casualty in the R.A.P., was completed for every patient admitted or transferred to the field ambulance and particulars of every patient were entered in the Admission and Discharge Book A.B. 27A.

On the A.F. W.3118 the following standard abbreviations were used:

A.T.S.

1000   Anti-tetanic serum 1,000 units administered

$M\frac{1}{4}$

1800   Morphia gr.$\frac{1}{4}$ given at 1800 hours

T

1820   Tourniquet applied at 1820 hours

U   Urgent case (marked in red ink or pencil)

(M. for morphia and T. for tourniquet were marked in indelible pencil on the forehead of the patient in the R.A.P.)

Deaths were reported as follows: officers by telegram to O.2E. at once, with confirmation by post the same day; O.Rs. by post to O.2E.

A weekly report on A.F. A.36 (nominal roll of patients in field ambulances) of all admissions, discharges, transfers and deaths of officers and O.Rs. was sent to O. i/c 2nd Echelon, the classification of battle casualties as given in Field Service Regulations Vol. I being observed.

The recording in the C.C.S. was similar to that in the field ambulance with the following addition. The personal numbers and names of officers and the army numbers, names and corps of O.Rs. on the dangerously ill list together with the nature and degree of the disability and any changes in their condition were telegraphed daily to the Casualty Section, the War Office and repeated to 2nd Echelon.

In the general hospital the A.F. I.1220 was prepared for each patient admitted or transferred and particulars of each case were entered in the A. and D. book. A daily report on A.F. W.3034 (nominal roll of patients in hospital) showing admissions, discharges, transfers and deaths of officers and O.Rs. was sent to O.2E. and a copy forwarded direct to the Casualty Section, The War Office. A weekly progress report on A.F. W.3034A of dangerously and seriously ill patients, officers and O.Rs., was sent to the Casualty Section, The War Office, with a copy to 2nd Echelon. A nominal roll on A.F. W.3034 of all those to be invalided and embarked was sent to 2nd Echelon.

At the beginning of the War of 1939-45 the statistical mechanism of A.M.D. consisted of a small section of the branch that dealt with the problems of hospital administration and to it no great importance was attached. It was far too inadequately staffed to be able to provide a 'fast news service' to the administrators and planners in the directorate. The admission of military patients to E.M.S. hospitals, which had a recording system of their own, led to much difficulty and greatly impeded the flow of statistical information into A.M.D. Even when A.F. I.1220 was taken into use in these hospitals and when military registrars were posted to them to take care of the records of military patients, these difficulties were not removed though lessened. Many batches of A.F. W.3118 and A.F. I.1220 from the Middle East were lost at sea and when a separate M.E.F. statistical section was set up in Cairo the flow of information of this kind arriving in A.M.D. became greatly diminished. In the Far East the commands were responsible to New Delhi and not to London so that the information received in A.M.D. from them was exceedingly slight and most incomplete. Early in the war A.F. A.31 was cancelled, in an attempt to cut down the amount of paper work, apparently, and though during the following years there was an almost endless succession of new forms, none of them really replaced this one. Overseas theatres developed the habit of producing army forms of their own, calling for this or that information of a statistical kind and these varied greatly in respect of usefulness.

These were the main reasons why the statistical data received by

A.M.D. during the war years remained so imperfect and so incomplete, why the administrators and planners were handicapped by the lack of the information that an adequate statistical service could have provided and why the data available at the end of the war cannot be used with any degree of confidence for the provision of a really valuable contribution to the Statistical Volume of the History. (*Admin.* I. p. 428.)

The Directorate of Medical Research undertook the reorganisation of the statistical section of A.M.D. in 1943–44 and a beginning was made to the introduction of a uniform system of documentation both in the United Kingdom and overseas. This was based upon two comprehensive returns, one relating to morbidity (A.F. W.3166(a) in the United Kingdom and A.F. W.3166 Overseas) and the other to bed-states (A.F. W.3167(a) in the United Kingdom and A.F. W.3167 Overseas).

After the war documentation in the field remained very much as it was before the war but with the following additions:

A.F. W.3210 (Label for patient) was prepared in duplicate in the A.D.S., the original being given to the A. and D. clerk for entry in the Admission and Discharge book A.B. 27A and the copy being put in the field medical card envelope A.F. W.3118A. When the casualty reached a rear medical unit the A.F. W.3210 was removed from the envelope for entry into the A. and D. book and thereafter returned to the envelope. For evacuation by air or sea A.F. W.3083 (Casualty Evacuation Label) was tied on to the clothing. It was in triplicate with detachable sheets. One of these was detached on embarkation or on emplaning, one when the casualty was disemplaned or disembarked and the third accompanied the casualty to hospital. The F.S.T. and the F.T.T. maintained an operation book A.B. 485. When the casualty was finally disposed of his A.F. W.3118 and A.F. I.1220 were sent to War Office, A.M.D. (Stats.).

The Evacuation Chain

The development of the aeroplane and of wheeled and tracked vehicles and the creation of new types of field medical units led to modification of the chain of evacuation from the front to the base. Figures 2 and 3 depict the chain as it was in 1935 and in the immediate post-war years respectively.

The three zones, collecting, evacuating and distributing, had given way to four areas, divisional, corps, army, and L. of C. and base. In each of these areas was an airstrip or airfield. In the divisional area the F.D.S. had taken the place of the M.D.S. of the field ambulance and among the field ambulance transport were light (2 stretcher or 6 sitting cases) and heavy (4 stretcher or 10 sitting cases) motor ambulances. The ambulance jeep, a standard 5 cwt. 4 × 4 car fitted with a frame designed to carry 2 stretchers longitudinally had amply proved its worth during the war (as indeed had all 4-wheel drive vehicles in the forward areas). When the necessity arose any type of fighting vehicle, e.g. armoured personnel carrier, was used for evacuation in this area. In Burma it was on occasion necessary to resort to pack ambulance transport, riding pony, mule litter, travois and cacolet.

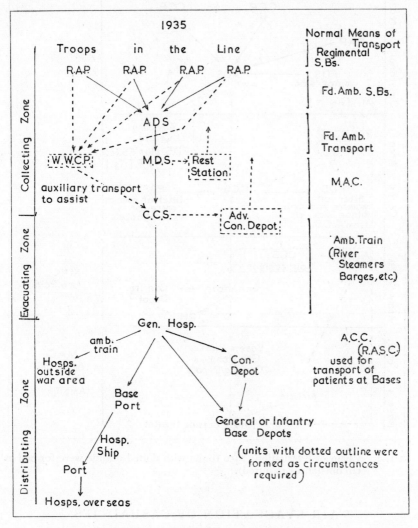

FIG. 2. Chain of Evacuation, 1935

In the corps area in the post-war scheme were the A.S.C. consisting of F.D.S., F.S.Ts. and F.T.T. and the corps medical centre composed of grouped C.C.Ss. and F.D.Ss. In the army area a C.C.S. was associated with the airfield.

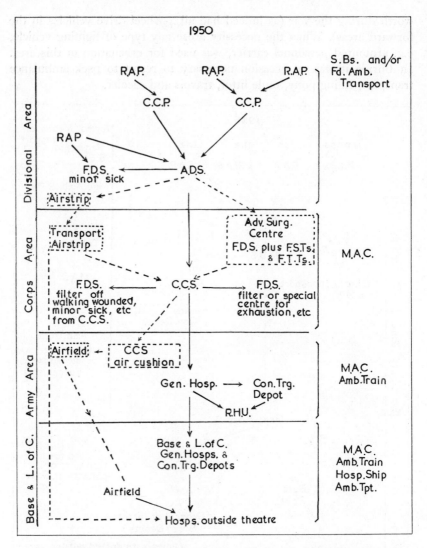

FIG. 3.   Chain of Evacuation, 1950 (units with dotted outline were formed as circumstances required).

AIR EVACUATION OF CASUALTIES

Soon after the outbreak of hostilities in the Middle East a request for five air ambulances was made by the War Office for use in that theatre. This had to be refused by the Air Ministry because of the shortage of aircrews, ground-staff personnel and of aircraft. The Secretary of State for Air, visiting the Middle East, suggested to the Foreign Secretary that twelve ambulance planes should be provided. This suggestion came to naught. In early 1941 the Secretary of State for War appealed once again to the Secretary of State for Air for twelve air ambulances and once again the request had to be refused for the same reasons as before. General Cunningham, in East Africa, appealed to the Chief of the Air Staff for six aircraft for the transportation of casualties from the front to railhead, some 300 miles to the rear. At this time it was quite impossible to find either the aircraft or the crews. In March 1941, however, the Australian Government decided to provide an Air Ambulance Unit for the Western Desert. About the same time the South African Government appealed to Britain for engines for two Lodestar aircraft that they intended to convert into air ambulances but even these could not be spared at that time. The same reply had to be given to a request for five Rapides to be used for the same purpose. The South African general public provided funds for the provision of one complete Lodestar air ambulance. Everybody, everywhere, was agreed that air evacuation was most desirable but shortages would not allow any aircraft or crews to be spared for this sole purpose.

So, the Royal Air Force began to develop the system whereby returning empty transport aircraft were used for the conveyance of Army casualties and in October 1942 the R.A.F. was given and accepted full responsibility for air evacuation. (*R.A.F.M.S. I. Admin.* Chapter 10.) It was during the campaigns in N.W. Europe (*Campaigns* IV. pp. 60, 604, 640) and in Burma (*Campaigns* V. p. 697) that the evacuation of casualties by air reached its peak. Indeed in Burma all the tactical planning in connexion with the second Chindit incursion into Japanese-held territory, the defence of the Imphal Plain and the swift southward advance towards Rangoon in the closing phase of the campaign was based upon the postulate that reinforcements and supplies would be ferried forward and that casualties would be evacuated to the rear, by air. This arrangement continued throughout the war years and was carried over into the immediate post-war period.

At all times during the war years it was the considered opinion of the senior administrative medical officers of the Army Medical Services that this arrangement was most unsatisfactory.

'Air Evacuation will never be satisfactory until the Army Medical Services have their own air ambulances as they have motor ambulances, ambulance trains and hospital ships. The aircraft is nothing more than another form of transport and whether it is a helicopter or a plane it must be wholly at the disposal of the Army Medical Services. The system of making use of "returning empties" is a relic of the past'. (A.H.)

'Ambulance planes will be essential for future wars. They should be marked with the Red Cross and international agreement for their protection should be reached. During the war, in spite of repeated applications for the allotment of special planes for casualty evacuation, these were not provided for the reason, it was invariably stated, that there were not enough aircraft available. This is a very old and hoary argument. In the Crimean War there were repeated requests for ships to be allotted to the Medical Department for hospital purposes. These were resisted by the Naval Authorities on the grounds that there were not enough ships. But public opinion, being aroused, ultimately forced the Naval Authorities to give way. In the South African War the evacuation of casualties from the forward areas was by returning empty wagons of the supply train. The Staff maintained that special transport for medical purposes could not be allotted for the reason that not enough vehicles were available. But ultimately the Ambulance Convoy had to be created and this it was that became the Motor Ambulance Convoy of World War I.

'When once the transport, be this a hospital ship or a motor ambulance convoy, is placed on the war establishment of an army in the field, it comes to be accepted as essential. Once ambulance aircraft are included in the war establishment of an army in the field they will surely be provided. The aeroplane will inevitably replace the hospital ship since it is far better, far cheaper and far more speedy.' (N.C.)

'The gradual growth of the use of aircraft for transport duties as well as in combatant rôles rapidly demonstrated the value of air transport for the wounded. It was unfortunate that so little support was given to the plea that the Army Medical Services should be given their own ambulance planes. The helicopter type is well suited for work with forward medical units. It is essential that the seriously wounded man should be transported rapidly and smoothly to a hospital as far as practicable outside the actual fighting zone where he can receive definitive treatment. The Army Medical Services must have their own air ambulance service, both for forward work and for long distance transportation of casualties.' (J.C.D.)

'The salient feature of this campaign (N.W. Africa) was the failure of air evacuation from First Army, although it was reported to have worked well on the L. of C. The main difficulty was to induce planes to be flown sufficiently far forward. The reason for the failure of this valuable method of evacuation was that whereas Eighth Army British planes were marked with the Red Cross and were accustomed to use very far forward landing grounds, U.S. planes were not. The conclusions drawn from this campaign were:

(i) that Army should be allotted a flight of Red Cross planes;

(ii) that these planes must be controlled by Army;

(iii) that a small holding unit of the nature of a field hospital should always be allotted to Army. This unit would hold casualties at ambulance air-head'. (*Campaigns* II. p. 384.) (D.D.M.S. First Army.)

'Air evacuation, however, will never be satisfactory until the Army Medical Services have operational control of ambulance aircraft in a manner similar to that of the motor ambulance company, R.A.S.C.' (E.P.)

'Air evacuation proved to be most satisfactory when a definite number of aircraft was allotted for casualty evacuation. The "Sparrow Flight" which was controlled by the P.M.O., Second Tactical Air Force and used for the shuttle back from forward areas so successfully, was always more reliable than the utilisation of Transport Command aircraft which arrived at uncertain times and in varying numbers.

'The holding unit for casualties awaiting air evacuation was best formed by an Army unit close to the airfield concerned. It could be provided with surgical or other specialist facilities and would cater for patients held up by delays in evacuation much more easily than could the R.A.F. unit on the airfield (C.A.E.S.). The R.A.F. unit need only be of waiting-room type, holding for an hour or two.' (*Campaigns* IV. p. 640.)

'During the war years it was not uncommon for D.D.G.A.M.S. (Ops.) to be required urgently to furnish the Secretary of State for War, through the Adjutant-General's department, with the numbers of casualties that had been evacuated from the various fronts by the R.A.F. Because D.D.G.A.M.S. (Ops.) was unable to procure such information from the Air Ministry without considerable delay, he attracted to himself much undeserved and adverse criticism. Since such information is important to the highest levels of the War Office, it is both desirable and necessary to devise a system of intercommunication whereby it could be transmitted without delay.' (W.E.T.)

That the Army Medical Services should have wished to have had ambulance aircraft of their own, or, alternatively, to have had aircraft allotted to them and placed under their control by the R.A.F. is understandable. The system had developed whereby they shouldered responsibility for the care of the wounded man from the time when he was evacuated from the R.A.P. to move along the chain C.C.P.–A.D.S.–C.C.S. or F.D.S.–general hospital. They used the ambulances of the field ambulance and also those of the M.A.C., belonging to the R.A.S.C. and manned by R.A.S.C. personnel but placed under the operational control of the R.A.M.C. Since there was no separate R.A.S.C. medical service the question as to where responsibility for the medical care of the casualty in transit lay did not arise. The aeroplane was regarded merely as another form of transport vehicle. It was to the motor ambulance what that had been to the horsed ambulance; it could move more quickly between two points. The air ambulance could reduce the time interval between the moment of being wounded and the time when definitive surgery or other treatment could be carried out; it could increase the chances of survival by enabling the casualty to avoid the pain, the discomfort and shock caused by passage over rough ground; it could ease the strain on road and rail communications and it could create a situation in which the numbers and varieties of medical units in the forward areas could be considerably reduced. But, since evacuation by air could only be safely undertaken in suitable flying weather and when superiority in the air was maintained, it followed that although this was the most efficient and most desirable method of casualty evacuation it had to be regarded as being ancillary to evacuation by land and sea.

It was because the R.A.F. had medical services of its own that complications arose. To the R.A.F.M.S. it seemed reasonable that, since the vehicles belonged to the R.A.F. and were manned by R.A.F. pilots, when Army casualties were being transported they should be cared for by R.A.F. medical and nursing officers. To the A.M.S. this point of view did not appeal. The attributes, personal and professional, of R.A.F. medical and nursing officers were not to be distinguished from those of the A.M.S. medical and nursing officers and there was nothing very unusual in being transported in an aircraft. To have two distinct medical services involved in casualty evacuation along the Army evacuation chain certainly increased the risks of breakdown and encouraged the development of unnecessary duplication.

Transport aircraft did not stand in a kind of cab-rank waiting to be summoned forward; they were not available at all times and so quite inevitably there were many delays and much frustration.

Since it is quite certain that in the future air evacuation will be the method of choice and will undergo considerable development, it is desirable that this question of divided responsibility for the care of Army casualties during evacuation should be settled. Possibly the integration of the medical services, as has been suggested, is the answer.

During the war years there was much discussion concerning the desirability or otherwise of displaying the Red Cross on aircraft carrying casualties. The Geneva Convention demands that such aircraft should be painted white. But transport aircraft could not be distinguished in this way for they would give away the location of a general purpose airfield all too readily. The Red Cross on a background other than white is not easily recognised and could be mistaken for some other emblem. Both the R.A.F. and the Luftwaffe reached the conclusion through experience that it was not worth while marking these transport aircraft when they were to be used for casualty evacuation.

In the immediate post-war period the system of air evacuation was as follows. It was understood that the evacuation of Army casualties was a joint responsibility of the Army and the R.A.F., the A.M.S. being responsible for the collection of casualties in the field and for their delivery at airfields, while the R.A.F.M.S. were responsible for the provision and control of transport aircraft and also for the professional care of casualties from the time they were handed over by the A.M.S. at airfields until they were deplaned at their destination. It was agreed that close liaison between the two medical services was essential to ensure that whatever facilities were available should be fully employed.

The R.A.F.M.S. provided medical and nursing personnel for the professional care of casualties during the flight and also medical equipment including oxygen, food and fluids. The transport used (helicopters and light, medium and long-range planes) were equipped with supports capable of carrying the service stretcher (Mark II); when these were not in use they could be stowed away in the plane. The planes were used to carry personnel and stores forward and to evacuate casualties on the return journey. Emplaning and deplaning facilities were provided at:

Advanced Airstrips which could quickly be improvised and located in divisional areas near advanced dressing stations. Casualties from the divisional field ambulances were collected at these strips and flown therefrom by helicopter or light aircraft to:

Advanced Air Transport Airstrips which usually were located in corps areas and were capable of providing landing facilities for helicopters, light and medium aircraft. The aircraft plying between the advanced airstrip and the advanced air transport airstrip picked up stretchers and blankets at the advanced air transport airstrip to replace those left behind with the casualties. At the advanced air transport airstrip a Casualty Air Evacuation Squadron (R.A.F.) was stationed to unload casualties and to hand them over to the A.M.S. for treatment in the corps medical centre or elsewhere. On the other hand, casualties from the corps medical centre fit for further evacuation rearwards, were handed over by the A.M.S. to the C.A.E.S. for emplaning in medium range aircraft *en route* for:

Main Transport Airfields located in army areas and within reasonable distance of general hospitals. On these airfields both medium and long-range aircraft could land. The C.A.E.Ss. on these airfields deplaned casualties arriving in medium range aircraft from the advanced air transport airstrips and emplaned patients from the general hospitals for rearward evacuation by long-range aircraft to:

Base Transport Airfields at the base or in the United Kingdom and capable of receiving the heaviest types of long-range aircraft. The C.A.E.Ss. on these airfields unloaded the casualties arriving from the main transport airfields and handed them over to the A.M.S. for distribution among general hospitals and special medical units. The C.A.E.S. contained both medical and nursing officers, nursing orderlies, clerks, cooks and other administrative personnel. Each C.A.E.S. was capable of manning 4 light aircraft airstrips or, 2 advanced transport airstrips or, 1 main transport airfield. The allotment of these units was, as a rule, 1 per army in the field.

EVACUATION OF CASUALTIES BY SEA

'The problem of evacuating transportable casualties, after primary treatment, from the beaches of Normandy was the cause of considerable anxiety. Hospital ships and carriers existed but there was no satisfactory method of loading them except in port. At sea, where they must necessarily be in an assault landing, there was no method of transferring casualties to them in bulk. Consequently, it was clear that some other method of sea transportation was required to deal with the hundreds of casualties to be expected in an assault upon Fortress Europe. At this juncture (1943) the D.U.K.W. put in an appearance—an amphibious godsend. Here was a six-wheeled vehicle capable of running on land or in water, capable of carrying up to 25 wounded with comfort, including 10 stretcher cases, from inland right out to sea. But the problem still remained how and where to embark them at sea. The answer was provided by the L.S.T. This remarkable sea-going vessel had an enormous hold, primarily designed for the carriage of tanks, with a wide ramp at the bow which was lowered for loading or off-loading operations.

'Once the L.S.T. had discharged its cargo it presented a picture of a ship with a vast hold, large enough to accommodate 300 stretcher cases, with a loading ramp laid down in the most inviting manner for vehicles to enter. It was at once obvious that if we could drive D.U.K.Ws. bodily into the belly of the ship, the problem would be solved. It was so solved. The D.U.K.W., loaded on the beach, could be driven right into the L.S.T., lying at anchor two miles out at sea and in a moderate swell. No difficulty was experienced in getting over the ramp; once inside, the D.U.K.Ws. unloaded their passengers and had the choice of backing out or of turning round, for though the D.U.K.W. was over 33 ft. long, the hold of the L.S.T. was so wide that the D.U.K.W. could turn round inside it. The problem of embarkation of casualties at sea was thus solved by a combination of D.U.K.Ws. and L.S.T., a completely satisfactory solution. All that remained was to supply a loading ramp for the D.U.K.Ws. and to equip the L.S.T. with stretcher-fittings and a surgery.' (R.D.C.)

The development of the L.S.T., the D.U.K.W., the L.C.I. and L.S.I., the L.V.W. and the L.V.T. during the war years led to many improvements in the system of evacuation across water.

In an opposed assault landing the hospital ship anchored in the open roadstead was exceedingly vulnerable and unless the sea was calm loading was difficult and slow since the casualties had to be hoisted aboard. These difficulties could be overcome in temperate waters by making use of the landing ship, tank (L.S.T.), instead of the hospital ship or carrier for short voyages up to 36 hours' duration. The tank hold of such a ship could accommodate up to 300 stretcher cases if stretcher-racks in tiers along the inside of the hold were provided. A small surgery had to be built in and medical and nursing staff provided. In favourable circumstances the L.S.T. could be beached so that casualties could be embarked dryshod at low tide. L.S.Ts. were not suitable for casualty evacuation when the sea passage was long because they pitched a great deal. They were not suitable for use in casualty evacuation in a tropical theatre for the reason that the hold temperature became very high.

The landing ship, infantry (L.S.I.), could be used instead of the L.S.T. if necessary while minor cases could be accommodated in the landing craft, infantry (L.C.I.), for short voyages.

Between shore and ship the best form of transport was the D.U.K.W., the $2\frac{1}{2}$ ton lorry made water-borne and one of the landing vehicles, wheeled (L.V.W.). The type of D.U.K.W. used in the Second World War had 6 wheels for use on land with a speed of up to 50 m.p.h., and a propeller for use in water with a speed of 6 knots. It could carry 10 stretcher cases plus 12 sitting cases without any modification. A loading ramp had to be constructed. It could be driven into the tank hold of the L.S.T.

Another form of the amphibious wheeled vehicle capable of carrying stretcher cases (2) was the jeep made water-borne.

Several types of landing vehicles, tracked (L.V.T.), were developed. They were all general purpose vehicles and not specially designed for casualty evacuation work, though in certain circumstances, particularly useful for this purpose. Sometimes a number of them would be allotted specifically for medical use in a particular operation; at other times they were used to carry stores and reinforcements forwards and casualties on the return journey. The later models were partially armoured.

The 'Buffalo' had a land speed of 27 m.p.h. and a speed of 6 knots in the water. It could carry without modification 5 stretcher and 20 sitting cases. A smaller type was the 'Weasel' which could be adapted to take two stretcher cases. The tracked amphibian had the advantage over the wheeled in that it could clamber up the steep sides of a ditch or up a river bank. The great advantage of these amphibians was that they could transport casualties across country with ditches and rivers and launch themselves from the beach into the sea to deliver their loads to the ships.

The Assault Landing

From the seaborne operations with opposed landings on enemy-held shores—Narvik, Dieppe, Algiers, Abadan, Ambararata Bay, Pantellaria, the Pachino headland in Sicily, Reggio Calabria, Salerno, Anzio and the most ambitious of them all, the Normandy beaches—much was learnt and with the passing of time and the accumulation of experience the techniques of the assault landing were perfected. In so far as the medical services were concerned the main lessons that were learnt were:

Complete co-ordination between the three medical services is essential. The Navy should be responsible for the care of all casualties occurring at sea and in transit between the beaches and the casualty carrying ships, craft or barges, with the exception of the casualties in the amphibians and in the water ambulances of the hospital ships and carriers. The Navy should also accept responsibility for the care of casualties embarked in landing ships or craft which have been specially adapted for the transport of casualties.

The Army should accept responsibility for (a) the collection and evacuation of all casualties on land across the beaches and for loading them into landing craft, barges and ships; (b) the loading and transporting of casualties in amphibians and (c) the care of all casualties on land and in vessels staffed by the A.M.S.

The Royal Air Force should be given the responsibility for (a) loading casualties into aircraft used for casualty evacuation and (b) the care of the casualties emplaned.

One of the most useful creations of the war years was the beach group. (*Campaigns* III. p. 6.) Included in this group was the beach medical unit consisting in the early post-war unit, of 3 M.Os., 3 non-medical officers and 69 O.Rs. with a small number of vehicles including 3 amphibians. The function of this unit was to provide one or more beach dressing stations (B.D.Ss.) and a casualty embarkation point (C.E.P.). The collection of the casualties was undertaken by pioneers or infantry of the beach group, trained as S.Bs. and in first aid.

A beach brigade consisted of two beach groups together with brigade troops. The brigade had two F.D.Ss., each of these having attached to it two or more F.S.Ts. and one F.T.T. Each brigade had a field ambulance and a section of this unit was usually attached to each of the battalions, landing with the brigade. The H.Q. of the brigade field ambulance landed with brigade H.Q. and opened an A.D.S. well clear of the beach. (*See* also p. 117.)

The ideal plan for the landing of the medical units and personnel in relation to the time when the first assault craft struck the beach (H hour) was as follows:

H + 30 minutes. Assault battalions ashore accompanied by their R.M.Os. and one section of the assault field ambulance to each assault battalion.

H + 60 minutes. Beach development parties ashore including elements of the beach medical units to open the B.D.S(s).

H + 90 minutes. Beach dressing stations fully open.

H + 120 minutes. H.Q. of assault field ambulance ashore with A.D.S. open in vicinity of assault brigade H.Q.

H + 240 minutes. The F.D.Ss. with the F.S.Ts. and F.T.Ts. ashore. An A.S.C. open about one mile inland. The C.E.P. open.

The first of the C.C.Ss. came ashore with the second tide.

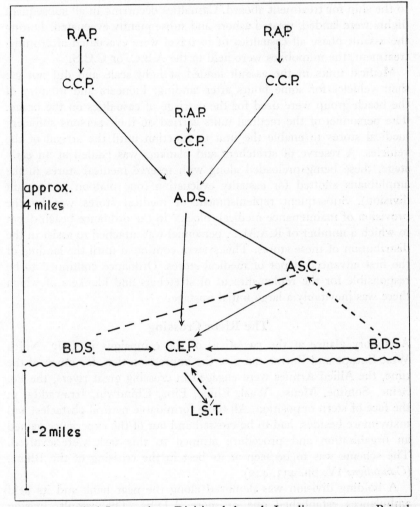

FIG. 4. Medical Layout in a Divisional Assault Landing on a one Brigade Front. H + 4 hours.

The section of the field ambulance attached to the assault battalion held its casualties until the opening of the B.D.S. when they were transferred thereto so as to restore the property of mobility to the section of the field ambulance. The B.D.Ss. and the A.D.S. of the assault field ambulance held their casualties until the arrival of the A.S.C. when cases unfit for immediate evacuation were transferred thereto and those fit to move were sent on to the C.E.P. after initial treatment. The C.C.S. on its arrival opened up near to the A.S.C. Casualty evacuation across the beaches continued until a port was opened or until it could be replaced wholly or in part by air evacuation.

Casualties occurring in the first flight landing craft were returned to the ship for treatment aboard. Casualties occurring in all subsequent flights were landed, treated ashore and subsequently evacuated. During the assault phase all casualties fit to travel were evacuated after initial treatment, the immobiles were held in the A.S.C. or C.C.S.

Medical units in the assault landed at light scale and did not get their vehicles for some hours after landing. Pioneers and infantry of the beach group were used for the carriage of casualties on the beach. The personnel of the medical units carried on their persons sufficient medical stores to enable the unit to function until the arrival of the vehicles. A reserve of stretchers and blankets was landed at an early stage, these being preloaded along with reserve medical stores in the amphibians allotted for casualty evacuation (one platoon per assault division). Subsequent replenishment of medical stores was by the provision of maintenance medical 'blocks' in the ordnance beach depot to which a number of R.A.M.C. personnel was attached to assist in the distribution of these stores. This system continued until the landing of the first advanced depot of medical stores. Ordnance continued to be responsible for the replenishment of stretchers and blankets of which there was inevitably a large initial wastage.

The River Crossing

A cursory glance at the narratives of the campaigns in Italy, North West Europe and Burma can give the impression that, for much of the time, the Allied Armies were engaged in crossing great rivers, the Po, Seine, Somme, Meuse, Waal, Rhine, Elbe, Chindwin, Irrawaddy, in the face of stern opposition. All these formidable natural obstacles, and many more besides, had to be crossed and out of the experience gained an organisation and procedure attuned to this task were evolved. The scheme was to be seen at its best in the crossing of the Rhine. (*Campaigns* IV. pp. 433, 449).

A holding division was deployed along the near bank and its field ambulances established one or more A.D.Ss. The assault division advanced through the holding division. A bank control group, the equivalent of the beach group in the assault landing, was detailed to give assistance to the assault division. A medical unit—the field ambulance of a division not involved in the operation, or the corps field ambulance, or an army field ambulance—was attached to the bank control group and its task was to free the medical units of the assault division from responsibility for the disposal of casualties of the assault division in the assembly

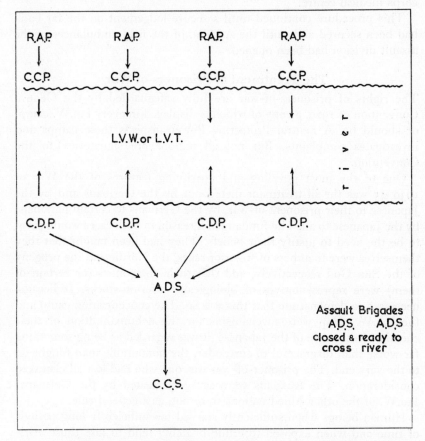

FIG. 5.   Medical Layout in a Divisional River Crossing on a two Brigade Front. (C.D.Ps. formed by medical unit allotted to bank control. A.D.S. formed by field ambulance from another formation or from reserve brigade of division.)

and marshalling areas on the near bank of the river. Amphibians were allotted for casualty evacuation across the river.

The medical unit attached to the bank control group set up casualty disembarkation points (C.D.Ps.) at suitable points along the river bank. The assault division's field ambulances, having crossed the river, established a number of casualty collecting posts (C.C.Ps.), casualty evacuation posts (C.E.Ps.), at suitable points along the far bank. The casualties of the assault division on the far bank were evacuated through the R.A.Ps. into the C.C.Ps., ferried across the river in amphibians, received by the C.D.Ps., transferred to ambulance cars, jeeps or 'weasels' for conveyance to the A.D.S. of the holding division (or of some other formation not involved in the operation) or to the C.C.Ss. in the corps medical centre.

This procedure continued until a secure lodgement on the far bank had been secured and until the A.D.Ss. of the field ambulances of the assault division had been opened.

The Treatment of Prisoners-of-War

The rights of prisoners-of-war are fully safeguarded by the Geneva Convention of 1929, a copy of which is displayed in every P.o.W. camp, or should be. A neutral Protecting Power inspects these camps and investigates complaints. But not all nations are signatories to the Convention.

One of the most puzzling and horrifying features of the War of 1939–45 was the ill-treatment meted out by the Germans and by the Japanese to their prisoners-of-war, by the Germans to certain nationals, by the Japanese to all. The fundamental reason in both cases would seem to be the need to justify their beliefs. They had been taught that they themselves were members of superior races, the Nordic and the progeny of the Sun God respectively, and that their antagonists (or certain of them) were representatives of biologically inferior stocks. It became necessary to demonstrate that this was so. The concentration camp and the P.o.W. camp were mechanisms for the dehumanisation of their enemies. In the case of the Japanese, it was regarded as being something far worse than disgraceful to surrender, the honourable man fought on to the very end. The prisoner-of-war was one who had lost all claims to consideration. The Russians were savagely treated by the Germans; P.o.W. of the other Allied nations were not, as a general rule.

Human beings when sufficiently starved for sufficiently long periods of time and when exposed to crude brutality tend to lose those attributes which are admirable in civilised man, compassion, kindness, consideration for others, self-care, self-respect and modesty and to become craven, crude, sycophantic, physically repulsive and entirely self-centred. When this happens it becomes easily possible for the immaculate, the comfortable and the powerful to despise them and to feel superior. One of the commonest methods of enlarging oneself is to belittle one's opponent.

Much of the cruelty of the P.o.W. camp stemmed from false biological doctrine concerning the relative worth of certain geographical varieties of mankind.

'It is only fair to say how much everyone appreciated the magnificent work done by the doctors in these P.o.W. camps (*on the Thailand–Burma railway*; *Campaigns*. II. p. 141.) They saved countless lives, working under the most appalling conditions, and having to rely on their own resources all the time. No drugs reached them in useable quantities until the end of 1944, and they performed operations that would have made the medical world shudder. On several occasions wood saws were used to amputate limbs, razor blades did duty as scalpels, old pieces of clothing were the only available material for bandages. Ordinary medical dressings were in short supply in most of the larger camps and non-existent in the small jungle camps.

'Many of the medical officers were quite young with little practical experience, and yet dozens of them found themselves pitchforked into the middle of the Thailand jungle and made responsible for the health of hundreds of men. This in itself was bad enough, but when it is remembered that they had to deal with tropical sicknesses without even a reference book, some idea can be formed of the task they faced.' (Barnard, Capt. J. T. *The Endless Years*. Chantry Publications Ltd. 1950)

To make war against Japan in 1940 was a very different adventure to fighting the Germans, for the former were not signatories to the Geneva Convention and were not bound by its rules. With very few exceptions they were largely indifferent to the requirements of the sick and wounded and made no effort to provide adequate medical facilities for their P.o.W. Medical officers and O.Rs. R.A.M.C. were shot in cold blood by Japanese soldiers and nurses criminally assaulted. These are matters that require careful consideration for it is obvious that the hazards to be faced when the enemy is like the Japanese of 1940–45 are very different from those likely to be encountered when the enemy has undertaken to observe the rules. It was necessary to arm medical units in Burma for self-protection as well as for the protection of their patients. In such circumstances is there not a place for the male S.R.N. in the A.M.S. when the enemy is not a signatory to the Convention?

IMPROVISATION BY PRISONERS-OF-WAR AND
INTERNEES IN JAPANESE HANDS

The attitude of the products of Japanese culture towards their civilian internees and military prisoners-of-war was such that it led directly to the establishment of conditions in the camps in which the possibility of continued existence on the part of the captives often depended very largely upon their ability to make good in one way or another the gross deficiencies in respect of the quantity and the quality of the rations that were issued and to find adequate substitutes for the many and varied medical supplies—anaesthetics, drugs, instruments, appliances—that were systematically withheld from them. It is quite certain that the ingenuity, inventiveness and resolution displayed by the captives did a great deal to conserve health and to save life among those who were subjected to what can only be described as barbarous and inhumane treatment.

In the large permanent camps the inmates were so numerous and their skills so varied that it was possible to develop an efficient organisation and to undertake the production of many of the things that were needed. But elsewhere, in the camps along the route of the Thailand-Burma railway, for example, this was much more difficult and the deficiencies were the cause of much suffering and of much untimely death.

Food

In Changi Camp an Allied Nutritional Advisory Committee, which included several men well versed in nutritional science, was formed and was continually active in recommending all kinds of supplements to the ration and in devising simple methods for their production. 'Changi-mite', a local substitute for Marmite, was obtained as a by-product of the manufacture of surgical alcohol from sweet potatoes and gula malacca and a small amount of yeast.

Gnawing hunger quickly overwhelms food fads, preferences and prejudices and slow starvation is a great promoter of experimentation. It was said that in one camp there was no living creature that ran, flew, swam, crawled or wriggled, and could be caught, that one prisoner or another had not at some time tried to eat. Snakes were boiled or fried; the weevils and other insect pests that infested the rice ration were skimmed off the water in which the rice was soaked, boiled in clean water and the resulting liquid strained off for the sick as a substitute beef-tea.

In the Stanley Internment Camp, Hong Kong, fish-heads from the very infrequent issue of fish were greatly prized and were equitably distributed among the captives in strict rotation. The crisp rice that gathered round the boiler when the rice was cooked was carefully collected and given to the infants and toddlers to chew. Meat bones, rich in calcium, were ground to a powder and given to the children.

In most camps bamboo roots, rice polishings, ground nuts, soya beans, green gram, towgay and kang kong grasses and many kinds of leaves were widely used as substitutes for vegetables. Extracts of various grasses and leaves were produced as were also small quantities of liver extract and of an injectable vitamin-B from rice polishings. An infusion of papaya leaves—'jungle juice'—was made and was thought to have a diaphoretic action. Jam was made from the rind of papayas and pomelos, ginger root and any sugar available.

Instruments and Appliances

In all the camps everybody was urged to hunt continually for anything that might be useful—scraps of cloth, bits of leather, rubber, wire, rope, string, solder, screws, nails, tin cans, lengths of bamboo, etc. Working parties employed outside the camps seldom returned empty-handed. There were black marketeers in most places, among the guards as well as among local civilians, who were always ready and eager to do business. Much was obtained illicitly from Japanese military stores. In one camp surgeons would describe the type of instrument needed, the black marketeer would use his own intelligence sources and then his agents would remove from some Japanese store either the required instrument, or something similar, or sufficient material for an improvised instrument to be made by a camp craftsman.

Proctoscopes were made out of tin with inbent edges; by reflecting sunlight from a mirror good vision as far as the three rectal valves could be obtained. Strictures in the healing stages were often seen and usually responded to stretching with graduated bamboo dilators. In one camp a scalpel was made out of the steel ribs of a woman's corset.

Spectacle frames were made out of the handles of tooth brushes and artificial eyes out of mah-jongg pieces. Dark spectacles for eye diseases were obtained by cutting lenses in half and fitting them in extemporised frames made from tin cans. A primitive still was used to distil water for eye drops. Experiments were made with grass extracts in the treatment of corneal lesions.

Dental instruments were fashioned out of pieces of fencing wire. Dentures were moulded out of raw rubber latex and riveted pieces of aluminium from a mess tin were used to repair broken dentures. Semi-permanent dental fillings, using oil of cloves and zinc oxide as a base, were successfully used until proper conservations could be made. Tooth powder was made from fine sifted wood-ash from the cookhouse, 5 parts, mixed with 1 part of rolled rock salt, the rolling being done by means of a bottle on a board. An obdurator to close off a syphilitic perforation of the palate was made out of a piece of Stent's Composition. Washers for dental syringes were cut out of pieces of leather from an old boot.

A kind of Brookes' truss for a patient with inguinal hernia was constructed with wood and sorbo rubber with rubber belts made out of the inner tubes of motor tyres.

In Changi Camp it was possible to open and staff a workshop for the manufacture of artificial lower limbs. The earliest types were made from Thomas' knee splints and leather from the seats of ambulance cars; they served their purpose well. But the craftsmen became more ambitious and began to make use of the 3/64 inch steel plates from discarded motor vehicles, wood from rubber trees, wrought iron from splints, rubberised fire-hose and copper wire. The shape and size of the stump were moulded by a copper wire cage and from this a wooden mould was made. The joints were welded and hinges made out of iron. The first of these artificial limbs was of the peg-leg variety but the second had a metal foot, hinged at the ankle, its positioning being controlled by means of a spring. A corset to fit the upper part of the limb was made out of fire-hose. Artificial limbs for higher amputations had knee hinges stabilised by means of a spring fixed to the rear of the true axis of the knee. Continual improvements of these limbs were made.

Physiotherapy apparatus was improvised from odds and ends of rope, board, bamboo and leather straps. Bamboo provided many things, crutches, washing bowls, mugs, trays, boxes and tubes of various calibres.

In Changi the only source of artificial light at night were lamps burning Malariol or Dieseline; in the camps along the railway route operations often had to be performed by the light of candles and bonfires.

Drugs and Therapy

In Changi with its exceptional facilities there was much activity of a pharmaceutical nature. Magnesium carbonate was made from sea water and soda ash; sodium iodide from iodine, old nails and soda ash; calcium carbonate from wood ash; sodium salicylate from salicylic acid and ash; surgical alcohol was produced by the fermentation of sweet potatoes and gula malacca—three pounds of each of these, a little yeast being added, yielded a pint of absolute alcohol. Cassia was grown to provide a laxative of the senna type; stramonium was grown to serve the needs of the asthmatic; derris root solution from local plants was used in the treatment of scabies. Soap was manufactured from fat from palm or coconut oil and alkali from potash in wood ash; glycerine was obtained as a by-product and magnesium hydrate derived from the sea water used in this soap factory was used in the treatment of peptic ulcers. In Kranji Camp also, magnesium hydrate was obtained from sea water.

In Thanbyuzayat Base Camp Hospital, on the railway route, there happened to be among the captives a Dutch chemist of considerable ability; among the many drugs he produced were emetine from ipecacuanha and novocain from some cocaine that the Australian senior surgeon was carrying. In this hospital, as elsewhere on this railway route, tropical ulcers were a very common cause of admission. No grease base was available for the making of ointments and so axle grease from Japanese motor vehicles was used, unknown, of course, to the Japanese. To it a small amount of an antiseptic was added. Bandages and dressings were made from rags, odd bits of clothing and the bottoms of mosquito nets. The bandages were held in place by liquid rubber obtained by tapping local trees. Rubber latex treated with a few drops of ammonia was used for making bandages for these leg ulcers in Changi. In several of the camps spoons and pieces of bent tin were used to scrape the ulcers. In many instances these ulcers were so deep and extensive that the Australian senior surgeon had to amputate the leg to save the patient's life. No general anaesthetic was available in Thanbyuzayat Camp Hospital and repeated appeals to the Japanese authorities were disregarded. The operation had to be performed under a local anaesthetic —the novocain produced by the Dutch chemist—and with a butcher's saw borrowed for the occasion from the camp cookhouse. In many camps hot rice poultices were used to promote inflammation in indolent tropical ulcers.

Minor operations, such as amputation of a finger or toe, were carried out without any anaesthetic and with a pair of strong scissors. Surgical gut was prepared from the entrails of cattle slaughtered to provide the meat ration.

In 'A' Force, one of the large groups of prisoners-of-war drafted for work on the Thailand-Burma railway, saline solution was administered to cholera patients by means of a wide bore needle made out of copper tubing that was 'found' and hidden. In 'F' Force also saline was given intravenously. A 300 ccm. ampoule was connected with stethoscope tubing to a thermometer case and thence to a bamboo cannula.* In the camp at Hintok distilled water for use in countering the extreme dehydration in cholera was produced in improvised stills made from purloined petrol piping surrounded by bamboo jackets and fed with water from a spring by way of bamboo pipes.

In 'A' Force surgical alcohol was distilled from Burmese 'brandy' and emetine was obtained from the liquid extract of ipecacuanha by the action of ether (from half-empty Japanese ampoules), sodium carbonate and alcohol. The technical difficulties were overcome and a product that could safely be used for intra-muscular injection was obtained. A tinea paint was manufactured from sulphur and slaked lime and used for the treatment of both tinea infections and scabies. In 'K' Force boiled strips of clothing removed from the dead had to be used for surgical dressings; there was nothing else that could be used. In 55-Kilo Camp, table knives were used for amputations, bent forks for retractors and a soldering iron for a cautery.

Appendicostomy and ileostomy, as methods of intestinal irrigation and drainage respectively for amoebic dysentery, were pioneered in prison camp hospitals with success as a life-saving measure. Charcoal and other local remedies were extensively used in diarrhoeal disturbances and amoebic dysentery when nothing else was available.

In the best of conditions the lot of the prisoner-of-war is an unhappy one. In the worst, such as obtained in the camps under Japanese control,

---

* These cannulae, made on the spot, were tied in the vein and proved to be preferable to the steel needles that were available.

it was one calculated to humiliate and degrade. The loss of liberty, accompanied as it was by so many deprivations, could have resulted in a much more serious sacrifice of human lives and greater incapacity among the survivors had it not been for a striking example of man's courage, ingenuity, determination and spirit to withstand and overcome misfortune. (See also Australia p. 640.)

The Biological Quality of an Army

The total size of the armed forces of a nation that are to be employed in a war and their actual composition in respect of the relative strengths of their component arms and services, are matters that are determined by considerations of general strategy. Decisions concerning them are made along with others that relate to the size and composition of the man-power requirements of industry and agriculture geared to a war-time economy and of the various services necessary for the maintenance of the social life of the country at a war-time level. In the ultimate analysis, however, the size and composition of the armed forces are not determined by purely military needs but by the demographic structure of the population from which these armed forces are derived and by the social structure of the country to which they belong. Manifestly, the very possibility that one nation can go to war with another in these modern days, with any hope of success, is largely determined by the relation of the total sizes of the two populations and by the relative degrees of the industrialisation of the two countries. Thermo-nuclear and bacteriological weapons tend to render large armed forces and large supporting industrial forces unnecessary for the conduct of war, but these newer instruments of war and their descendants are, and will continue to be, the products of the large and most industrialised populations.

In 1939 the estimated population of the United Kingdom was 47,762,000, 22,962,000 males and 24,800,000 females of all ages. By 1945 it was estimated that it had become some 49,182,000, including 23,725,000 males. Of the age-groups within this population the 20–49 range provided the intakes for the armed forces. Of these there were about 9 million males. Many were found to be unfit for military service, the percentage of the unfit increasing progressively with the age-groups of those examined, being four times greater among the age-groups 36–40 than among the youngest, the under-twenty-ones. The older the individual the less likely was it that he would pass the test. This is as would be expected.

The Army expanded nearly sevenfold during the first year of the war, by 34 per cent. during the second and thereafter more slowly, to reach its maximum strength in 1945, but even then its numbers were not twice what they had been in 1940. The annual intakes were

415,600 in 1939 and 1,544,100 in 1940, progressively diminishing thereafter to 301,900 in 1945.

This vast expansion in total size was no haphazard affair; it was a carefully planned enlargement up to pre-determined maximum size, having reference to the nature and complexities of unfolding military strategy and being limited only by the competitive demands of industry, agriculture and the various civilian services upon the very same range of age-groups, for this was a time when the whole of the available man-power of the nation was mobilised. But when the age-structure of the Army is examined and the changes in this structure with the passing years is noted, it becomes clear that this enlargement was achieved and maintained only by extending the range of the age-groups liable for military service and by replacing men by women in an ever-increasing range of occupations within the Army.

As the war continued there was a steady progressive fall in the proportion of the youngest age-groups and a concomitant fall in the proportions of the oldest (45 plus). The age-groups that showed the largest proportional increase were those between 28 and 42, this being made possible by the replacement of men by women in a variety of civil occupations.

The significance of these observations lies in the fact that the peak of physical efficiency in terms of output of the average male is reached well under thirty years of age. After this it levels off and then begins to decline. Training for modern warfare involves the rapid acquisition of a wide variety of new skills. Weapons assume an ever increasing complexity and for their efficient use much ability of a general kind is demanded of the soldier. The experience of industry has shown that it is more difficult for a man of 35, of little technical education and of set ways, to adapt himself to new conditions and to acquire new skills than it is for a man in his early twenties. A rising mean age of an army must necessarily have its repercussions upon weapon design and utilisation, on training and on tactics.

It also is attended by changing patterns of morbidity and mortality. It was observed (*Statistical Review of the Health of the Army 1943–45*, 1948 H.M.S.O.) that (*a*) among the youngest age-groups the major causes of wastage were psychiatric disorders and tuberculosis; (*b*) among the middle age-groups the major causes were psychiatric disorders and peptic ulcer and (*c*) among the oldest age-groups the major causes were bronchitis and psychiatric disorders. As the mean age rises tuberculosis loses its importance as a cause of wastage and peptic ulcer takes its place, while the incidence of bronchitis increases.

Tuberculosis is a disease that, under the conditions that existed in the United Kingdom before the war, affected, by primary infection, about 80 per cent. of the urbanised population. The fate of the young adult so attacked is determined in part by the degree of resistance he has acquired from previous attacks. This resistance is reinforced by the general vigour of the individual, who, as a result of favourable standards of living, enjoys robust health. It is diminished when the individual is exposed to conditions which lower his general well-being and to circumstances that cause severe emotional stress. Life in the Army in time of war can be very strenuous, thoroughly testing a young man's capacity to cope successfully with the tubercle bacillus. This is the reason why this disease was one of the major causes of wastage among the youngest age-group. The same result was seen in the First World War.

Bronchitis in the ageing is very commonly a sign of physical degen-ration, and, indirectly, of developing inefficiency of the cardiovascular system. The stress of army life is a test of the efficiency of this system in the oldest age-group.

The fact that psychiatric disorders and peptic ulcer figured so largely among the major causes of wastage in a national army and in a war such as that of 1939–45 is of peculiar significance. The forms of psychiatric disorder that made the greatest contributions to this wastage were anxiety neurosis and hysteria, diseases which can be displayed by all who are exposed to severe stress. Every man has his breaking-point under stress, although individuals differ markedly in respect of the degree of stress they can endure without loss of resilience. To large numbers of men service in the armed forces in war is a cause of severe inner conflict. They are the products of a peace-time nurture, inherently creative and productive and valuing human life; service in the armed forces demands of them a profound repression of their codes; in it they find no abiding satisfaction. Because of this conflict they are unable to adjust themselves to the circumstances of army life and they become ill, for illness can be a means of escape from the unendurable.

Peptic ulcer is a disease into the causation of which psychological factors enter. To it individuals of the O blood-group are especially prone. It seems that worry and anxiety and grave discontent are as knives that cut a hole through the wall of the stomach of a man through which he can crawl away from the disagreeable and dangerous towards the comfort of the congenial and safe. The circumstances of battle make extortionate demands upon the ability of many men to suppress their emotions, demands that in many an instance are too great. Unless he can be reassured and rested it becomes probable that he will break down and seek refuge in neurosis or hysteria, which can be the signs of the complete exhaustion of the individual, or an expression of his deep desire for survival. Together with the incidence of self-inflicted wounds, the incidence of these mental disturbances can be a measure of the extent to which the individuals of a group are unable to resolve the conflict between their private doubts and the identification of themselves with the group. It is an inverse measure of the completeness and of the permanence of the psychological preparedness to which they were exposed.

According to some, a rising incidence of these conditions in a succession of wars or a high incidence in a war following a long peace is to be accepted as an indication that the national group concerned is becoming effete. By others it is regarded as a sign of a gathering distaste for war as a method of solving disputes. Still others hold that it is merely an indication that the weapons of war have become increasingly terrifying. It seems probable that the second and third of these interpretations most closely approach the truth.

The Army of 1939–45 was a highly complex organisation that demanded from its component members a constellation of intelligence, dexterity, agility and skill of a quality not less than that required of the worker in a highly mechanised industry. It is established that individuals of the same age differ very markedly among themselves in respect of native ability, aptitudes and acquired skills. It was accepted that the needs of the Royal Navy and of the Royal Air Force in respect of these attributes exceeded those of the Army and so it was that from the available reservoir, those called-up for service and passed by the recruiting boards, the Army received a disproportionate share of the dullards, the illiterates, the unskilled and the frail. As early as 1940 it had become apparent that not less than 4 per cent. of the Army intakes were such as could never be moulded by the existing systems of training into efficient soldiers and that in every command there were very large numbers of men who, because of their poor physical development or their educational backwardness, constituted a severe drag upon the attainment of efficiency by the units to which they belonged. It came to be recognised that, in the vast task of creating a national army out of the raw material that was being allotted to it and in which the standards of pre-selection were necessarily low as compared with those of a small peace-time regular army maintained by voluntary enlistment, new procedures would have to be adopted.

The Adjutant-General introduced the basic principle that in allotting personnel within the Army no man should be employed on work that was definitely above, or on the other hand definitely below, his capacity to perform it. (*Admin.* II. p. 478.) The acceptance of this principle produced profound changes in many spheres—medical categorisation, personnel selection, training and posting, particularly. So long as there was a wide variety of talents to match with the wide variety of tasks to be performed this deliberate attempt to counteract the more obvious causes of inner conflict in the minds of men and to produce a state of equilibrium between the individual and the conditions and circumstances of his external world was successful. But inevitably, as the war dragged on, the numbers of men in the higher categories of fitness progressively dwindled while those of the men in the lower categories steadily enlarged. In 1943 and 1944 it was already noticeable that the numbers in the A categories were dwindling, that those in the B categories were increasing slightly and that those in the lower categories were showing a heavy increase. During these years there was much wastage from transfers from high to low categories. (*Admin.* II. p. 138.) Increasing difficulty was encountered in finding replacements and reinforcements for first-line formations while the numbers of those found fit only for base and garrison duties mounted to yield an ever-expanding surplus. Standards of fitness had to be lowered and training methods had to be modified as the composition of the Army in respect of the relative numbers of men in the different categories of fitness for service underwent a progressive change for the worse. In the later years of the war the numbers of the mentally sub-normal among the intakes grew larger. These are they who contribute so largely to the psychiatric casualty lists of an army in the field and who constitute so great a burden to their units, being continually transferred from one unit to another, attending sick parade with unfailing regularity and making no contribution of any worth to the war effort. It came to be recognised that such men should never be admitted to an army.

THE EFFECT OF LENGTH OF SERVICE OVERSEAS UPON THE MORBIDITY-RATE

In the early phase of overseas service the sick-rate in a well-disciplined and well-cared-for unit is low. Morale is high and the novel conditions and circumstances are such as to absorb the interest of the vast majority of the troops. But, with the passage of time their thoughts become detached from their immediate surroundings and begin to focus themselves nostalgically upon home, relatives and the joys that used to be. Conflicts and disorganised reactions begin to fester in the mind and, as they grow, become revealed in a rising sick-rate.

If for a period of three years or so the sick-rates from such diseases as malaria, dysentery and gonorrhoea, in the avoidance of which personal effort and self-care are demanded, are examined it is found that whereas during the first eighteen months or so of overseas service they are well below the monthly average of the whole period, at about the half-way stage they begin to rise steeply above this average. The exact point at which they begin to rise is influenced by a number of factors. It is delayed under conditions in which there is much successful activity and advanced under conditions of seemingly pointless inactivity. The main causes of this rise would seem to be a progressively developing *ennui* and mounting anxiety concerning domestic affairs (especially if there are troops of an Allied nation in the homeland). An increase in careless behaviour and a disregard for the ordinary simple rules of disease avoidance are to be observed. There is a deterioration of discipline and of military efficiency.

Among the main measures for the prevention of a rising sick-rate due to this cause are victory, leave, regular mail and increased care in the field of man-management. It would seem that, as a general rule, overseas service (without leave at home) should ideally be restricted to about eighteen months.

THE MILITARY VALUE OF ACQUIRED IMMUNITIES

Different ethnographical stocks serving in the same theatre and exposed to the same hazards showed significantly different sickness rates from many of the diseases which affected them all. Certain of these differences were reflections of differences in respect of acquired immunities, for example, the acquired immunity of the African to malaria, due to his successful reactions to frequent attacks during infancy could have been expected to have given African formations in Madagascar and in Burma a great advantage over the British formations that were fighting alongside them. Any such advantage was nullified, however, by the co-existence in the African, hospitalised on account of malaria, of other disabling diseases, so that the actual duration of stay in hospital was generally about twice as long in the case of the African as it was for the British soldier hospitalised for the same reason.

PSYCHOLOGICAL CONTRIBUTIONS TO THE PREPARATION OF AN ARMY FOR BATTLE

The stress of warring has become such that by it all but the very exceptional sooner or later become 'burnt out'. The speed of the development of this exhaustion varies greatly in different individuals, in different units and in different situations. Individuals differ among themselves in respect of endurance and resilience. The indoctrination of the individual and his training can be complete or otherwise. The battle can be long drawn out or brief. The terrain can be desert or close rocky country. The weapons of the enemy can include the most feared. Dullards and the mentally backward tend to break quickly, so also do the emotionally unstable. Should a battle remain undecided for four days or more a trickle of psychiatric casualties is likely to become a flood. Swift victory yields very few such casualties, defeat begets many. Competent resolute leadership is rewarded with a low psychiatric casualty-rate, poor leadership with a high one. All these matters need to be carefully considered when a formation is being prepared for battle.

The pattern of this preparation varies with the national constitution of the troops and with the personality of the commander, as well as with the general military situation. The preparation for the battle of El Alamein provides an example of one method. The coming battle was presented as though it were a contest of skill between two professional groups. The confidence of Eighth Army in its commander was sedulously sought. He was presented as a symbol of unity, seeking the intelligent co-operation of his colleagues. The tactics of the forthcoming struggle were made widely known. The manifest superiority of the might, the armament and the equipment of Eighth Army over those of its opponent was emphasised. Tired units were rested and raw ones 'blooded' and habituated to the enemy's tactics and weapons. Experienced formations were reminded of their prowess and flattered by being allotted special and peculiarly important tasks. Victory was promised.

It has to be recognised that the procedures adopted in Eighth Army are not without their dangers. When this army moved to Italy there to become part of a much larger force, its members were required to develop another loyalty—to a larger group and to another commander. It ceased to remain a closed community and from it personnel and units were transferred to other formations. The result in one formation was mutiny.

The success of the exercise of this art is determined by the extent and quality of the knowledge of the craft of man-management possessed by the commander and his advisers and by the skill with which this knowledge is exploited under the circumstances that obtain. The psychiatrist has much to offer concerning the nature of the raw material out of which soldiery is fashioned and concerning the provision of those things which this nature requires if its needs are to be satisfied. The knowledge that in the coming battle adequate medical cover is to be provided contributes greatly to the morale of the troops who are to be called upon to face very considerable risks.

BIOLOGICAL CONTRIBUTIONS TO THE DESIGN AND UTILISATION OF WEAPONS

A weapon is the extension of the arm of the man who uses it to magnify his powers. It is a tool which in the hands of one set of men produces effects upon another set of men, and the military value of a weapon is determined by its physical and mental effects upon those who use it and upon those against whom it is used. The value of an artillery bombardment is not to be measured only by the number of those whom it kills or wounds or by the amount of material damage it causes, but by the kind and the degree of the change it causes in the behaviour of those against whom it is directed. The scream of the dive-bomber can be as effective an agent in determining the actions and the attitudes of men as can the lethality of the bomb that it carries. The reputation that a particular weapon attracts to itself can come to be as important to those against whom it is directed as its actual precision. The creation of anxiety was no less important an attribute of the schu mine or of the V.1 rocket than was their ability to inflict grievous physical hurt.

The individual in battle is torn between two desires; that of sharing to the full in the interests and activities of the group of which he is a member and that of avoiding personal annihilation. A weapon is an instrument that is deliberately used for the purpose of detaching the individual from the group and of encouraging him to think only of self-preservation; it must therefore possess, or seem to possess, the power to kill.

This being understood, biological considerations have their part to play in the design and in the utilisation of weapons. Thus far the contributions of the biological sciences have been largely restricted to the sphere of psychological warfare in which the object is to erode the morale of the enemy and so speed the process of deterioration of resistance. Subtle, disturbing notion and reiterated word are the seeds of doubt which, flowering, can be expected to detach the loyalty of individuals from the group to which they belong.

During the War of 1939–45 with its deliberate and systematic bombing of cities and with the use of the V.1 and V.2 rockets and the atomic bomb, all discrimination between soldier and civilian, between combatant and non-combatant disappeared. Of the weapons used in that war only the atomic bomb produced a sufficiently profound effect upon the minds of those against whom it was directed to persuade them that further resistance was useless. The uranium and plutonium bombs dropped at Hiroshima and Nagasaki killed some 120,000 people and injured about the same number out of a total population of around half-a-million. Death was the fate of 95 per cent. of all those who were directly exposed to the action of the bomb within 1,000 yards of the point above which it exploded in the air. Serious burns were endured by people two and a half miles away from this point. Even if the heat and the blast did not kill, the gamma rays produced illness within a period of from one to five weeks. About 85 per cent. of all the injuries received consisted of trauma and burns while radiation deaths comprised 15 per cent.

But these effects, appalling as they are, fade into insignificance when contrasted with the possible effects of this energy upon the germ plasm of those exposed to it. This energy is known to be mutagenic, evoking changes in the genes that are resident in the chromosomes of the nuclei of the cells that give rise to the ova and the spermatozoa. The mutant genes, for the most part, yield abnormal, pathological characterisations in the offspring of those who have been exposed to the

Military Psychiatry

By R. H. Ahrenfeldt, M.R.C.P., M.R.C.S.

CONTENTS

THE ARMY PSYCHIATRIC SERVICE

INTRODUCTION

WITH the ever increasing emphasis in medicine on the fundamental importance of 'positive health', psychiatry has, in more recent years, evolved and expanded in scope, with greatly enhanced efficiency, in close co-operation with the psychological and social sciences, and also with other specialised medical fields— its orientation being directed towards an eventual psychosomatic synthesis and collaboration throughout the entire range of medical practice. It has therefore properly become the function of the psychiatrist not only to treat mental illness and maladjustment, but to study individuals and societies alike, and their mutual and respective reactions and adaptability, in the interests of psychiatric prophylaxis and the promotion of mental health.

In the light of this dynamic concept of psychiatry and its social implications, it is perhaps not irrelevant, in the first place, briefly to enquire how far the psychiatric lessons of medical history are in fact learnt, and applied in the future (whether in war or in peace), on the basis of that previous historical experience which has been reliably recorded; and how far it is, on the other hand, subsequently necessary for generations and individuals to re-learn such lessons the hard way, i.e., solely as a result of personal experience—obviously, a most wasteful process so far as society is concerned. 'If man is to progress,' as Ginzberg[14] observes, 'he must learn from experience. It is the only way. World War II was a most costly experience.' Unfortunately, the student of medical, as of general, history is all too often led by incontrovertible facts to agree with Hegel[17] (whose significant words may perhaps here be quoted, for once, in accurate translation): 'What experience and history teach us, however, is this: that peoples and governments never have learnt anything from history, or acted according to lessons that should have been derived from the latter.'

That the history of military psychiatry in the Second World War, both in this country and in the United States, proved no exception in this respect is evident from the facts that have been duly recorded and fully documented in recent years.[1] Detailed accounts and appraisals of the most important and vital lessons derived from the disastrous experiences of the First World War were indeed available[18, 37, 39] for all who would, to read, mark, learn and inwardly digest. In fact, as noted by Brigadier J. R. Rees,[32] there was thus a considerable amount of material

175

to aid us in planning, before the outbreak of the Second World War, and many experiences of the First World War were repeated in the Second. How many such documents have, however, in the past been generally ignored, or else have suffered the fate of Cassandra's prophecies! While it is also, no doubt, very largely true, as Brigadier-General Menninger[26] stated with regard to American experiences early in the last war, that 'the psychiatric profession as a whole . . . permitted the military to forget almost all the lessons' that had been learnt in the First War, it is, to say the least, difficult to see how psychiatrists, had they been sufficiently aware of the situation, might effectively have prevented the development of this retrogade amnesia and functional amblyopia which afflicted military and administrative authorities (medical and non-medical) between the two wars.

In this country, Dr. C. S. Myers[30] observed that his account (published in 1940) of psychiatric experiences in the First War might 'perhaps raise a doubt in some minds as to how far the present senior administrative officers of the Army Medical Service and the Adjutant-General's Department will be prevented from repeating the same mistakes— errors of commission, omission, and especially of wasteful procrastination—as arose during the last war.' Similar warnings were given by Dr. Emanuel Miller[27] and others.

In the shadow of such disturbing historical facts as are here outlined, there can be no room for complacency; and, however fashionable the administration of ataractic drugs may have become, it would be unrealistic and delusory to attempt, from any but the most critical point of view, the task of evaluating the contributions and vicissitudes of military psychiatry in the Second World War, and of deducing the lessons that are there to be learnt by those who might be so disposed. It is hoped that the present analysis of past difficulties and problems— that might well, whether in war or peace, become future ones—will be judged and weighed in the same objective spirit in which it is proffered.

It is of the greatest importance, at the outset, clearly to understand the range and interrelationship of individual and social influences, conflicts and adjustments involved, which are not only of medical and psychiatric, but indeed of general military, significance in time of war. Essential and indispensable as they are, a stringent medical examination at intake, and adequate selection and allocation procedure, are primarily concerned with the physical and mental health, intelligence, aptitudes and quality of the individual, although these must necessarily affect to a considerable extent the mental health and stability of the entire military social organism; but the basic psychiatric problems that have so great an impact on the general morale and efficiency of an army in war-time are ultimately dependent upon the adaptability of the individual, and his potentialities for satisfactory integration in a new and exotic social environment* which makes very special and exacting demands upon him, and in particular, for a maximum degree of adjustment and optimum performance, in a minimal period of time. It is also of considerable importance to provide, where required, adequate social rehabilitation, whether for further effective (even if restricted) military service, or for return to a useful and self-supporting place in civilian life.

Thus, these several essential problems arising within the military organisation, in total war and with general conscription, resolve themselves very largely into applied 'social psychiatry', i.e., the preventive and curative measures which are directed towards the fitting of the individual for a satisfactory and useful life in terms of his particular social environment.[46] How these social implications of psychiatry are applicable and relevant in the military context, is well shown by the following observations of Ginzberg *et al*[14]: 'The multi-dimensional approach goes beyond the individual, his strengths and weaknesses, and includes a consideration of how the demands and pressures, the opportunities and supports in his environmental situation are likely to affect his performance. There is no way of assessing performance adequately except by making room for these situational forces. This lesson is embedded in the many cases of breakdown in the Army. The pressure that war exerts on men is unique and sooner or later even the strongest may break under the strain . . . Since no man lives or works alone, his performance will be affected by the quality of his relationships with the individuals to whom he looks for support and leadership. Among the disturbing effects of war is the disruption in personal relationships, first when a man is separated from his family and friends, and later if he sees those with whom he has established new bonds injured or killed.'

Undoubtedly, at the beginning of the Second World War, one of the most serious deficiencies on the part of psychiatry as a whole was its emphasis on the individual, almost as an isolated unit independent of group dynamics, and its relative neglect of 'social psychiatry'. Just as medicine is, however slowly, coming to realise the basic significance of psychosomatic concepts, and that neither psyche nor soma may be ignored, whatever the nature of the illness, without detriment to the patient, so also it is (in the 'physical' as in the 'psychological' field) gradually coming to accept the fact that the individual cannot be treated *in vacuo*, or 'society' considered in the abstract, but that the two are necessarily interrelated and interdependent. Indeed, the dichotomy is, in both cases, entirely artificial and meaningless, and factors which have

---

* 'It should be remembered that an army is, in the words of Freud,[13] a "highly organised . . . and artificial group"—and all the more "artificial" for civilian conscripts, who do not, as a rule, altogether take for granted this specialised type of social structure —"who are not soldiers . . . by profession: and who never wanted to be".'[29]

so often been regarded as opposed and conflicting are seen to be essentially complementary.* The aim of medicine, in this respect, must therefore be to ensure, or re-establish, a harmonious equilibrium— 'the reconciliation of the opposites', on which Jung has wisely placed so great an emphasis.

Thus, referring to American experience, Menninger[26] rightly stated that few psychiatrists 'had thought in concrete terms of which methods were applicable to the Army. We often failed in orientating our own medical officers, including psychiatrists, to the specific needs of the military, in which one must accept the group aim . . . as of paramount importance instead of that of the individual.' And, as noted by Braceland,[7] 'most psychiatrists entered the military services with insufficient knowledge of the normal reactions to the vicissitudes of everyday life and the slight deviations of young adults under stress, and thus they were unprepared for most of the situations which they were to encounter.' These comments are equally true, in general, of the psychiatric profession in our own country at the beginning of the war.

It is in fact the function of the psychiatric and allied services, in the Army as in civilian life, to direct their activities towards the integration of the individual in the social environment in which he must, at any given time, live and work, thus preventing so far as possible wastage of man-power through mental breakdown, maladjustment and inefficiency, and ensuring the fullest utilisation of the limited human resources available.†

It is ultimately on the extent to which we have succeeded or failed in achieving this aim, that the evaluation of the psychiatric contribution in any sphere must be based. As recorded by Sutherland and Fitzpatrick,[35] 'In the course of the war, the psychiatrists in the British Army were confronted with a number of problems which were appreciated by them

---

* This is, of course, far from saying that psychiatry is not properly concerned in essence, as Masserman[25] has rightly emphasised, with 'the study of individual motivations and adaptations, whether or not these need to be regarded from a "social" standpoint. . . Actually there exist only human beings with needs, strivings and variously acquired patterns of adaptation to each other and their "environments" as they conceive them. In the study of the individual then, lie the problems of social interaction.' It was only through the study of individual adjustment and maladjustment, largely on the basis of psychoanalytic orientation, that it was possible for the concepts and practical results of 'social psychiatry' and group dynamics to evolve, in the Army[35] as in other fields.

† Extensive research on the factors responsible for 'the ineffective soldier', and the wastage of man-power through psychiatric disability, defective selection and allocation procedure, etc., in the U.S. Army in the Second World War, as also on such matters as civil resettlement after discharge, was undertaken at Columbia University by the Conservation of Human Resources Project, under the direction of Professor Eli Ginzberg. The results of this detailed study and re-appraisal of war-time experience have been published,[14] and are deserving of the most careful consideration by all those whose responsibility it should be to concern themselves with these essential problems, whether in this country or in the United States: they most certainly provide a very clear and significant illustration of the lessons to be learnt in this connexion.

to belong to the institution of the army as a whole or to groups within it and which accordingly could best be treated by methods dealing with the dynamics of the group in its total setting. These problems were new to the psychiatrists who therefore had to tackle them without previous direct experience of what was involved. As successive tasks were dealt with, a degree of clarification accompanied the increasing and widening experience. While the measures taken were spoken of at the time as "psychiatric", it was realised that the traditional frontiers of psychiatry had been greatly extended and that the psychiatrists, and the psychologists who later joined them, were in fact in new rôles in relation to the groups they were treating.'

It would be highly desirable that the following words of the late Dr. Alan Gregg[15] (then Director, Division of Medical Services of the Rockefeller Foundation) should be constantly borne in mind by all whom they may concern: 'The lessons of the war are clear enough. . . Many . . . are humiliating—a powerful reason for repressing them. Many call for unremitting work if the mistakes are not to be continued and repeated. . . The greatest unpleasant surprise of the war for medical men was the importance of psychiatry and psychology. And yet so inconstant, evasive, or preoccupied are the majority of men that this greatest lesson can be disputed, evaded, and soon forgotten.'

These lessons, which are so far as possible summarised below, are derived from the arduous, and sometimes disastrous, experiences— errors, failures, needs and also successes—of two major world wars without historical precedent, separated by less than a mere quarter of a century. They have surely been 'tried in the fire', and have in consequence established beyond doubt the essential contribution of psychiatry to the mental health, morale and efficiency of the Army, when it has been necessary to mobilise our country's entire, but limited, resources in total warfare.*

Before proceeding to an evaluation of the application of psychiatric techniques to specific military problems during the war, it is important to note the following facts concerning the basic requirements for the adequate organisation of Army psychiatry. Experience has shown that, in order to co-ordinate the various important prophylactic and therapeutic activities of Army psychiatry in war-time, and to maintain necessary liaison with the several branches and departments of the War Office, it is absolutely essential for functional efficiency that there be an independent central organisation (Directorate of Army Psychiatry) as a part of the Army Medical Department. Equally important from the psychiatric point of view is the establishment of a separate, specialised

---

* A comprehensive bibliography of the subjects discussed in the following sections has been compiled by Ahrenfeldt.[1]

psychological department, in charge of personnel selection (Directorate of Selection of Personnel) as part of the Adjutant-General's branch of the War Office. It is also essential that these departments receive the active co-operation and support of the Director-General, Army Medical Services, and the Adjutant-General, respectively and collectively (such as was provided, in the Second World War, by Generals Sir Alexander Hood and Sir Ronald Adam).

THE MAGNITUDE OF THE PSYCHIATRIC PROBLEM

As stated by Lt.-Gen. Sir Neil Cantlie,[40] formerly D.G.A.M.S., the *Statistical Report on the Health of the Army*, 1943–1945, 'draws attention to the magnitude of the psychiatric problems of modern Army medicine and presents a much needed record of the contribution made by Army psychiatry.'*

Psychiatric disorders constituted the largest single cause (one-seventh) of man-power wastage from disease in the British Army. They were also the largest cause, comprising nearly one-third (31 per cent.), of medical discharges from the Army.†

In addition, more than 2 per cent. of all men medically examined prior to national service were rejected for psychiatric reasons—which represents one-eighth (12 per cent.) of all medical rejections at intake.

It should therefore be realised that, of over 5·5 million men of military age examined by Ministry of Labour and National Service medical boards in 1939–45, one man in every forty was either considered unfit for military service, or subsequently discharged from the Forces on medical grounds, on account of psychiatric disability.

In the United States, psychiatric rejections at intake amounted to 10 per cent. of all men examined (32 per cent. of all rejections), and psychiatric discharges from the Army comprised 45 per cent. of all medical discharges. With reference to the U.S. Armed Forces in the Second World War, Ginzberg[14] states: 'Of the 18 million young men who were screened for military service, 2·5 million were either rejected or prematurely separated because of a mental or emotional defect . . . No society can afford to ignore the fact that one out of every seven men was judged to be mentally or emotionally incapable of serving effectively

---

* The statistics here quoted are derived from the official Report,[40] an article by Brigadier A. E. Richmond,[34] and a comparative analysis of the available data for the U.K. and U.S. (cf. Ahrenfeldt,[1] Appendix C, pp. 276 ff.—where references are also given to the relevant literature of both countries).

† These figures, therefore, refer only to discharges on medical grounds, under *King's Regs.*, 1940, ¶390, (xvi)(b); they do not include administrative discharges, under ¶390, (xviii) (a), of 'psychopathic' and chronic delinquents, many, if not indeed all, of whom were psychiatric cases at least in so far as they could, for the most part, have been detected and rejected at intake by adequate psychiatric screening.—(Cf. *Queen's Regs.*, 1955, ¶503, sub-paragraphs as above.)

in its armed forces in time of war; or that a significant, if much smaller, proportion cannot support themselves in time of peace. The cost of failure not only to the individual but to his family . . . and to the larger community is too high to be tolerated by a responsible democracy.'

In assessing the significance of the fact that one man in forty in the United Kingdom was considered at the outset, or subsequently proved, to be psychiatrically unfit for military service, as compared with the American figure of one in seven, it should be borne in mind that there is ample evidence that, in this country, the number of psychiatric rejections at intake were far too low. Indeed, psychiatric examination at intake was to all intents and purposes non-existent, and it was not until the belated introduction of a comprehensive system of personnel selection, that a second, more thorough screening procedure for mental capacity and emotional stability became available.

PERSONNEL SELECTION AND ALLOCATION

As early as 1922, the Southborough Committee[39] had expressed their views clearly and unequivocally in the following terms: 'As far as it is possible to foresee the conditions of any future war on a large scale, it seems probable that the circumstances are likely to make even greater demands upon the mental and nervous resources of the personnel of the fighting services than the events of 1914–18. If this should prove to be the case, appropriate measures designed to admit into the services only those who are possessed of at least an average degree of mental and nervous health and stability will be a factor of prime importance in the successful conduct of the war.'

It might have been hoped that the experience of the Armed Forces of our own and other countries in the First World War, and in particular the experiments undertaken in the U.S. Army in 1917, would have been accepted as sufficient evidence and warning of the need for an active and comprehensive policy of personnel selection in the British Army, and particularly, in a conscript army in war-time. Unfortunately, Hegel was once again proved right. Nothing at all was done at the beginning of the Second World War, and a pre-war attempt in April 1939 (in a memorandum submitted by Dr. J. R. Rees and Mr. Alec Rodger to the medical authorities at the War Office), to initiate a scheme of selection testing in the Army, failed to receive any support, or understanding of its immense significance, on the part of the authorities concerned.[32] It was only after much discussion, and some two years later, that methods of personnel selection such as had previously been commonly employed in civil life (in industry) and in some foreign armies, were eventually accepted in principle, and received official recognition with the formation, in June

1941, of a Directorate of Selection of Personnel under the Adjutant-General.

As a result of this 'wasteful procrastination'—to use Dr. Myers' pertinent phrase—in introducing scientific selection into the Army in the Second World War, there is no doubt that, as Brigadier Rees[33] observed in 1945, 'many horses were out of the stable before the door was shut. It is sad but true that no force has yet gone overseas from Great Britain, every man of which has gone through selection procedures'. A leading article in *The Lancet*,[3] in 1941, spoke of our 'tardy recognition . . . of the fact that the soldier's mental qualities are at least as important as his physical, in estimating his efficiency, or placing him in a job where he will be most useful'. It also referred to the organisation then being set up in the United States on the principle that the Army needed men sound in mind and body, with the comment that this 'is flouted by those misguided patriots among examining doctors who can't see why "a bad hat should get away with it".'

In July 1942 the General Service Corps intake scheme was eventually introduced and all men entering the Army were subjected, during their period of basic training, to selection and allocation procedures in which specially trained Personnel Selection Officers worked in co-operation with psychiatrists and psychologists.

A thorough preliminary medical (physical and psychiatric) examination and a most stringent initial selection procedure, are essential, and indeed indispensable, for they are designed to eliminate from intake into the Army those who are mentally and emotionally unfit and unstable, and those whom it is possible, within attainable limits, to predict as liable to break down under relatively minor stress, or to prove a source of inefficiency, delinquency, wastage, etc., or otherwise to exert an influence deleterious to group morale—i.e., those who may be regarded as 'poor psychiatric risks' for an Army in war-time. Very much more than this cannot reasonably be expected of the preliminary medical and selection procedures at intake, however adequate and thorough these might be.* Ginzberg[14] gives a timely warning of the limitations in this respect: 'Selection is a useful and . . . necessary facet of a comprehensive personnel programme, but training and assignment must be relied upon to fit the individual into an organisation so that he can perform effectively. The Army was faced with a truly herculean task in World War II because it had to convert in the shortest possible time such large numbers of peace-loving civilians into efficient soldiers.'

---

* It has already been noted that, during the war, notwithstanding the rejection by the U.S. Army at intake, for psychiatric reasons, of 10 per cent. of all men examined, and in spite of effectively organised initial selection procedure, the number of cases subsequently discharged on psychiatric grounds nevertheless amounted to 45 per cent. of all discharges for mental and physical disabilities.

Psychiatrists and psychologists had indeed drawn attention to the acute man-power situation and the urgent need for employing every man in the Army on work most suited to his medical category and aptitude; and, in particular, to the fact that men whom it subsequently became necessary to place in lower medical categories were in many cases transferred to other duties with little regard to their individual aptitude or to the man-power requirements of the several arms of the Service. They pointed out that the morale of soldiers in low medical categories had been allowed to suffer as a result of unsuitable employment, although experience had shown that, appropriately employed and trained, such men could not only render useful service, but release others in higher categories for more active duties. Such reallocation was eventually undertaken by Army Selection Centres, established early in 1943, although these were open to criticism in several respects.[1]

Experience proved beyond doubt the fundamental importance for the efficiency of the Army and the conservation of man-power, of providing adequate procedures not only for selection but for correct allocation at intake, and also facilities for suitable reallocation where this might subsequently become necessary. In this connexion, two comments by Ginzberg *et al.*[14] may here be noted, which are as highly relevant to British Army experience as to that of our American allies in the Second World War: 'Since policy changes always create problems, especially in an organisation which is forced to rely on relatively inexperienced personnel, the Army would have been in a better position had it had a clearer understanding earlier of both its requirements and the characteristics of the man-power pool. Such knowledge would have enabled it to avoid many of the sudden shifts in selection policy which did so much to confuse the examiners and to lower their effectiveness.'— 'The Army's inability to make maximum use of the assignment and reassignment system was undoubtedly costly.'

In general terms, it may be asserted that it is essential, and particularly so when it is necessary to mobilise the country's total resources of man-power, that all those men who have been found fit for full or limited military duties should be subjected on enlistment to thorough scientific selection, on the basis of intellectual capacity, vocational aptitudes and experience, etc., in order that they may be allocated to duties in such a manner as to make full use of the limited skilled man-power available, to ensure maximal efficiency and to avoid psychiatric breakdown or serious demoralisation as a consequence of inappropriate allocation. It is equally essential that facilities should exist at all times for expert reallocation of men who have been wrongly allocated, of those who through subsequent impairment of their physical or mental condition become fit for limited duties only, or in cases where the

G*

exigencies of the military situation require a widespread redistribution of man-power.

SELECTION OF OFFICERS AND PARACHUTISTS

There can be few subjects that have caused greater emotional controversy, aroused more prejudiced and misinformed criticism, and encountered such determined and misdirected opposition, as the introduction into the British Army, in the Second World War, of a scientific system of officer selection in which psychiatrists and psychologists played an essential part. The vicissitudes of this most thorny passage of military psychiatric history have been fully described and discussed elsewhere.[1]

It is, however, our sole concern here to provide a few basic facts which have clearly demonstrated the value of the more scientific methods of selecting officers, and to place on record the essential nature of the psychiatric contribution to this procedure, for it must be emphasised that the experimental research in this field, in the British Army in 1941, was in fact initiated and developed by psychiatrists (T. F. Rodger and E. Wittkower). A battery of written tests was devised, by psychologists and psychiatrists working in close co-operation. Selection Boards were established in 1942–43 throughout the United Kingdom and with the Forces in all the principal theatres overseas. Each Board consisted of an experienced senior regular officer (as president) who interviewed each candidate and, together with a specially selected regimental officer (Military Testing Officer) evaluated performance in military tests; and also, a psychiatrist. Psychological tests and a psychiatric interview were included in the procedure.[1]

A most interesting and valuable additional technique was provided by the Leaderless Group tests, developed by another psychiatrist, W. R. Bion,[5] which enabled each member of the Board to obtain a far more complete and integrated picture of the candidates' personality and character: 'The essence of the technique which was evolved, and has since become the basis of selection techniques in many different fields,* was to provide a framework in which selecting officers, including a psychiatrist, could observe a man's capacity for maintaining personal relationships in a situation of strain that tempted him to disregard the interests of his fellows for the sake of his own.' The purpose of this technique was, therefore, to investigate and test the quality of the man's social relationships with his fellows.

---

* The Leaderless Group principle was successfully applied by Bion and Rickman,[5, 6] Main[22] and others, to the treatment and rehabilitation of neurotics in a military psychiatric hospital; and by Wilson, Doyle and Kelnar[41, 42] to resettlement problems of repatriated prisoners-of-war. (*See* also, Sutherland and Fitzpatrick.[35])

It should be noted that, from the start, the psychiatrist had two main and essential functions at the W.O.S.B. As technical adviser, he had to give an expert opinion on the psychological aspects of the military tests (in co-operation with the psychologists). As medical examiner, he originally interviewed every candidate, and was, therefore, in a position to assess personality and stability in each case.[11]

Follow-up investigations proved that it is possible, with the W.O.S.B. procedure as developed by psychiatrists, greatly to decrease the rejection rate of suitable officer candidates. The old, traditional system of officer selection is extremely wasteful in that it rejects at least one out of three of the best candidates appearing before the Selection Board. In one large sample of men who had been selected for Officer Cadet Training Units (O.C.T.Us.) by the respective methods, the proportion of candidates passing out of the O.C.T.Us. who were graded as 'above average' was 22 per cent. with the old methods and 34·5 per cent. with the W.O.S.Bs.[1]

Modified W.O.S.B. techniques were later successfully applied to the selection of candidates for several other specialised services, in this country and elsewhere, and notably for the Civil Service.

Thus it is apparent that, at a time when the number of officers required far exceeded the number of those normally available to the Army and of regular officers available on completion of their training, the introduction of scientific methods of selection rendered possible the fullest and most economical utilisation of suitable officer material. Experience has established beyond doubt that such methods of selection, provided that they are efficiently organised and include a skilled psychiatric personality assessment as well as psychological and military tests, can at least increase by one-third the number of suitable officer candidates discovered by the conventional, unscientific methods.

Another significant example of the successful adaptation of selection techniques for specialised purposes was the procedure initiated by Army psychiatrists early in 1943, for the screening of paratroop volunteers with a view to reducing the wastage rate. Indeed, it was found that, of those volunteers accepted by the methods in use at that time, nearly one-quarter failed during parachute training, and that among those who succeeded in qualifying as parachutists there had been a heavy wastage during collective training in the battalions.

The psychiatrists who undertook the enquiry had, themselves, first been fully trained as parachutists. A screening process similar to that employed by the W.O.S.Bs. comprising a series of written tests, made it possible to select cases for individual psychiatric interview, and each volunteer received a psychiatric 'predictive' grading. Follow-up studies showed that psychiatric grades provided effective prediction of all forms of training wastage other than through accidental injuries.

As a result of this new method of selection, about 20 per cent. of paratroop volunteers were rejected at the initial selection stage, the great majority of these being rejected by the psychiatrist and by the medical officer. About 70 per cent. of all candidates arriving at the Airborne Forces Depot completed the course successfully, and the training wastage did not rise above 10 per cent. Thus, more than four-fifths of the total wastage was eliminated from the training period by selective methods.[1] It is therefore clear that, in this specialised field also, the application of scientific selection proved of very great value and achieved its purpose of reducing wastage of specifically trained personnel.

PROBLEMS OF MENTAL DEFECT AND DULLNESS

It is certain that the stresses and increased *tempo* of modern warfare, and the duties of the infantryman today, which demand a technical knowledge of a number of specialised weapons and the mastery of many skills, require not only emotional stability, but at least an average degree of intelligence; they present an impossible task to the dull man. Whereas he may have been self-supporting and capable of carrying out some simple job in civilian life, the dullard, placed among men of relatively higher intelligence in the Army, often became maladjusted and developed feelings of inferiority and anxiety. Being slow to learn, he held back the squad or class during training and aroused antagonism and impatience in his comrades and instructors—a state of affairs which was detrimental both to his personal morale and to that of the group.

A great problem was, therefore, created by the introduction of such men into the Army when it became necessary to make the fullest possible effective use of men of low intelligence, because of the considerable and urgent demands of the Fighting Services, civil defence, industry and agriculture, on our limited resources of man-power.

The maladjustment of men of low intelligence in the Army very soon began to manifest itself in many ways; particularly so because of the complete lack of any adequate psychiatric examination or selection procedure at intake in the first years of the war and the absence of administrative provision for the special allocation, or for discharge, of dullards who had been taken into the Army. It gave rise to mental instability and breakdown; it was a frequent cause of military delinquency, particularly absenteeism, and the dullard often became a disciplinary problem in his unit through failure to understand the nature of regulations and the reason for them. There is also most positive evidence that the incidence of venereal disease, scabies and pediculosis and the general sickness rate, were appreciably greater among dullards than among men of average intelligence.[1]

With the introduction of adequate selection procedure, which eventually rendered possible the posting of recruits in the lowest intelligence groups from Primary Training Centres direct to the appropriate section of the Pioneer Corps, it was found that the morale and performance of dullards so allocated showed considerable improvement, with a corresponding decrease in the incidence among them of the various manifestations of maladjustment that have been mentioned. Living and working together with men of like capability, and with the benefit of special assistance in matters of education and welfare, they became better adjusted to their new environment, more efficient, and definitely far less of a problem than when they had been distributed throughout the Army. Nevertheless, it is hardly surprising that the Pioneers remained a greater liability than other units to the medical and disciplinary authorities.

There were, unfortunately, many changes in administrative policy concerning the disposal and allocation of dullards, their employment in arms of the Service other than the Pioneer Corps, and the organisation and functions of the latter (and of its armed and unarmed sections). These administrative deficiencies and, worse still, the vacillating inconsistencies in policy, could not but provide a considerable body of evidence (if this were needed) as to the futility of attempting to employ on more skilled duties men who, as a result of selection tests and psychiatric examination, had been found suitable only for service in armed or unarmed units of the Pioneer Corps.[1]

It was not until January 1942, that adequate provisions were made, in an Army Council Instruction (A.C.I. 84/42), for the discharge or allocation of dull and backward soldiers: *viz.*, (*a*) the medical discharge of all those (unstable dullards) whose mental backwardness rendered them permanently unfit for any form of military service; (*b*) the transfer to an unarmed unit of the Pioneer Corps of those who were emotionally stable, but so dull and backward that they were not fit to bear arms, though fit for routine manual work; and (*c*) the transfer to an armed company of the Pioneer Corps of those who were emotionally stable, but had a capacity to learn which was much below average (and, it was somewhat unnecessarily added, were therefore unlikely to benefit by advanced training), though fit to bear arms.

It is therefore evident (as was indeed to be expected) from experience in the Second World War, that men of low mental capacity are of limited military value. Where, however, it is imperative to make the fullest possible use of available man-power, the Army can employ stable dullards on simple labouring duties, provided that they are organised into separate units, according to their fitness to use arms in self-defence or, alternatively, for an unarmed unit only. Thus segregated, stable dullards maintain a high level of morale and do not constitute an appreciable disciplinary, medical and psychiatric problem, or a threat to the morale and efficiency of men of higher intelligence, as is in general the case when they are present as misfits in an ordinary military unit. Furthermore, their employment on simple labouring duties releases men of higher intelligence for more skilled work. Unstable dullards, on the other hand, are not fit for any form of military service, and any attempt to employ them in the Army on the specious grounds that they should not be permitted to 'evade' military service inevitably results in the placing on the military medical and non-medical authorities of a burden out of all proportion to the numbers, and practical value to the Army, of these men, who may nevertheless be employed in some limited, but socially useful and personally beneficial, capacity in civil life.

PROBLEMS OF MORALE

The fact should be recorded, as one of the lessons for military medicine derived from the war, that it was the senior officers of both 'A' and 'G' Staffs who very soon became aware of the importance of the contributions which could be made by Army psychiatry to the understanding and management of many problems relating to morale; whereas the medical administrative authorities, on the other hand, frequently showed by their decisions and attitudes throughout the war that they had failed to appreciate the immense potential value of applied psychiatry in this field.

In order to evaluate the essential significance of psychiatry in this connexion, it is, in the first place, necessary fully to understand the complex nature and extensive ramifications of a matter of such fundamental military importance as morale. It is to the exceptional insight of Field-Marshal Montgomery[28, 29] into the problems concerned, that we are largely indebted for a clear and comprehensive exposition of the several factors which require to be taken into consideration, correctly assessed and carefully weighed, by the commander, if he is to build and maintain a high morale and fighting efficiency in a modern army at war. This itself necessarily demands for its practical realisation an informed and inspired leadership.

It has already been emphasised that the individual must needs be considered in relation to his social environment. Consequently, individual and group morale are also inevitably interdependent, and cannot be regarded as isolated states. It must ever be borne in mind that—in the words of Field-Marshal Montgomery—'an army is not merely a collection of individuals, with so many tanks, guns, machine-guns, etc. . . . . The raw material with which the general has to deal is men.'[29]* 'Man is still the first weapon of war. His training is the most important consideration in the fashioning of a fighting army. All modern science is directed towards his assistance, but on his efforts depends the outcome of the battle. The morale of the soldier is the most important single factor in war.'[28]

Just as, in Pascal's phrase, 'man is but a reed, of all nature the weakest; but he is a thinking reed', so it may be that the soldier in war is but a pawn, but it should never be forgotten that, constituting as he does the 'raw material', he is for all that a thinking pawn. The following appraisal by Field-Marshal Montgomery[29] is highly relevant in this respect: 'It is essential to understand that battles are won primarily in the hearts of men. When Britain goes to war the ranks of her armed forces are filled with men from civil life who are not soldiers, sailors or airmen by profession, and who never wanted to be.' The young man today, by means of the knowledge he acquires from newspapers, cinema, radio and television, 'can now measure his everyday environment in a way which was impossible in the Victorian era . . . He can think, he can appreciate, and is definitely prepared to criticise. He wants to know what is going on, and what you want him to do—and why, and when. He wants to know that in the doing of it his best interests will be absolutely secure in your hands.' There is no room in the modern Army for the Tennysonian concept, 'Theirs not to reason why'. The soldier today will in general be prepared to do whatever is required of him, so long as it is understood that he reserves the right to 'reason why'. If he is thus kept informed, and has the inspired leadership that is based on personal contact between the men and their officers and commander,—provided always that, in the first place, he is emotionally stable, well trained, and not suffering from campaign exhaustion—his morale, and consequently his military efficiency, will be of a very high order, and 'the greatest achievements become possible.'[29]

Men will not normally, and certainly should not, go into battle either like the suicidal, instinct-driven lemmings, or as the possessed Gadarene swine. Attempts in Battle Schools in 1942, to inculcate in fighting men an artificial, synthetic impetus of 'hate', once again, as in the First World War, were proved to be not only ineffective, but very definitely harmful to morale and efficiency, because they undermined one of the foundation stones of morale—human self-respect. What is required for efficiency in battle, as General Montgomery observed, is the building of a true offensive spirit combined with the will-power which will not

---

* ' . . . for it is the men that make a State, not walls nor ships devoid of men.'
(Thucydides, VII, p. 77)

recognise defeat[1]*—and this, of course, is dependent on morale and its constituent factors. The whole army should go into battle 'knowing what is wanted and how it is to be achieved . . . It is the spoken word which counts, from the commander to his troops; plain speech is far more effective than any written word.'[29]†

The part played by 'welfare' in relation to morale in a fighting force, should here be mentioned. The term 'welfare' has been widely and frequently used to include a number of different matters: e.g., the 'social welfare' concerned with a man's individual and family problems, the regular supply of mail and information about the home front; and, on the other hand, the provision of various amenities (canteens, entertainments, sporting equipment, etc.). These matters must not, however, be confused, as their relative importance to morale, and thus to individual and group efficiency, differs very greatly. The position has been well stated by Field-Marshal Montgomery,[28, 29] whose views are entirely supported by the considerable body of psychiatric and other evidence available concerning the conditions in the theatres overseas at different periods of the war: 'A man's ordinary day-to-day life must be well organised. Thus, hard conditions imposed on him in training to inculcate discipline do not rule out the desirability of good living-quarters; and in the line a soldier's morale will be much improved if the administrative arrangements are good and if he is assured of proper conditions,

---

* It should be noted that what is here referred to is the type of 'hate training' based on the encouragement of uninhibited, primitive instinctual and sadistic trends, and blood-lust, which are as 'unnatural' as they are undesirable manifestations in emotionally mature citizens of contemporary societies in Western civilisation; it is in this sense that they must be regarded (in the words of General Montgomery) as foreign to our national character.[1] These considerations are quite distinct from the need, in war-time propaganda, for representing the enemy as the 'bad object', and for 'dehumanising' and 'depersonalising' him, so far as possible, so that killing then loses some of its emotional impact for the civilised man who must learn to act in a way that conflicts with normally firmly established, and rigidly enforced, ethical and legal codes, and the consequently developed inhibitions affecting social patterns of behaviour. In war-time, it is obviously necessary to 'build' the true offensive spirit: 'The troops. . . must enter the fight with the light of battle in their eyes and definitely wanting to kill the enemy.'[29] To remove such (normally) socially desirable and fundamental inhibitions, and yet control and canalise them for a specific and vital purpose and subsequently, after a lengthy period in adult life, firmly to re-establish and re-enforce, them, is without doubt one of the most difficult problems in human psychology with which a civilised society may have to contend.—Cf. Ginzberg et al.[14] (2: 102 ff.), on the 'Conflict of Cultural Values'.

† The quality described by Max Weber as 'charismatic leadership'—and the ability to speak 'as one having authority' (*Matthew* vii. 29)—appears to have been possessed by some individuals, almost from the first 'syllable of recorded time'. In the military context, ancient history provides notable examples of certain commanders who were able to lead their men—who were far from being 'all unspotted soldiers'—in arduous campaigns and in adversity, even when medical science and logistics were extremely inadequate, if not indeed non-existent; and this, solely through a general intuitive appreciation of morale, and specifically, because they well knew how, and when, to address their forces.—Cf. especially, the account of the Peloponnesian War by Thucydides; also, Xenophon (*Anabasis*), who had so great an understanding of his men, that he was reproached with being 'too much a friend of the ordinary soldiers' (VII, 6); and, e.g., Caesar's speech to his troops (*Bellum Gallicum*, I, p. 40); etc.

with a reasonable amount of leisure and comfort when he leaves the front. But here a warning must be given. . . . Welfare by itself will not produce good morale because it is essentially soft; and . . . morale cannot be good unless it contains a quality of hardness. . . . Men will endure great hardships if they know why and are convinced of the necessity.'[28] 'Men dumped in some out-of-the-way spot in the desert will complain less of boredom, because they have to shift for themselves, than those surrounded with a wide choice of amenities.'[29]

The 'thinking soldier', not unnaturally, requires to be informed of the situation at home, to hear from his wife, family and friends, and to feel assured that he has been relieved (so far as possible) of any current domestic and financial worries; and also, that everything possible is being, or will be, done for his family, in the event of their being 'bombed out'. He is then in a far better position to adjust himself to the urgent military situation with which he is required to deal, without being distracted from his immediate and essential task, or 'driven to distraction', when it is necessary for him to concentrate on fighting the enemy, fulfilling to the best of his ability his particular rôle in the military plan and organisation, and maintaining a relative—and, in general, somewhat precarious—balance in his military environment, under considerable stress, from day to day. Referring to the mental health of a fighting force, Main[21] stated: 'The sense of separation from home, from its security and its comforting permanence and its familiar reassurance of one's personal status, is a permanent stress. A camaraderie is the only human recompense for a threatening sense of impotence in the face of death and the waywardness of elemental forces and the decisions of the mighty who use soldiers like pawns.'

It is highly relevant here briefly to refer to certain specific problems of morale, in the last war, which are of considerable importance from the military, psychiatric and 'educational' points of view.

The events which eventually led to the so-called 'Salerno mutiny' in September 1943, and were subsequently the subject of a careful investigation by an Army psychiatrist (T. F. Main), provide a most significant lesson that should not be allowed to be forgotten, as to the serious, and potentially disastrous, military consequences of ignoring certain principles essential to morale, and in particular, the fundamental importance to group morale of divisional loyalty and identification of individual soldiers with a specific unit, based on the development of mutual trust between the men and their own officers, and a spirit of comradeship. The circumstances of this incident, so far as they concern the subject of Army psychiatry, have been recorded in some detail elsewhere.[1] It may here be recalled, however, that the very great majority of those involved in this 'mutiny' were experienced fighting men of previously high morale—men willing and glad to face whatever the future might hold for them in the unit and community to which they felt they belonged, with their familiar officers and comrades; all were men who together had been through past battles and campaigns, and had been led to believe in a common prospect of rejoining in the field a division, brigade or battalion to which they were attached by bonds stronger than paper.*

There was, on the part of the local military authorities at the time, a total disregard (whether avoidable or not) of these well established group loyalties, in attempting to draft these men as reinforcements to other divisions, in the complete absence of any clear direction, precise information, or firm leadership throughout. And when, in addition to their initial bewilderment and their feeling of having been abandoned, on being charged with mutiny and taken into custody they were further demoralised by the humiliation of being subjected to ridicule by German prisoners-of-war and the contempt of their comrades in arms, their self-respect was badly—and very nearly, irreparably—damaged. The effect of these serious errors in man-management and leadership, was a gradual disintegration, first of carefully built-up and well tried group morale, and then of individual morale.

It should be emphasised that, in such unfortunate and avoidable incidents as the 'Salerno mutiny', and the 'Airborne mutiny' (in Malaya, 1946), these 'lesions of group morale' are almost invariably a direct consequence of disregard for, or ignorance of, basic principles essential to morale, as also of mismanagement, on the part of certain officers; and a result of neglect of one of their most important and elementary duties— that of attending to the welfare of their men.† Where officers fail in this respect, the men are at a serious disadvantage, in that no satisfactory means are available, through official administrative procedures, whereby other ranks may put forward, in however orderly and proper a manner, collective complaints or representations.[1] This is a matter of considerable importance, in so far as suitable provisions to this end would enable grievances, where these might be partly or wholly justified, to be redressed. Where the grievances were shown to be baseless, an opportunity would nevertheless have been provided to bring into the open, and disperse, unjustified and irrational complaints (which, however, might well be symptomatic of a low group morale). As Francis Bacon observed, 'To give moderate liberty for griefs and discontentments to evaporate (so it be without too great insolency or bravery), is a safe way; for he that turneth the humours back, and maketh

---

* As stated by an Army psychiatrist, A. T. M. Wilson, 'Officers and men cannot be attached and removed like articles of equipment. A unit is a living organism in which grafting is as difficult as in trees.'[1]

† Referring to the 'Salerno mutiny', General Montgomery stated (in 1944) that, where soldiers get into trouble of this nature, it is nearly always the fault of some officer who has failed in his duty.[1]

the wound bleed inwards, endangereth malign ulcers and pernicious imposthumations.'

In either case, the existence of adequate and well defined provisions for collective complaints would reduce to a minimum the risk of such regrettable and unnecessary incidents—most harmful to group morale and military efficiency—as those mentioned above. It would require careful consideration to decide whether this purpose could best be fulfilled by close and frequent personal contact, from day to day, between C.Os. and other officers, and their men; or whether it might be advisable, in addition, to institute some form of free and open group discussions, at regular intervals, of any matter that was considered of importance by the men of a given unit, where other ranks would be suitably represented, and which would be attended by the C.O. and (or) other experienced officers, and possibly also the unit medical officer (if he were adequately trained in this respect). Such discussions should, of course, be as informal as is possible in the military setting (where officers and other ranks are present), and yet be conducted with due regard to the necessary requirements of military discipline and propriety.

It is also important here to mention that the futility of the death penalty for desertion in war-time—a punishment so frequently and irresponsibly advocated as an alleged deterrent—has been demonstrated beyond doubt by a comparison of the incidence of desertion in the British Army in the two World Wars. Discipline is an integral part of morale, and in the absence of the latter will most certainly break down. Indeed, from the abundant evidence available, it should be clear and indisputable that morale depends not on threats, nor on driving, but on leading men.*

In summary, then, 'An army must be as hard as steel in battle and can be made so; but, like steel, it reaches its finest quality only after much preparation and only provided the ingredients are properly constituted and handled'.[29] It may be said that there are three essential requirements, representing the successive evolutionary stages in the building of morale in an Army at war.

First, it is clear that the 'raw material'—the human resources—must be basically sound. This is dependent upon adequate psychiatric and psychological screening, in order to ensure, so far as possible, the rejection at intake, or, where this has for some reason failed or not been

---

* Cf. Ahrenfeldt[1], Appendix B, pp. 271–5.—'In a word, it is. . . a mark of extreme simplicity for anyone to imagine that when human nature is wholeheartedly bent on any undertaking it can be diverted from it by rigorous laws or by any other terror. We must not, therefore, so pin our faith to the penalty of death as a guarantee against revolt as to make the wrong decision. . . "For he who is wise in counsel is stronger against the foe than he who recklessly rushes on with brute force." ' (Thucydides, III, pp. 45–48.)

practicable, the early segregation or discharge, of those men who, it can quite certainly be predicted, will exert a deleterious effect on group morale by reason of emotional instability, low mental capacity, inherent inadequacy, or of psychopathic, asocial or antisocial trends. Experience in the Second World War demonstrated conclusively that such psycho-social maladjustments in a fighting force manifest themselves sympto-matically, as psychiatric breakdown (under relatively minor stress), delinquency, absenteeism and desertion, alcoholism, frequent minor illness, a high incidence of V.D., or abysmal inefficiency or obstructive-ness;[1] and these must obviously result in a very considerable wastage of available man-power and a serious impairment of efficiency, which cannot be afforded by a nation such as ours, with necessarily limited human resources, engaged in total defensive warfare. It cannot too often be repeated, that 'the Army is an organisation for the defence of the nation and is not to be considered as a corrective institution'. [38] It is, however, possible, and indeed imperative, to eliminate at the outset important basic causes of low individual and group morale, by the removal of the potential 'misfit', and also, through correct scientific allocation procedure, by preventing the wasteful and demoralising effects which must inevitably ensue from the employment of men on unsuitable jobs.

Secondly, having thus ensured, by adequate methods of selection and allocation, the quality of the 'raw material', the latter can, and must, then be tempered by thorough training based on sound psychological, as well as military, principles (including, e.g., the correct use of 'battle inoculation', and the avoidance of any such primitive, exotic and delusory methods as 'hate training').[1]

Thirdly, such 'raw material' of good quality, thus tempered by sound training, and so brought to the highest point of individual efficiency, can then—as Field-Marshal Montgomery[28] has expressed it—be welded into a cohesive whole. This is achieved by the development of group loyalty, singleness of purpose and a common, well defined aim, and true discipline, under the influence of informed and inspired leadership. But, however great the leader's ability, this end will yet be no more attainable than some alchemical transmutation, if the individuals concerned prove to be basically poor material, either because of defective selection and allocation procedures, or as a result of inadequate and insufficient training.

FORWARD PSYCHIATRY

From the large amount of available evidence concerning the Second World War,[1] there can be no doubt as to the value of forward psychiatry, in such matters as the relationship between morale, emotional stability and mental capacity, and desertion during fighting; and the fundamental importance of adequate selection and allocation in drafts proceeding overseas, in preventing psychiatric breakdown and ensuring the maintenance of high morale and optimal military efficiency among soldiers under conditions of stress in battle, or after prolonged service abroad and separation from home. Circumstances demonstrated all too clearly the serious consequences of the absence of any scientific selection procedure at the outbreak of hostilities, and their subsequent repercussions throughout the war. It was also found, as psychiatrists and psychologists had predicted, that certain formations, where the commander had insisted upon very careful sorting of his men, proved highly efficient in battle and showed an outstandingly low rate of psychiatric casualties. On the other hand, in those units whose personnel was far below the necessary standard of selection, and which contained, in consequence, a large proportion of men of low intelligence, precarious mental stability, 'misfits' and incorrectly allocated individuals, and too many dull N.C.Os.,* there was a very high incidence of psychiatric disorders.

In discussing the basic problems of forward psychiatry, Main[21] well observed that 'The mental health of a fighting force is not the same thing as the mental health of a nation at war. With the differing functions, different standards are needed. If a sergeant can recover his poise for one month, it can be regarded as a satisfactory therapeutic result in an Army fighting for its very life, though such a result would not be worth having in civilian life. Then the stresses which such a man must be capable of withstanding are very different from those which would operate upon him in civilian life—and they must be fully understood by the psychiatrist. Lastly, the positive factors which will support the mental health of such a man are different in the forward area from those in the rear areas. The job of the psychiatrist, in fact, demands a grasp of the social as well as the medical variants which influence treatment and disposal.' It was necessary for Army psychiatrists to modify and adapt their techniques in forward areas to the incidence, treatment and disposal of psychiatric casualties under widely varying conditions of environment and warfare in the several theatres of operations overseas, at different periods of the war. It is not, therefore, surprising that 'one campaign does not seem to train a psychiatrist automatically for another.'[21]

It is unfortunately necessary to recognise the fact that, even today, intelligent and educated laymen and medical men alike not infrequently adopt the pharisaic and facile attitude, that no man should break down, nor indeed be 'allowed' to break down, in battle. In effect, they labour

---

* One important field of research in which little was done in the last war, and which would deserve most careful study and attention, is the selection of N.C.Os., especially in war-time when very large numbers are required.

under the delusion 'that somehow courage and cowardice are alternative free choices that come to every man, overriding all emotional stress, and that a man... can be courageous if he is told he must be.'[33] Such wishful thinking is in part due to a regrettable ignorance of well established psychological principles; but it is, more specifically, referable to an affective myopia, or hemianopia, which itself is but a precarious defence against deep-seated personal anxiety and insecurity that has not been permitted to enter the restricted conscious range or field of vision.

It has been established beyond doubt that, however successful may be the prophylaxis of psychiatric breakdown (including adequate initial selection and allocation), and however effective the promotion of positive mental health and morale, wherever fighting is in progress psychiatric casualties will nevertheless inevitably occur; and that when the fighting is severe the number of these casualties becomes such as to constitute a military problem. In the British Army in the Second World War, psychiatric casualties comprised on an average some 10 per cent. of total battle casualties. Depending on the type of battle—and therefore the nature and degree of the specific stresses—figures varied from 2 per cent. to 30 per cent.*

On the basis of experience derived from a study of over 12,000 cases in three theatres of war during $4\frac{1}{2}$ years with the British Forces in the Second World War, Palmer[31] considered that a psychiatric service for a task force required five subsidiary organisations. The aim of psychiatrists with the armies overseas was, wherever possible, and subject to necessary local modifications according to the specific type of warfare, to provide a psychiatric service on these, or similar, lines:

(*i*) *and* (*ii*) *The Filtration Units:*

(i) the Forward Filtration, or Corps Exhaustion Centre, attached to a C.C.S.;

(ii) the Main Filtration Centre, or Advanced Psychiatric Wing of a forward general hospital.

(*iii*) *The Rehabilitation Centre.*

(*iv*) *and* (*v*) *The Base Psychiatric Units:*

(iv) the Base Psychiatric Wing of a base general hospital;

(v) an Evacuation Unit, which should ideally be attached to the main evacuation hospital for the command.

---

* As Main[21] has recorded, 'When the numbers are high during a big battle, you may imagine the alarm in high places, the increase in diagnosis of "cowardice" by administrative staffs, and the reluctance to recognise the problem as a psychiatric one... One popular view at such times—popular in rear areas at least—is that access to the psychiatrist will discourage the fighting men who are sticking it out. This may be so, but I have yet to meet a regimental medical officer who knows of a single instance of a good man being discouraged by the knowledge that if he became a casualty of any sort he would get looked after.'

The first four of these constituent units were to be regarded as providing the means of restoring the psychiatric casualty by a process of rehabilitation (which included an immediate phase of psychiatric first-aid). The fifth unit was intended for the ultimate disposal of the residual casualties who were permanently unfit for further military service with the force.

As summarised by Kenton,[19] the military problem arising from this type of battle casualty resolves itself into the following several objects: first, to prevent psychiatric casualties from impeding actual fighting operations, or the evacuation and treatment of the wounded; secondly, the selection and treatment of those casualties who would be capable of early return to further effective combatant duties; thirdly, the prevention of deterioration in those unable to return early, or at all, to further combatant duty; and finally, due consideration of the factor of long-term conservation of man-power.

With adequate triage at R.A.P. and M.D.S., and a properly constituted 'Exhaustion Centre' at C.C.S. level or its equivalent (e.g., one F.D.S. taken over for the purpose), it is possible to return the majority of men to their units within a week (in the Second World War, the proportion varied from 70 per cent. to 56 per cent.—and only some 5 per cent. of these broke down again in the same battle). It must be emphasised that the whole success of forward psychiatry depends on early treatment, the essentials of which are adequate sedation by the regimental medical officer immediately after the breakdown, and continuance of this sedation at the M.D.S. and Corps Exhaustion Centre. (The results were as good as those quoted only when treatment could be given first within a matter of hours.) Cases of poor prognosis alone should be evacuated to the base. It is also essential that patients from psychiatric rehabilitation units should proceed direct to their future unit without an intermediate period of waiting in R.H.Us. if they are to avoid subsequent deterioration. It requires a high degree of morale, and also of mental stability, to withstand boredom and inaction. Men recently recovered from a psychiatric breakdown are obviously not fit to endure this negative kind of strain. Indeed, it must be emphasised that the best therapeutic results can be obtained only where it is possible to ensure that the whole progress from breakdown to final return to active, effective duty shall be continuous.[1]

In the light of experience in the Second World War it is certain that modern mechanised warfare imposes on the individual a strain so great that men involved in active fighting, however basically stable they may be, will ultimately break down, in direct relation to the intensity and duration of their exposure to the stress of battle (i.e., if they do not, within a sufficient time, obtain relief from such stress, either in the matter of its intensity or of its duration). Thus, psychiatric casualties of the type described as 'campaign exhaustion' are as inevitable as gunshot and shrapnel wounds in modern warfare.

Detailed American investigations by Appel and Beebe[4] in the Italian Campaign in the Second World War, showed that for the infantryman, who is exposed to the greatest danger and the greatest stress, the point at which complete breakdown occurred and the soldier became ineffective was, at the most, in the region of 200 to 240 'aggregate combat days' (10 combat days being taken, in this instance, as equivalent to 17 calendar days), and in the majority of cases, very much earlier. By the end of this period in the line the average soldier was 'worn out' and had either developed an acute incapacitating neurosis, or else become 'hypersensitive to shell fire, so overly cautious and jittery that he was ineffective and demoralising to newer men.' The number of men who were still on duty after this amount of consecutive combat experience was small and their value to their units was negligible. 'From the Sicilian Campaign onward, it was noted that an increasing number of the psychiatric patients being sent back from the lines were not "weaklings" who had merely broken down after a short exposure to combat but experienced veterans . . . with excellent combat records'—for the most part, N.C.Os. Many of the line officers were emphatically of the opinion that, in this campaign, a man reached his peak of effectiveness in the first 90 days of combat, after which his efficiency began to fall off and he became progressively less valuable, until finally he was useless. Most men, in their experience, were ineffective after 140 to 180 days. As compared with the acute psychiatric breakdown under stress in battle, the soldier who suffered from campaign exhaustion and was 'worn out' was subsequently useless as a combat soldier, and at least six months would have been required to make him once more effective for this purpose (although, of course, he still might be very usefully employed on non-combatant duties).

These authors made the following interesting and significant observations on comparative American and British experience in this respect, in this same campaign: 'The effective combat life of the average infantryman appears to depend largely on how continuously he is used in combat. The British, for example, estimate that their riflemen in Italy will last about 400 regimental combat days, about twice as long as U.S. riflemen in the heavily used U.S. divisions in Italy. They attribute the difference to their policy of pulling infantrymen out of the line at the end of twelve days or less for a rest of four days. The American soldier in Italy, on the other hand, was usually kept in the line without relief for twenty to thirty days, frequently for thirty to forty and occasionally for eighty days. Although tactical requirements may have required this policy, the fact that a man wears out in combat has apparently been insufficiently recognised by command.'

Similarly, Swank and Marchand[36] noted that, in the Normandy Campaign, from D-day until the break-through, when the stress of combat was continuous and severe and rests were infrequent and usually for no longer than one day, combat exhaustion in U.S. infantrymen occurred, in the majority of cases, in about 30 days, and otherwise, in from 15 to 50 days. 'One thing alone seems certain: practically all infantry soldiers suffer from a neurotic reaction eventually if they are subjected to the stress of modern combat continuously and long enough.'

Experience has shown that Corps and Divisional Psychiatrists are of proved value in the field in an advisory and supervisory capacity, and the latter in particular serve an essential function in theatres of war where local conditions make it necessary for divisions to operate independently.* Another very important aspect of divisional psychiatry, apart from tactical considerations in a specific theatre at a given time, is the fact that, as Field-Marshal Montgomery[29] has pointed out, all divisions are different, because the men of which they consist are themselves—as a group—very different (e.g., according to the region from which they have been recruited, and consequently, their particular character and abilities): 'In the 1914–18 war, if ten divisions were needed for an offensive, the staff would take the ten most easily assembled. But a division develops an individuality of its own, which the higher command must study and thus learn the type of battle each is best at.'†

In order to ensure effective measures of psychiatric prophylaxis and therapy in units and in the field, it is necessary to supply sufficient numbers of Command and Area Psychiatrists, and, in overseas theatres, Corps and Divisional Psychiatrists, as well as Psychiatric Consultants and Advisers, who must, together with the nucleus of a psychiatric organisation, accompany any force which is being sent overseas.‡

* In January 1918, the U.S. War Department created the position of divisional psychiatrist, and this—its first recognition of the utility to the Army, in the field, of psychiatric specialists—'proved of the utmost importance.'[37] In the British Army in the Second World War, Divisional Psychiatrists were of fundamental importance in the Burma campaigns. Similarly, in the C.M.F., at a late stage of that campaign, divisions changed their corps frequently and at relatively short notice, thereby very considerably reducing the efficacy of forward psychiatry based on a corps structure, and the undoubted advantages, in these circumstances, of a system involving the use of Divisional Psychiatrists very soon became apparent.[1]

† The 'Salerno mutiny', which has been mentioned above, provides an example of the importance of divisional 'individuality', and consequently, group loyalty, and the danger to morale and military efficiency of ignoring these essential factors.

‡ Because of intense hostility and opposition on the part of both medical and non-medical administrative authorities with the First Army in North Africa, it was impossible to arrange for an adequate psychiatric organisation in the B.N.A.F. during the Tunisian Campaign. The medical authorities had therefore made no arrangements and had sent out no hospital for the treatment of psychiatric casualties when the Force landed early in November 1942. The consequent serious and avoidable psychiatric difficulties which arose during this campaign provide sufficient evidence in this respect, should it be required. The absence of a psychiatric organisation, through similar administrative opposition, in Malta during the siege (June–November 1942), is yet another notable example (and it might be hoped, a 'lesson') of unnecessary suffering and disability, as well as military inefficiency, resulting from the lack of essential specialised medical personnel at such a time.[1]

REHABILITATION (FOR MILITARY AND CIVIL LIFE)

It has already been mentioned that some of the most significant advances in Army psychiatry, during the Second World War, were in the field of 'social psychiatry'. This was particularly true of certain experiments which led to the development and application of techniques of rehabilitation.

In an excellent survey of the general principles here involved, Main[24] observed that 'Rehabilitation is not . . . a process which concerns only the individual, but an interreactive relationship between a dynamic environment and a dynamic individual. It is a two-way process and implies mutual adaptation between two dynamic structures.' Given the capacity for adaptation in the individual, rehabilitation techniques must be directed towards the 'provision by the environment of the opportunities to adapt to it.' Similarly, Bion and Rickman[6] stated that 'psychology and psychopathology have focused attention on the individual often to the exclusion of the social field of which he is a part. There is a useful future in the study of the interplay of individual and social psychology, . . . and war-time makes this study an urgent issue.'

These experiments were principally concerned with the military or civil rehabilitation of men suffering from psychiatric disorders, military delinquents, the civil rehabilitation and resettlement of repatriated prisoners-of-war, and of soldiers with severe physical disabilities.

The most important lesson that is to be learnt in this connexion from the experience of the Second World War is that so far as is possible, it is absolutely essential to decide in every case, at the outset, whether it is proposed to rehabilitate the individual in question for further effective military service, or alternatively, for a self-dependent, useful and adequate place in civilian life. The importance of making such a decision from the very start, and of segregating and rehabilitating these two groups according to their respective, and necessarily divergent, needs, cannot be over-emphasised.

There is no doubt whatsoever, in the light of medical experience, that, in mixing these two groups and adopting a temporising policy of 'wait-and-see', the very best techniques designed for military and civil rehabilitation respectively, will quite certainly fail. A man with any disability (whether physical, mental, or both) requiring rehabilitation cannot be left suspended between military and civil life, and yet be expected satisfactorily to adapt himself and return to one or the other of these very different environments. The situation encountered (whatever the type of disability) is well illustrated by the two following examples, which refer to the rehabilitation of neurotic soldiers in the British and American Armies, respectively:—

When psychoneurotic soldiers who required to be discharged to civil life were mixed, in a military hospital, with those whom it was intended to return to the Army (and, therefore, to transfer, after medical treatment, to a military 'Training Wing'), it was found—as stated by Foulkes[12]—that 'the contrast posed for all the problem of the future and showed the unwilling soldier his first target, namely, to remain sufficiently ill and unserviceable to the Army to avoid his transfer to khaki and the Training Wing.'

On the other hand, in the case of those men whom it was necessary to discharge to civil life, Ginzberg[14] has noted: 'Many of the soldiers who broke down because they could no longer cope with the demands that the military situation made on them were on their way to recovery as of the moment they received their discharge papers. The Army found that its elaborate efforts to rehabilitate soldiers prior to discharge were frequently ineffective because many men remained depressed and despondent as long as they continued to be in uniform.'

The experiments in the rehabilitation of the several categories mentioned above, in the British Army in the Second World War, are briefly summarised below.

(a) REHABILITATION AND DISPOSAL OF PSYCHIATRIC CASES

In general, experience in the last war tends to show that military psychiatric hospitals are best suited to deal with patients whom it is proposed to rehabilitate for further service in the Army. The maintenance of a modified military organisation and atmosphere not only is essential to bring about the greatest possible degree of re-adaptation to military life, but also greatly facilitates the continuity of treatment, rehabilitation, and subsequent appropriate reallocation according to the individual's capacities and limitations. This was clearly shown by the experience derived from the gradual evolution of the Northfield Military Hospital in dealing with psychoneurotic cases.[1] In particular, specialised techniques of group discussion and group psychotherapy were successfully adapted to the treatment and rehabilitation of these cases, by Bion and Rickman,[5, 6] Foulkes,[12] and Main[22] and his colleagues.

Where the value of such a hospital, when correctly organised, for the military rehabilitation of neurotic soldiers, became clearly apparent, was with the opening of the Second Front, in June 1944. The majority of patients admitted at that time were not chronic, inadequate neurotics, but young, active soldiers who had broken down in battle. As a result, in November 1944, a new phase—the so-called 'Northfield Experiment' —was initiated. A military staff was selected who had acquired positive understanding of the psychiatric point of view, and, in particular, of group-psychological orientation, through experience with the War Office Selection Boards. The Hospital was gradually allowed to develop into a self-responsible community, with some degree of self-government in so far as the organisation and activities of the community were concerned. The former dichotomy between chronic neurotics requiring to be discharged from the Army, and others who became fit for return to military duties, as also between the 'Hospital Wing' and 'Training Wing', no longer existed, and the 'Training Wing' was replaced by a Convalescent Depot through which most patients passed who were returning to the Army.[8, 12, 22]

A highly important factor in the successful military rehabilitation of psychoneurotic patients was their suitable disposal and employment after discharge from hospital. In the earlier part of the war, it was found that many such patients, who had responded well to treatment, relapsed after they had returned to their original units and duties—a situation which was largely remedied as a result of later experience at Northfield and elsewhere. The procedure ('Annexure' Scheme) that was introduced first in 1941, largely at the suggestion of Professor Aubrey Lewis, made possible the reallocation of these men to the most appropriate type of employment (whether in a restricted or a full capacity).[45] The employment recommendations were originally made by psychiatrists, and subsequently by the Personnel Selection services when these had become more generally available (at the end of 1943). The importance of this procedure is shown by the fact that some 60 per cent. of men who had suffered from neuroses and would otherwise have been considered suitable only for discharge, were thus retained in the Army, at a time when the man-power situation was acute. About five-sixths of these (50 per cent. of the total) continued to give satisfactory service in their new work, were contented and had made an adequate adjustment. This experiment was thus proved to be fully justified.[1]

Where it is apparent, on the other hand, that a patient is unfit for further effective military service, and requires either prolonged psychiatric treatment in hospital, or to be discharged from the Army as soon as possible and rehabilitated for civil life, it would seem that these functions can be best fulfilled by civil psychiatric hospitals, which also have, in general, greater facilities with regard to staff, the more complex forms of therapy, and after-care. As already mentioned, the civilian orientation of therapeutic and rehabilitative activities in these hospitals will be most likely to benefit the Serviceman who requires to be discharged from the forces and rehabilitated for a useful and adequate rôle in a civilian environment.

As stated by Main,[24] 'There is increasing recognition that the "results of treatment" cannot safely be judged by the clinical state of the patient after "treatment", but only by the extent to which he makes a good subsequent adaptation to his domestic, social and industrial environment. . . . The life performance after illness is, of course, the criterion of biological adaptation, and plainly a cure that is not succeeded by rehabilitation is no cure at all.' It is apparent that, in the Second World War, our efforts, whether in military or in civil (E.M.S.) hospitals, to rehabilitate for civil life psychoneurotics who were discharged from the Army, did not meet with that measure of success which might have been anticipated. Two significant and detailed follow-up investigations were undertaken by psychiatrists and psychiatric social workers, of the readjustment in civil life of men who had been discharged from the Army, after treatment in military or civil hospitals between 1941 and 1943, on account of neurosis. Lewis[20] found that, in 120 soldiers so discharged, after an average period of some 6 months in civilian life (at a time of full employment) one-half were earning less than their usual civilian wages, one-third were experiencing domestic or social difficulties, and one-half had been under medical care; one-third of the potential working days of the group had been spent in unemployment. Guttmann and Thomas,[16] investigating a series of 382 soldiers thus discharged, found that 75 per cent. of these men received medical attention during the next 15 months; nearly all of them lost working time through illness (the absence rate was 13 per cent. of the time at risk); and about 10 per cent. showed signs of serious domestic and social maladjustment. Lewis[20] found that, in his series, approximately 6 months after discharge from the Army, 12 per cent. were unemployed, and only 50 per cent. could be classed as socially satisfactory in respect of work and general adjustment. On the other hand, Guttmann and Thomas[16] noted, in their series of cases, that, after 15 months, 6 per cent. of the men were unemployed, i.e., only half of the incidence found by Lewis at a shorter interval after discharge—which 'shows a gradual process of adjustment.'

While there was, therefore, an obvious relative effectiveness in a number of these cases of the *vis temporis medicatrix*, aided, no doubt, by previous therapy, removal of situational stresses and change of environment, this process of 'natural readjustment' could hardly be relied on for a permanent and universal 'cure'. Some of the difficulties involved, in this connexion, have been well stated by Ginzberg[14]: 'Since so many who had broken down had succumbed to pressures in the military situation, they started to recover as soon as they had . . . received their discharge. But leaving a burdensome and traumatic situation was only half the story. Many soldiers soon discovered that civilian life was also full of problems and pressures, many of which would tax them to the utmost. Some came back to family situations that had greatly deteriorated during their absence and found that their hopes and plans for the future which had helped to sustain them during many difficult periods while they were in the Service would have to be radically revised.' It is not surprising also, because it was an index of the stability and maturity of the individual, that 'The quality of a soldier's performance in the Army prior to discharge was found to be an important predictor of his performance after his return to civilian life.'[14]

It should be noted that the difficult problem of the rehabilitation and disposal of psychoneurotic soldiers not only was a matter of experiment and of trial and error, but was also necessarily determined to some extent by the changing man-power requirements of the Army consequent upon the exigencies of the military situation at a given time. It was, however, very wisely decided by the authorities (at the end of 1943)—and all the more so because of the need to utilise to the fullest advantage the limited available military medical resources—that admissions of neurotics to military hospitals would be restricted to cases in which there was a high probability of return, after treatment and rehabilitation, to full regimental duties.[1]

In general, it may be said that all available evidence tends to support the opinion expressed by J. R. Rees,[33] after five years' experience in the Second World War, that 'probably over all it would be better to have any man whom it is hoped to send back to the Army under care in a military hospital all the time, and only use civilian hospitals for the necessary rehabilitation of those who are going back to civil occupations.'

(b) REHABILITATION AND DISPOSAL OF DELINQUENTS

In general, the question of the rehabilitation and disposal of delinquents has not been dealt with adequately or realistically by the Army, any more than by the civil authorities. Nevertheless, two significant and enlightened experiments were carried out during the Second World War in the social rehabilitation of military delinquents whom it was considered necessary to retain in the Army for reasons of man-power policy: i.e., the formation of Special Training Units (S.T.Us.) for young soldiers (up to the age of 21 years), and of Command Labour Companies for older men who were 'habitual bad characters', chronic absentees, etc. These experiments, which were undertaken between 1942 and 1945, and have been described in some detail elsewhere,[1] suffered, particularly in the early stages, from inadequate selection of the cases which it was proposed to rehabilitate in these units. An attempt was, however, made to grade these men in broad groups, and to allocate each group accordingly to a specific unit; and, so far as they were available, psychiatrists and Personnel Selection teams gradually sorted out the men to be sent to these units, and eliminated the dull and unstable individuals who required to be discharged from the Army. It was, of course, the purpose of these units, through non-penal methods of modified military training, etc., to rehabilitate the delinquents for military service. There were, inevitably, considerable difficulties in obtaining suitable staff for the units, as is indeed the case in civil and military penal establishments, even when the nation's man-power is not principally committed to the urgent exigencies of a major world war.

The S.T.Us. constituted an important and promising experiment in social rehabilitation, which came to an end while still in its early stages. With the average offender it was found that the methods of modified military training in a special unit produced very satisfactory results; in spite of certain limitations, it was estimated that over 75 per cent. of the trainees made a good adjustment on returning to their ordinary units. With the more complex anti-social individual, rehabilitation by this system was not so readily achieved; it is in the treatment of these latter cases, as well as in the selection of trainees, that psychiatrists, had they been available, could have made a valuable contribution to the experiment.

Experience with the Labour Companies showed that the chronic absentee is frequently a military misfit who is 'redeemable', i.e., able to give efficient service in a non-penal unit, but only if the latter is specially staffed; otherwise, the mistakes of previous units will tend to be repeated. It was found that such Companies can save C.Os. much administrative and training time and that they also contribute to the morale of normal units by disposing of the impression that the chronic absentee obtains his discharge through his offences. In practice these non-penal Companies proved a successful experiment and justified the imaginative outlook of those who planned them; they rehabilitated at least one-third of the men sent to them.

In summary, it may be said that experience suggests that the only satisfactory method of dealing with military delinquents, from the point of view of economy of man-power and money, is to subject them to a thorough scientific process of sorting principally based on a psychiatric personality assessment (and, of course, routine intelligence tests, etc.), in order that their further potential usefulness to the Army may be accurately determined. Men who, on the basis of personality and military record, are regarded as redeemable for further useful military service should be rehabilitated by the Army in suitable units or institutions, which must, however, be such as to foster in the men who are sent there high individual and group morale. Chronic offenders, men with long and serious criminal records in civil life, unstable and anti-social psychopathic types with severe personality disorders, are useless to the Army, exert an adverse effect on morale and efficiency out of all proportion to their numbers, and involve the Service in a completely unjustifiable expenditure of money and man-power which it can ill afford. Such individuals, who are irredeemable for military service, would better be dealt with, as regards detention and rehabilitation for civil life, by the civil authorities (who, it may be hoped, will gradually develop more progressive, constructive and scientific methods in their penal system). It is, in any case, essential that the Army should cease to be regarded by many—(not only by civilians, but even within its own organisation)—as a suitable penal colony upon which may be unloaded such social misfits, on the specious grounds that the latter should not be permitted to 'evade' military service and that the Army can, or indeed has the time and resources to 'make men of them'.[2]

(c) CIVIL RESETTLEMENT OF REPATRIATED PRISONERS-OF-WAR

It was already a well recognised fact from experience in the First World War that repatriated prisoners-of-war show evidence of considerable psychological instability and maladjustment, and have great difficulty in resocialisation and reintegration in the community. As an ever increasing number of such men returned to the United Kingdom during the Second World War (from 1943 onwards), and at the end of hostilities, it soon became apparent that their basic problems in this respect were in no way different from those encountered in the previous war.* Preliminary investigations and experiments confirmed the view that it is essential to provide special units with the specific function of aiding the psychological rehabilitation and civil resettlement of these men, if they are not subsequently to become social misfits and a burden to the community. Between 1945 and 1947 special Civil Resettlement Units (C.R.Us.) established by the Army for this purpose, successfully carried out the rehabilitation of a large number of repatriated prisoners-of-war. (Although attendance was voluntary, a total of some 19,000 ex-European, and 4,500 ex-Japanese, prisoners-of-war passed through the C.R.Us. in the period of approximately 2 years during which these units functioned.)[1]

The basic problem which had to be faced was that of the soldier's transition from the authoritarian military community, where his individual responsibility and initiative had been limited, and he had necessarily become dependent (or, indeed, over-dependent) on authority for the provision of his needs and the direction of his activities, to civil life in a democratic community, where he was expected suddenly to assume an appreciable degree of personal responsibility and initiative, and himself to become the figure of 'authority' who must direct and provide for himself and his family. It was thus almost inevitable that the Army's decision—however right it may have been—to undertake the responsibility in this unaccustomed rôle of rehabilitating repatriates, should lead to difficulties in fitting civil resettlement into a military framework; for the function of the C.R.Us. was not to make or train soldiers, but

---

* 'This evidence. . . was strongly supported by the abundant testimony offered at this time by ex-Ps.O.W. of World War I, many of whom gave accounts of distress and difficulties of an unusually pervasive kind which had over a period of many years influenced wide areas of their behaviour and disturbed personal relationships of the greatest importance to them.'[10]

to create good and effective civilian citizens, and reintroduce the returned soldier to civil life. The C.R.Us. were, therefore, transitional, but 'democratic', communities, and their atmosphere was necessarily largely civilian. Although the majority of men elected to wear their uniform, and the officers on the staff were for the most part military, the usual discipline and routine of Army life were excluded from these units.

The aim of the C.R.U. was to enable men not only to learn about post-war civil life and receive such specialist advice as they required, but to live as members of a free society while they were in the unit, and to reintegrate themselves within the civilian community in general, and their home environment in particular. They received vocational guidance, had the opportunity of practising former trades or acquiring new skills and were given expert assistance and advice on their many domestic and financial difficulties.[1]*

The most important aspect of all, however, was the resocialisation of the individual, principally by the application to the specific problems with which the C.R.Us. had to deal, of techniques of group therapy (Wilson, Doyle and Kelnar[41, 42]), aided where necessary by individual psychotherapy.

A carefully controlled and representative follow-up investigation was undertaken of socially comparable samples (in the same area) of re-patriated prisoners-of-war who had attended C.R.Us., and others who had not done so, some months after demobilisation, both in relation to each other and in relation to a control group of families representing the civilian norm (at the same socio-economic levels). It was found that, of the men who had attended C.R.Us. 26 per cent. showed evidence of 'unsettlement' (i.e., social maladjustment at home, at work, or in the community), as compared with 64 per cent. of those who had not had C.R.U. training. Through the application of criteria of social participation, it was found that the level of adjustment of the C.R.U. sample was not only superior to that of the non-C.R.U. sample, but also, that it was in fact superior to that of the control group (in spite of the fact that persons reputed to be 'unsatisfactory' or 'difficult' had been excluded from the latter).[10]

Discussing the significance of these findings, Curle and Trist[10] stated: 'In the less obvious forms of unsettlement, not only is the man's own life, and particularly his family life, reduced to a far lower plane of efficiency and enjoyment, but the whole of the society to which he belongs will suffer by his withdrawal from active social participation. Such unsettled men are dead weights in society and, if their external situation deteriorates, through sickness, unemployment or anti-social

---

* The civil resettlement scheme was the subject of a detailed and important sociological study by Curle and Trist.[9, 10]

activity, they may become actual casualties to the community and liabilities to the state. This is all the more serious in view of the fact that unsettlement of this kind does not appear to be much reduced as time goes on, but rather to harden into a rigid and intractable mould. . . . The man who had been to a C.R.U. had one advantage. . . . He had learned, chiefly through group discussion, to understand the nature of the tensions which are almost bound to arise in resettlement and had some idea of how they might be dissipated. He appreciated the fact that unsettlement is not one-sided, and that even if he himself felt perfectly well integrated, the domestic balance achieved by his wife and children during his absence would inevitably be thrown out of gear by his return. . . . The significantly higher proportion of well-adjusted men in the sample who had attended a C.R.U. emphasises the worth of the C.R.U. as a therapeutic community.'

It should, finally, be noted that, as Main[23] and others have pointed out, ex-Servicemen who have been for long periods in overseas theatres, present essentially the same basic problems as those encountered by repatriated prisoners-of-war, in their readjustment to civil life, and especially, to family life. While they would, consequently, in many cases undoubtedly benefit by similar provisions, it was, of course, not possible to create Resettlement Units for this purpose—and, indeed, the numbers of ex-Servicemen returning from service overseas were too large for such a scheme to be practicable.

(d) REHABILITATION OF THE PHYSICALLY DISABLED

Detailed investigations by an Army psychiatrist, E. D. Wittkower,[43, 44] concerning the problem of the civil rehabilitation of Servicemen with severe physical disabilities, emphasises the fact that, although such disablement was commonly regarded as merely a surgical and financial matter, psychological factors were of the greatest importance in determining the course of the subsequent social adjustment, as well as the vocational re-adaptation and working capacity, of such men. Three large groups of disabled men were studied, in this connexion: those suffering from loss of a limb, loss of vision in one eye, and total blindness, respectively. These investigations clearly demonstrated that, in many, if not indeed the large majority of such cases, a successful result in physical, psychological and social rehabilitation can only be achieved by the fullest co-operation between surgeon, physician and psychiatrist, in a combined psychosomatic approach.

SUMMARY AND CONCLUSIONS

The fundamental lessons in military psychiatry, derived from experience in the Second World War, may be summarised as follows:—

Central Organisation. In order to co-ordinate the prophylactic and therapeutic activities of Army psychiatry in war-time, and to maintain effective liaison with other administrative departments of the War Office, it is essential to establish at the outset a separate, central psychiatric organisation (Directorate of Army Psychiatry) as a part of the Army Medical Directorate. It is also of the utmost importance that a separate administrative psychological section (Directorate of Selection of Personnel), in charge of personnel selection and related matters, be formed simultaneously as a part of the Adjutant-General's branch of the War Office. The work of these two central departments—psychiatric and psychological, respectively—must at all times be closely co-ordinated and receive the active support of the D.G.A.M.S. and the A.G., acting in full agreement and co-operation on matters of policy which should necessarily be of mutual concern.

Medical Examination before Enlistment. The magnitude of the psychiatric problem in a modern Army in war-time emphasises the absolute necessity for a most thorough psychiatric examination and screening procedure in the general medical examination prior to enlistment. During the Second World War in the United Kingdom, one-eighth of all medical rejections by National Service Boards before enlistment were for psychiatric reasons (and psychiatric examination and rejection by these medical boards were not nearly stringent enough); and in the British Army, psychiatric disorders constituted the largest single cause of man-power wastage from disease (one-seventh), as also of medical discharge (one-third of all cases).

Personnel Selection and Allocation. It is essential, particularly when it is necessary to mobilise the country's total resources of man-power, that all those men who have been found fit for full or limited military duties should be subjected at intake to thorough scientific selection, on the basis of intellectual capacity, vocational aptitudes and experience, as well as physical standards, in order that they may be allocated to duties in such a manner as to ensure maximal efficiency, morale and mental health. It is equally important that facilities should exist at all times for expert reallocation, where this may be necessitated by physical or mental disabilities, or where the military situation requires a widespread redistribution of man-power.

Selection of Officers and Specialised Personnel. Where it is necessary to obtain, as efficiently and rapidly as possible, large numbers of officers or of other specialised personnel, it is essential to employ scientific methods of selection specifically devised for the required purposes. Such methods, provided that they are efficiently organised and include a skilled psychiatric personality assessment as well as psychological and military tests, can at least increase by one-third the number of suitable officer candidates discovered by the conventional methods (and eliminate an appreciable number of unsuitable candidates, who would otherwise have been accepted and subsequently have proved unequal to their responsible task). Similar methods can also, for example, eliminate from the training period more than four-fifths of the total wastage in para-troop volunteers. It is, in this way, possible to reject in the early stages the majority of unsuitable candidates, with obvious advantage to military efficiency, morale and mental health.

Military Employment of Dullards. Men of low mental capacity are of limited military value. Where, however, it is imperative to make the fullest possible use of all available man-power, the Army can employ stable dullards on simple labouring duties, provided that they are organised into separate units (Pioneer Corps), according to their fitness to bear arms in self-defence, or, alternatively, for an unarmed unit only. Thus segregated, stable dullards maintain a high level of morale and do not constitute, as would in general otherwise be the case, an appreciable disciplinary, medical and psychiatric problem, or a threat to the morale and efficiency of men of higher intelligence in ordinary units. Unstable dullards, on the other hand, are not fit for any form of military service (although they may frequently be employed in some limited, but socially useful and productive, capacity in civil life).

Morale. From the psychiatric point of view, essential factors in the maintenance of high individual and group morale are: adequate selection and allocation (including the rejection or segregation of the immature, inadequate, unstable, anti-social, and mentally backward); thorough training based on sound psychological, as well as military, principles (including, e.g., the correct use of 'battle inoculation', and the avoidance of primitive and artificial 'hate training'); good leadership based on wide experience and on insight into human problems and group situations (especially under stress); and attention, wherever possible, (particularly in overseas theatres) to such matters as good welfare facilities, regular mails, and the provision of frequent and adequate information about the war in general, the home front, and the local military situation. It has been clearly established that morale is the only real and permanent basis of discipline, and that there is a definite and direct relationship between low morale and a high incidence of military disciplinary and social problems, such as absenteeism and desertion, sexual promiscuity and V.D., etc.

Forward Psychiatry. However successful and effective may be the methods of preventing psychiatric breakdown and promoting positive mental health and morale, it is an incontrovertible fact that wherever fighting is in progress psychiatric casualties will occur, and that when fighting is severe their number becomes such as to constitute a military problem. (In the British Army in the Second World War the incidence of such psychiatric casualties was, on an average, 10 per cent. of total battle casualties—varying from 2 per cent. to 30 per cent. according to the type of battle). The military problem, in this respect, resolves itself into: (i) preventing psychiatric casualties from impeding actual fighting operations, or the evacuation and treatment of the wounded; (ii) selection and treatment of those among them who are considered (psychiatrically) capable of early return to effective combatant duties; (iii) preventing deterioration in those unable to return early, or at all, to combatant duties; and (iv) due consideration of long-term conservation of man-power. The whole success of forward psychiatry depends on early treatment (first within a matter of hours), the essentials of which are adequate sedation by the regimental medical officer immediately after breakdown, and its continuance at other levels. With adequate triage and sedation at R.A.P. and M.D.S., and a properly constituted 'Exhaustion Centre' at C.C.S. level or its equivalent (e.g., a F.D.S.), it is possible to return the majority of cases to fighting within a week— (70 per cent. to 56 per cent. in the British Army in the last war—of which only 5 per cent. broke down again in the course of the same battle). Cases of poor prognosis alone should be evacuated to the base. It is essential that the whole progress from breakdown to ultimate return to active duty should be continuous if the results of treatment are to be good; patients from psychiatric rehabilitation units should proceed direct to their future unit without an intermediate, demoralising period of waiting in R.H.Us., etc., if subsequent deterioration is to be avoided.

Modern mechanised warfare imposes on the men involved in active fighting a strain so great that, however stable, well trained and experienced they may be, they will ultimately break down, in direct relation to the duration and intensity of their exposure to the stress of battle. Casualties of this type ('campaign exhaustion') are as inevitable as gunshot and shrapnel wounds; in particular, the infantryman—who is exposed to the greatest danger and stress—reaches a peak of effectiveness within a certain number of days of combat experience, after which he becomes progressively less valuable, until finally he is 'worn out' and useless for further combatant duty (and cannot then be rehabilitated for this purpose at relatively short term, as is possible in many cases of acute psychiatric breakdown in battle). The point at which 'campaign exhaustion' occurs, depends on the stresses involved, and the frequency and duration of the periods when infantrymen are pulled out of the line. (In the U.S. Army during the Second World War, it occurred, on an average, after 180 combat days in the Italian Campaign; and after 30 days in the Normandy Campaign during the severe and continuous stress from D-day until the break through).

Corps and Divisional Psychiatrists are of proved value in the field, in an advisory and supervisory capacity, and the latter in particular serve an essential function where local conditions make it necessary for divisions to operate independently (as in the last war, e.g., in the Burma Campaigns, and in the later stages of the C.M.F. Campaign). Corps or Divisional Psychiatrists, together with an experienced Consultant and the nucleus of a psychiatric organisation, must accompany any force proceeding overseas. (Where this did not occur, in the course of campaigns in the Second World War, the consequent impairment of military efficiency and wastage of essential man-power proved as disastrous as it was unnecessary, and their repercussions on general morale and mental health were both extensive and serious.)

Rehabilitation (Military and Civil). To ensure the successful rehabilitation of Servicemen—whatever the disorder or disability from which they suffer—it is essential that this be undertaken, from the outset, with a view to their return, respectively, to effective military service, or to useful civil life and employment. A temporising or vacillating policy of dealing collectively with the respective groups, will fail to achieve adequate and effective readjustment for either purpose, and will be of service neither to the community nor to the individual.

(a) *Psychiatric Cases*. In general, military psychiatric hospitals are best suited to deal with the rehabilitation of patients for further service in the Army. A modified military organisation and atmosphere not only are essential for successful re-adaptation to Army life, but also greatly facilitate the continuity of treatment, rehabilitation, and subsequent appropriate reallocation according to the individual's capacities and limitations. Where, on the other hand, a patient is unfit for further effective military service, and requires either prolonged psychiatric hospitalisation, or to be discharged from the Army as soon as possible and rehabilitated for civil life, these functions can be best fulfilled by civil psychiatric hospitals, with a civilian orientation of therapeutic and rehabilitative activities, and for the most part, greater facilities with regard to staff, the more complex forms of therapy, and after-care, for this purpose.

(b) *Delinquents*. It cannot be reiterated too often, that the Army is an organisation for the effective defence of the country, and is not a penal colony for psychopaths, chronic delinquents, and other social misfits. To ensure the utmost economy of man-power and money, it is essential that military delinquents be subjected to a thorough scientific process of sorting, specifically including a psychiatric personality assessment and routine psychological tests, in order that their further potential usefulness to the Army may be accurately determined. Men who, on the basis of personality and military record, are regarded as redeemable for further effective military service, should be rehabilitated by the Army in suitable units or institutions which must, however, be such as to foster in the men who are sent there high individual and group morale— (e.g., the S.T.Us. and Labour Companies, in the last war). Chronic offenders, men with long and serious criminal records in civil life, unstable and anti-social psychopaths with severe personality disorders, constitute a pernicious, onerous and parasitic element in the Army; they are irredeemable for military service, and consequently would better be dealt with, as regards detention and rehabilitation for civil life, by the civil authorities. (It is hoped, eventually, by truly progressive, constructive and scientific methods of penology).

(c) *Repatriated Prisoners-of-War.* In view of the well-known psychological and social difficulties in readjustment of repatriated prisoners-of-war, it is essential to provide special units (such as the highly successful 'transitional communities'—Civil Resettlement Units—organised at the end of the Second World War) with the specific function of aiding the psychological rehabilitation and civil resettlement of these men, if the latter are not subsequently to become a chronic burden to society. Ex-Servicemen who have been for prolonged periods in overseas theatres frequently present similar problems in their readjustment to civil life, and would also in many cases benefit by provisions of this kind.

(d) *Physically Disabled Servicemen.* The results of research and practical experience have clearly demonstrated the considerable importance of psychological factors in determining the course of the subsequent adjustment of the physically disabled. In the majority of such cases, a successful result in physical, psychological, social and vocational rehabilitation, can only be achieved by the fullest co-operation, in the first place, between surgeon, physician and psychiatrist, in a combined psychosomatic approach.

REFERENCES

1. Ahrenfeldt, R. H. 1958. *Psychiatry in the British Army in the Second World War.* London (Routledge and Kegan Paul).

2. Ahrenfeldt, R. H., and May, P. R. A. 1958. Practical considerations on the disposal of delinquents in the Army. *Ibid.*, Appendix A, pp. 260–70.

3. Anon. 1941. Mental fitness of U.S. recruits. *Lancet, 2:* 103–4.

4. Appel, J. W., and Beebe, G. W. 1946. Preventive psychiatry: an epidemiologic approach. *J. Amer. Med. Ass., 131:* 1469–75.

5. Bion, W. R. 1946. The Leaderless Group project. *Bull. Menninger Clin., 10:* 77–81.

6. Bion, W. R., and Rickman, J. 1943. Intra-group tensions in therapy: their study as the task of the group. *Lancet, 2:* 678–81.

7. Braceland, F. J. 1947. Psychiatric lessons from World War II. *Amer. J. Psychiat., 103:* 587–93.

8. Bridger, H. 1946. The Northfield Experiment. *Bull. Menninger Clin., 10:* 77–81.

9. Curle, A. 1947. Transitional communities and social reconnection; a follow-up study of the civil resettlement of British prisoners-of-war; Part I. *Human Relations, 1:* 42–68.

10. Curle, A., and Trist, E. 1947. Transitional communities and social reconnection; Part II, *Human Relations, 1:* 240–88

11. Fitzpatrick, G. A. 1945. War Office Selection Boards and the rôle of the psychiatrist in them. *J.R.Army Med. Cps, 84:* 75–8

12. Foulkes, S. H. 1948. *Introduction to Group-Analytic Psychotherapy.* London (Heinemann).

13. Freud, S. 1922. *Group Psychology and the Analysis of the Ego;* (transl. J. Strachey). London (Hogarth Press); p. 41.

14. Ginzberg, E., et al. 1959. *The Ineffective Soldier: Lessons for Management and the Nation.* 3 vols. New York (Columbia University Press). (Cf. especially: vol. *1:* pp. 194–203; vol. *2:* pp. 199–201, 268–75; vol. *3:* pp. 141–59, 190–1, 216–8, 271–314.)

15. Gregg, A. 1947. Lessons to learn: psychiatry in World War II. *Amer. J. Psychiat., 104:* 217–20.

16. Guttmann, E., and Thomas, E. L. 1946. *A Report on the Re-adjustment in Civil Life of Soldiers discharged from the Army on account of Neurosis. Rep. Publ. Hlth. Med. Subj.* (Ministry of Health), No. 93, London (H.M.S.O.).

17. Hegel, G. W. F. 1840. *Philosophie der Geschichte.* 2nd ed. Berlin; p. 9.

18. *History of the Great War: Medical Services.* 1923.—*Diseases of the War,* vol. *2.* London (H.M.S.O.); Neurasthenia and War Neuroses, pp. 1–67.

19. Kenton, C. 1946. *In:* Discussion: forward psychiatry in the Army. *Proc.R.Soc.Med., 39:* 137–40.

20. Lewis, A. 1943. Social effects of neurosis. *Lancet,* 1:167–70.

21. Main, T. F. 1946. *In:* Discussion: forward psychiatry in the Army. *Proc.R.Soc.Med., 39:* 140–2.

22. Main, T. F. 1946. The hospital as a therapeutic institution. *Bull. Menninger Clin., 10:* 66–70.

23. Main, T. F. 1947. Clinical problems of repatriates. *J.Ment.Sci., 93:* 354–63.

24. Main, T. F. 1948. Rehabilitation and the individual. *In: Modern Trends in Psychological Medicine,* ed. N. G. Harris. London (Butterworth); pp. 386–411.

25. Masserman, J. H. 1948. Psychological medicine and world affairs. *In: Modern Trends in Psychological Medicine*, ed. N. G. Harris. London (Butterworth); pp. 412–4.

26. Menninger, W. C. 1947. Psychiatric experience in the War, 1941–1946. *Amer.J.Psychiat.*, *103:* 577–86.

27. Miller, E. (ed.). 1940. *The Neuroses in War.* London (Macmillan).

28. Montgomery, B. L. 1946. Morale in battle. *Brit.Med.J.*, *2:* 702–4.

29. Montgomery, B. L. 1958. *Memoirs.* London (Collins); pp. 83–5, 88–90.

30. Myers, C. S. 1940. *Shell Shock in France*, 1914–18. (Cambridge University Press).

31. Palmer, H. A. 1945. Military psychiatric casualties: experience with 12,000 cases. *Lancet*, *2:* 454–7, 492–4.

32. Rees, J. R. 1943. Three years of military psychiatry in the United Kingdom. *Brit.Med.J.*, *1:* 1–6.

33. Rees, J. R. 1945. *The Shaping of Psychiatry by War.* London (Chapman and Hall).

34. Richmond, A. E. 1947. Positive health: its attainment in the soldier and the Army's contribution to it in the civilian. *J.R.Army Med. Cps, 89:* 274–89.

35. Sutherland, J. D., and Fitzpatrick, G. A. 1945. Some approaches to group problems in the British Army. *Sociometry, 8:* 443–55.

36. Swank, R. L., and Marchand, W. E. 1946. Combat neurosis: development of combat exhaustion. *Arch.Neurol.Psychiat.*, *Chicago, 55:* 236–47.

37. U.S. Surgeon General's Office. 1929. *The Medical Department of the United States Army in the World War:* vol. *10, Neuropsychiatry.* Washington, D.C. (U.S. Govt. Printing Office).

38. Von Storch, T. J. C., Pratt, G. O., *et al.* 1941. Observations and suggestions concerning neuropsychiatric examinations for the Army of the United States. *New Engl.J.Med.*, *224:* 890–7.

39. War Office. 1922. *Report of the War Office Committee of Enquiry into 'Shell-Shock'* (Cmd. 1734). London (H.M.S.O.).

40. War Office. 1948. *Statistical Report on the Health of the Army, 1943–1945.* London (H.M.S.O.).

41. Wilson, A. T. M. 1946. The Serviceman comes home. *Pilot Papers, 1,* No. 2: 9–28.

42. Wilson, A. T. M., Doyle, M., and Kelnar, J. 1947. Group techniques in a transitional community. *Lancet*, 1: 735–8.

43. Wittkower, E. D. 1945. The war-disabled: their emotional, social and occupational situation. *Brit.Med.J.*, *1:* 587–90.

44. Wittkower, E. D. 1949. Psychosomatic medicine. *In: Modern Practice in Psychological Medicine*, ed. J. R. Rees. London (Butterworth); pp. 126–34.

H*

45. Wittkower, E. D. and Lebeaux, L. 1943. The Special Transfer Scheme: an experiment in military psychiatric vocational re-employment. *Med. Press*, 209: 366–8.

46. World Health Organisation. 1959. *Social Psychiatry and Community Attitudes: Seventh Report of the Expert Committee on Mental Health. World Health Org. Techn. Rep. Ser.*, No. 177; p. 3.

The Royal Air Force Medical Services

By Wing Commander S. C. Rexford-Welch, M.A., M.Sc.,
M.R.C.S., L.R.C.P.

CONTENTS

THE ROYAL AIR FORCE MEDICAL SERVICES

Introduction

The Royal Air Force Medical History of the Second World War comprises three volumes entitled *Administration, Commands* and *Campaigns*. It aims to cover the whole field of aviation medicine, the scope of which broadened considerably over the war years. A historical record of this size necessarily includes accounts of trial and error, of the use of new discoveries in medicine and of the application of scientific research to aviation medicine. Some of the recorded facts relate to pre-war history or are of special interest to relatively few specialists; or they may refer to matters which are not of major medical significance. It is desirable, therefore, that the important lessons of the war in respect to medicine, and especially aviation medicine, should not be submerged or overlooked in a wealth of detail and an effort has been made to select and present the highlights in succinct form.

It is recognised that during the war many lowered standards had to be adopted, shortages accepted and approval given to conditions which would not have been tolerated in peace-time. Criticism has been made of these conditions in the hope that similar mistakes may be avoided in the future and the lessons learnt, often through painful war experience, put to the most practical use. It is beyond doubt that many of the difficulties could have been avoided by simple forethought and better use of the resources available. Some of the criticisms were recorded by the junior medical officer in the field as he saw the situation, often without knowledge of the relevant circumstances, such as world shortages or lack of man-power, or other factors known only to those with full knowledge of the position and able to see the picture as a whole. From the medical point of view, however, conditions were either right or wrong and they were judged accordingly.

Finally, adverse comment on any particular point does not necessarily imply general condemnation. A number of such criticisms may be based on single incidents, but it should also be borne in mind that one instance of failure or carelessness, particularly in the field of hygiene, could result in widespread infection, costing a vast amount of work and expenditure and invalidating all the preventive measures which had been laboriously built up.

Accommodation

Living conditions have such far-reaching effects on morale and play such an important part in the production of high or low standards of hygiene that the whole subject of accommodation in the R.A.F. is being dealt with first in this review.

In 1939 the total number of personnel, men and women, in the R.A.F. was approximately 140,000, housed with few exceptions in first-class brick built stations possessing all the amenities of a small town in which even the most ardent hygienist would have found it difficult to suggest anything but very minor improvements; furthermore, the personnel were regulars who had chosen the R.A.F. as their career. By 1944 the position was vastly different; the strength of the force had increased to well over one million personnel employed in over 200 trades; the majority were housed in non-permanent buildings and even tents, the well laid out stations were few in relation to the strength and the austerity of total war was abundantly evident. (Vol. I. Chap. 7.)

Between 1939 and 1944, therefore, the R.A.F. had to find living quarters for nearly a million additional personnel, male and female, in a country where there were many other claims on existing accommodation and on building materials, where there was a shortage of man-power and where the threat of dislocation by enemy action was always present. In these circumstances it was inevitable that much occurred which was not acceptable medically nor even consistent with the most elementary ideas of preventive medicine.

The responsibility of the Medical Branch with regard to accommodation was laid down, indirectly, in King's Regulations and Air Council Instructions (para. 1485)* which stated, with reference to a medical officer's duties, 'He will advise the C.O. of the station on sanitary matters, and will, as necessary, instruct the sanitary detachment in their duties, but it will be the responsibility of the C.O. to ensure that these duties are carried out.' This regulation offered little difficulty of interpretation in peace-time when its provisions were observed as a matter of course, but in war-time it assumed much greater importance and the manner in which it was carried out could make all the difference between a unit with a high medical standard and one in which conditions were dangerous to health.

The regulation quoted above was the link between the Executive and Medical branches as far as responsibility for living conditions was concerned. A good station commander and an experienced medical officer could achieve high standards of hygiene in the most primitive

---

* Where King's Regulations and Air Council Instructions are quoted the reference is to the 1942 edition as typical of the war period.

conditions, but difficulty could easily arise where there was any lack of harmony between C.O. and M.O., and particularly when the latter was new to the Service. In practically every instance a station medical officer found himself virtually in charge of the hygiene detachment (or sanitary squad, as it was usually known) and adviser on a host of subjects far removed from the average medical curriculum and demanding an awareness of the problems associated with many trades outside the scope of medicine.

SITING

Obviously the main building programme of the R.A.F. was directed to the construction of airfields and not only did the provision of living quarters for the personnel to operate them have to receive secondary consideration, but the actual geographical location of the accommodation was dictated by operational requirements. Unavoidably, therefore, many of the sites where new buildings had to be erected were not those which would have been chosen as medically desirable.

In some cases airfields were sited in low damp areas, with little in the way of wind breaks, and usually in regions enjoying a high degree of isolation. Two problems immediately come to mind—the difficulty of providing healthy living conditions in low-lying, damp, wind-swept country, and the question of morale in places where recreation for leisure hours would be non-existent apart from anything which could be arranged by the personnel themselves.

The siting of airfields caused even greater difficulty overseas, where there was the additional hazard of tropical disease likely to occur in just those areas which were most suitable for the construction of airfields. Such important details as the siting of domestic quarters in relation to the prevailing wind and swamps or other mosquito breeding grounds were often overlooked, while the site chosen might adjoin a native village which, although providing a ready source of labour, would also menace an unseasoned R.A.F. population with highly dangerous disease.

Not until late in the war was medical advice sought, as a routine procedure, before deciding on the siting of airfields; up to that time, many instances are recorded of two sites being available but the poorer of the two, from the medical aspect, being chosen.

DISPERSAL

In peace-time, R.A.F. stations were constructed as compactly as their functions allowed, but during the war the policy was to disperse all buildings as much as possible to lessen the effects of bombing. The domestic site, working site and headquarters unit were thus often separated by distances that could be measured in miles, while the sick quarters were frequently so isolated from all other sites that there was more than a grain of truth in the saying that 'you have to be fit to go sick!'

The basic idea of dispersal was good, but it was sometimes carried to such lengths that it interfered with economic working, both because of the time needed to move from one part of the station to another and because it precluded the economic use of piped water, sewerage systems and electricity. Criticism of the policy was general—particularly in places where the weather was especially inclement—but dispersal was undoubtedly necessary on many of our airfields and if the latter had been attacked in a major degree there would no doubt have been far more favourable comments on the policy as a whole. Where attack was unlikely or units were of insufficient size to warrant attention from the enemy, it would probably have been better if dispersal had not been used, particularly as it was on these small units where transport was normally scarce, that the worst effects were felt.

On many airfields, in addition to the dispersal described above, large numbers of aircraft were also dispersed, using natural cover such as woods as camouflage. Airmen servicing the aircraft had considerable distances to cover between, for example, the aircraft on which they were working and the domestic site where their meals were taken. Normally, the distance between domestic site and aircraft did not affect the air crews as transport was provided to take them to the 'dispersal'; in certain Commands, however, where aircrew were required to do 'stand-by' duty at the dispersals, and wherever night operations were carried out, the difficulties were increased both for the men who serviced the aircraft and for the crews themselves. In relatively few instances was authority given for huts to be erected on these sites, although much was done on an unofficial basis to provide some kind of shelter.

The most serious problem caused by the policy of dispersal was that of sanitation and although medical officers gave constant attention to the subject an entirely satisfactory solution was never found. Frequent and most vigilant sanitary rounds were essential if a reasonable standard of hygiene was to be maintained. As far as the aircraft dispersals were concerned, bucket latrines were the only solution, although these always gave rise to inevitable difficulties of cleaning and maintenance.

TYPES OF ACCOMMODATION USED AT HOME AND ABROAD

The problem of housing personnel in the rapidly expanding air force was met by (i) the use of existing accommodation to its fullest capacity; (ii) the requisitioning of hotels and private houses; (iii) billeting; (iv) erection of various types of huts; (v) tents—both in the British Isles and abroad.

Use of Existing Buildings. As already mentioned, the pre-war R.A.F. Stations were good and for a few months after the outbreak of war it was possible to absorb into them the recruits being drafted into the Service. This was done by increasing the numbers permitted in messes, dormitories, barrack rooms and workshops and by the use of tiered sleeping bunks and, later, the introduction of cafeteria-type messing. Medical officers were uneasy about the whittling down of the authorised 60 square feet of space per man, but the reduction was unavoidable and by 1942 the allowance had been cut to 32 square feet per man.

At certain periods of the war, some of the larger stations were accommodating as many as four times the number for which they had been designed. The most serious problems which arose from such overcrowding concerned the station utilities, particularly sanitation, but little could be done to increase their capacity because of the considerable structural alterations which this would have entailed, coupled, in many instances, with war-time shortages of materials.

On the purely medical side, respiratory epidemics on a large scale were an ever-present possibility, and to combat this danger 'gargling parades' were instituted, men slept 'top-to-tail' and N.C.Os. ensured that windows of sleeping accommodation were kept open at night; despite these precautions, however, the situation was a constant anxiety to medical officers.

Requisitioned Buildings. The method of housing R.A.F. personnel in requisitioned buildings was used extensively throughout the war period. Large country houses strategically situated in relation to R.A.F. units were adapted as headquarters or taken over as mass dormitories or sick quarters. Such alterations were carried out as would enable the fullest use to be made of available space, but requisitioned buildings were naturally less economic than those built specifically for R.A.F. use. Here again the most serious difficulties arose over the sewerage system, which was often old-fashioned and never designed, even in hotels, to cater for such large numbers of people. Improvements were made wherever possible, but the extensive structural alterations which were desirable were out of the question owing to shortage of labour and materials.

Apart from the sanitation problem hotels were very suitable for mass billeting with a minimum of alteration. Quite a number of hotels were taken over for conversion to R.A.F. hospitals, notable examples being the Station Hospital, Morecambe (the Midland Hotel), the Officers' Hospital, Torquay (the Palace Hotel), and the Officers' Hospital, Blackpool (Cleveleys Hydro). All these hotels did yeoman service as hospitals, although their conversion presented some difficulty and they were rarely easy or economical to run. The main obstacles were the lack of lifts big enough to take stretchers, lack of sanitation facilities and such additional requirements as sluice rooms, and the unavoidable use of many small rooms instead of large wards, this being wasteful of nursing staff and making supervision by ward sisters difficult. (Vol. I. Chap. 5.)

Billeting. This took two forms—first, where billeting was used as a temporary measure to supplement R.A.F. accommodation until further construction could be carried out, and, secondly, where billeting was the main method of accommodating large numbers of personnel, such as at Blackpool and Morecambe. The problems which arose were similar in both types of billeting. (Vol. II. Chap. 9. p. 578.)

Most householders looked on their obligation to accommodate Service personnel as a way in which they could assist the war effort and the trouble they took and the kindness they showed went far beyond what was officially required of them. There were of course exceptions, but perhaps with some justification in that the billeting fee paid by the Service was barely adequate and the presence of Service men and women could become a burden financially as well as in other ways.

The main problems for the air force authorities were that close supervision of personnel and the enforcing of R.A.F. regulations were impossible and that it was difficult to obtain the usual Service 'atmosphere' in a civilian environment—this applying particularly to recruits on their initial entry.

For the medical officer, billeting added considerably to his normal duties, for he had to endeavour to inspect all billets and ensure that they remained of the required standard, visit sick personnel unable to leave their billets and arrange for their transfer to a Service hospital—often in a strange neighbourhood, sometimes in blackout conditions and over such a wide area that merely getting from place to place occupied a considerable amount of his already overcrowded time. In short, in such circumstances it was impossible to ensure adequate medical supervision.

It would appear that billeting is undesirable, except for short periods, and should only be adopted when all other methods of accommodating personnel have been explored.

Huts. Most of the new construction which took place during the war made use of semi-permanent wooden or pre-fabricated huts. Over a dozen designs were accepted, although they were usually all referred to by Service personnel as 'Nissen' huts, after the well known huts of the First World War.

Most of these huts were so designed that they could, in theory, be erected rapidly by semi-skilled labour, and if necessary, dismantled and re-erected elsewhere; unfortunately, this did not always work out in practice and the combination of flimsy construction and rough unskilled handling meant that on re-erection the separate parts rarely fitted or were so damaged that they were often useless.

The huts were of two basic sizes, those for domestic and small office accommodation measuring 16 feet by 36 feet and those for communal rooms, such as messes, 30 feet by 24 feet. It was possible to combine several huts of the same or different sizes to produce spacious messes and dining halls, and when tastefully decorated they became very pleasant buildings, despite their forbidding exterior appearance.

All huts were erected on a concrete base and most of them had double-skinned, un-insulated walls of various substances—wood*, compressed wood shavings, concrete blocks and a number of proprietary substances. Some huts had a few courses of bricks, rarely more than three feet high, on the side walls, above which they curved gradually into a roof section resembling a Roman arch; windows with either metal or wooden frames were let into the curved sides and doors were normally in the end sections—the latter usually made of wood and often ill-fitting.

Though of simple construction these huts were far from cheap and this fact, together with the many medical problems they created which are described below, suggest that serious consideration needs to be given to the provision of improved means of accommodation if widespread expansion should ever again become necessary.

(a) *Heating†*. Central heating was installed in a few locations but the normal method of heating was by slow combustion stove. It is interesting to note that throughout the war period no good word was recorded of these stoves.

There were usually two stoves located centrally in each hut, with asbestos flue pipes running up vertically through the roof. They were uneconomic both in fuel and man-power, required continual adjustment and were easily affected by wind changes as cowls were fitted rarely. The heat produced was usually inadequate, men near the stoves being too hot and exposed to fumes, while those at a distance felt no warmth. These stoves were also used in nearly all dispersed station sick quarters, but were so dirty that they were quite unsuitable for use in a medical establishment, with its requirement for a high standard of cleanliness.

(b) *Sanitation*. The principle was to construct communal ablution blocks serving a number of huts in order to economise in plumbing, but this resulted in very considerable discomfort for those using them. Many of the huts were some distance from ablution

---

* Wood was used progressively less as the war went on, owing to its scarcity and the fact that what was available was rarely seasoned.

† *See* also Note on Heating of Buildings, at end of Section.

blocks and this was not conducive to cleanliness, particularly in winter on bleak unprotected sites. The majority of huts had a latrine compartment with either an Elsan or bucket latrine for use at night.

(*c*) *Condensation*. A great disadvantage of the metal type huts was the amount of water that collected on the inner surface, for heating and cooling conditions were often such that the whole building acted as a huge condenser. Paint with anti-condensing properties was used in an attempt to combat this and sometimes the hut was given a further lining of hardboard or similar material, but the difficulty was never really overcome.

(*d*) *Lighting*. Electric lighting was eventually installed in nearly all huts for there were few stations which were never on mains supply. Until the electricity was connected various forms of lighting were used—mainly pressure and hurricane lamps—but these were unsatisfactory because they produced small pools of light around the lamp while the remainder of the hut was almost in darkness.

(*e*) *Weathering of Huts*. On many sites huts were exposed to constant strong winds, often combined with driving rain or sleet, so it was not surprising that the huts often leaked. Wooden end sections, often constructed of unseasoned wood, tended to warp, leaving large gaps through which water was driven in considerable quantities. Later in the war porches were added in an effort to overcome this difficulty.

(*f*) *Mud*. Because of the urgent need for accommodation personnel were drafted to stations as each section was built, so that a camp might have quite a large R.A.F. population before it was completed. Apart from other problems, considerable difficulty arose over the initial lack of paths, for the new sites were invariably muddy, especially in winter, and in spite of Wellington boots being worn much dirt was carried into buildings and especially the domestic huts. Duck boards were put down wherever possible, but their use was limited, and the only other solution—that of removing boots before entering huts—was seldom practicable. In summer, a problem was created by dust being blown into huts.

(*g*) *Global Use of Nissen Huts*. Huts were used in all theatres abroad, except in operational areas where the fluid nature of the fighting precluded any form of permanent or semi-permanent building, but there were not enough designs. It could not be expected that huts suitable for a climate such as that of Iceland would be equally acceptable in India and their world-wide use was not entirely successful. Little could be done to make the huts warmer in very cold conditions, while in the Tropics they were too hot and had the additional disadvantage of being difficult to make mosquito-proof.

Undoubtedly the various kinds of huts did excellent service in providing semi-permanent accommodation which could be erected relatively quickly and simply, but they left much to be desired. Rigorous trials of all types of hut should be carried out in peacetime instead of leaving the lessons to be learned in war.

Many improvements were made, such as the additions of porches in wet climates and provision of thatch or insulating roof layers to combat strong sun; personnel who were prepared to use initiative and self-help could make very habitable buildings out of the otherwise austere huts, particularly where they were backed by an energetic Commanding Officer and sound medical advice. Nevertheless, in medical opinion the poor conditions offered by certain hutted camps were responsible for an increase in the rate of sickness.

Tents. In the early days of the war tents were used for sleeping accommodation, being erected on stations where it was possible to use some if not all of the permanent utilities and other amenities. It is to the credit of the executive staff and Works Departments that relatively few men had to pass the first winter of the war under canvas and medically no epidemic occurred which could be traced to the tented accommodation. Until 1942 tents were used extensively in Technical Training Command, where at one time tented accommodation was needed for more than 20,000 personnel. (*See* Vol. II. p. 573.)

NOTE ON HEATING OF BUILDINGS

One important observation was made—namely, that sometimes the destruction of glazing through bombing was sufficient to necessitate the evacuation of an otherwise habitable hospital, owing to the impossibility of keeping patients warm. It would be of value to include as basic equipment rolls of transparent plastic material which could be fixed easily and rapidly in such emergencies and allow the building to continue to function.

The R.A.F. in the Field

GENERAL SURVEY

The R.A.F. was in many respects a static force compared with Army formations, but in the Campaigns highly mobile R.A.F. units were developed—e.g., in the Western Desert, in Normandy and in Burma—with the consequent problems of living in the field. As already mentioned, on some permanent R.A.F. stations at home large tented camps were erected to supplement existing accommodation and personnel lived under conditions very similar to those prevailing in the field (*see* 'Tents', above).

R.A.F. field formations ranged from large units such as the Second Tactical Air Force or the Desert Air Force down to small radar sections living, often under canvas, in complete isolation. The most important R.A.F. medical field units were the Mobile Field Hospitals, Mobile Dental Units and Casualty Evacuation Sections. Often a number of units were encamped together for considerable periods, allowing communal use of facilities, while, at the other extreme, many units operated in isolation, relying entirely on their own resources and ingenuity and depending on air supply for the necessities of life. This distinction is important for it explains why units had to carry what might appear at first sight to be a rather formidable range of equipment— for example, such things as carpentry tools could be vital to an isolated unit and their absence could prevent the rapid construction of the majority of 'home made' sanitary and cooking appliances. The problem demanded a balanced judgment, for if the unit was under-supplied it became ineffective, but if over-stocked it lost the mobility which was a vital part of its function. The best 'scales' were usually discovered by a method of trial and error, units ruthlessly discarding or 'acquiring' the equipment as they went along. 'A week of operational camping was worth a year of non-operational exercise.'

A further point of very great importance from the medical point of view was the global nature of the Campaigns. Men found it hard to realise that apparently minor errors of hygiene in tropical climates could have such serious consequences and that one man's indiscretion could be responsible for the infection of a whole unit.

TRAINING

Wherever possible the training of units in the art of field craft was carried out under conditions approximating as nearly as possible to those in overseas theatres. It was difficult to simulate some of the conditions which would be met—i.e., the climate in Burma or Iceland and operational activity on battle fronts—and judging from the early records of the M.F.Hs. in Normandy (1944) the training given, though helpful, had not been fully assimilated by the units. Many gross indiscretions were committed in the early days of this Campaign and these encouraged the rapid spread of a serious outbreak of enteritis in the beachhead.

Apart from personnel in units which were formed and trained before going into action, it is of some interest to note how ill-prepared was the average officer or airman sent as a reinforcement to an overseas area in which tented accommodation was the rule—for example, forward areas in the Western Desert or Burma. The airman's basic training had covered general R.A.F. matters such as discipline and marching and more specialised instruction in the trade of his choice, but the curriculum made no provision for realistic training in field conditions. More often than not an airman made his first acquaintance with camping when he was shown a large, bulky bag and ordered to pitch the tent it contained —a task which, understandably, completely baffled all except those who had once been boy scouts. On most units a 'new' airman learned the rudiments of camp craft from his companions, but if a large number of reinforcements suddenly joined a busy operational unit their instruction was often protracted and knowledge painfully acquired.

To those in the forward areas expert camping knowledge was as necessary as experience in the use of firearms, for personnel had to be ready to move at a moment's notice, irrespective of the time of day or state of the weather, and to re-erect their camps in any kind of territory with the utmost speed and with all their equipment intact. Practical experience gave this vital knowledge, and men learned to live in health in the Burmese jungle—those who did not learn often became medical casualties.

THE UNIT MEDICAL OFFICER'S RESPONSIBILITY IN THE FIELD

All medical officers entering the Service attended a course at the School of Hygiene and Sanitation, Halton, where they were given a basic training, including field hygiene. The course was excellent in theory, but almost completely failed to consider many of the practical difficulties which would be encountered in the field. Unless experienced instructors can be provided such courses are not justified.

The medical officer was responsible, under the commanding officer, for the health of the men, for the setting up of a medical inspection room, for liaison with neighbouring medical officers and the nearest hospital and for supervision of hygiene. He was also adviser and prime mover in a number of matters not strictly medical, as in the construction of field sanitary apparatus or the improvisation of spraying plant.

SOME DIFFICULTIES REFERRED TO IN MEDICAL OFFICERS' REPORTS

In the following paragraphs it is proposed to deal very briefly with subjects which appeared again and again in medical officers' reports, for although some problems were due to war-time conditions, others could have been solved either completely or partially, beforehand.

Tentage. Those commonly in use were the familiar bell tent, the 160 lb. ridge tent and marquees of various sizes. The first two types were found to be easily erected and capable of standing up to comparatively rough handling, but the marquees were, without exception, difficult to erect, poor in regard to both lighting and ventilation and deteriorated rapidly with each move; in addition, they were very difficult to stow when wet, camouflage was a problem as the numerous guy ropes were almost impossible to conceal from the air, and they fared badly in high winds owing to their square design.

Certain specially designed tents used as operating theatres in the Second Tactical Air Force were adversely criticised by surgeons during the training period, but it was not possible to replace them with a more suitable type because of the large stocks which existed.

There was high praise for the German type tents used in the Western Desert. These were double-skinned, the outer skin acting as the fixation for tent pegs, and units who captured them found them easy to work and particularly easy to camouflage owing to the absence of tell-tale guy ropes.

The units which suffered most owing to unsuitable tents were undoubtedly those in Burma, where the frequent moves combined with the heavy rains induced a very high rate of wear and tear—units which had been in the field for any length of time being easily distinguished by their patched and bedraggled tents.

Sanitary Apparatus. The construction of urinals and latrines was usually left to the units concerned.* Efficient urinals could be made quite easily from waste fuel tins and caused little difficulty, but the field latrines constructed left much to be desired, conditions often reaching a state of dangerous and culpable neglect.

In many theatres Service-made latrine seats were issued which were designed to fit the top of 5 gallon fuel tins, the latter being nearly always available in unlimited quantities in all areas. These seats were made of unseasoned wood, the separate pieces having large cracks between them which made cleaning and drying very difficult; a heavy lid was attached by small ungalvanised hinges which were usually torn off after the first day's usage. These seats did not stand up to wear, could not be easily cleaned and the wood quickly warped and rendered fly-proofing an impossibility. The issue of seats of light metal construction, sufficiently robust, simple to clean and allowing easy fly-proofing, would have been more effective.

Elsans were issued in some areas, but they were found to be too flimsy for Service use; in any event the chemicals they required were rarely available; the apparatus usually degenerated into an ordinary bucket latrine, without the robustness of the latter.

Apart from inadequate apparatus, many difficulties occurred because some units were not sanitary minded. A common fault was that a unit would take over a camp site and, thinking they would only be staying one day, make either no latrine provision or use completely inadequate and poorly sited shallow trenches. If the unit did not move the following

---

* In certain large camps sanitary apparatus was constructed by army engineers.

day, and this often happened, the ground was rapidly fouled and conditions went from bad to worse. Not infrequently another unit would camp on the same site at a later date and the risks to its personnel if the ground was already fouled, can well be imagined.

Sanitary Squads. Though not technically his immediate responsibility the M.O. usually found that from a practical point of view he was in charge of the sanitary squad. These squads were usually manned from lower intelligence grades, for C.Os. were reluctant to allocate their more intelligent airmen to sanitary duties, not appreciating that the health of the entire unit might be at stake. Medical officers had to be firm and outspoken in their requests for suitable personnel to be picked out for sanitary squad duties.

Malaria Control. This was normally under the control of the sanitary squad, but it was not until the later years of the war that the necessity for good control was fully appreciated by the executive. There was frequently a shortage of spraying apparatus and suitable fluid. When D.D.T. began to be used more generally in the later years of the war, there was rarely enough to meet the need.

Mosquito nets, normally a personal issue, were always in short supply and immediate replacement in the forward areas often impossible. The conscientious always mended holes and the careless caught malaria. Personal anti-malaria precautions were clearly laid down and frequently repeated in routine orders, but the executive was slow to ensure that the precautions were fully carried out and in the early days of the campaigns a poor example was sometimes set by those in authority. The Allied Air Commander-in-Chief, South-East Asia, found it imperative to issue a stern directive to all commanding officers which left them in no doubt as to their responsibilities or the fate of those who continued to shirk them, in this and other fields of hygiene.

Water. The provision of adequate safe water supplies presented a big problem in the field and one that was never properly solved. In the Desert Campaign, where from a hygiene point of view camping was relatively clean, the problem was not so much to render the water pure as to obtain any supplies at all, owing to the distances involved. In areas such as West Africa, on the other hand, plenty of water was available but supplies were liable to be contaminated, with consequent risk of intestinal diseases.

In India and Burma, where the problem was greatest, water was usually collected from Army water points by R.A.F. water bowsers; normally, such supplies were already sterilised, but there were many occasions on which it was necessary for the R.A.F. field units to do their own sterilising. The normal R.A.F. water bowsers were heavy units of 300 or 500 gallon capacity; the larger of the two was a highly complex piece of apparatus which was designed to purify water electrolytically. In practice the mechanism was too complicated for field use and it was very difficult to obtain spares to deal with the breakdowns which occurred. Their weight was a further drawback and in wet areas or in places where they had to be filled from streams with marshy banks it was not uncommon for them to become deeply bogged. These bowsers were, in fact, generally condemned in all theatres and finally became no more than unwieldy water tanks on wheels, whose contents were treated by hand dosage with sterilising powder.

The greatest need, especially on small units, was for a water tender of 50 or 100 gallon capacity. Where none was available makeshift arrangements had to be made or one of the larger bowsers had to be used in an obviously uneconomical manner. Difficulty arose over moving the larger bowsers from site to site for although the 300 gallon bowser was self-propelled, the large 500 gallon bowser had to be towed and it was often not easy to provide a vehicle sufficiently powerful to do this over difficult terrain.

Laundry. There were no R.A.F. field laundries and although Army units assisted wherever possible this could only be a chance arrangement. Personal laundering in the field was usually the responsibility of the individual and hence in the less fastidious the cleanliness of clothing left much to be desired. Units such as M.F.Hs. had a very considerable amount of hospital laundry and usually local labour was enlisted and paid by barter. The drying of linen created another problem in areas subject to enemy air attack, for washing hanging out to dry provided an excellent guide to the whereabouts of units and in such circumstances lower standards of cleanliness had perforce to be accepted.

Field Cooking. Most field units contrived to construct efficient field ovens, but many field kitchens were not clean, particularly when native labour was employed and supervision poor—as was often the case owing to the shortage of R.A.F. cooks throughout the war.

Although their training included lessons in field cookery, many of the cooks who arrived on field units were, in practice, completely ignorant of this art and the standard of meals varied considerably; many cooks lacked imagination in the preparation of field rations and presented this food in the most unappetising and dreary forms.

Food safes were not issued generally by the Service. Though rations were mainly tinned, fresh meat was often available, even in the hardest campaigns, and the storage of this and other perishable food always created a problem. Safes were sometimes improvised, but most medical officers felt that the risks of food contamination were so great that a light, strong, portable safe should have been a standard issue to field units. The additional protection afforded would have more than justified the expenditure involved.

Mechanical Transport. Because of the shortage of all types of vehicles during the war many smaller units had only the bare minimum of mechanical transport, which meant that an accident or mechanical failure immediately gave rise to difficulties.

The scarcity of transport was felt particularly by sanitary squads working at a distance from the main camp, for the man-handling of heavy drums of spraying fluid and other such apparatus was difficult and caused much loss of time; the deficiency was usually made good by the use of medical transport, but such misemployment of the latter was undesirable and should not have been looked upon as the normal procedure.

Responsibility of Commanders. It was often not realised by commanders that ill-health could jeopardise operations as surely as unserviceability of machines, and that they held heavy responsibilities to maintain health. Too often this was left entirely to medical officers without sympathetic executive co-operation.

The Highway of the Air

It requires only a very cursory knowledge of history to recognise the pains taken by successful generals in the past to ensure that their troops could be moved rapidly from place to place and that there should be an adequate supply system. The Romans built their roads to suit the needs of the legions; in more recent times Napoleon attached very great importance to his horse transport and commissariat.

When the Second World War began our ideas, though indeed more up to date than the examples quoted, proved in a sense to be just as outmoded. In many respects we still thought in terms of the static War of 1914–18, relying on road, rail and sea for transport on a large scale, and we had, from a practical point of view, disregarded the air. Allied planning was soon disillusioned when the full impact of German *blitzkrieg* fell on the Allied Forces—fast moving armoured divisions and motorised troops all covered, and often entirely supplied, from the air. Hitler had learnt his lesson in the training ground of Spain—we still had ours to learn.

In the early days of the war aerial travel was used mainly by senior officers and those intimately connected with aircraft. By the end of the war air transport was in many theatres the main or only method of movement for all.

This changeover was not effected quickly or easily, nor was the new method of air transport without disadvantages, and it is now proposed to discuss the more important medical difficulties which were encountered in opening up and maintaining these military highways of the air.

FERRYING OF AIRCRAFT

Early in the war the Allies' need for aircraft of all descriptions was acute and as British industry could not supply all the immediate and urgent requirements the method of 'lend-lease' was invoked. This necessitated aircraft being sent from Canada to the United Kingdom, either crated and shipped or flown direct (with or without stops). Both methods were used. In the latter case, aircraft often carried as passengers Service or civilian personnel travelling on business of urgent national importance. The medical problems involved, whether passengers were carried or not, are outlined briefly below. (Vol. II. Chap. 4.)

Crew. The majority, in the early stages, were Canadian bush pilots, Britons and members of the Commonwealth too old for operations, and Americans sympathetic to the Allied cause. Medical examination initially was either waived entirely or so sketchy as to be of little value and it was not until the Assistant Chief Medical Officer of the Canadian National Railways set up the necessary organisation, later to be absorbed into Ferry Command itself, that medical examinations became in any way effective.

The Aircraft. These were mainly medium and heavy bombers and freighters, often fitted with overload tanks for the purpose of ferrying. They were ill-suited to the carrying of passengers and were not even comfortable for the crew on the very long Atlantic flights. From these basic facts sprang the main medical difficulties.

(*a*) *Oxygen.* During the flights it was often necessary to ascend to oxygen heights in an attempt to avoid bad weather and, in particular, icing. Although the aircraft carried oxygen for the crew it was often insufficient for the very long flights and if passengers were being carried the position was even worse. The medical authorities set up an organisation to examine all who were about to cross the Atlantic, to instruct them in the correct use of oxygen, to ensure that sufficient was available and that the apparatus was in working order.

(*b*) *Heating.* Though the aircraft were normally heated in the crew positions little or nothing was or could be installed for passengers. This constituted a major hazard as cold conditions were almost invariably encountered *en route*. Modifications to the aircraft were usually not feasible and such makeshift methods had to be adopted as the issue of flying clothing and extra blankets and the use of Wood's Arctic Robes. When aircraft were used to return Ferry crews to Canada, a necessary alternative to the slow sea convoys, it was possible to adapt a few aircraft, in the United Kingdom, to ensure heating for these passengers.

(c) *Escape*. The chances of survival if an aircraft came down in mid-Atlantic were not good; nevertheless, all possible safety precautions were taken and everyone boarding the aircraft was made aware of the correct procedure for ditching in that type of aircraft and the method of entering and means of surviving in a dinghy. The medical authorities in Canada, in conjunction with the executive officers, ensured that in every aircraft taking off the crew and passengers had been adequately briefed.

(d) *Fatigue*. The crews responsible for ferry work were at all times at a premium and it was necessary to put a limit on the hours flown and the number of flights undertaken in a given time. Little thought had been given to such problems before the war, when very few long flights had been undertaken, and it was not until 1942 that a good solution was found. However urgent the operational requirements for aircraft might be, it cannot be over-emphasised that the use of tired crews involves unjustifiable hazard and this was one reason why priority of accommodation at night stops was given to the crew and not to the passengers.

FERRYING OF PASSENGERS AND FREIGHT

At the beginning of the war the Allies had few facilities for carrying passengers or urgent freight from one place to another by air, but by the end of hostilities they boasted an air transport system which can truly be termed global. Such feats as the movement of an Indian Division from the Arakan in Burma to Imphal in India were well within the compass of this organisation, which was represented in the R.A.F. by Transport Command.

The medical difficulties inherent in such an organisation will be briefly outlined below.

Staging Posts. To allow for refuelling, night stops and maintenance of aircraft, it was necessary to set up considerable numbers of staging posts at strategic positions strung out literally round the globe. These posts varied in size from those manned by 20 men to large terminals with over 2,000 personnel on the staff. Each post had its own problems which varied mainly according to the climate and the operational situation. A further difficulty experienced particularly by the smaller posts was that they were often lodger units and therefore under the dual control of the host formation and their own Transport Command—with co-operation on both sides this arrangement was quite acceptable, but difficulties did occur at times.

Accommodation. The greatest problem centred round the provision of accommodation. The smaller staging posts were designed mainly for refuelling and their modest facilities were inadequate for crew and passengers if aircraft had to stay overnight owing to mechanical failure or adverse weather. In temperate climates the result was only perhaps inconvenience, but there were areas in which it was a serious hazard and was responsible for a toll of illness among passengers and crew, dysentery and malaria being the chief enemies. If crew became sick during the flight replacement was both difficult and time-consuming and a valuable aircraft was rendered non-effective; it was therefore only common sense to reserve the best accommodation for the crew rather than for the passengers.

Provision for Health and Comfort.
  (i) *Mosquito Nets.* The policy varied, but mosquito nets were normally a personal issue, and staging posts could not always supply sufficient numbers if crew or passengers were unable to produce their own. As transit buildings were rarely proofed, considerable numbers of crew and passengers contracted malaria in transit.
  (ii) *Messing.* The smaller posts could not provide 'round the clock' catering facilities for the unexpected arrival or early departure of aircraft and passengers were usually provided with packed meals from base; apart from being unappetising and monotonous only a limited amount of food could be carried and this supply was soon exhausted if the stops were of any duration. Liquid refreshments were also carried but in hot climates drinks were in great demand and replenishing at brief stops was not without risk, as water was often obtained, unwittingly or through carelessness, from contaminated sources.
  (iii) *Clothing.* Problems arose, particularly for the crews, in that personnel might begin their journeys from a cold country and find themselves, within a few days, in a completely different climate. The baggage allowance of about 60 lb. was sufficient to allow the prudent and experienced traveller to pack the necessary changes of clothing, but very many instances were recorded of personnel not having the correct clothing readily available, in spite of warnings given before the beginning of a flight; this again contributed to the sick rate.

Civilians flying as passengers, not realising the inherent operational difficulties, often and understandably complained about the conditions under which they had to travel or to spend time *en route*.

Sanitary Difficulties. In most of the medium and larger aircraft Elsan toilets were provided and in theory the used containers should have been exchanged for clean ones at staging posts; in practice, however, this created many difficulties and although every attempt was made to maintain a high standard of hygiene a completely satisfactory system was never evolved. The chief problems were the unpredictability of aircraft arrivals, the flimsiness of the containers and a shortage of the Elsan fluid.

Invalids in Transit and Medical Facilities at Staging Posts. Only on rare occasions were sick persons sent by normal flights (*see* 'Casualty Air Evacuation' p. 251), but often elderly persons or those who had recently recovered from illness and were thought to be fit for a normal passenger flight became ill or relapsed if conditions were rigorous and involved unexpected hardship. There were also occasions when sudden illness occurred among fit passengers. Small posts were in some difficulty in such circumstances as they might have only a nursing orderly immediately available and the smallest of sick quarters or M.I. rooms. The only solution was to send the patient to the nearest hospital—often a very long way in the case of a small isolated unit. At the larger posts a sick quarters and a doctor were available, but even then there were difficulties, for the size of the sick quarters was related to the permanent establishment and did not allow for illness of any extent among transients as might happen, for example, in a sudden outbreak of gastro-intestinal disease.

DISEASE AND AIR TRAVEL

This presented two problems: the possibility of passengers or crew acquiring diseases *en route* and the danger of diseases being transmitted to 'safe' areas.

DISEASES OF IMPORTANCE TO PERSONNEL

From the individual's point of view, the most serious diseases were dysentery and malaria, because of their prevalence abroad and because they could be contracted easily.

Dysentery. Both bacillary and amoebic forms were acquired by numbers of crew and passengers in transit. There were two main causes of infection, the first being poor hygiene at the staging posts, often due to the employment of native labour in the cookhouses and to lack of supervision. The second and most common cause was indiscretion on the part of passengers who, despite warnings, ate at native cafés, drank water which was not safe and, in fact, generally disregarded the most elementary principles of hygiene for hot climates. Many were young Servicemen abroad for the first time, but ignorance cannot be pleaded as an excuse as pre-flight lectures always stressed, in simple but emphatic language, the extreme importance of hygiene abroad.

Malaria. As with dysentery, the major factor responsible for the considerable number of personnel who contracted malaria was the disregard of common methods of protection shown by travellers, both Service and civilian; shorts and short sleeved shirts were often worn after sundown, mosquito nets were not carried or incorrectly used and many forgot or deliberately omitted to take suppressive drugs. It is true that the accommodation used was often unsuitable, but here again the prudent man could take personal precautions which were usually effective if carried out in a commonsense manner. Slack unit discipline, not only at junior levels, was a potent cause of infection and bad examples were recorded on units large and small.

DISEASES OF IMPORTANCE TO HEALTH AUTHORITIES

Before the advent of the aeroplane the best protection against transmission of disease from one country to another lay in the relative slowness of sea travel, which usually covered the incubation period of the more serious diseases and allowed the sufferer to be removed at the port of entry and those in contact to be put in quarantine or otherwise kept under observation. The use of passenger transport aircraft meant that this safeguard no longer existed and it was necessary for the authorities to take other steps to ensure that the transmission of diseases by air did not become a universal menace.

In this connexion the Sanitary Convention for Aerial Navigation* served a useful purpose and allowed the health authorities of the interested countries, in conjunction with those responsible for the control of the aircraft routes, to discuss and standardise the precautionary measures to be adopted. There was still considerable local variation in health requirements and in certain localities the by-laws and policies were continually changing to meet new contingencies, with consequent difficulties if all parties concerned were not given reasonable notice of impending changes, but the measures outlined below were generally accepted and indicate the modifications which were made to meet the war-time situation.

The most important diseases which had to be considered by both Service and Civil authorities were smallpox, cholera, typhus, plague and yellow fever—all of them diseases which, if transmitted to non-endemic areas, might be responsible for wholesale infection of a non-immune population. Yellow fever was the disease which gave most concern as its transmission and introduction into such countries as India and Egypt did not appear beyond the bounds of possibility. The authorities in both these countries were well aware of the danger and strictly enforced the various measures to combat it.

Yellow Fever. The main difficulties arose in connexion with the reinforcement routes over which aircraft were flown to aid our forces in the Western Desert. Briefly, aircraft were flown from the United States of America *via* South America to West Africa, both yellow fever

---

* Originated in 1933 and revised periodically.

areas, and then across that Continent to base airfields in Egypt. In addition, crated aircraft were shipped from the United Kingdom to West Africa, where they were assembled ready for flying to Egypt.

Considerable discussion, sometimes acrimonious, took place between the authorities concerned, but every control measure adopted depended for its efficiency on local arrangements and these, not surprisingly in such a vast undertaking, varied in the strictness of observance. The main precautions are summarised in the diagram below. Further and fuller details will be found in *R.A.F. Medical Services.* Vol. I. (p. 391 ff.), where a critical survey of the problem has been made. Volumes II. p. 404, and III. pp. 92, 292, 373, deal with the problem in relation to the various Commands which were affected by it. (*See* also '*Medicine and Pathology*' in this Series. p. 212.)

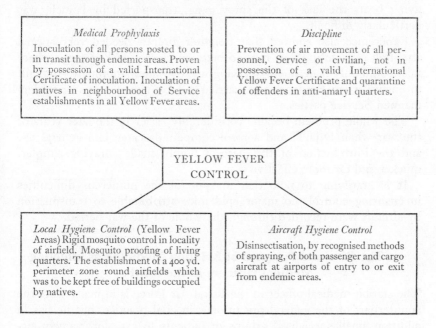

Medical Prophylaxis	*Discipline*
Inoculation of all persons posted to or in transit through endemic areas. Proven by possession of a valid International Certificate of inoculation. Inoculation of natives in neighbourhood of Service establishments in all Yellow Fever areas.	Prevention of air movement of all personnel, Service or civilian, not in possession of a valid International Yellow Fever Certificate and quarantine of offenders in anti-amaryl quarters.

YELLOW FEVER
CONTROL

Local Hygiene Control (Yellow Fever Areas) Rigid mosquito control in locality of airfield. Mosquito proofing of living quarters. The establishment of a 400 yd. perimeter zone round airfields which was to be kept free of buildings occupied by natives.	*Aircraft Hygiene Control* Disinsectisation, by recognised methods of spraying, of both passenger and cargo aircraft at airports of entry to or exit from endemic areas.

Difficulties Encountered in Medical Prophylaxis. In the early days of the war certain technical difficulties were encountered both in the production of yellow fever vaccine and in its administration. On one occasion a batch of faulty vaccine was held responsible for a considerable number of cases of hepatitis which occurred in troop drafts some time after their arrival in the Mediterranean theatre. Following this incident, different methods of production were adopted and there were no further occurrences of this degree, although occasional cases of hepatitis were sometimes, rightly or wrongly, attributed to yellow fever inoculations.

Inoculation was carried out only at certain recognised centres in the

United Kingdom. This was necessary in order to ensure a standardised technique of administration with vaccine known to be stored under the special conditions required.

Difficulties in Aircraft Hygiene Control. One other major precaution which was instituted was the spraying of aircraft to rid them of mosquitoes acquired in an endemic area. (See *R.A.F. Medical Services.* Vol. III. West Africa. pp. 373–379, for full description of requirements and experiments to gauge the effectiveness of such spraying). Difficulties arose through shortage of personnel, lack of spraying equipment and transport for the spray gangs, and the relatively large area of airfields and dispersals. Passengers and crew were impatient of delay on either landing or take-off, and if the delay was protracted tended to disemplane or take off before the spray gang arrived. In the special instance of flying boats the task of the spray gang, transported by launch, was particularly difficult.

Experience also showed that freighter aircraft needed very special attention as 'safe' pockets formed between closely packed cargo where mist could only penetrate if spraying was extremely thorough—difficult to ensure when the work was carried out by native gangs or under-manned Service parties.

The whole problem became considerably easier in the later years of the war when D.D.T. and aerosol compounds came into general use and the introduction of the 'aerosol bomb' made spraying simpler, quicker and far more effective.

It is gratifying to note that in spite of the numerous difficulties in ensuring control, no major epidemics attributable to transmission by aircraft were recorded through the whole of the war period.

The Rise and Progress of Aviation Medicine as affecting Medical Officers in the R.A.F.

The station medical officer in the Royal Air Force is in many ways the counterpart of the general practitioner in civil practice, but he has in addition small specialised groups of patients to care for, namely aircrew. All 'trades' in the Royal Air Force are important in 'getting aircraft into the air', but the striking power of the force rests ultimately on its flying personnel and consequently their health is vital if the force is to carry out the task for which it is designed.

In the early days of aviation, and indeed into the late 'thirties, the physical demands made on the body by the performance of aircraft were not severe and medical problems were consequently few, judged by present-day standards. Attention had been given to such matters as flying clothing and oxygen, but with the relatively short flights and the low altitude at which they were carried out these were not serious problems. Not until the rise of Hitler's Germany, with her *blitzkrieg* methods of warfare, was serious attention given to the medical implications of aircraft development, upon which our survival depended. Even today, there still remain aero-medical problems which must be solved if continued progress in aviation is to be made. In fact, it is probably true to say that the whole future of very high speed and altitude flight depends on the help which medical science can give to the human body subjected to an environment in which it was in no way designed to exist or to function.

During the six years of the war there were marked advances in the development of aircraft. Enhanced performance and the growing complexity of the mechanism placed greater responsibilities on the aircrew as well as increasing the hazard to the human frame as it attempted to keep up with the performance of the machine. Every new development brought its problems and these in turn led to advances in aviation medicine on an unprecedented scale.

The following paragraphs describe, firstly, how aircrew were made aware of the help medical science could give them in the discharge of their flying duties and, secondly, how those medical officers who were also qualified pilots investigated aero-medical problems. A final section gives a brief résumé of the main advances in aviation medicine during the period 1939–45.

THE MEDICAL OFFICER/AIRCREW RELATIONSHIP

This section may conveniently be divided into two parts, dealing respectively with the 'general duties' station or squadron medical officers and with the work of those officers employed wholly on medical/ flying duties and known as 'Flying Personnel Medical Officers'.

(1) *Station and Squadron Medical Officers.* On entry to the R.A.F. all medical officers were required to attend a course at the Institute of Aviation Medicine, Farnborough, which provided them with what might be called the A.B.C. of aviation medicine. From then onwards they were left to broaden their knowledge by close association with squadron members, ground crew and instructors. Upon the medical officer's own personality and drive depended success in his professional care of flying personnel. Aircrew were delighted to find him genuinely interested in flying and if he thus proved himself acceptable they would look on him as an essential and valued member of the squadron.

Time spent in the hangars, workshops and briefing rooms acquainted the medical officer with the actual problems encountered by aircrew in their duties and ultimately a successful medical officer would find himself occupying the position of consultant and confidant on a large number of subjects not normally associated with medicine, but often having more than a passing bearing on the medical problems of aircrew.

A medical officer was required, as part of his duties, to lecture to his squadron on such subjects as the use of oxygen, physiology of the ears and sinuses, elementary first aid, aircrew clothing, night vision and frostbite. If these lectures were delivered by a medical officer who was known by his audience to have flown and experienced these hazards himself, his words carried considerable weight. The majority of medical officers were enthusiastic young men who welcomed the opportunity to mix with aircrew and to fly whenever possible and from such M.Os. aircrew were prepared to accept any medical instructions; they were obviously less ready to listen to advice given by a M.O. who only emerged from his sick quarters to deliver lectures or issue medical instructions which were not backed up by personal flying experience.*

The influence of a popular medical officer could be invaluable to his squadron. Most of the aircrew were young, fit men who were, not surprisingly, inclined to be boisterous and adventuresome; although this was a desirable trait in the air it could be carried too far on the ground, with such consequences as intemperance and a high venereal disease rate. In such circumstances the example and tactful guidance of a well-liked medical officer could be of immeasurable value. Again, by intimate personal knowledge of his squadron a medical officer could see, at an early stage, the member who was beginning to break down under the strain of war-time operational flying; by a tactful approach to those in authority he could obtain a timely lightening of the load for one who might otherwise have been lost to the R.A.F.

The personality of a good medical officer gave added confidence to aircrew. They saw the efficiency of his sick quarters, the good management of his crash room and the speed with which ambulances and fire tenders reached crashes. Though such subjects were rarely discussed by aircrew, they were very much aware of the professional efficiency of their medical officer—a factor which could do much to assist morale, particularly if a squadron was suffering heavy operational losses.

(2) *Flying Personnel Medical Officers and their Relationship to Aircrew.* For station and squadron medical officers aviation medicine was only a part of their everyday work. They were the 'G.Ps.' of aviation medicine. The Flying Personnel Medical Officer, on the other hand, was concerned only with aviation medicine in theory and in practice; he was the 'specialist'.

It became evident early in the war that considerable advantage was to be gained by obtaining critical observations from someone who was not only well versed in medicine, but also an accomplished pilot; such a person was in a position to understand and to speak authoritatively on

---

* K.R. & A.C.I. para. 1483 made provision for Medical Officers to be given flying training.

the subjects both of medicine and flying. Furthermore, aircrew person-nel were more willing to take their problems to a man who could, if necessary, himself take up the aircraft in question and actually experience and investigate the problem in the air. With the steady increase in aircraft performance aviation medical problems loomed larger each year and F.P.M.Os. were able to render invaluable aid in seeking to resolve the difficulties upon which medicine or physiology had a bearing.

It was found that aircrew often accepted discomfort or even hazard without official complaint as they did not realise that their complaint would be welcomed by authority and that a remedy might be possible. In such circumstances the F.P.M.O. was able to bring forward sug-gestions which, if found valid, could be implemented at once with very considerable benefit to aircrew in general. Again, if a Command H.Q. was anxious over a certain problem on which aviation medicine had a bearing, the F.P.M.O. could visit squadrons in that Command and obtain first hand information from the aircrew concerned. Such an arrangement led to a very profitable liaison, for aircrew were usually prepared to discuss problems with the F.P.M.O. with a frankness which could not always be obtained if other channels were used.

During visits to squadrons the F.P.M.O. was often able to deliver lectures containing the most recent information from aviation medicine research with which he himself was in close contact, and to give some idea of the coming trends; in this way aircrew were kept as up to date as possible in both theory and practice. In such matters as ensuring that aircrew were using the latest types of clothing and safety equipment these visits by F.P.M.Os. were invaluable.

INSTITUTE OF AVIATION MEDICINE

The Institute of Aviation Medicine (I.A.M.), previously the R.A.F. Physiological Laboratory, South Farnborough, in the grounds of the Royal Aircraft Establishment, was well situated for liaison with the various scientific branches of flying located at the Establishment.

The scope of the Institute's interest was very wide, but its main functions can be summed up as follows:

(i) Production of F.P.M.Os. highly qualified in aviation medicine and instruction of all R.A.F. medical officers generally in aviation medicine.

(ii) Investigation of aero-medical problems and difficulties.

(iii) Research and development work in the aero-medical field.

(iv) Liaison with other Services and friendly countries so that common problems might be discussed.

This bare summary does less than justice to the volume of work conducted at the Institute, for its attitude has always been that no problem or idea is too trivial for serious investigation and the many very varied requests for assistance are too numerous to tabulate.

PRINCIPAL ADVANCES IN AVIATION MEDICINE 1939-1945

In this section only advances of major importance and interest will be mentioned to give an indication of the type of problem which had to be dealt with by F.P.M.Os. generally and the I.A.M. in particular.

Oxygen. In 1939 relatively few of our aircraft operated consistently above obligatory oxygen levels (approx. 14,000 ft.) and those that did, such as fighters, employed a simple system of continuous flow oxygen, delivery being at the same pressure during both inspiration and expiration.

The amount of oxygen which could be carried by aircraft when using this system was not sufficient for the longer flights being undertaken by such aircraft as the Blenheim bomber. This difficulty was met by the invention of the 'economiser', which while supplying a small constant flow, responded in quantity only to inspiration. A given amount of oxygen lasted about twice as long with this system as with the old continuous flow equipment.

Early in 1940, the need for portable oxygen apparatus became apparent. On some of the longer flights crew members had to move about the aircraft at oxygen heights, but whenever they left their normal position they were cut off from the aircraft's oxygen supply. Suitable portable oxygen sets were devised and issued towards the end of that year.

Parallel with the increased use of oxygen came the need to impress on aircrew the vital importance of taking oxygen to avoid the serious consequences of anoxia. Strangely enough, this was not an easy task, and much time had to be spent in making aircrew 'oxygen conscious'. Lectures and posters played their part and valuable lessons were taught by the use of the decompression chamber, in which personnel experienced for themselves, while on the ground and under supervision, the reality of anoxia, and learned the dangers of incorrect oxygen drill.

Before the war, static decompression chambers were only available at a few centres, but the need for teaching oxygen drill was so great that mobile chambers were devised and these toured the country with great benefit to all aircrews.

Heating. It became apparent early in the war that aircrew comfort, one of the main interests of the I.A.M., was a subject which would need considerable attention. With aircraft flying at greater heights and for longer periods, the comfort of the crews was vital if they were to maintain the efficiency on which depended not only the success of their mission but their very lives.

One of the major enemies was cold, which was responsible for a general speeding up of many undesirable physiological processes, such as anoxia, fatigue and anxiety. With the advice of I.A.M., aircraft were fitted with cabin heaters and heated suits, gloves and other equipment were provided, many improvements being the result of criticisms and suggestions made by the F.P.M.Os. who had flown, as observers, on operational sorties.

The greatest difficulty was experienced in the rear gunner position because the mobility of the rear turret made it impossible to provide supplementary aircraft heating and electrically heated clothing only could be used. The bombing position was another which caused difficulty, as it was often necessary to open panels to obtain a clear view.

Considering how often aircraft were damaged by flak, with consequent breakdown of heating apparatus, cases of frostbite were surprisingly few. Those that did occur were often due to carelessness or to disregard of orders concerning the wearing of protective clothing; one of the most common causes of frostbite of the hand, for example, was the wearing of gloves with holes, or the removal of gloves to handle equipment.

Night Vision. The connexion between sufficient oxygen and good night vision was emphasised during oxygen training. Much experimental work was carried out to discover other ways in which night vision could be improved. Findings were disseminated by a special Night Vision School established at R.A.F. Station, Upper Heyford, excellent practical results being obtained. Later, additional centres were set up at Commands and Groups and a mobile van was made available for touring. The entire project continually expanded throughout the war years, as the importance of good night vision standards for crews became more pressing.

Clothing. Here the assistance given by the I.A.M. was considerable. The Sidcot flying suit, issued at the beginning of the war, consisted of an outer suit of Grenfell cloth and a lining of artificial fur. In 1940 thermally insulated flying clothing was introduced, comprising leather jacket and trousers, both lined with fur. Though warm and comfortable this had the serious disadvantage that in the event of a crash and subsequent fire the wearer was liable to be severely burned through the leather and fur becoming saturated with petrol.

After this came an electrically heated lining made of Union twill and flameproofed poplin and incorporating electrical elements, this design being followed, in 1941, by a new pattern flying suit of light-weight gabardine with a separate quilted kapok-filled lining. This suit proved satisfactory.

The I.A.M. was also responsible for safety equipment and did much to promote safety in such matters as seat and parachute harness and in improving the design of goggles and helmets. When operations began in such theatres as the Middle and Far East further changes in the design of flying clothing became necessary and new problems, particularly in respect of ventilation, had to be considered.

The designing of protective clothing was often fraught with difficulty, the production of flying boots being an example of the kind of problem which had to be faced. Flying boots were required to perform two entirely different functions. They had, first, to be completely satisfactory for flying, allowing easy and sensitive operation of the rudder bars and providing adequate warmth; secondly, they had to be boots in which, if the aircraft had to be abandoned, crew members could walk inconspicuously for considerable distances through enemy territory. The difficulty was eventually overcome to a great extent by the design of boots with a detachable upper section.

Finally, it must be mentioned that the now familiar pressure suit came into being during the war. The first one introduced was the Franks anti-'G' suit (see *R.A.F. Medical Services.* Vol. II. p. 626), which was tested operationally before D-day, but was not considered practicable for general use in the Second Tactical Air Force.

Survival. The many medical implications of survival were closely studied by the I.A.M. The chief aim was to provide, in a very small space, equipment and medical supplies which would not only enable the crashed or stranded airman to survive but assist him in reaching help or escaping from enemy-held territory.

Much of the equipment suitable for survival in the Atlantic would be useless in the jungle of Burma, and it was necessary to teach members of aircrew the principles of survival appropriate to the areas over which they were flying. Special attention was paid, both in provision of supplies and in instructions, to the avoidance of malaria and dysentery and advice on 'living off the country' was given.

Fatigue. In aircrew, impaired efficiency due to fatigue is of major importance, for errors due to fatigue at the end of a long trip could result in crashes and consequent wastage of precious aircraft and crews. The I.A.M. helped considerably in minimising the occurrence of fatigue, again basing their recommendations on the reports of F.P.M.Os. who put forward suggestions from their own observations. The pooling of many ideas led to great advances in this vital subject in aviation medicine.

The problems described above were only a few of those investigated at the I.A.M., but they give some idea of the diversity of work undertaken and, most important, they show the intimate connexion which was established between the Flying Branch and this specialised section of the Medical Branch. This liaison continues today and is growing still closer and more vital as aircraft make yet further demands on the human frame.

Casualty Air Evacuation

The lot of a casualty in a battle area has for generations been unenviable. The War of 1939–45 produced one of the greatest advances in solving the problem of dealing with the wounded—the use of air transport to bring large numbers of casualties speedily under highly skilled medical care. By the end of 1945 over one and a half million Allied sick and wounded had been carried by this means from the front lines of the various theatres to adequate base medical facilities. The story of how this near-miracle was accomplished is outlined briefly below.

Before 1939 the possibility and desirability of carrying wounded in aircraft had been recognised and small lifts had, in fact, been successfully carried out. Nevertheless, at the beginning of the war there was no air evacuation plan. Germany, on the other hand, had made good use of the Spanish Civil War to try out new ideas, one of which was the bulk evacuation of wounded by air. This had proved very successful and it was not surprising to find plans for the air evacuation of casualties an integral part of German strategy, for its economies and benefits were appreciated by the German commanders in the field and their supporting medical services.

For the Allies, the evacuation of casualties by air, as we now understand it, began in the Western Desert. The Germans were flying ambulance aircraft, painted and marked as laid down by the Geneva Convention, early on in the Desert Campaign, and the absence of similar facilities for our troops caused no small comment. The official answer to such criticism was 'lack of aircraft' but while discussions on the matter at a high level had reached deadlock, unofficial action was being taken by medical officers in the forward areas who found themselves swamped with casualties. With the co-operation of the sympathetic aircrews, they were loading the wounded into freighter aircraft returning empty after unloading their supplies in the forward areas. For a time only a small proportion of casualties were returned to base areas in this way, but very soon considerable numbers of wounded were being transported by air and special arrangements had to be made in the Cairo area for their reception.

Up to this time, the official attitude had been, quite understandably, that the operational situation and general shortage of supplies made it impossible to allot aircraft for a purely ambulance rôle; once the principle had been accepted of 'supplies forward—casualties back', full advantage was taken of this life-saving and economical measure. Wounded men who previously would have had to endure long and harrowing journeys by ambulance and train were now being cared for at base hospitals within a few hours of being injured and the justifiable enthusiasm of patients and glowing press reports did much to bring field commanders to the acceptance of air evacuation as a normal routine.

It was quickly realised that there were other advantages to be gained by returning wounded to base rapidly and smoothly. The policy had always been for medical units to be established as near to the front line as possible and either to operate on their patients or, after improving their condition sufficiently, to send them by ambulance or train to base hospitals for final surgery. This necessitated numerous medical units in the forward areas and in addition to creating problems of supply, tied down large numbers of medical personnel, ambulances and all the equipment for the running of a big field medical network. Following the introduction of rapid air travel only operations and treatment of immediate urgency were undertaken and the entire forward medical establishment could be reduced to very much smaller proportions. Early doubts on the wisdom of flying dangerously ill patients were soon removed and it was found, with some surprise, that even such injuries as severe gun-shot wounds of the abdomen travelled exceptionally well by air, the risk indeed being greater after operation.

With the diminished need for these medical units in the front line it was possible to provide much better medical facilities in the base area and to open special wards or even hospitals to deal with certain types of casualties—for example, head injuries. This greatly influenced the formation of the Special Centres (orthopaedic, head injury, burns, neuro-surgery, etc.) which later, during the Invasion of Europe, were responsible for the saving of many lives as a result of their accumulated surgical and nursing experience.

It must not be thought, however, that in the development of air evacuation everything went smoothly. The organisation was built up in the hard school of trial and error and in the following paragraphs the main difficulties will be discussed briefly.

AIR SUPERIORITY

Transport aircraft flew unarmed and as it was often impossible to provide a fighter escort, there had to be a reasonable margin of air superiority. In certain stages of the war (e.g., the Invasion of Europe) such air superiority was present, but when C.A.E. began it was some-times necessary to balance the risks of enemy air attack against the advantages of speedy evacuation; it says much for the skill and judg-ment of Allied pilots that on only a few occasions were freight/ambulance aircraft shot down. It was soon realised that the aircraft were at greatest risk while on the ground and for that reason the speedy loading of casualties was vital. To ensure this it was necessary to set up special medical units.

CASUALTY AIR EVACUATION UNITS

These were medical units, completely self-contained and fully mobile, which could be set up quickly on any airfield at which it was known that freighter aircraft would be arriving to discharge cargo. The usual strength of such units, which comprised medical and administrative sections and were commanded by a medical officer, was about thirty. The unit would arrive at the airfield, set up camp and notify local medical units that casualties could be flown out at a stated time and that the unit would be responsible for marshalling the flow of ambulances, sorting out cases unsuitable for flight (e.g., sucking chest wounds) and above all ensuring a rapid loading of casualties on to the waiting freight aircraft. It was the usual practice to attach these 'C.A.E. units' to Mobile Field Hospitals (usually two to each M.F.H.) which acted as parent unit. This liaison was of particular value in that if the C.A.E.U. became swamped it could call on the M.F.H. for assistance—in fact in the Invasion of Europe the normal work of M.F.Hs. was so reduced by air evacuation that a number of them were employed solely as large C.A.E.Us. These small units became remarkably efficient and often over 200 patients, walking and stretcher, were loaded in less than 20 minutes.

The greatest difficulty arose when bad weather or sudden operational changes of plan diverted transport aircraft to another airfield at the last moment, for if communications were bad, as was often the case, the C.A.E.U. might be unaware of the change until it was too late to move the casualties to the new loading point. More commonly, delay in the arrival of aircraft created the problem of having to hold seriously ill patients for a longer period than was catered for by the necessarily modest accommodation. It was this difficulty which led to the formation of special, larger units known as Holding Units.

THE HOLDING UNIT

These were enlarged C.A.E. units equipped with sufficient tented accommodation to house 50 or more casualties, depending on the ingenuity of the unit personnel in improvising shelter beyond their official capacity if the need should arise.

Holding units were always located in immediate proximity to the airfield, with good road access for ambulances and easy outlet on to the airfield. They had sufficient equipment to provide meals and continuation treatment such as chemotherapy and transfusions and also prepared the patients for flight. It was thus possible for the unit to summon patients preparatory to air lift and hold them in adequate surroundings, overnight if necessary, when take-off was delayed for any reason. If, exceptionally, a holding unit became overloaded with casualties, assistance was requested from local Army medical units and R.A.F. Field Hospitals and this was always willingly given.

As the war progressed Field Commanders came to regard evacuation by air as an integral part of military operations and numbers approaching 1,000 in one day were not unusual.

CASUALTY AIR EVACUATION CENTRES

During the Invasion of Europe the numbers of wounded being evacuated made it necessary to establish a large unit of field hospital size as the holding and despatching unit for air evacuation. Casualties were flown to this unit by shuttle air services from a number of other holding units and overnight accommodation for a minimum of 200 patients was guaranteed. Such units were known as Casualty Air Evacuation Centres.

RECEPTION CENTRES, UNITED KINGDOM

With such a system working on the Continent it is not surprising that the numbers arriving in the United Kingdom were large—for example, in August 1944 a total of 12,106 invalids were flown out, of whom 8,955 were stretcher cases. The Reception Centres in the United Kingdom had, therefore, to be specially organised to allow a ready flow of casualties.

They had to undertake three main tasks: sorting all wounded into categories of urgency, operating as quickly as possible on certain selected cases and distributing the remainder to other hospitals and special centres all over England.

The three airfields chosen as Reception Centres were Down Ampney, Blakehill Farm and Broadwell. A system of multiple admission and medical checking was evolved which allowed for fast handling of casualties and at no time was there any hold-up in the air lift due to 'blocking' at the reception end of the line. The two main casualty clearing stations were R.A.F. General Hospital, Wroughton, and E.M.S. Hospital, Stratton St. Margaret, both near Swindon in Wiltshire.

To summarise, the evacuation of casualties by air was virtually non-existent at the beginning of the war, but by the end of hostilities over 1½ million wounded or sick personnel had been carried by the Allied Air Forces, with such notable feats as 200,000 lifted out of the difficult Burma terrain, often at the rate of 600 a day. It was accepted that freighter aircraft should be used for casualties on their return journeys and that aircraft should not generally be earmarked for ambulance duties alone. It had been found necessary to establish special medical units to ensure that evacuation was carried out efficiently and safely and that continual modification of such units was necessary to meet the changing war situation.

This account is necessarily brief, but various full accounts appear in the three volumes of the R.A.F. Medical Services in this series. The following will be of particular interest: Volume I, pp. 252–259 and 476–536; Volume III, Middle East pp. 136–141, Italian Campaign pp. 413–415, and Invasion of Europe pp. 502–506.

AIR AMBULANCES

As indicated above, it was rarely possible to allot aircraft solely for the rôle of evacuating casualties from battle areas, and returning freighter aircraft were generally used for this purpose. There were, however, limited numbers of ambulance aircraft available for specific duties.

Air Ambulances in Scotland. In Scotland, particularly the Hebrides, there were some small, very isolated stations for which medical cover could only be provided if a civilian medical practitioner was within reasonable distance. Sudden illness demanding, for example, surgical intervention, presented a major problem which was overcome, to some extent, by the allocation of an Anson aircraft to each of two strategically placed R.A.F. stations, namely Abbotsinch and Wick.

These ambulance aircraft carried over 300 patients between late 1941 and 1944 and were greatly appreciated not only by Service personnel but by civilians, for whom they were also used on occasion.

Light Ambulance Aircraft. In Burma very considerable use was made of the Stinson light aircraft for detecting enemy movements in the jungle, for the L.5, as it was better known, could land and take off from small jungle strips. It was found possible to fit a single stretcher into these aircraft and individual casualties could be lifted out of jungle terrain from such units as advance patrols which had no medical cover. Pilots were unarmed, subject to Japanese air attack and, although they had had no medical training, were virtually responsible for the patient throughout the flight. Such was the morale value of these lifts that the authorities saw the wisdom of permitting a number of L.5's to be used wholly on ambulance duties.

Emergency Air Ambulances. On occasion emergencies arose where it was imperative to remove a patient immediately to a special centre. For this purpose the nearest flying unit was asked to provide an aircraft, such a request only being refused, and then with great reluctance, in the face of the most vital operational necessity.

In the early summer of 1942 during an outbreak of poliomyelitis in the Azores, a Flying Fortress was 'borrowed' to fly ten men, critically ill with incipient respiratory paralysis, to the United Kingdom as no 'iron lungs' were available on the island; seven of these patients survived.

Finally, the use of float and amphibious aircraft was not overlooked, for in certain circumstances these offered the only means of removing patients to medical care.

Venereal Diseases

During the period 1937–45, R.A.F. medical statistics show that 59,396 R.A.F. officers and airmen* contracted one or other of the venereal diseases. The period of treatment per case ranged from 74 days in 1937 to 10 days in 1945.

The loss of working hours and efficiency due to V.D. was needless as well as serious, as the avoidance of this disease is within the control of the individual. The most conservative estimate suggests that over half a million working hours were lost.

The steps taken, officially and unofficially, to prevent and control V.D. may be grouped under three broad headings:

(i) Executive and disciplinary control;

(ii) Medical advice, together with the provision of certain facilities for prevention and early treatment, and propaganda;

(iii) Moral approach through padres and other interested voluntary bodies.

EXECUTIVE AND DISCIPLINARY CONTROL

Prior to the Second World War a member of the R.A.F. who contracted venereal disease was considered to be suffering from a 'disease due to his own fault' and was thus liable to pay a hospital charge towards his treatment, but this payment was abolished in the war years as accounting was unworkable and the practice was likely to encourage concealment.

The responsibility of officers and others with regard to V.D. control was laid down by K.R. & A.C.I. paras. 938—'Warnings of Venereal Disease' and 1102 'Concealment of Venereal Disease' which are summarised below:

K.R. 938. The C.O. of a P.D.C., in conjunction with the M.O., was responsible for seeing (i) that all drafts going abroad were warned of the prevalence and virulence of V.D. abroad, the special dangers that existed at sea ports and that over-indulgence in alcohol led to risk; (ii) that draft officers were aware of their responsibility for the men under their control if the draft was delayed in towns while in transit.

K.R. 1102. Every unit was to have a standing order that airmen suffering from V.D. must report sick immediately. This order to be read on unit parade at not less than three monthly intervals

---

* W.A.A.F. statistics: total cases for 1939–1945 = 1,511 or 2·36 per 1,000 per annum.

and special care taken to ensure that it was brought to the attention of recruits on joining.

Such was the bare outline of an executive officer's obligations regarding the control of V.D. But into the actual words may be read the spirit of the regulations, which was that an officer should 'take care of his men', and the majority of officers and N.C.Os. acted on this implication in using their influence and taking various steps to prevent V.D. in their unit. Good relations between officers and men and the example set by the former were of the utmost value and in fact, where leadership was good, the V.D. rate was usually low; unfortunately, however, the reverse was equally true. Much was done by fostering unit pride and by providing entertainment and recreational facilities.

RESPONSIBILITY OF MEDICAL OFFICERS

In K.R. 1490 it was stated that a medical officer 'will deliver lectures from time to time to officers and airmen . . . on the subjects of venereal disease and personal hygiene.' This was the only specific mention of a medical officer's responsibility with regard to V.D., but his obligations were extended indefinitely by K.R. 1477, which stated that a station medical officer must act in an advisory capacity to the Commanding Officer of the station on the physical efficiency and well-being of airmen and in prevention of sickness and maintenance of health.

The majority of medical officers carried out their duties conscientiously and to the best of their ability, but on a number of stations conditions left much to be desired. In some units regular lectures were not given, and it was always difficult to obtain full attendance. The Service offered some guidance in the matter of lecture material, but this in itself constituted a danger for a stereotyped lecture delivered by a medical officer with no flair for public speaking would, in the end, become so boring that personnel would treat the whole subject with contempt.

Medical officers had as their audience young men of varying moral standards and intellectual ability; many were singularly ignorant of the facts of life and a medical officer who used any but the simplest terms in speaking to them was rewarded by blank faces and a complete failure of his lecture. A method which gave good results was for the M.O. to lecture for a maximum of half an hour, devote a similar amount of time to questions and finish by inviting men to come to sick quarters and discuss with him privately any matter on which they were in doubt. This last point was of particular importance in that it gave an easy opening for the frightened youth who, rightly or wrongly, thought himself to be suffering from a venereal infection.

METHODS ADOPTED TO CONTROL VENEREAL DISEASE

MORAL APPROACH AND PROVISION OF ENTERTAINMENT

As regards the moral approach much devolved upon the station padres, who did their utmost to bring the moral issue before personnel by all possible means. It is probably true that the best approach was the indirect one of taking an interest in welfare in its broadest aspect and by entering into as many of the station functions as possible. The contribution made by padres in the field of organised recreation was very great and all efforts in this direction were appreciated by station commanders and medical officers alike. Service clubs, staffed by voluntary organisations, such as the Red Cross, provided an attractive alternative to the more dubious forms of civilian entertainment.

Issue of Condoms. In the latter two-thirds of the war period authority was given for condoms to be available for Service personnel serving overseas. They were usually made available through the S.S.Q. or guard room, distribution being arranged as informally as possible so that the aim would not be defeated by causing embarrassment. Though never officially sanctioned an issue was also arranged privately on several stations in the United Kingdom. This policy was, in the opinion of many medical officers, justifiable in that it conferred a fair degree of protection.

Early Treatment Rooms. In all permanent and semi-permanent units, and where possible in mobile formations, an E.T. Room was set up and personnel made aware of its exact location and purpose. Light, running water and privacy were desirable, but in many instances these were not attained and the rooms were consequently little used. In any case, the time elapsing between exposure in a town and return to camp lessened their usefulness and to overcome this E.T. rooms were set up in many cities for the use of Service personnel; this also provided a facility for personnel on leave in the particular area. (See *R.A.F. Medical Services.* Volume I. pp. 401–402.) Abroad the provision of adequate E.T. rooms was even more important than in the United Kingdom.

Early Treatment Packets. These were made available, as a free issue, to all personnel, and were usually obtainable from the guard room. If correctly used they were of value, but often were either forgotten, remembered too late or used incorrectly.

Prostitution. Known prostitutes were not accepted into the women's services although instances are recorded of such women gaining admission.

As far as control of prostitutes was concerned in the United Kingdom, Defence Regulation 33B which provided for the compulsory treatment of contacts who were known sources of infection was of great value when co-ordination with the civil authorities was close.

The 'amateur' constituted a greater danger than the professional prostitute, as the latter was aware of the risks and took some kind of precautions for her own sake. The 'amateur' was usually an unthinking, pleasure-seeking girl who took little trouble over personal protection and was slow to realise that she had contracted an infection and equally slow to seek medical advice. The problem of the 'amateur' was particularly great in the industrial cities and was very difficult to solve.

Vice Squads, Civil Watch Committees. These bodies facilitated discussion between Service and civil authorities; such discussions were of value in assessing the moral aspects as well as the gravity of the particular situation in a given locality.

Free From Infection (F.F.I.) Inspections. These inspections, carried out at regular intervals, had a very limited immediate value in detecting V.D.; it was impossible to ensure that the inspection was complete and as far as females were concerned infection was rarely discovered in this way. But it is believed that some sufferers were led to seek early medical advice, rather than risk discovery at a routine parade.

Propaganda. Medical officers not only gave lectures on V.D. at varying intervals, but used their influence to ensure that no opportunity was lost of publicising the dangers of the disease. Films on the subject were available and were shown regularly, but these were open to criticism in that they were not of a particularly high technical standard and that, if seen more than once, they did little good and probably harm, through familiarity.

Posters depicting the dangers of venereal disease were shown in many public rooms on stations and other suitable places such as transit camps and P.D.Cs. It was often difficult to get posters produced quickly (see *R.A.F. Medical Services.* Volume III. p. 672) and here again familiarity bred contempt, while sometimes the impact was lessened by the poster appearing among half a dozen others on various subjects.

Penicillin. This drug was not produced in quantity until late in the war. Two dangers were associated with its use; the first was that its efficacy as a specific became so well known that personnel treated the acquisition of V.D. with lighthearted contempt; the second was that personnel might obtain treatment with small doses of penicillin, from unofficial sources, which though perhaps effective against neisserian infection, would cloak a concurrent syphilitic infection. (*See also* page 268. Supply of Important drugs.)

Dental Branch

Between 1939 and 1945 over two and a quarter million members of the Royal Air Force were rendered dentally fit. During this period over seven million fillings, two and three quarter million extractions and work involving over half a million dentures was carried out by a force of rarely more than 900 dental surgeons. From such a mass of work and organisation many lessons were learnt.

DENTAL OFFICERS

To meet war-time expansion an organisation called the Central Dental Emergency Committees (later to become the Dental War Committees) was set up under the aegis of the Ministry of Health in 1939 to undertake the call-up of dentists to the Forces and to ensure, as far as possible, that civilian and Service needs were equitably met. In this way it was possible, on the whole, to provide minimum requirements for each of these commitments throughout the war years, although at times individual Commands and areas had their difficulties. The employment of women dental officers was, surprisingly, never fully implemented.

DENTAL CLERK ORDERLIES

If the provision of dental officers caused relatively few problems, that of finding the necessary orderlies to assist them gave rise to difficulties which increased as the war progressed. In August 1939, W.A.A.F. personnel were admitted into this trade (at a ratio of 3 W.A.A.F. to 2 R.A.F.). This experiment was initially successful largely because the first entrants had had peace-time experience but this reservoir was soon exhausted. In an effort to increase the numbers of orderlies the training period was decreased and men of lowered medical categories were admitted to the trade. This proved a mistaken policy for a high proportion of these men were unfit for service overseas, where W.A.A.F. substitution was often not permitted. The difficulty could have been met and time saved if the General Service training had been shortened and if sufficient dental instructors had been available.

DENTAL MECHANICS

In September 1939 the R.A.F. had only 20 dental mechanics, but by the end of the war this number had increased to 325. Considerable difficulty was encountered in attaining this figure, largely owing to training difficulties and the relatively poor standard of qualified mechanics drafted into the Service. To deal with the problem a special shortened course was introduced by the R.A.F. Dental Branch. The successful entrant was designated Dental Mechanic under Training and worked under careful supervision until considered fit to be regraded as a fully trained dental mechanic. This improvisation proved most satisfactory and without it the work of the Dental Branch would have been almost impossible. It is interesting to note that although the trade was open to women only two ever qualified as dental mechanics.

DENTAL HYGIENISTS

In 1941, when dental officers were being hard-pressed with ever-increasing arrears of work, it was suggested that some of the minor treatment such as scaling and polishing could be undertaken by suitably trained W.A.A.F. personnel. This suggestion was in direct conflict with the terms of the Dental Act of 1921, but the latter was not binding on the Services. After considerable discussion at a high level, it was agreed that W.A.A.F. personnel might be employed in this manner after special training (12 weeks) and then always working under the supervision of a dental officer. The first Dental Hygienists were trained and started work early in 1943 and immediately proved a boon to the overworked dental officers. The benefits of this scheme so far outweighed the possible hazards that it was felt it should have been introduced earlier. There is little doubt that it was due to the work of these hygienists that no major outbreaks of ulcerative gingivitis were encountered during the war, while their employment played an important part in making Service personnel dentally minded.

OVERSEAS SERVICES

At first, responsibility for R.A.F. dental fitness overseas was undertaken, in most areas, by the Army Dental Corps. With expansion it soon became evident that this arrangement was unsatisfactory and impracticable and R.A.F. dental officers and staff were accordingly posted abroad.

The work overseas was hampered by the shortage of dental officers in relation to the wide distribution of personnel and the inevitable difficulties of transport. The formation of Mobile Dental Units and the attachment of dental officers to Mobile Field Hospitals somewhat eased the problem but the services available fell below those obtaining in the United Kingdom, where reciprocal arrangements between commands and civilian services were more easily and advantageously arranged.

In war-time the posting of dental officers overseas in proportion to numbers of personnel must be on a generous scale to allow for the inevitable geographical difficulties.

CIVIL CONSULTANT IN DENTAL SURGERY

In 1941 a dental specialist of international repute was appointed as the first Civil Consultant to the R.A.F. His services proved invaluable not only in regard to overall guidance, but also because he commanded the respect of the dental profession as a whole and was able to foster a beneficial liaison with the Ministry of Health and civilian hospitals.

EQUIPMENT

Early in the war dental equipment became progressively scarcer until in 1941 the position was acute. This was chiefly due to the inadequate reserves of equipment to meet the rapid expansion of the Force, the lack of standardisation of equipment among the manufacturers and the call-up of civilian tool makers into the Forces. The position improved when all dental manufacturers were brought under the direct control of the Ministry of Supply, who ensured as complete a measure of standardisation as possible, and when the R.A.F. Dental Branch formed an instrument repair section under the direction of a specially trained N.C.O.

The supply position was even more difficult overseas due to the combined factors of distance, irregularity of supply, damage resulting from inadequate packing or excessively rough handling and poor tropicalisation of fragile apparatus. The position was eased by the introduction of storage sub-depots and advances in the science of tropicalising instruments and electrical apparatus. Relatively portable apparatus was designed and issued, but it was still bulky and caused difficulty in air transport. It is clear that if dental officers are, in the future, to form part of highly mobile and airborne forces their equipment must be light and robust; dental X-ray equipment may be given as an example of apparatus of which a portable type was never satisfactorily evolved during the war.

ADMINISTRATION

At the outbreak of war it was clear that decentralisation of command was essential for the smooth running of the Dental Branch and accordingly senior dental officers were appointed to certain commands and formations. A somewhat similar organisation was set up to cover overseas commands, but here it was often more convenient to establish officers on a geographical basis to minimise the difficulty of travelling.

As regards dental arrangements for campaigns it was noted that S.D.Os. were often not supplied with sufficient information as to the scope of proposed operations to allow them to make the necessary arrangments for adequate and effective dental coverage of the force, a situation similar to that noted by some medical officers in like circumstances.

ACCOMMODATION

In the United Kingdom excellent dental facilities in respect of surgeries, store rooms and plaster rooms existed in nearly all sick quarters on permanent stations and although the standard was considerably lower on the war-time-built prefabricated stations, workable accommodation was usually achieved after certain minor alterations had been made to the often ill-conceived basic design. Abroad matters were less well arranged and many of the war-time-constructed facilities showed that their designers had little knowledge of dental requirements; even after necessary alterations this accommodation was often not conducive to either good or economic work.

MOBILE DENTAL UNITS

In common with the rest of the R.A.F. the Dental Branch had to adapt itself to mobile warfare in many theatres. The first mobile dental surgery and laboratory was constructed (at the Cairo base) in 1942, utilising the chassis of an Albion ambulance, and was attached to No. 21 Mobile Field Hospital in the Western Desert. From this small beginning many mobile dental vehicles and trailers were introduced with varying success.

Certain principles emerged from experience of these mobile dental units. Although trailers (caravans) had certain advantages they were not generally suitable (except in the United Kingdom) for operational usage as they were entirely dependent on another vehicle for movement and were never sufficiently robust to stand up to cross country work. The ideal pattern was considered to be a converted four-wheel drive chassis of standard Service pattern so that 'cannibalisation' was possible to avoid a valuable vehicle being out of commission for any length of time. In certain difficult terrain, such as jungle, specially devised light-weight tentage will always be necessary and should be constructed with a view to its ease of transport by light aircraft.

TRAINING

Dental Officers

All dental officers entered the Service with a civilian qualification acquired before call-up and consequently little was needed to supplement their professional armamentarium. It was necessary, however, for all dental officers to attend a brief course to familiarise them with the ways of the Service and the running of their own branch. The length of this course varied but was usually about six weeks; it might well have been shortened.

Specially picked dental officers were given training in the treatment of maxillo-facial injuries and were then usually attached to special centres; however, so essential was this subject that short courses were also arranged for other dental officers, particularly those who were either going overseas or being attached to Mobile Field Hospitals. Many dental officers also attended courses on anaesthetics.

Dental Clerk Orderlies

Training of these personnel was one of the main difficulties encountered throughout the war.

In order to fill the many vacancies training was speeded up and divided into two sections—the first of approximately three weeks allotted to theory and the second, lasting five weeks, devoted to supervised practical work on certain large stations and centres; at the end of this course candidates were trade tested. On the introduction of W.A.A.F. orderlies difficulties were encountered in finding suitable accommodation and it was some time before their training was parallel with that outlined above.

The main difficulties encountered were poor quality entrants which entailed a high examination failure rate with a consequent waste of valuable training time, the necessity for relatively small classes (16 being considered the desirable maximum) and the difficulty of providing enough suitable instructors, and finally, the lowered medical standards which precluded many orderlies from serving overseas.

Dental Mechanics

Candidates for this trade had of necessity to possess a very high degree of skill and few were obtained by direct entry. In view of the shortage a compromise was reached whereby men were initially trained and then worked at big stations or centres as Dental Mechanics under Training for a further period of what was virtually apprenticeship. Although by this means the need was met, it would appear that very careful planning should be made in peace-time to ensure that if the need arises sufficient numbers of these key tradesmen will be available to a rapidly expanding Dental Branch.

Dental Hygienists

A 12 weeks' course of instruction was given covering a wide range and a very high pass rate was the rule, no doubt due to the careful pre-selection of W.A.A.F. candidates. The introduction of hygienists must be considered one of the most important advances during the war years.

Women's Services

Before the official conscription of women under the Defence Regulations of 1941, a number of women had been admitted to serve with the R.A.F. as volunteers. The numbers were small, being just over 2,000 at the outbreak of war, but although it had been hoped to increase the strength to 20,000 by 1940 it was soon clear that the necessary recruits were unlikely to be forthcoming.

In 1941 single women became liable for service in the Armed Forces and from that date onwards the number of women in the R.A.F. rapidly increased until in early 1944 over 178,000 women were employed in over 60 different trades.

The figures quoted above are of particular interest for two reasons. First, it is extremely unlikely that any planner in the initial war years would have contemplated that so many thousands of women would eventually be absorbed into the R.A.F., for in those early days it was considered that the employment of women—the 'weaker sex'—would be strictly limited and confined to service in the United Kingdom. Secondly, women were initially employed in the R.A.F. in three trades only, as drivers, cooks and clerks, it being considered that this was the limit of their use to the Service. How very different was the picture in 1944 when women had equal responsibility with men in over 60 different R.A.F. trades, including such arduous and technical work as balloon operators and engine fitters and vital posts such as those in operations and control rooms.

DIFFICULTIES ENCOUNTERED—GENERAL

The difficulties which arose were remarkably few, the majority of women recruits adjusting themselves quickly and easily to Service life. Initially the authorities laid down very stringent rules to ensure that women were neither overworked nor asked to carry out physical tasks beyond their capacity. These rules, which seemed reasonable enough at the time, had been largely abandoned by the end of the war; women had shown that they could undertake the majority of R.A.F. ground duties equally as well as their male counterparts and in certain trades—for example, radar screen interpreters—their efficiency surpassed that of the airmen.

EXECUTIVE/MEDICAL DIFFICULTIES

Accommodation. R.A.F. buildings had, with few exceptions, been designed to house men only and the recruiting of women in large numbers gave rise to certain basic difficulties, such as the lack of privacy and inadequate sanitary provision on living and working sites. It was sometimes possible to augment existing facilities, but the war-time shortages of labour and materials often made it impossible to enlarge sewerage plants or to carry out other alterations.

In the standards of accommodation laid down for women, the floor area per person was larger than that allotted to airmen and consequently, when substitution took place on a numerical basis, the original buildings could not provide sufficient accommodation. Dispersal of accommodation also created special problems and these were accentuated when they involved women.

MEDICAL DIFFICULTIES

General. These were much as predicted and for this reason the medical authorities were to some extent prepared. Medical accommodation was the main problem, for pre-war sick quarters were not designed to accommodate both sexes. The simplest solution as far as sick parades were concerned was to hold these at different times, while the same facilities for the treatment of minor ailments and for medication could be made available for both men and women; beds for women were more difficult to provide, for sick quarters already had to segregate airmen from officers, but it was usually possible to find a small room in which at least two beds could be erected. In some cases, pre-war married quarters were used and later specially designed Nissen huts were constructed on W.A.A.F. sites.

Sickness Rates. Women reported sick for minor complaints more frequently than men. Incidence of gynaecological conditions was low.

One matter which calls for special mention was the prevalence of pediculosis capitis among recruits on entry. Over 25 per cent. of intakes were found to be infested and an elaborate organisation for initial treatment and follow-up had to be instituted to deal with this surprising situation. It was thought that girls who had had expensive hair treatment were unwilling to wash their hair. If the occasion should again arise for large-scale recruiting of women, one of the first amenities to be installed in a W.A.A.F. depot should be a hairdressing centre where recruits could be examined and if necessary immediately disinfested.

ROYAL AIR FORCE NURSING SERVICE

No mention has been made of the part played by members of Princess Mary's Royal Air Force Nursing Service and by W.A.A.F. nursing orderlies. This omission is intentional for there was nothing exceptional about women undertaking nursing in the Services and the conditions, except in some overseas areas, were very similar to those experienced by their civilian counterparts. It is of interest to note, however, the considerable numbers of women employed on nursing duties in the R.A.F.—1,390 Nursing Sisters (all possessing the S.R.N. qualification before enrolment) and over 5,000 W.A.A.F. nursing orderlies (nearly all trained by the Service after enlistment).

No particular problems arose and no praise is too great for the work they did. In the forward areas particularly the presence of a nursing sister had a beneficial effect upon morale which could only be gauged by those able to note the effect on wounded and apprehensive men of finding a woman so near to the 'firing line'.

Advances in Special Medical Fields

In the Second World War very definite advances were made in certain specialties, both in Service and civilian medicine and in the Royal Air Force, most notably in the treatment of burns, in plastic surgery and in rehabilitation.

BURNS

All three Services encountered a high proportion of burns among their operational personnel. Aircrew were greatly at risk; crashes were so often accompanied by fire.

During the Battle of Britain burned aircrew were admitted to civilian and Service hospitals all over the country. Treatment was uneven and indeed often unsatisfactory owing to the use of methods not appropriate to the type and extent of injury, particularly the coagulation technique. Medical authorities advised, whenever possible, the transfer of burns cases to hospitals where specialist attention and facilities were available. This led to the introduction of the Burns Centres, with a highly skilled staff. From these centres the major advances came, such as the saline bath technique and early coverage with skin grafts.

Medical officers, burns specialists and appropriate executive officers also directed their attention to the preventive aspect and among a number of notable achievements were the introduction of the self-sealing petrol tank, more effective fire-proof bulkheads and semi-fireproof flying clothing. These measures, combined with a drive to make aircrew aware of the steps that they themselves could take to minimise burns in crash landing, did much to lessen the risk of this type of injury.

Other causes of burns, particularly in the Campaigns, were due to such dangerous practices as lighting a fire with 100 octane as the fuel or using it as a 'disinfectant' in field latrines.

PLASTIC SURGERY

Considerable advances were made in the treatment of disfiguring and disabling injuries, particularly among flying personnel. The R.A.F. was fortunate in having Mr. A. H. McIndoe (afterwards Sir Archibald McIndoe) as Civil Consultant and it was largely due to his advice and foresight that special centres were set up, often in conjunction with Burns Centres, for those who required plastic surgery. By the end of the war such treatment had reached a very high standard and new plastic techniques and applications of skin grafting had been evolved. The centres were staffed by specially trained surgeons and carefully chosen nurses and orderlies who had similarly undergone special training.

The patient's morale and mental outlook also received careful attention. The 'Guinea Pig Club', the Ministry of Health and Branch P.5 of the Air Ministry relieved, as far as possible, any social and financial hardships during the often protracted periods of treatment.

REHABILITATION

During the Battle of Britain it was found that many airmen after discharge from hospital were still far from fit to resume duty or to be discharged to seek other employment. In considering how their return to full function could be hastened, it was apparent that the normal hospital could offer neither the necessary remedial treatment nor a satisfactory environment suitable for rehabilitation.

It thus became essential to set up special centres for rehabilitation. The first, at the R.A.F. Officers Hospital, Torquay, evolved the pattern for this type of unit, previously unknown in the Royal Air Force. Service discipline was cut to a minimum and every effort was made to encourage patients to 'assist themselves to a return to full function.' It was found advantageous to adopt an indirect approach such as competitive games, dancing, and swimming, while mental stimulus was provided by talks, discussions and the production of a unit 'magazine'. Even a bar was permitted!

So successful was the initial experiment that other centres were opened and small rehabilitation departments attached to existing hospitals. Every effort was made to encourage patients to carry out remedial exercises, for which specially designed apparatus for specific disabilities was available and it was found that few patients failed eventually to resume their R.A.F. career or find useful and profitable employment in civilian life.

It was found essential to employ specially trained staff, both medical and non-medical, who could be relied on to encourage patients at all times and yet ensure that they did not overtax their strength; well-known sporting personalities were ideal for this purpose. These were invariably popular and understanding, as might be expected from men of their proved quality.

Supply of Important Drugs

The commonly known drugs which rapidly became scarce in Britain were the Bitters Group (Gentian, etc.) and quinine, the former being supplied mainly from the Marseilles area and the latter from the Dutch East Indies. Small quantities of Cinchona were obtainable from South America throughout the war, but from a practical point of view it became unobtainable after the Japanese overran Malaya.

MEPACRINE AND MALARIA

The seriousness of the losses sustained by the Allies from malaria cannot be over-emphasised, as medically it must be looked on as a preventable disease. In West Africa in 1942 the rate was 844 cases per thousand in a total R.A.F. population of just over 5,000 and in India in 1944 the yearly rate was roughly 157 cases per thousand in a population of nearly 100,000.

The fact that supplies of quinine had been virtually cut off posed a difficult problem. Existing reserves in the United Kingdom (in hospital dispensaries, practitioners' surgeries, etc.) were mobilised, but fortunately before these supplies were exhausted the problem was solved by chemical elaboration of the anti-malarial drug known as mepacrine, which was to become one of the main medical factors in assuring Allied success in the Far East. This drug had a supressive efficiency much greater than quinine.

Slight initial difficulties were met in the general use of this drug due to sensitivity, demanding adjustment of dosage, and also, surprisingly enough, to personal opposition occasioned by rumours that the drug had sterilising effects; although these rumours were unfounded, they persisted throughout the war. At first mepacrine was not issued to aircrew engaged on operational flying as it was thought that the drug might adversely affect the oxygen-carrying power of haemoglobin; following a careful investigation at Farnborough, however, these fears were proved to be groundless and all aircrew used mepacrine from July 1944 onwards—approximately one year after it had been introduced for personnel in ground trades.

Difficulty was sometimes experienced in making executive officers realise, not only the undoubted value of the drug, but also that if adequate protection was to be maintained there must be no interruption to the daily dosage. The majority of cases of malaria encountered after the introduction of mepacrine were due to disregard of orders specifying the daily dosage. Only very rarely were true cases of non-absorption of mepacrine encountered.

The Japanese suffered severely from malaria; they had no drug equivalent to mepacrine and although they held large stocks of quinine they never used it generally as a suppressant and only rarely for treatment.

SULPHAGUANIDINE AND DYSENTERY

Next to malaria the greatest hazard to our forces in overseas campaigns was dysentery and enteritis, two clinical entities which could not easily be distinguished in most forward areas as laboratory confirmation was rarely available. Amoebic dysentery remained one of the great dangers of tropical service and one in which little advance was made either in easy clinical diagnosis or treatment; the R.A.F. alone suffered over 10,000 cases during the war years.

For the commoner form, bacillary dysentery, sulphaguanidine, introduced just before our re-entry into Burma, had a rapid and specific effect on most types of the disease; it was easily administered and did not involve a risk of anuria.

In forward areas it was customary and expedient to treat all precipitant forms of diarrhoea as being bacillary in origin and a standard régimen for the administration of sulphaguanidine was introduced which usually allowed the sufferer to return to duty within about a week without hospitalisation. The effect of this drug on the operational situation was very great, for prior to its introduction it had often been necessary to send patients to hospital for treatment—a most time-consuming procedure in forward areas.

The R.A.F. suffered over 32,000 recorded casualties from bacillary dysentery. The true figure, however, must have been much greater, for after the introduction of sulphaguanidine a large number of cases were simply labelled enteritis and treatment was so effective and rapid that patients never showed the clinical signs of dysentery.

The widespread use of the drug, however, had one distinct disadvantage in that, because it was now unnecessary to send patients to hospital, stool tests were no longer carried out. This meant that, in patients with the dual pathology of amoebic and bacillary dysentery, the former was often missed and became chronic, not being diagnosed for months or even years.

D.D.T. (DICHLORO-DIPHENYL-TRICHLORETHANE) AND MOSQUITO CONTROL

Although the introduction of mepacrine greatly minimised the risks of malaria, the basic principle of the hygienists was to remove the vector and this was the purpose behind all Service field prophylaxis. In the early stages of the war many insecticides were issued, traditional larvicides, and insecticides having pyrethrum as the active principle, but supplies were short and the success attained only limited.

When D.D.T. was introduced it was found to be one of the most powerful weapons available to the hygienists, for whole areas could be brought under control both quickly and with economy of labour. D.D.T. was applied either from the ground by a variety of hand and mechanical sprays or by aerial dispersion, the latter being a most valuable method of treating areas such as swamps which were difficult or impossible to reach in any other way.

Unfortunately, it was not until towards the end of the war that D.D.T. was available in sufficient quantities. Its earlier introduction would have been of immense value in such areas as West Africa, Sicily and Burma.

In connexion with mosquito control, the use of personal repellents must be mentioned because their limitations tended to outweigh their efficiency. Several types of repellent were in use, some having a grease base and others being liquid preparations, but none was popular, the greasy type being the least favoured. It is only fair to say that the repellents available during the greater part of the war generally gave very little protection and in some instances appeared to attract rather than repel mosquitoes.

WATER STERILISING TABLETS (CHLORAMINE AND SODIUM THIOSULPHATE) AND DYSENTERY

These tablets were issued to personnel unable to obtain safe water, when bulk sterilisation was impracticable. They were widely used in forward areas and proved a reliable safeguard; they were also included in escape and evasion packs.

HYOSCINE AND MOTION SICKNESS

The problem of motion sickness was one that affected all three Services. It was, of course, if a persisting disability, a permanent bar to aircrew training, and aircrew could not be 'drugged'.

Many substances were tried out, but it was generally agreed that hyoscine in small doses was the most effective drug. It produced imbalance, however, in many persons if the dosage was too high. The anti-histamine groups were little used as, at that time, their development had not reached an advanced stage.

PENICILLIN

Penicillin was not generally introduced in the R.A.F. until late in the war and its use never became widespread. R.A.F. trials began in 1942, the small supplies available being administered under the direct supervision of Senior Consultants on specially selected cases. The drug was first used in quantity in the treatment of casualties from the D-day landings, but there was considerable difference of opinion as to what should constitute standard dosage. The first official Air Ministry publication giving guidance on the subject (Air Ministry Pamphlet 186) was issued in July 1945 and this stated that use of the drug was to be confined to general hospitals and special centres, sick quarters using it only with special Air Ministry permission.

The uses and advantages of pencillin are well known and R.A.F. medical personnel rapidly became aware of the value of the drug, particularly in burns and 'dirty' accident cases. Its very efficiency, however, had one serious consequence, which became evident very quickly after the introduction of the drug. It soon became common knowledge among Service personnel that the drug was a panacea for venereal disease, and this engendered an attitude of carelessness among some who would otherwise have refrained from exposure because of a fear of V.D. and the difficulty and uncertainty of effective treatment.

The problems which presented themselves in Medicine, Psychiatry and Surgery are discussed in other contributions to this volume. Fuller accounts are to be found in *Medicine and Pathology* and *Surgery* in the United Kingdom Official Medical History of the Second World War.

The Emergency Medical Services

By

Sir Arthur S. MacNalty, K.C.B., M.A., M.D., F.R.C.P., F.R.C.S.

and

Lieutenant-Colonel C. L. Dunn, C.I.E., I.M.S. (Ret.)

CONTENTS

THE EMERGENCY MEDICAL SERVICES
The Civil Defence Casualty Services

UP TO December 1938 all Air Raid Precautions (A.R.P.) Services, including the Casualty Service, were under the control of the A.R.P. Department of the Home Office. Control of the first-aid post and ambulance service was then transferred to the Ministry of Health, but that of the first-aid party (and stretcher party) service remained with the Home Office, which also continued to be responsible for the recruitment of personnel and their preliminary training in first aid. Early in 1939 Mobile Units (later Mobile First-Aid Units) were added to the Casualty Service to supplement first-aid posts (fixed), and doctors were allocated to every one of these (mobile and fixed). The administration of the Casualty Service was now placed under the control of the Director General, Emergency Medical Services at the Ministry of Health.

In the Regions medical officers of health of local authorities were made responsible for the local administration and operational control of these services, subject to general direction by the A.R.P. Controllers and acted as agents for Regional Hospital Officers, who were in turn responsible to the D.G.E.M.S.

On the outbreak of war the Ministry of Home Security was set up for the co-ordination of civil defence throughout the country. In December 1939 responsibility for the technical oversight of first-aid training for first-aid parties was transferred to the Ministry of Health.

THE CIVIL DEFENCE CASUALTY SERVICES IN SCOTLAND AND NORTHERN IRELAND

These services were under the direction of the same central authority as the Emergency Hospital Services, thus bringing all sections of the Emergency Medical Services under the control of one Minister. In England and Wales the first-aid party service remained under the central control of the Home Office throughout the war.

UNITS OF THE CASUALTY SERVICES

FIRST-AID POSTS

Where possible these were based in hospitals, especially in areas most exposed to attack; otherwise, they were provided in protected buildings on a scale of six posts per 100,000 population, and in urban areas not more than one mile apart. A typical first-aid post, with gas cleansing section, consisted of a building with lateral and overhead protection, staffed by a doctor, a trained nurse and twenty-five nursing auxiliaries (including a lay superintendent and two men) with special first-aid equipment. Many posts were set up in schools, public halls, etc., but where they were not available *ad hoc* buildings were erected to a special design by the Ministry of Home Security and the Ministry of Health. Their purpose was to deal with lightly injured and mentally disturbed persons who would otherwise flood Casualty Receiving Hospitals and impede their work, provide supervision and classification of casualties by a doctor, give necessary immediate treatment and shelter, comfort, warmth, food and drink, and have cleansing facilities for persons contaminated by persistent gas in the event of this form of attack being used by the enemy, an event which did not occur. At the beginning of the war, 1,912 First-Aid Posts of the 2,180 which had been approved, were ready; 150,000 personnel had been enrolled for first-aid posts and mobile units, 10,000 men and 35,000 women being whole-time, the rest part-time.

FIRST-AID POINTS

In the early days of the war some 6,500 first-aid points were established in rural and semi-rural districts as small emergency treatment centres. Each point had a box of first-aid equipment kept in some convenient house where volunteers could meet and train in first aid. No doctor or trained nurse was attached to a point.

MOBILE UNITS

Each consisted of a motor vehicle with first-aid equipment. The staff was composed of a doctor, a trained nurse who travelled in the vehicle and a personnel of 18 nursing auxiliaries (which could include two men) who worked in three shifts of six persons and travelled separately. Two men drivers were attached to each unit. These mobile units went to an incident and set up a first-aid post either in some convenient and previously selected building or even in the open air, to which casualties could be brought; they reinforced an overworked first-aid post or took over from one damaged or destroyed; they provided supervision, classification of injuries and skilled treatment on the spot; or acted as a temporary Casualty Receiving Hospital, where a hospital had been damaged or destroyed. At the beginning of the war 783 of these units were approved and most were ready.

AMBULANCE SERVICE

This comprised (*a*) the large ambulances usually improvised from single decker omnibuses taking up to ten stretcher cases, and (*b*) small ambulances with two to four stretchers for picking up casualties or clearing first-aid posts. These were improvised from light cars by local authorities. Each standard A.R.P. ambulance carried four stretchers and had a driver and attendant, both trained in first aid. On the outbreak of war, 1,600 whole-time and about 150 part-time local authority ambulances were ready in the London Region and 5,300 whole-time and 5,200 part-time in the provinces. The total personnel in England and Wales was 80,889 (of which London Region provided 17,344). The total number of whole-time men and women was 26,887 against 54,002 part-time.

SITTING CASE CARS

On December 31, 1939 there were 2,332 whole-time and 12,524 part-time sitting case cars for the conveyance of lightly injured casualties unable to walk to first-aid posts.

FIRST-AID PARTY SERVICE

First-aid parties (in London, called stretcher parties) consisted of four men with a car and a driver. They were stationed in depots, and went out in their own transport with first-aid equipment when summoned by the local Control Centre, or, exceptionally when called directly by wardens, police, etc. (the Control Centre being notified). Four stretchers and eight blankets were carried in each party car. As the result of experience, parties were allocated on a scale of sixty-six per 100,000 population in most vulnerable areas, thirty-three in highly vulnerable areas, twenty-six in less vulnerable areas and twenty in least vulnerable areas. In August 1939 the total strength was roughly 66,000 available personnel.

THE RESCUE PARTY SERVICE

Rescue parties each consisted of six or eight men with their own transport under the control of the local authority Engineer or Surveyor. Eventually, heavy and light rescue parties were constituted and allocated on a scale of six heavy parties of nine men each and twenty-four light parties of seven men each per 100,000 population in most vulnerable areas, three heavy and twelve light parties in highly vulnerable areas, one heavy and nine light parties in less vulnerable areas and one heavy and six light parties in least vulnerable areas. Their main duties were the extrication of casualties from damaged buildings, in demolition work and the removal of débris. They were based on depots similar to those of first-aid parties. In January 1943 the Rescue and First-Aid Party Services were amalgamated as 'The Civil Defence Rescue Service' and combined the functions previously performed by the two constituent services. This helped to release whole-time personnel for industry.

K*

THE INCIDENT DOCTOR

The desirability of the presence of a doctor at every incident was realised early in the war, and this was officially recognised in May 1941. Rotas of doctors, who were not members of the Casualty Service Organisation but were willing to attend at incidents, were maintained by medical officers of health, generally at Control Centres and sometimes at Wardens' posts.

CIVIL DEFENCE

In 1941, the name 'Civil Defence' was substituted for 'A.R.P.', with new service markings and a national system of badges of rank. Uniforms were sanctioned for doctors at first-aid posts. The name 'Civil Defence' was prefixed to each unit of the Casualty Service (e.g., Civil Defence Ambulance Service). In April 1942, the total number of whole-time personnel of the Civil Defence Services was reduced by one-third throughout the country, to release persons in these services to contribute to the war effort in industry.

THE RIVER EMERGENCY SERVICE

This service was designed by the Port of London Authority as a casualty service in 1939 to co-operate with the Civil Defence Casualty Service on land when required. It operated between Hammersmith and Canvey Island. The ambulance ships carried doctors, nurses and stretcher bearers and were in constant communication with Civil Defence Controllers on land. The Service dealt with casualties caused by enemy action and with all other types of casualty met with on the river. Equipment and replacement of medical stores was done by the Ministry of Health, whose Regional Medical Officers made frequent inspections of the ambulance ships. The River Emergency Service did good work during the raids, especially in those of the latter part of 1940 and early part of 1941.

CONCLUSION

The Civil Defence Casualty Services and their work throughout the war are described in *The Emergency Medical Services*. Vol. I. Chapters 7 and 8. The Civil Defence organisation stood up nobly to the enemy's repeated aerial onslaughts by piloted and robot bombing on this country. Much of its preliminary work had been devoted to arrangements for dealing with aerial gas attacks. Gas was not used, but the precautions taken, including the distribution of gas masks to the civilian population provided an insurance against this inhuman form of warfare. Through the provision of shelters and the precautions taken for their healthy conditions, by the provision of rest centres, national fire service, first-aid centres and transport by ambulance, the effects of the bombing raids were minimised as far as possible. The public health and medical work done by medical officers of health, doctors, nurses, sanitary inspectors, health visitors and others was beyond all praise. The Women's Voluntary Service rendered great assistance. A high tribute must be paid to the efficiency of the ambulance service and to the courage, zeal and resourcefulness of the drivers, many of whom were young women. Countless epic stories are related of their heroism and exploits. Some died at the wheel; others carried on when wounded, thinking not of themselves but of the patients they were conveying to hospital. All concerned in the Civilian Casualty Service, as in the Emergency Medical Services, were imbued throughout with the spirit of patriotism and self-sacrifice.

The Hospital Services

EARLY STEPS TO ESTABLISH A CASUALTY HOSPITAL SERVICE

The Committee of Imperial Defence soon after the War of 1914–1918 inquired into the question of air-raid precautions in the event of air attack from the Continent in a future war (*see* Introduction to *E.M.S.* Vol. I). A standing sub-committee was set up in 1921, which in 1925 requested the Ministry of Health to draw up a scheme for the collection and medical treatment of air-raid casualties, for hospital accommodation and the evacuation of the wounded. The Ministry submitted a preliminary report in 1926. Then an inter-departmental committee, on which the Ministry of Health, the Home Office, the War Office and the Ministry of Transport were represented, was appointed to devise a scheme for the medical services of London. From 1927 this Committee issued a number of reports culminating in a comprehensive scheme in 1934 for the first-aid treatment of casualties and their removal to hospital.

In May 1935 the Air Raid Precautions Department of the Home Office was set up. Local authorities were asked to make provisions for mobilising the medical and first-aid resources of each area, for ambulances, casualty clearing hospitals, for hospitals for more extended treatment and for efficient anti-gas precautions.

As the German menace grew more threatening, in May 1937 the Committee of Imperial Defence appointed the MacNalty Committee to give further consideration to the measures necessary for the hospital treatment of casualties. As a result of the recommendations of this Committee the organisation of 'base' hospitals was assigned to the Ministry of Health.

The Ministry at once made a comprehensive survey of the hospital accommodation in England and Wales. From this survey the Ministry was able to grade the hospitals in accordance with their capabilities, size and geographical distribution. The artificial separation between casualty clearing and 'base' hospitals was abolished with the consent of the Home Office. That Department retained responsibility for the ambulance and first-aid services administered by the local authorities. On June 1, 1938 the Ministry of Health accordingly assumed control of all hospitals in England and Wales and the Department of Health for Scotland assumed a similar responsibility for that country. From this date regional organisations were constituted. Central committees were set up to provide for the recruitment of medical, nursing and technical personnel to expand the staff of the existing hospitals included in the scheme, for hospitals to be converted, up-graded or newly constructed and for the ancillary medical services of the hospitals. The co-operation and help of the administrative and medical staffs of both local authority and voluntary hospitals were essential for the Emergency Hospital Scheme, and it is a tribute to their public spirit that it was freely given and that many personal sacrifices were made and irksome restrictions accepted in the interests of national defence. (The measures taken to establish an Emergency Hospital Service are detailed in *E.M.S.* Vol. I. Chaps. I and II.)

REGIONAL ORGANISATION

The Ministry then set up an organisation for the Emergency Medical Services. In doing so, account had to be taken of the question of evacuation of school children, young children, pregnant women, cripples, blind, etc., from crowded centres of population particularly exposed to aerial bombardment —the main problem for both hospital and civilian evacuation being London, that unwieldy large collection of buildings that stretches out its tentacles in so many directions. For many reasons a regional organisation was required in time of war and it was also possible that communications might be temporarily severed with the central seat of government. The Government therefore divided England into ten regions, each of which was under the charge of a Civil Commissioner. A Commissioner was also appointed for Wales. If central communications had been severed, for the time being the Commissioner would have acted for the Government. He had working with him in each region officers who represented the different Government Departments, including a regional office of the Ministry of Health, with a representative staff. In each region a Hospital Officer or Officers appointed by the Ministry of Health worked on the preparation and development of the hospital scheme in co-operation with the local authorities (who controlled the County and municipal hospitals) and the voluntary hospital authorities.

There were other medical and public health problems of much complexity and variety. To cope with these a medical organisation was planned in five larger regions by a redistribution of part of the existing medical staff of the Ministry of Health, at the head of which was a Principal Regional Medical Officer. Such an organisation had already been for many years in force for Wales. The Principal Regional Medical Officer and the Hospital Officer formed part of the Departmental Staff at the Regional Commissioner's headquarters town, and worked in close co-operation. The medical officers of health of all counties and county boroughs also closely co-operated. Through the Principal

Regional Officer and the Hospital Medical Officer the Ministry of
Health in Whitehall was kept in close touch with the work of the local
authorities and of the voluntary hospitals in dealing with air-raid
casualties and the evacuation or reception of women and children.
Before and throughout the war these officers were continually advising
local authorities and local organisations. The regional organisation was
the basis of the war-time scheme.

CENTRAL ORGANISATION

Centrally, a special department of the Ministry of Health was established
for the Emergency Medical Services. On the administrative side there
was a Principal Assistant Secretary with an Assistant Secretary,
Principals and clerical staff. On the medical side a Director General of
Emergency Medical Services was appointed under the general supervision of the Chief Medical Officer of the Ministry of Health. The
Emergency Medical Services departments directed and organised the
hospital services. In this, as already indicated, the hospital medical
officers in the Regions were of great use.

ORGANISATION OF THE VOLUNTARY HOSPITALS

The hospital organisation of London presented problems of its own,
owing to the heavy concentrations of population, the wide area over
which movements of patients had to be arranged and the number and
diversity of hospital authorities. Accordingly the London Region was
divided into ten sectors each radiating from an apex in the centre out into
the Home Counties. Nine of the sectors were based on one or more of the
teaching hospitals, while the tenth (the Essex sector) was based on the
large hospitals in East Ham, West Ham, Romford, Stratford and Ilford.
At the wide ends the sectors extended beyond the boundaries of the
Metropolitan Police District, and included parts of Essex, Hertfordshire,
Buckinghamshire, Berkshire, Surrey and Kent which strictly belonged
to other Defence Regions. This wider area was essential for the evacuation
of casualties from London.

A 'Group Officer', who was the Dean or other senior member
of the medical staffs of the teaching hospitals, was appointed
for each of the ten sectors. These officers, in co-ordination with the
general plan laid down by the Ministry of Health, arranged the precise
use to which each institution was to be put and the distribution of
casualties and medical personnel to hospitals in the outer part of the
sectors. The Hospital Officers were responsible for co-ordinating the
operation of the emergency scheme over the whole region. In order
further to co-ordinate the work of the group officers and to solve any

difficulties as they arose the Director General of Emergency Medical Services kept in close and continuous touch with them, and additional medical officers were appointed to his staff to facilitate this work. A Lay Sector Officer and a Sector Matron were also appointed for each sector, the first to organise the various non-medical matters involved in the dispersal of the London hospitals, the second to deal with the distribution of the nursing staff. The Group Officers and Lay Sector Officers were able to meet the Permanent Secretary of the Ministry in Committee, and could make any necessary representation through him to the Minister of Health.

The Government was responsible for determining which hospitals were to receive casualties, and for equipping hospitals to enable them to carry out the work allotted to them. It was an important principle in the Emergency Organisation that the individual hospitals should continue to manage their own affairs and that there should be no interference by the Departments in the internal affairs of any hospital.

AFFILIATED HOSPITALS

In the provinces it was not found necessary to divide any other towns in England and Wales into sectors as was done in London. The Hospital Officers, however, arranged to affiliate a number of the hospitals and institutions outside the larger towns in England and Wales to the inner hospitals, and Group Officers were appointed for these affiliation schemes in eighteen towns, who undertook, as in London, the organisation of the medical personnel among the affiliated hospitals.

MEDICAL PERSONNEL

The British Medical Association's Central Emergency Committee before the war asked all the medical practitioners of Great Britain to register with it, on a voluntary basis, for a national emergency. The response was general. The doctors on this register were classified into their appropriate services, so many for the Navy, so many for the Army, so many for the Air Force, so many for specialist services, so many for hospitals, so many to continue in official posts or in general practice. This work was aided by local committees. A scheme was also devised by the Association whereby a doctor's practice was carried on in his absence on war work by another practitioner.

In London the Royal College of Physicians and the Royal College of Surgeons set up a Committee of Reference for the medical staffs of London hospitals on similar lines. For additional hospital officers the Government called up the doctors they required from these committees and remunerated them. For first-aid posts they obtained the services of local medical practitioners in the same way.

The dental profession was dealt with in the same way through the Dental Emergency Committees for England and Scotland and their District Committees, while Central Committees were also set up for registration for national service of pharmacists and opticians.

NURSING PERSONNEL

The shortage of trained nurses in peace-time had already given rise to anxiety and in 1937 the Inter-Departmental Committee on Nursing Services under the chairmanship of the Earl of Athlone had been appointed to advise how recruitment could be improved. The question of providing reserves of nurses for the Defence Services in time of war had already been considered by sub-committees of the Committee of Imperial Defence in 1927 and 1936. In October 1937 the Nursing Sub-Committee was reconstituted under the chairmanship of Sir Arthur MacNalty, Chief Medical Officer of the Ministry of Health, and reported in September 1938 as follows:

(1) That in March 1938 there were 89,254 trained nurses on the register; there was no information as to the numbers of unregistered trained nurses; and it was a vital necessity to appoint a co-ordinating body for the nursing profession.

(2) That the College of Nursing be asked to compile a register of all nurses and assistant nurses; that the British Red Cross Society and the Order of St. John be asked to compile one for auxiliary nurses prepared to offer their services; and that the W.V.S. should deal with all hospital auxiliaries other than nurses.

(3) They recommended that a Central Emergency Committee for the nursing profession similar to that of the Central Medical War Committee for the medical profession should be set up.

The Central Emergency Nursing Committee was duly constituted in December 1938 to carry out the duties contained in these recommendations.

This Committee maintained the organisation and supply of Civil Nursing Services in war-time with zeal and efficiency. (For an account of its work see *E.M.S.* Vol. I. Chap. 15.)

MEDICAL SERVICES
FIRST-AID POSTS

The provision of first-aid posts was the responsibility of local authorities (Air Raid Precautions Act, 1937). The approval of these schemes was transferred from the Home Office to the Ministry of Health in December 1938. Every Region had a certain number of first-aid posts.

They were generally supervised by the local medical officer of health and were controlled by a local medical practitioner (usually part-time). He was remunerated by Government. The staffing was by volunteer personnel. Wherever possible these posts were situated at existing medically equipped buildings e.g., out-patient departments and health clinics.

Mobile ambulance parties went out after air-raids to collect casualties and to render first aid. (See *E.M.S.* Vol. I. Part I.)

ANTI-GAS PRECAUTIONS

Much time and attention was devoted to this subject. *Ad hoc* cleansing stations in public baths or other suitable buildings and decontamination stations in the grounds of hospitals were provided by local authorities. It was probably the knowledge of these precautions and of the fact that the Government were in a position to retaliate with potent gases that decided the enemy not to employ this cruel weapon in the Second World War.

THE ORGANISATION OF MEDICAL SUPPLIES

The Ministry of Health, conjointly with the Home Office (later with the Ministry of Home Security), supplied hospitals and first-aid posts with adequate medical, surgical and domestic equipment, needed to enable them to carry out the additional services required of them under the E.M.S. and A.R.P. This being an entirely new and national service the cost of providing all medical and surgical equipment and replenishing consumable supplies was borne by the Exchequer. At first the London County Council acted as purchasing agents for the Ministry of Health, the Ministry of Home Security and the Department of Health for Scotland until November 1941. By then the Directorate of Medical Supplies had been established in the Ministry of Supply and was able to combine the purchasing of medical and surgical supplies for E.M.S. and A.R.P. services with those required by the Armed Forces. Considerable gifts of equipment were received from friends overseas, particularly in Canada and the U.S.A. The channels of these gifts were, on the other side, the Canadian and American Red Cross Societies and, on this side, the British Red Cross Society and Order of St. John.

The passing of the Lend/Lease Act, provided a further means of procuring medical and surgical apparatus from the U.S.A.

AMBULANCE TRAINS. INTER-HOSPITAL TRANSPORT

The E.M.S. made provision for thirty-four Casualty Evacuation Trains. They were intended for the transference of large numbers of casualties from one area to another and to supplement the military ambulance trains for the transport of Service sick from ports of disembarkation, etc. Standard stretchers were used instead of cots for the transportation of stretcher cases. Each coach on the train accommodated thirty lying cases. Later, coaches for sitting cases were added. The staff comprised a medical officer, three nursing sisters, ten auxiliary nurses and eight nursing orderlies. These trains were little used during the war for the transportation of air-raid casualties, being mainly used for military casualties.

OMNIBUS AMBULANCES

In addition to the ambulance trains, 1,090 omnibus ambulances, each capable of carrying eight to ten cases on the standard stretchers, with fitments, were provided at the outbreak of hostilities. In the London Region 220 omnibus ambulances were stationed at appropriate depots under the Chief Ambulance Officer, London District. In the provinces the ambulances were usually stationed in large centres of population. They transferred sick from vulnerable areas to hospitals in the outer zone, and later transported military casualties from ambulance trains to hospitals and from ports of disembarkation to adjacent hospitals. The number of these ambulances was considerably reduced as the result of experience but a reserve was maintained for use at short notice.

In 1940 a generous organisation in the United States, called the American Ambulances (Great Britain), provided and maintained a number of well-equipped ambulances, each for four stretcher cases, and cars for sitting cases. These proved useful for carrying small numbers of patients at a time and especially for the transfer of urgent cases and of cases which had to be taken a long distance.

CASUALTY RECORDING ORGANISATION

Casualty bureaux were set up in every provincial region by each scheme making authority i.e., county councils and county borough councils and a few large non-county boroughs. A form, E.M.S.105, was drawn up, on which to record the cause and nature of the injury for each civilian and Service casualty admitted to hospitals. In London casualty bureaux were set up at the headquarters of each of the ten sectors instead of by the scheme making authorities. For the purpose of medical statistics, for use in clinical treatment on transfer, and for the payment of pensions, the Ministry of Pensions supplied all hospitals with a series of Ministry of Pensions' forms M.P.C.42–47, which recorded details of all civilian and Service casualties and Service sick from the time of first treatment at a first-aid post or hospital until final discharge or death. These records were forwarded to the Casualty

Recording Offices of the Ministry of Pensions. (For further details see *E.M.S.* Vol. I. p. 87.)

THE HOSPITAL LABORATORY SERVICE

The Hospital Laboratory Service established during the war organised pathological and bacteriological work in the E.M.S. Hospitals and provided laboratories staffed by skilled pathologists in hospitals where such facilities had hitherto been incomplete or lacking. The Service worked in close accord with the public health laboratory service. It owed much to the initiative and direction of Sir Philip Panton, Consultant Adviser to the Ministry of Health and has remained an essential part of the National Health Service. (For an account of the Emergency Hospital Pathological Services, see *E.M.S.* Vol. I. Chapter 10.)

MOBILISATION

At the time of the Munich Crisis in 1938 there had been a dress rehearsal of mobilisation in the E.M.S., but by the actual outbreak of war in 1939 a year's breathing-space had enabled the organisation of the E.M.S. Hospital Services to be much more advanced. The 'clearance' of hospitals by restricting admissions, accelerating discharges and transferring civilian patients to convalescent accommodation by stages began on September 1, 1939. In London 3,600 patients had been transferred from thirty-four hospitals to the provinces in twenty-one improvised ambulance trains; and about 1,900 children had been evacuated to children's hospitals in outer areas in 10-stretcher omnibus ambulances. In the provinces 18,000 patients had been evacuated from the hospitals in large towns. These moves and the clearance of hospitals provided 163,500 beds for casualties on September 3, of which 51,000 were in the London Sectors. Each doctor to be employed whole-time had received an intimation as to what he was to do in the event of a state of emergency being declared, and full instructions to doctors were also broadcast. To reach places where enemy attacks would be most severe, it was necessary to form mobile surgical teams. These were based on the large hospitals and consisted of a surgeon, a sister trained in theatre duties, an anaesthetist and a male assistant or orderly. A rota of these teams was kept so that the teams next for duty on any particular day would always be available. The hospital authorities requiring the services of one or more mobile surgical teams were instructed to communicate with the hospital officers, who would be responsible for deputing a team from one of the hospitals on which they were based. Although normally available within a region or sector, these teams could be called upon for duty outside their region or sector. Transport, if not available from ordinary sources, was obtained from the nearest A.R.P. ambulance depot.

TREATMENT OF THE CIVILIAN SICK

In the absence of casualties due to enemy action, towards the end of September, all hospitals were allowed to admit civilian sick up to seventy-five per cent. of their normal capacity. The beds available for casualties which had reached 187,000 by September 7, thus gradually decreased to 181,000 by the end of the month. Subsequently, all restrictions on admissions were removed, provided that one bed per 1,000 of the population remained available for casualties in each of the areas concerned. As the 'upgraded' hospitals and the large base hospitals were rapidly coming into use during the autumn, the admission of ordinary civilian patients reverted to normal.

TRANSFERRED SICK

In order to ensure an adequate number of beds for the reception of casualties being available at all times, considerable numbers of ordinary civilian sick had to be transferred from the large centrally situated hospitals in the London Sectors to the fully equipped hospitals in the outer zone. Similar transfers were necessary also from the large provincial towns. Later on, a considerable number of civilian sick was transferred from hospitals situated in the Coastal Belt during the period when invasion by sea was a possibility and admissions to these hospitals had to be greatly restricted. The number of civilian cases transferred for these purposes was very considerable throughout the period of hostilities. The transfers were effected by omnibus ambulances of the Inter-hospital Transport Service for stretcher cases and in coaches for the sitting cases. The Ministry of Health accepted full financial responsibility for the treatment of all the transferred sick, as well as for police sick, police casualties, casualties among Civil Defence workers while on duty and for unaccompanied evacuated children. Additions to the list of categories entitled to treatment in E.M.S. hospitals were made from time to time and by the end of the war included many classes of civilian war workers.

TREATMENT OF SERVICE SICK

When war began the E.M.S. became responsible for the treatment of all Service sick and casualties where admission to Service Hospitals was not practicable, with the exception of patients with infectious diseases (including tuberculosis and venereal disease) and mental diseases. These were admitted to special hospitals under the peace-time procedure. By the end of October 1939, 3,600 Service sick and casualties occupied beds in E.M.S. hospitals and over 16,000 by the end of January 1940.

The Army Council considered that for the preservation of discipline, distribution of pay and avoidance of unduly prolonged detention in hospital, definite blocks of beds for Service patients were essential. Early in November 1939 blocks of 300 beds were allotted in six large base hospitals. These blocks of beds were termed 'military wings' of the E.M.S. hospitals or 'convoy' hospitals, and R.A.M.C. registrars, a clerical staff and a staff of military police were appointed to each hospital. Later on, owing to the increasing shortage of medical personnel, the medical registrars were replaced by Army Officers (non-medical).

As the number of convoy hospitals increased, in order to effect economy in personnel, registrars were allotted to groups of hospitals, including convalescent hospitals, for Service patients and had their headquarters in one of the large hospitals in the group. These hospitals were afterwards called 'registrar hospitals' and, as far as possible, all Service patients were concentrated in them. If Service patients requiring treatment for more than a few days were in the first instance admitted to other hospitals, e.g. in the case of Service sick from home stations, they were transferred to registrar hospitals.

EXPANSION OF THE CONVOY HOSPITALS

By the end of January 1940, 16,000 beds were occupied by Service patients. The War Office's peace-time provision of some 3,000 beds had been expanded to 10,500 and was expected to reach 15,000 apart from 3,500 beds in camp hospitals and reception stations. Special provision had been made for cases of psychosis in certain military hospitals and in portions of civil mental hospitals taken over from the Board of Control and also for venereal diseases. The War Office authorities anticipated further casualties in the near future which in a peak period might amount to 16,000 a week. The Ministry of Health, therefore, had to provide additional accommodation for Army casualties by the building of *ad hoc* hospitals. Authority was given in February for the construction of hutted hospitals with 45,000 beds. The Ministry of Pensions was also authorised to extend its hospitals by 2,500 beds. In March 1940, 100,000 beds were available for Army sick and wounded and in April the War Office was supplied with a list of 112 hospitals providing 75,000 beds suitable and available for military patients. The special treatment centres were fully available to the Services.

SPECIAL CENTRES

An important part of the E.M.S. Organisation was the establishment at certain suitably placed institutions of treatment centres specially staffed and equipped to deal with patients requiring certain forms of specialist treatment. Special centres were established for the treatment of the following conditions:

Injuries requiring orthopaedic surgery	20
Peripheral nerve injuries	3
Injuries of the spine and cauda equina	4
Injuries to the chest	10
Head injuries	11
Maxillo-facial injuries	12
Burns	3
Neurosis	14
Rheumatism	2
Effort syndrome	1
Skin diseases	20
Children's diseases (London Sectors)	13
Amputations (Ministry of Pensions Hospitals)	7

The number of beds in each of the centres was variable and no difficulty was found in accommodating all the cases requiring treatment.

CONSULTANT ADVISERS AND REGIONAL ADVISERS

The consultant advisers at headquarters, appointed by the Minister of Health, advised in the arrangements necessary to provide efficient treatment for the difficult types of cases admitted to these centres and regional advisers were appointed also.

GROUP ADVISERS

In December 1940 the E.M.S. hospitals, including auxiliary hospitals, were formed into groups. To each of these medical officers of consultant status, resident in the group, were appointed on a part-time basis in order to ensure that all the facilities provided by the Emergency Hospital Scheme for the efficient treatment of patients should be used, and that no case requiring treatment in special hospitals was being unduly detained in the receiving hospital.

FRACTURE DEPARTMENT

In addition to the special centres for orthopaedic surgery, there were many hospitals specially equipped and staffed for the treatment of fractures and others were added for this purpose. Where necessary the special equipment for remedial and occupational therapy was provided.

No special centres were set up for ophthalmology, ear, nose and throat cases or dental surgery. Class I hospitals had fully equipped departments for these cases. St. Dunstan's provided for military and civil patients who had been blinded.

ACCOMMODATION FOR CASUALTIES

By May 1940 the numbers of hospitals in the Emergency Medical Services were as follows:

	Hospitals	Total Beds	Casualty Beds
Class IA Hospitals	667	281,985	189,184
Class IB Hospitals	104	6,814	4,746
Class II Hospitals	436	117,813	68,929
Totals	1,207	406,612	262,859

This shows an apparent diminution of 1,163 hospitals and 85,958 beds since September 1, 1939, but many beds included in the early estimates were in institutions which through lack of staff and equipment could not have provided full and effective treatment.

After the invasion of Holland and Belgium on May 10, 1940, the E.M.S. were prepared to accommodate up to 173,000 casualties in beds immediately available, while provision for others could be made at any time by 'clearing hospitals'. There was also the following accommodation available in Service and Ministry of Pensions Hospitals:

	Hospitals	Total Beds	Occupied Beds	Vacant Beds
Royal Navy	7	4,485	2,225	2,260
Royal Air Force	13	2,674	1,604	1,070
Army	66	8,991	6,389	2,602
Ministry of Pensions	8	2,244	995	1,249

EVACUATION OF THE BRITISH EXPEDITIONARY FORCE FROM FRANCE

The evacuation of the British Expeditionary Force from Dunkirk and other ports in France (end of May 1940) resulted in a sudden flow of casualties into Service and E.M.S. hospitals. This ceased by June 10, by which date 28,354 Army and 3,487 Navy casualties had been admitted to E.M.S. Hospitals from 47 ambulance trains. An additional number of casualties was received in the London Sector hospitals in the South-East of the London area, from coast towns from which they were conveyed by ambulances.

On May 29, the influx of casualties into Dover was so great that the staff of the local emergency hospitals had to be reinforced; a mobile surgical team, extra nurses and equipment were sent. In the hospital 190 operations were performed, while 1,873 patients were dealt with in the sector hospitals. Although nearly half of these patients had received no previous treatment, other than first aid, and had travelled in ambulance coaches from between 30 to 60 miles, only 33 or 1·7 per cent. of all the patients died.

ARRANGEMENTS TO MEET ENEMY INVASION

By June 1940 enemy preparations for an attack on Great Britain by air and by sea were evident and it seemed likely that increased accommodation for casualties would be required. Accordingly, the Minister of Health appointed an Emergency Hospitals Commission with wide terms of reference to advise him on this subject. The Commission's important recommendations were implemented as follows:

HOSPITAL ANNEXES

After inspection and selection of buildings by the Regional Officers some 10,000 extra beds were provided, the majority in large country houses and some in schools.

'SHADOW' OR 'RESERVE' HOSPITALS

Other buildings, not necessarily near hospitals, were also selected after inspection. Of these, 68 designated 'key' hospitals, were at once adapted and equipped. Other buildings eventually selected were 339 in number. Thus the total number of reserve hospitals was 407, accommodating 9,778 beds.

AUXILIARY HOSPITALS

Convalescent homes for Service personnel as an intermediary stage between their discharge from Class I hospitals and their return to duty were required. As part of the E.M.S. Hospital Scheme, 10,000 beds in suitably placed country houses were adapted and equipped for this purpose by the Joint War Organisation of the British Red Cross Society and the Order of St. John. The organisation also provided a part-time medical officer and Red Cross and St. John personnel. These hospitals were included in groups under the group system for military registrars. They fulfilled a useful purpose. Later, some of them were used for civil convalescents.

MEDICAL ARRANGEMENTS IN THE COASTAL BELT

It was the Government's scheme to evacuate the whole of the civil population, except 10 per cent. engaged in essential services, from the coastal belt. In the first place, the aim was voluntarily to evacuate 60 per cent. of the population in an area roughly 20 miles deep stretching from Great Yarmouth to Southend-on-Sea and from Margate to Hythe. As part of the scheme special measures were taken to evacuate the sick from all E.M.S. hospitals in the area, and also domiciliary chronic sick.

Under the voluntary evacuation scheme out of a total population of 493,935 in 19 towns, 304,375 persons were evacuated. Of the remaining 189,560 persons, 50,665 were essential workers. Seventy-three doctors remained in these towns to attend at hospitals and on domiciliary sick. The E.M.S. evacuation was from June to August 1940; 2,352 patients were transferred from hospitals in 15 civil evacuation trains. An extension of the scheme to other towns was prepared but it was never required. As the threat of invasion diminished restrictions were relaxed; in 1941 hospitals were required to keep only 25 per cent. of their beds vacant for emergencies. Later on these restrictions were removed altogether.

ACTIVE OPERATIONS IN BRITAIN

THE 'BATTLE OF BRITAIN'

The prelude to the Battle of Britain began in May 1940, when the enemy dropped some 100 bombs of various calibres on England, but only three serious casualties were caused. During June, July and August the estimated weight of bombs dropped, mostly by daylight, was 9,820 tons, which caused 1,410 fatal casualties and resulted in 1,858 casualties being admitted to E.M.S. hospitals. These raids were mainly directed at ports and aerodromes in Southern England.

THE NIGHT RAIDS

In September 1940 heavy raiding by night on London and later on the larger provincial towns, began. In this month 9,980 tons of bombs fell in England and Wales, causing 6,964 deaths and 9,472 casualty admissions to hospitals. Thus about the same weight of bombs when directed against thickly populated areas caused approximately five times the number of casualties as compared with those dropped in the daylight raids. This month was the peak period in weight of attack and casualties, both of which gradually decreased until February 1941, rose again slightly from March to May 1941 and died away to negligible figures in June and July. The heaviest attack was made on London on the night of April 16–17, 1941, when 1,179 persons were killed and 2,233 admitted to hospitals; the next heaviest being the night of May 10–11 when 1,452 were killed and 1,792 admitted to hospitals. In the provinces the heaviest recorded single attack occurred on the night of November 14–15, 1940, when 554 were killed and 865 seriously injured in Coventry.

DAMAGE TO HOSPITALS

A large number of hospitals were damaged by direct hits or near misses, but few were put completely out of action, although some were rendered untenable for varying periods. The number of hospitals damaged in the London Sectors was 175. St. Thomas's Hospital, situated by the Thames, received six direct hits.

WORK OF THE HOSPITALS

The number of civilian air-raid casualties in hospital rose from under a hundred in May 1940 to 7,181 on December 1, after which it fell progressively to 3,516 on July 1, 1941. It fell again to an average of about 1,000 for the period ending December 1942, but rose again slightly in 1943 and again in 1944. The occupied beds in E.M.S. hospitals (ordinary civilian patients, civilian casualties, Service sick and casualties) which were about 160,000 in May 1940, gradually rose to 175,834 on March 1, 1941, then fell to 166,000 by July 1, 1941 and remained, approximately, at that figure to the end of 1942. The numbers of beds still available for casualties never dropped below 120,000 during the whole period, and no reduction in the admissions of ordinary civilian patients was necessary.

EVACUATION OF THE CHRONIC SICK

In 1940 evacuation of the chronic sick and shelter derelicts from the London area was decided upon. Between October 10 and November 14, 7,612 chronic sick and infirm patients were evacuated primarily to large hospitals in rural areas. Similar evacuations took place in Southampton, Plymouth, Cardiff, etc. The cases were eventually transferred from these hospitals to more suitable accommodation.

BASEMENT OPERATING THEATRES

Emergency theatres in strengthened basements in order that operations on urgent cases could be performed, were set up during the raids at St. Bartholomew's, St. Thomas's, Guy's, The Middlesex and other hospitals, including one at Birmingham and another at Aston. They were also set up in certain other large towns and proved of great value.

DISPERSAL SYSTEM

In this system, introduced by the Coventry authorities after the first heavy raid there, casualties occurring in the central area were taken direct to peripheral or advanced based hospitals instead of to the highly vulnerable hospitals in the centre of the city.

LIMB FITTING CENTRES

These were established by the Ministry of Pensions for the supply of artificial limbs to Service and civilian casualties. (See *Civilian Health and Medical Services*. Vol. II. Chap. V.)

REHABILITATION

With the progress of the war the demand for man-power gradually increased, which necessitated every effort being made to render all Service patients fit to return to duty as soon as possible. This necessity applied also to civilians engaged on essential war work—a large proportion of the population. In October 1941 the Ministry of Labour and National Service introduced a scheme for linking up the labour exchanges with hospitals; this provided for the interviewing of disabled patients in hospital before their discharge and endeavouring to find suitable employment for them. Attention was specially paid to patients suffering from medical as well as surgical disabilities. In 1942 it was arranged that vocational training centres (Ministry of Labour) could refer cases under training to certain E.M.S. hospitals for specialist opinion regarding suitability of the trainees for vocations by reason of their disabilities and, if necessary, for their out-patient treatment at these hospitals. These arrangements were extended to disabled persons training at technical colleges.

After receiving a report from the Ministry of Labour's departmental committee (The 'Tomlinson' Committee) in 1942 the Ministry of Health took the following action:

(1) Systematic visitation of the larger hospitals in order to consider desirable improvements in rehabilitation.

(2) Appointment of a medical officer in charge of rehabilitation in each selected hospital.

(3) Advice to medical staff to apply principles of rehabilitation from the beginning of treatment.

(4) Issue of E.M.S. Memorandum No. 6 on the organisation of a hospital rehabilitation department. As a result conferences between the Ministry's expert advisers and hospital boards of management and medical staffs were held in many parts of the country. The Ministry also provided courses on modern rehabilitation techniques for doctors and physiotherapists; on occupational therapy for students and auxiliaries; additional staff, equipment and apparatus, huts for gymnasia or occupational therapy; and gave permission to adapt existing buildings, where necessary, coupled with substantial financial grants. By 1945 the number of hospitals employing active rehabilitation was 333. For an account of the methods see Physiotherapy and Rehabilitation in Surgery, Chapter 22.

LATER AIR-RAID CASUALTIES

ENEMY ATTACKS, JULY 1941—DECEMBER 31, 1942

During the last six months of 1941, the Luftwaffe employed 'tip and run' raids, chiefly directed against the coastal areas in the East and

South-East. These raids resulted in 1,207 persons being killed and 1,424 being admitted to hospital, of whom 105 killed and 108 admitted to hospital were in the London Region. This type of attack continued during the whole of the year 1942, during which period the total casualties were 3,195 killed and 4,109 admitted to hospital. A considerable proportion of these casualties was caused by the 'Baedeker' raids on the Cathedral cities of Exeter, Bath, Norwich, York and Canterbury, which occurred between April 23 and June 7. (See *E.M.S.* Vol. II. Chap. 14.)

ENEMY ATTACK, 1943

During 1943 it was estimated that 2,320 tons of bombs were dropped by the enemy. Casualties were 2,273 killed and 3,350 admitted to hospital. Of these 542 were killed and 989 admitted to hospital in the London Region. In the rest of England and Wales the attacks were widely distributed, chiefly along the East and South coasts.

SERVICE SICK AND WOUNDED

During 1943 the following numbers of Service sick and wounded from units in this country and overseas were treated in E.M.S. hospitals:

Army, including A.T.S.	176,022
R.A.F., including W.A.A.F.	85,544
Canadian Forces	3,664
Allied Forces	2,790

In addition a number of sick and wounded from the Royal Navy (including W.R.N.S.) were also treated, and the routine admission of civilian categories continued.

RENEWED AIR ATTACKS, 1944–45

The early days of 1944 were marked by a slight increase in night raids, intended, presumably, to be regarded in Germany as comparable with the massive attacks then made by the Air Forces of the Allies. The Germans made a heavy attack in January over South-Eastern England and the Southern part of East Anglia, followed a week later by a heavy raid over the same area and extending as far as Hampshire and Oxfordshire. In both raids aircraft penetrated the London area in which 107 persons were killed and 270 seriously injured. In February a series of five brief concentrated attacks on London occurred in which some 600 civilians were killed and 1,300 seriously injured. Over 1,800 fires were caused, ninety-four per cent. in London, by incendiary bombs and seventeen hospitals were damaged. Casualties for February amounted to 962 killed and 1,713 seriously injured. Thereafter attacks by piloted aircraft were few and scattered, but by the end of May casualties had increased to 1,563 killed and 2,916 seriously injured.

FLYING BOMBS (V.1)

On June 13, 1944, the enemy launched robot high-speed flying bombs from the French coast against London and South-East England. Each bomb contained an explosive charge of less than one metric ton, the weight varying with the filling used. Casualties on the first day from this new form of attack were nine killed and 23 seriously injured. Attacks rapidly gained momentum. In a week casualties amounted to over 700 civilians killed and approximately 2,600 seriously injured. By the last week of August the casualties were some 5,500 killed, 16,000 seriously injured and 30,000 slightly injured. London was throughout the primary target, over 2,300 of some 8,000 bombs launched during the 80 day ordeal of the main attack having reached the London area where over 92 per cent. of all the fatal casualties occurred. Here, on average, 2·2 persons were killed and 6·3 seriously injured per flying-bomb strike, these rates being some twenty and fifteen times greater than those per incident in other regions, and double those for the country as a whole. Total casualties per incident were approximately ten times greater in London than elsewhere, a fact explained by London's high population-density. Of the flying-bombs launched, probably not more than two-thirds inflicted casualties. Comparisons with estimated weight of bombs despatched in previous air-attacks showed this new long-distance missile to be more destructive, weight for weight despatched or launched, than the bombs of earlier attacks.

Casualties were similar in type to those caused by the parachute bomb in previous raids and included a large number of lacerations and eye injuries, due to splintered glass and flying débris. Later, the habit of taking cover was accompanied by an increase in injuries and death from collapsing buildings. The E.M.S. hospital provision was ample for the number of admissions due to flying-bomb casualties.

DAMAGE TO HOSPITALS

Hospitals suffered greatly during the flying bomb ordeal. Several were hit in the first week and by the end of October no less than 100 hospitals had been damaged. In the London sectors alone 76 were damaged, involving the permanent loss of some 2,600 beds, the temporary loss of over 6,000 beds and the evacuation of approximately 8,000 civilian patients to other regions. Of the staffs only 24 were killed and 146 injured. Patients killed number 138; those injured were 1,155.

EVACUATION

The flying-bombs' toll in killed and injured would have been higher but for the resumption of officially arranged evacuation. Some 818,000 people left the London area, including 228,000 mothers and expectant mothers, 537,000 children and 53,000 old, invalid and blind persons.

END OF V.I ATTACKS

Towards the end of the summer of 1944, combined fighter, gun and balloon defences, which had brought down about one-third of the flying-bombs launched during the first week of the bombardment, became so efficient that on one day (August 28) out of 101 bombs which approached the English coast 97 were destroyed and only four got through to London. By the end of August the main fight against this form of attack was practically won. Concurrently with the Allied advance through France and into the Low Countries the attacks rapidly diminished in number and frequency although a few incidents occurred in East Anglia, Kent and London in the latter part of the year. Having lost their launching sites, the Germans were now adapting Heinkel aircraft as carriers for flying-bombs which were launched from over the North Sea. By the middle of January 1945 these attacks ceased for six weeks. Early in March they were resumed, apparently with a new type of increased range from land bases in Holland. They were short-lived and of little effect. The last attack was on March 29.

During the whole of the V.1 attacks, over 9,000 flying-bombs had been plotted, nearly 6,000 of them over land, and some 5,600 incidents had resulted, of which approximately 2,400 occurred in London and 3,200 in other regions. Casualties were some 5,837 killed, 16,762 seriously injured; 92 per cent. of the fatal casualties and 91 per cent of the seriously injured occurred in the London Region.

THE LONG RANGE ROCKET (V.2)

This new weapon, produced by the Germans, weighed 12 tons, contained an explosive warhead of 2,000 lbs., attained an altitude of 60–70 miles and had a range of over 200 miles. The projectile could not be intercepted in action and of its approach at a speed much greater than sound no warning could be given. It therefore produced higher casualty rates per rocket-strike than those of V.1. The first V.2 used against London and South-East England fell at Chiswick on September 8, 1944. The last rocket fell on March 27, 1945 at Orpington, Kent. During the 29 weeks of the attacks over 1,000 rockets inflicted 2,724 fatal, 6,691 seriously injured and over 15,000 lightly injured, casualties. Casualties treated in hospitals averaged 230 per week. In London 20 E.M.S. hospitals were damaged, resulting in 633 beds being put out of use temporarily and 260 permanently and necessitating the transfer of 386 patients to other hospitals. Except for a few slight injuries hospital patients had no casualties. Hospital staffs suffered three fatal, two seriously injured and 11 slightly injured, casualties.

CROSS-CHANNEL SHELLING

The people of Dover, Folkestone, Deal, Ramsgate and neighbouring

UNITED KINGDOM—CIVILIAN SERVICES 301

villages—the area known as 'Hellfire Corner'—endured shelling from the other side of the Channel from August 12, 1940 to September 30, 1944 when the German long-range guns were captured by the Allies. Although 2,500 shells fell and 6,000 properties were damaged the casualties were only some 150 killed, 250 seriously injured and 400 slightly injured.

MEDICAL ARRANGEMENTS FOR THE SECOND FRONT IN WESTERN EUROPE

In the summer of 1943, after discussions with the War Office, it was agreed that the treatment of all casualties from the Second Front should be undertaken by the Emergency Medical Services.

PORTS AND HOSPITALS

Certain ports were selected for seaborne casualties, namely, Southampton, Gosport, Portsmouth, Dover and Tilbury. Of these only Southampton and Portsmouth, and Gosport to a small extent, were eventually used during the first four months of the operation.

Hospitals of three categories were scheduled to receive these casualties:

(1) *'Coastal'* or *'Port'* *Hospitals* for the reception of casualties unfit for further travel after disembarkation. These were all close to the ports.

(2) *'Transit'* *Hospitals* reached from the port by road or short rail journeys, roughly corresponding to Casualty Clearing Stations.

(3) *'Home Base'* *Hospitals* in which the patients were retained and fully treated.

In the Portsmouth and Southampton areas seven 'Coastal' hospitals containing over 1,200 beds were prepared. The Queen Alexandra's Hospital, Cosham, with 450 beds, served the double purpose of transit and coastal hospital, while two hospitals in Winchester, with 350 beds, served as transit hospitals only; these hospitals were all served by road transport. Thirteen transit hospitals, reached by railway at distances up to about 40 miles from the ports, with about 6,550 beds, were selected. The area could accommodate nearly 8,000 cases in transit, the required figure estimated by the General Staff, but the greatest number of beds in actual use at any one time never exceeded about 4,000. Some of the excess transit hospitals were closed owing to their being in the danger area for flying-bombs. By October 1944 the Royal South Hants Hospital, Southampton was the only port hospital in use, while the Royal Hants Hospital, Winchester, Park Prewett Hospital, Basingstoke, Botley's Park and Horton Hospital, Epsom were retained as transit hospitals.

REINFORCEMENTS FOR THE PORT AND TRANSIT HOSPITALS

To provide adequate surgical and nursing service, 48 surgical teams, 29 general duty medical officers, 31 radiographers, 120 medical students and 727 nurses were sent from London on June 5, the day before D-day The Army also provided 12 surgical teams during the early weeks of the fighting. The coastal hospitals were more heavily reinforced than the transit hospitals as they dealt with the most severe cases.

RECEPTION AND DISTRIBUTION OF THE CASUALTIES

The unloading of tank carriers and other vessels, as well as road transport, was the responsibility of the Army. The E.M.S. took over at ambulance trains or hospitals.

The selection of cases was highly important; this was done by Army surgical specialists from 21st Army Group. Admissions to port hospitals at the beginning amounted to 8·3 per cent. of the cases, instead of the estimated 10 per cent. Later, the figure became much lower, when active surgery could be done overseas. The selection was excellent. Six civil evacuation trains were berthed near the ports of disembarkation for the transport of the cases selected for the transit hospitals. The normal staffs of these trains were strengthened by extra nurses and by medical students. Penicillin was provided for the treatment of patients in the trains so as to ensure the continuity of treatment with this drug when necessary.

WORK OF THE TRANSIT HOSPITALS

At first a considerable number of cases admitted to Transit Hospitals had perforce to be sent on to the Home Base Hospitals after examination and re-dressing, but soon nearly all cases had their definitive wound treatment carried out in the transit hospitals. There was a wide and equal distribution of cases through England and Scotland so that no hospital area became overloaded. Up to October 23, 1944 Southampton was the main port of disembarkation and some 70,000 cases had passed through the transit hospital system. From October 24 the main port of disembarkation became Tilbury. From that date also the system of primary admission to transit hospitals was found unnecessary and was abandoned, all patients fit to travel proceeding direct from the ports to the Home Base hospitals. From October 24 to December 31, 1944, about 10,500 further cases arriving by sea were admitted to E.M.S. hospitals, bringing the total to that date to 80,500.

HOME BASE HOSPITALS

These were situated north and west of a line from the Wash to Lyme Regis. There were 97 hospitals with a total accommodation of 50,000 beds of which 23,000 were vacant on D-day. Casualties arrived by ambulance train at 23 railheads which were served in rotation to avoid overcrowding. From these hospitals, when their condition permitted, patients were transferred to secondary accommodation. The number of secondary beds in this area was 58,000, of which 13,500 were available on D-day. There were also 13,000 reserve beds which could have been used in an emergency. When a suitable stage of recovery was reached, patients went to the Joint War Organisation Auxiliary Hospitals and to convalescent depots.

THE RECEPTION AND DISTRIBUTION OF AIRBORNE CASUALTIES

Airborne casualties were brought to three aerodromes near Swindon in planes which were used for outward goods transport. Cases began to arrive on D-day + 7, beginning with an average of 300 a day, the peak number being 934 on one day. The general scheme for reception and distribution was the same as for seaborne casualties. Cases unfit for further transport were admitted to two hospitals near Swindon which could receive about 1,200 patients; the rest were taken by train direct to Home Base hospitals. The selection of cases for transport was a R.A.F. responsibility, while the Army transported the patients to the ambulance trains.

From D-day to October 23, 1944 about 40,000 cases were transported by air and admitted to E.M.S. Hospitals. Subsequent to this date four-fifths of all the casualties arrived by air. By December 31, 1944 airborne admissions totalled 51,500.

SPECIAL CENTRES

Special arrangements were made for the road transport of urgent cases (both seaborne and airborne) to the special centres; head and spine cases went to St. Hugh's Military Hospital, Oxford, The Royal United Hospital, Bath and the Canadian Neurological Hospital, Hackwood Park, Basingstoke. Chest cases went to Kewstoke and burns and maxillo-facial cases to Rooksdown House, Park Prewett, Basingstoke.

Additional special centres were established in the Home Base Hospitals area as follows:

Neurosurgery	Derby Royal Infirmary, Cardiff Royal Infirmary
Plastic and Jaw Surgery	St. James's Hospital, Leeds
Thoracic Surgery	Leicester City Isolation Hospital.

The medical arrangements for the reception of casualties from the Second Front were well planned in advance and the organisation worked admirably. Great credit is due to all concerned. This successful work was the last great development of the Emergency Medical Services, for the war ended in 1945. The Emergency Hospital Scheme provided an example of a system in which the interests of the State, the hospital authorities and above all the patients, were as fully provided for as war conditions would permit.

THE EMERGENCY HOSPITAL SERVICES IN 1945–1946

ACCOMMODATION IN HOSPITALS

During 1945 further reductions were effected in E.M.S. hospital accommodation. By the end of June the total beds in E.M.S. hospitals, exclusive of 20,207 reserves, amounted to 157,048, of which 118,205 were occupied. By the end of the year hospitals had been reduced to 528, and beds (including 18,979 reserve) to 137,176 of which 104,602 were occupied. At the end of August the auxiliary hospitals had been reduced to 198, containing approximately 12,100 beds.

CLASSES OF E.M.S. PATIENTS

By the end of June the number of E.M.S. in-patients in hospital was 49,727, of whom 34,411 were members of the Fighting Services—injured and sick—and 10,232 transferred civilian sick. Civilian casualties, including police, amounted to 2,027; fractures among civil defence workers and certain categories of industrial workers amounted to 1,082 cases. Thus the chief responsibilities of the E.M.S. were for three classes of cases: (a) military sick and injured; (b) transferred civilian sick and (c) air-raid casualties.

In addition, transferred war workers, special classes of workers, evacuees, refugees and civilian fracture cases were treated by the E.M.S.

The policy in the E.M.S. was to release hospital beds and medical and nursing staffs to meet the urgent requirements of the civilian population as soon as this could safely be done, while still retaining adequate accommodation for the treatment of Service personnel and for the estimated number of casualties. Such was the flexibility of the organisation that this policy could be put into force and also reversed at very short notice as the operational situation indicated.

With the end of hostilities in Europe, the release of beds and hospitals continued; and when Japan surrendered in August 1945, the pace of release was considerably increased. At the end of the year 1946, 35,132 beds, out of a total of 116,128 in 366 suitably distributed hospitals were available for E.M.S. patients. Many of these were long-stay civilian and Service patients for whose accommodation the Ministry of Health continued to be responsible. This arrangement enabled patients to be treated near their homes and avoided the need to retain any special E.M.S. medical and nursing personnel. Some of the special centres were retained in certain hospitals pending the establishment of the National Hospital Service in 1948.

THE EMERGENCY HOSPITAL SERVICES IN SCOTLAND AND NORTHERN IRELAND

The plans for the Emergency Hospital Services in Scotland and Northern Ireland, having been drawn up in close collaboration with the Ministry of Health in England and Wales, were similar in policy and principles. Certain minor differences were, however, inevitable owing to differences in the Central and Local Systems of Government. In England and Wales all E.M.S. hospitals, including annexes either newly constructed or adaptations of existing buildings, remained under the administration of the authorities controlling them in peace-time. Newly constructed *ad hoc* hospitals were administered by the authority in whose area of jurisdiction they were built. All auxiliary hospitals were administered by the Joint War Organisations of the St. John Ambulance and the British Red Cross Society. In Scotland, however, all *ad hoc* newly acquired or constructed hospitals were administered directly by the Department of Health for Scotland, as were all buildings used as auxiliary hospitals.

In Northern Ireland all hospitals were administered as in peace-time, but under the direction of Government. As there was no Ministry of Health, the whole of the Emergency Medical Services were at first under the direction of the Public Health Division of the Ministry of Home Affairs, then under the Ministry of Home Security and finally, in 1944, they were transferred to the newly formed Ministry of Health and Local Government.

These Ministries were thus enabled to acquire, as in the case of England and Wales, a considerable amount of valuable experience in the direction and control of National Hospital Services.

OFFICIAL TOTAL OF CIVILIAN CASUALTIES

The following table gives the official total of civilian casualties during the Second World War. It will be seen that the total number of killed and wounded amounted to 146,760. Of these 60,585 were killed and 86,175 were injured and retained in hospital. In London the total number of killed and wounded amounted to 80,387, so that the densely populated metropolis had nearly four-sevenths of the casualties. It is a justifiable conclusion that had it not been for the arrangements for dispersal of the population and the efficiency of the Civil Defence Casualty Services and the Emergency Hospital Services the total number of civilian casualties would have been much heavier.

*Official Total of Civilian Casualties
during the Second World War*

Killed

Men	26,920
Women	25,392
Children	7,736
Unclassified	537
	60,585

Injured and Retained in Hospital

Men	40,736
Women	37,816
Children	7,623
	86,175

Total number of killed and wounded amounted to 146,760.

London Area Casualties

Killed	29,890
Badly Injured and Retained in Hospital	50,497
	80,387

London therefore had nearly four-sevenths of the casualties.

THE LESSONS TAUGHT BY THE EMERGENCY MEDICAL SERVICES

INTRODUCTION

The inception, growth and functioning of the organisation to deal with civilian casualties caused by enemy air raids on this country during the Second World War are described fully in *Emergency Medical Services*. Vols. I and II.

A general summary of the work of the Emergency Medical Services has been given here in order to give the fruits of war's experience. The applicability of some of these lessons concerns those engaged in the organisation of Civil Defence and Hospital Services in the event of a future war.

The development of nuclear weapons in the megaton range has considerably altered the post-war plans for war-time first-aid and hospital services which were based primarily on the knowledge, experience and practice of the Emergency Medical Services in the War of 1939–45 and modified on the experience gained by the use of the atomic bomb in Japan and in subsequent experiments made in the United States, the Pacific Ocean and Australia. It is true that the advent of the megaton nuclear weapon by its very power of destruction may be a deterrent against war and, provided the deterrent is maintained, the likelihood of nuclear global war decreases. Nevertheless, if war should come it would entail both human and material destruction on an unprecedented scale, and to enable the hospital service to fulfil its function, not only in saving life but also in sustaining public morale, some of the lessons of the Second World War may be of service.

THE CIVIL DEFENCE CASUALTY SERVICE

The further experience gained during the later years of the war only served to emphasise and strengthen the opinions already expressed by the great majority of those chiefly concerned with the work of the civil defence services after the extensive air raids which ended in July 1941. These may be summarised as follows:

FIRST-AID SERVICE

1. The first-aid posts should be considered as advanced dressing stations of the hospitals, staffed by them and controlled by the same chain of authority under the Ministry of Health.

2. The fixed aid posts should be reduced in number and staffed by the personnel of mobile medical units based on the hospitals.

3. The mobile units should establish temporary aid posts when necessary in any suitable premises in the vicinity of major incidents.

4. All premises equipped as fixed aid posts should be underground, protected and adapted according to the needs of such units.

5. The personnel should consist of a nucleus of trained whole-time members and of part-time volunteers trained in the hospitals, who are prepared to serve by rota in the hospitals and the aid posts when called upon to do so.

6. The appointment of 'Incident Doctors' proved most valuable in the Second World War.

CIVIL DEFENCE SERVICE

1. The civil defence service should be a service partly whole-time and mobile and a part-time service whose members have volunteered for tours of duty in their local areas.

2. The whole-time mobile service should be a National Service with a disciplinary code, whose members are prepared to serve in any area to reinforce the local services when required. The local service should be administered by the local authorities under the control of the central authority.

3. The personnel of the civil defence services should be fully trained in first-aid, rescue and decontamination duties. They should be males only.

4. The part-time members of the service must be prepared to undertake tours of duty when called upon to do so for training and in emergencies.

5. Their depots being in vulnerable areas should be in underground premises and fully protected. The accommodation should provide all the necessary facilities for rest, meals and suitable recreation during periods of inaction.

THE LOCAL AMBULANCE SERVICE

1. The local ambulance services should be, as in the last war, administered by the local authorities under the control of the central authority.

2. The personnel, which may consist either of men or women should, like the other civil defence services, consist of whole or part-time members.

3. Their living accommodation and the garages for their vehicles will require the same degree of protection as that provided for the other civil defence services whose duties must be carried out in the vulnerable areas. They should therefore be underground and their exit facilities should be protected. Many suitable premises of this description which would require little alteration are available already in most industrial areas.

The organisation of this service would therefore require little change, except in the matter of garaging, from that which rendered such noble service in the last war.

It should be emphasised (a) that Air Raid Precautions and the provision of first aid throughout the country have demonstrated that the most efficient war injury and accident services depend on the rapid and easy transport of accident cases to a hospital which should be adequately protected and situated underground, if possible, and competent to provide resuscitation and efficient plenary treatment; (b) that first aid on the spot should be of the simplest kind to save life and enable the patient to be transferred to hospital, and (c) that for this an efficient ambulance service throughout the country is essential. This service must operate over wider districts than those of a local authority, and cover both urban and rural needs.

It is of course of the greatest importance to ensure that the closest possible liaison should be established between the various branches of the civil defence service and the central control. There was little fault to find with this organisation in the Second World War. It seldom failed, and then only as the result of enemy action, and alternative methods of communication were usually efficiently and rapidly established. It may, however, be found to be much more difficult to attain in the future in view of the increase in the destructive effect of the weapons which may be used.

THE EMERGENCY HOSPITAL SERVICE

The organisation, development and work of the Emergency Hospital Service has been summarised in the preceding narrative.

Under the compulsion of war, from 1939 to 1945, a great experiment was made in working a hospital system on a national basis. It was a successful experiment and provided valuable lessons which did much to prepare the medical profession and the general public for a State Hospital Service, which was one of the first constructive tasks of peace.

It demonstrated the advantages of a unified service with a large measure of decentralisation. In the first place this decentralisation was delegated to Regional Authorities; from them it passed to Hospital Groups each provided with centres for special treatment, adequately staffed by specialists and consultants and equipped with the means of applying the latest advances in medical knowledge to the diagnosis and treatment of disease. It provided full treatment for Service casualties from home or overseas units at all stages of their treatment and met the special requirements of each of the Services.

All this knowledge, experience and practice of the Emergency Medical Services were utilised and applied by the Ministry of Health in launching the Hospital Service of the National Health Service. It is a service which could readily be organised and adapted to serve war conditions. The adaptability, mobility and flexibility fostered in the Emergency Medical Services, the pooling of resources and the large measure of decentralisation and autonomy achieved by the Regional and Group systems are basic principles. Successfully applied, they might enable the National Hospital Service to function in a future emergency with suitable modifications in view of the great advance in the destructive power of the war weapons which might be employed in attacks against this country.

A wide dispersal of fully equipped hospitals to areas considered to be beyond those likely to be rendered untenable by the destructive and contaminating effect of atomic weapons would be essential.

Even in the absence of weapons of such devastating destructive power, one of the lessons of the Second World War is that the efforts made to protect medical installations in thickly populated areas by reinforcing portions of them as protection against blast were largely ineffective, and gave no return commensurate with the large expenditure entailed.

In any future war, as far as is possible and practicable, all casualty receiving units and centres for emergency surgical treatment must be constructed in adequately protected underground buildings in which accommodation for the staff on duty, as well as for the estimated number of casualties, is provided. The approaches to such units should have adequately protected space for loading and unloading casualties. In all places where improvised underground units were provided, they proved to be wholly justified and continued to function even when the buildings above them were put out of action. Many more such units could have been provided in existing underground accommodation—which in many cases required little additional protection. Malta provided an example of what could be done in this way, with highly satisfactory results. All other hospitals should be dispersed to sites beyond the vulnerable areas. In London this policy was partially followed by evacuating the top storeys of some of the large hospitals but failed by not providing adequate underground facilities. The result was that large numbers of avoidable casualties occurred in the abnormal proportion of the partially evacuated hospitals which were more or less seriously damaged by direct hits.

As regards the organisation and planning of an Emergency Hospital Service and a Civil Defence Casualty Service the general principles set out fully in *Emergency Medical Services*, Vols. I and II will doubtless be carefully considered and applied to meet the needs of future warfare so far as it is possible to forsee them. *Si vis pacem, para bellum*—and all mankind should wish for peace.

Editorial Note. The above account purports to do nothing more than to complete the historical narrative by setting out the chief lessons which emerged from experience of the Emergency Medical Services in the Second World War. It is beyond the scope of this History to indicate to what extent these lessons are realistic and applicable to defence against the development of nuclear weapons in the megaton range. Documents on Civil Defence issued by the Home Office and Scottish Home Department and by the Ministry of Health and Department of Health for Scotland should be consulted on this question.

The Civilian Medical Services

By Sir Arthur S. MacNalty, K.C.B., M.A., M.D., F.R.C.P., F.R.C.S.

CONTENTS

(95349)

L* 2

I—THE UNITED KINGDOM

PUBLIC HEALTH ADMINISTRATION IN THE WAR OF 1939–45

WAR IS the enemy of health. There are the risks of famine and under-nourishment, of infectious diseases and epidemics through overcrowding, lack of sanitary precautions, movements of troops and population, increased fatigue and mental overstrain and lowering of bodily resistance. Grave fears were expressed at the outset of the Second World War that the national health would be seriously affected. Some considered that enemy action might render the maintenance of the public health and social services difficult if not impossible. Much additional work was thrown upon the Ministry of Health and the local authorities in the organisation of an emergency medical service for the treatment of air-raid casualties and the wounded; and in the evacuation scheme, which included the transfer of school children, pregnant women, young children, cripples and blind persons from urban centres to other areas less exposed to enemy air raids. Yet by selfless devotion to duty, medical officers and their depleted staffs succeeded in maintaining the essential health services during the war at a high level of efficiency. Intelligent anticipation in preparation went a long way to secure this, but rapid improvisation to meet sudden emergencies was repeatedly necessary. These administrative arrangements together with good team work and high civilian morale enabled the United Kingdom to survive the long-drawn-out ordeal with its standards of health maintained and even in some respects improved.

CENTRAL ORGANISATION

The general preparations made from 1935 onwards to meet the calls of war on the civilian medical services were manifold, and the Government and their medical advisers were faced with totalitarian warfare involving for the first time in history the whole civilian population, for which no precedent existed. The estimates of air-raid casualties soared into astronomical figures which no hospital provision in the time allowed could have coped with. The only answer was to make use of the existing hospital provision in the country and to supplement it as far as possible by additional beds in the time allowed between the Munich crisis in 1938 and the outbreak of war in 1939. The 10 Civil Defence Regions of England were paralleled by regional organisations for the hospital service and a partial regionalisation of the public health side of the Ministry of Health. Centrally, a Director-General of Medical Services was appointed under the general supervision of the Chief Medical Officer of the Ministry of Health. The regional organisations were flexible, and were designed so that in the event of enemy action interfering with central direction, each region could maintain its public health and Emergency Medical Services as an independent unit for the time being.

In all this organisation there was close co-operation with the Medical Officers of Health who rendered great service to the war effort. Despite the added demands imposed by evacuation and civil defence, the local authority public health service had by 1943 spared 47 per cent. of its fit-recruitable male practitioners and 50 per cent. of its recruitable women practitioners for service with the Forces. The flow of new entrants ceased with the cessation of D.P.H. courses and a series of measures giving the Minister of Health control over medical appointments to the public health service was necessary. This control was partially relaxed in 1945 and finally ceased in 1946. The allocation of medical man-power was a difficult problem which called for special consideration by the Central Medical War Committee, the Medical Personnel Committee with its regional Committees etc. (See *Emergency Medical Services*. Vol. I. Chap. 14.) Much of the inspectorial work of the National Health Insurance Service had to be suspended. In 1944 30 per cent. of medical men and women were in the Services; in consequence in some places the ratio of general practitioners rose to 1 doctor to 4,500 civilian population. Port-health administration, water supplies, the Insurance Medical Service and the Dental Service also presented war-time problems, especially in relation to man-power.

THE EMERGENCY PUBLIC HEALTH LABORATORY SERVICE

To reinforce existing safeguards against epidemic disease in war-time, and to augment the laboratory services, which were inadequate in many areas, the Emergency Public Health Laboratory Service was set up, organised and managed by the Medical Research Council on behalf of the Ministry of Health. This service, planned by Professor W. W. C. Topley and subsequently directed by Professor G. S. Wilson, proved of immense value in preventive medicine and subsequently became an integral part of the public health service of the country.

THE HOSPITAL LABORATORY SERVICE

This service set up by the Emergency Medical Services under the guidance of Sir Philip Panton extended in a similar manner to that of the Emergency Public Health Laboratory Service diagnostic facilities in pathology to hospitals throughout the country. These two services promoted a closer association between clinicians and pathologists and marked another advance in preventive and curative medicine.

PUBLIC HEALTH IN WALES

In Wales the public health authorities faced the same problems as in England with equal competence and success. (See *Civilian Health and Medical Services*. Vol. I. Chap. 6.)

MENTAL HEALTH SERVICES

No less than 26,000 mental hospital beds were surrendered for the reception of war casualties. Overcrowding, the blackout, reductions in medical staffs, air-raid damage to mental institutions and the shortage of nurses raised many problems, but the death-rate in mental hospitals, despite an increase, almost inevitable in the circumstances, in tuberculosis, was much less than that experienced in the First World War. A remarkable feature was the co-operation of patients in war-time measures and the absence of panic and exacerbation of mental symptoms among them when exposed to air raids.

AIR-RAID SHELTERS

Before the collapse of France in the summer of 1940, it was not anticipated that public shelters would be used as dormitories, but with the intensification of the air attacks and particularly with the continuous night raids upon London, shelters not originally designed for sleeping began to be used every night as dormitories. There was a rush to the underground tube railway stations, which rapidly led to severe overcrowding, and the emergence of a serious public health problem. The Minister of Home Security and the Minister of Health appointed a Committee under the chairmanship of Lord Horder to inquire into the health conditions in air-raid shelters and a team of medical officers, selected from the staffs of the Ministry of Health and Board of Education, with other doctors, was appointed to visit shelters and co-operate with the local authorities. Attention was paid to overcrowding, to the provision of sanitary accommodation, to defective ventilation, to dampness, to cleansing, to disinfestation, to medical care of shelterers and to epidemiological conditions, including a careful watch on the incidence of infectious disease and body vermin and insect pests, especially mosquitoes. In these and other ways the health of shelterers was safeguarded as far as possible. Fortunately, neither major droplet infections nor epidemics of infectious disease of any magnitude occurred, in spite of many pessimistic prophesies. Medical aid posts were opened and staffed. Bunks were provided and shelters coded to indicate clearly their capacity both for dormitary purposes and casual shelterers. The management of the shelters was made part of the warden service of local authorities. Buildings were re-surveyed to find further shelter accommodation and a long term policy of deep tunnels, additional to the London tube railway system, was undertaken. Eight large tunnel shelters were constructed under the existing tube railways.

TYPES OF SHELTERS

(*a*) *Domestic*. These included 'Anderson' shelters, strutted basements, individual or communal brick surface shelters and, later on, indoor shelters such as the 'Morrison'. These presented no general public health problem.

(*b*) *Public shelters*. Basement shelters under public buildings, large blocks of flats and large shops; trench shelters in parks and open places (these were not popular, many being damp and cold); street surface shelters, again not popular; railway arches—the night population using the Tilbury Arches in Stepney at one time approached 15,000. London's extensive system of tube railways provided very popular ready-made shelters, with safety, easy access, warmth and lighting. The Chislehurst Caves in Kent and St. Clement's Caves at West Hill, Hastings were extremely popular in spite of their dampness. Tunnel shelters were constructed in some areas and use was also made of disused railway tunnels. Tunnels were made in the Chalk at Dover and Ramsgate. For further details see *C.H. & M. S.* Vol. I. Chap. 8.

COMMENTARY

If the United Kingdom should ever be involved in atomic warfare deep underground shelter provision will at once be demanded by the population, and the problem of such provision is no doubt engaging the attention of Civil Defence at the present time. It is therefore of importance to note how the public health problems of such deep shelters were dealt with in the Second World War. The supervision, medical care and public health precautions undertaken reaped their reward in that the health of the shelter population was maintained. That no major epidemics occurred may or may not be a proof of the efficacy of these preventive measures for they were never tested under epidemic conditions.

The view was advanced that some degree of natural immunity existed, which was due partly to age and 'herd' composition and partly, perhaps, to the psychological attitude of the shelterer and well-balanced rationing.

It can be said in conclusion that the public health measures planned and worked out in the war should be put into force in regard to deep underground shelters in the event of a future emergency, though naturally improved and modified in the light of relevant medical and scientific advances.

REST CENTRES

When the air attacks began, 'rest centres' were instituted where persons rendered homeless by enemy action could be received until they were billeted. In the Metropolitan area, 613 first line and 384 second line rest centres which could accommodate 132,000 persons were available. Even during the last nine months of the war some 117,000 were cared for in rest centres. It was soon found that while most of the homeless could be billeted, a certain proportion remained in the rest centres, either those waiting to return to their homes after repair, or after the removal of unexploded bombs, or aged persons whose relatives, with whom they had previously lived, were dispersed. In the early days these persons were retained in the rest centres until arrangements could be made for their disposal. Later on hostels were set up for both classes. Arrangements were made for medical and nursing care and if necessary hospital treatment. Hostels were set up for able-bodied aged persons and for the aged and infirm in the evacuation areas. Detailed arrangements, including public health, medical and nursing provision, were made for refugees and evacuees from abroad. (See *C.H. & M.S.* Vol. I. Chap. 9.)

THE VOLUNTARY SERVICES

A. THE WOMEN'S VOLUNTARY SERVICES

One of the outstanding features of the war was the notable part women played in civil defence. An organisation, known as the Women's Voluntary Services (W.V.S.), directed and planned by the Dowager Marchioness of Reading, not only provided workers for civil defence, but also helped to facilitate the smooth working of the national and local authority services. Among these services were included those concerning the maintenance of public health and the medical services. The Women's Voluntary Services was a Service devised for war-time needs. It proved so valuable and filled so great a national need that under the aegis of H.M. Government it has become a permanent institution in times of peace. It is a flexible organisation and in the unfortunate event of another war it would adapt itself to new conditions of warfare and once more play its part in civil defence. (See *C.H. & M.S.* Vol. I. Chap. 10.)

B. THE JOINT WAR ORGANISATION OF THE BRITISH RED CROSS SOCIETY AND THE ORDER OF ST. JOHN

The services of this organisation in the War of 1914–18 were set up under the provisions of the Geneva Convention as only the Fighting Services had then to be provided for. It was revived in September 1939 to carry out similar humanitarian and relief services during the Second World War. Its activities were extended to the relief of civilians injured by enemy action as well as to the sick and wounded of the Forces and prisoners-of-war. It rendered conspicuous services at home and abroad. Its multifarious relief activities at home for the benefit of the civilian population comprised services during the air raids, convalescent and welfare services, and services during evacuation. (See *C.H. & M.S.* Vol. I. pp. 240–242 and the *British Red Cross Society and Order of St. John of Jerusalem War Organisation Official History, 1939–47* by P. G. Cambray and G. G. B. Briggs, published in 1949.)

C. THE AMERICAN RED CROSS AND HARVARD FIELD HOSPITAL UNIT

In July 1940 Harvard University sent a group of field and laboratory workers to reinforce the staff of the Ministry of Health. The first comers of the team, which eventually numbered over 100 persons, were Dr. John E. Gordon, Professor of Preventive Medicine and Epidemiology in the University and his assistant, Dr. J. R. Mote. Their help was cordially welcomed by the Ministry and they were for a time attached to its medical staff. Eventually, through the American Red Cross and other institutions in association with the Harvard University, 22 buildings prefabricated in America were erected on a site near Salisbury. This institution which had 120 patient beds was with great generosity handed over by the United States to the Ministry of Health at the end of the war. Dr. Gordon's staff helped with air-raid shelters, emergency public health laboratories and actively co-operated with the Ministry's Medical Officers. Studies were made of typhoid and paratyphoid fevers, upper respiratory infections, scabies, trichinosis, cerebro-spinal fever, fibrositis, epidemic hepatitis, gastro-enteritis in infants, typhus fever and nutrition. (See *C.H. & M.S.* Vol. I. pp. 242–246.)

THE SCHOOL HEALTH SERVICE

The School Medical Service (now the School Health Service) carried on its work with a depleted medical and nursing staff under circumstances of great difficulty during the war. Problems and work in connexion with evacuation of school children occupied much of its time. In the evacuation areas the Service was entirely suspended and routine inspections of the children had to be suspended or curtailed. Nevertheless, the authorities did their utmost to keep the treatment services in full operation and for the most part succeeded in doing so. Certain forms of treatment, such as child guidance, speech therapy, clinics for the treatment of diseases of the eye and defective vision, for diseases of the ear and deafness and for orthopaedic defects, were either established or expanded in many areas. The nutrition of school children by the provision of school meals and milk was successfully maintained.

Amid the stress of war Mr. R. A. Butler, Minister of Education, brought in the Education Act of 1944 which introduced many desirable educational reforms and extended the school-age to 15 years. Provisions of the Act or of regulations made under it also concerned the use of the School Health Service for research, the qualifications of school medical officers and school nurses, the appointment of senior dental officers, the duty (previously a power) to provide milk and meals at all maintained schools and the power to prohibit or restrict the employment of children. The Act, obviously, had little effect upon school health during the war, but its provisions held promise for the future health and welfare of school children. It was one of the major constructive achievements of the nation at war. (For the full account of the School Medical Service in war-time see *C.H. & M.S.* Vol. I. Part II. Chap. 1.)

ADVANCES IN PREVENTIVE MEDICINE DURING THE WAR OF 1939–1945

VITAL STATISTICS

The chief vital statistics of England and Wales during the war years were as follows:

POPULATION

The estimated mean population in thousands of persons at all ages was 41,246 in 1939 and 37,785 in 1944. Taking into account men in the Services both at home and abroad in the middle of 1941, the rate of decennial increase in population since 1941 was 4·4 per cent. as compared with 5·5 per cent. from 1921 to 1931. Children under 15 years of age declined in number from 8·79 million in 1938 to the low level of 8·53 million in 1942, but increased again by 1944 to 8·67 million. There was an addition of half a million older persons during five years of war. This figure carried important implications for the provision of future health and pension services.

BIRTH-RATE

The birth-rate, rising from 1941 onwards, reached 17·7 in 1944, the highest it had been since 1926, and the effective reproduction rate (provisional 0·99) came within one per cent. of a full replacement standard.

DEATH-RATE

The death-rates did not notably increase. With the exception of a slight rise in 1941 to 2·79 per thousand total births, the maternal mortality rate (including abortion) fell gradually from 3·10 in 1939 to 2·62 in 1940, 2·47 in 1942, 2·30 in 1943 and 1·92 in 1944. This rate was still too high, but it was satisfactory that, despite the shortage of staff for both hospital and domiciliary midwifery services, the rate decreased during the war years, and that in the fifth year of war a new low level was attained. Through treatment by sulphonamides, there was a notable decline in deaths from puerperal fever and sepsis. In 1941 deaths from these causes reached the low level of 0·48 per thousand births. The decline continued with a fall to 0·42 in 1942, 0·39 in 1943 and 0·28 in 1944. The infant mortality rates rose a little up to 1941 but thereafter declined, and in 1944 the rate dropped to the record figure of 45. An outstanding feature was the low mortality of children from disease during the war years. Despite the loss of some 7,000 lives at ages under 15 as a direct result of enemy action and an increase in accidental deaths arising through war conditions, the mean annual death-rates during 1940–1944 were below the rates for any year prior to 1939 at every year of age from 1–5 and at 5–9 and 10 to 14. It is a remarkable fact that the year 1939, practically a year of peace, had produced new favourable records for mortality at every age-group under 15 years, the fall being specially great at ages between 1 and 10. It was thought unlikely that these favourable figures would be maintained during the war, much less that they would be surpassed. Yet new records of low mortality for the second and third years of life were seen in 1942, and for the first, second, fourth, fifth years and at 5–9 years in 1943. Further improvement followed in 1944, when new low levels were reached for neonatal mortality and for mortality at 1–12 months, in the second, third, fourth and fifth years of age, and at 5–9 years, a most favourable health record—the reasons for which will be discussed later.

INFECTIOUS DISEASES

EXPERIENCE GAINED IN THE WAR OF 1914–18

In the War of 1914–18, in Great Britain the death-rates of the acute infectious diseases were not exceptional apart from the high mortality of cerebro-spinal fever. At the same time the war brought its new diseases—*encephalitis lethargica*, trench nephritis and trench fever.

The amount of typhoid and paratyphoid in the campaigns overseas was lower in proportion to the number of combatants than in any past experience. This good result was ascribed to anti-typhoid inoculation and the insistence on chlorinated drinking-water. In this country, the care and purity of our water supplies, good sanitation, absence of contaminated shell-fish and prompt hospital isolation of the sick, helped to protect from the enteric group of infections.

In the latter years of the War of 1914–18, dysentery and malaria were introduced into England from Salonika and other Eastern theatres of war. A few outbreaks occurred among civilians but were quickly controlled. The most serious menace to the public health was the pandemic of influenza which swept its tidal wave of destruction throughout Great Britain in the winter of 1918–19. Apart from this unavoidable tragedy, the record of civil public health in this war was good.

Generally, the chief diseases which engaged attention during the previous war were watched for and prevented by the same means in the War of 1939–45. These means were the maintenance of the normal health services as far as possible; port sanitary control, which guarded against the introduction of infectious diseases from abroad; purity of the water supplies; notification of infectious diseases; hospital isolation; maintenance of adequate nutrition, and so forth.

INFECTIOUS DISEASES DURING THE SECOND WORLD WAR

Some account will now be given of those acute infectious diseases which were the object of special concern during the war.

Smallpox

In the six years, 1939–44, 28 notifications of smallpox were received for England and Wales, but in four instances the diagnosis was not confirmed. There were three deaths, all in 1944. In Scotland there were three main outbreaks. The first occurred in Glasgow during the months of June and July 1942. The total number of cases diagnosed as smallpox was 36, of whom eight died. The first group was directly due to infection of a severe type imported from the East on a ship which arrived on May 29 at the Port of Glasgow; it consisted of 11 cases with two deaths among the crew and passengers. The second, or city group, comprised 25 patients from among the general population. Several of the patients had severe illnesses and six died. A direct connexion between these two groups was never clearly demonstrated. The second outbreak occurred in Edinburgh in October–November 1942. Again there were 36 persons affected, of whom eight died, a fatality rate of 22·2 per cent. The source of infection in this outbreak was not traced. The third outbreak occurred in the County of Fife, October–November 1942, there being 29 cases with eight deaths. The three outbreaks were speedily controlled through vaccination of patients and contacts, hospital isolation and formalin disinfection of patients' homes. In Glasgow Sir Alexander Macgregor organised a scheme of general immunisation and it was estimated that approximately half a million persons submitted themselves to vaccination in less than a month. This provides an interesting illustration of the response of a population in the face of virulent smallpox, and Sir Alexander was of the opinion that the people themselves, by taking timely advantage of the advice given and the facilities provided, stopped the outbreak at its beginning. The city patients who contracted smallpox were either unvaccinated or had not been vaccinated or re-vaccinated successfully for upwards of thirteen years prior to the outbreak.

Scarlet Fever

The incidence of this disease declined in the period 1939–42; it then increased to epidemic proportions in 1943, with some regression in 1944. During the war the already low fatality-rate fell still lower and throughout compares favourably with any pre-war period.

Measles and Whooping Cough

As a measure of war precaution, and with special consideration for the control of epidemics in evacuated children, the notification of measles (excluding German measles) and of whooping cough became compulsory in England and Wales in February 1940.

Measles was severely epidemic in England and Wales in 1940 and 1941; a remission in 1942 was followed by a recrudescence in 1944 when the recorded prevalence was 158,479. The deaths in the epidemic years 1940 and 1941 were only 75 per cent. of the average number in the quinquennium 1935–39 and the mortality-rate generally in the war years was unusually low.

The deaths from both measles and whooping cough have considerably declined during the past fifty years. Female mortality is higher for whooping cough; male mortality higher for measles. The decline in the fatality of measles during the period in which it has been notifiable has been more rapid than that of whooping cough, but the fatality of whooping cough is about five times that of measles. Appreciation by local authorities of the serious nature of the complications of the two diseases, in particular broncho-pneumonia, of the need for protecting children under five years of age, the age period of highest mortality from infection by measles, the institution of health visiting of cases and the provision of nursing and medical care and hospital treatment of severe cases, have been most useful. These methods pursued for many years have undoubtedly resulted in an increased decline in mortality, although the incidence of these diseases remains high. Other contributing factors have been treatment by convalescent measles serum, oxygen therapy and improved standards of hygiene and nutrition. It is doubtful whether any lowering of virulence of the causative organisms has occurred. The recorded figures for whooping cough for 1940–45 indicate that the incidence of the disease was on the average much less than that of measles and little more than that of scarlet fever. The death-rates from whooping cough per million for the war years were as follows:

1939	1940	1941	1942	1943	1944	1945
140	78	279	94	129	121	79

Measures for protection against and the treatment of whooping cough were still not on an assured scientific basis. Serum therapy gave inconclusive results. Vaccine prophylaxis at this time seemed of little avail, though some held that vaccine treatment might modify the severity of the disease and its respiratory complications. Nevertheless, the Ministry of Health in 1942 decided to sanction the provision of free immunisation against whooping cough by local authorities. The choice and expense of the prophylactic were considered matters for the local authority.

Diphtheria

A striking success was achieved in the prevention of diphtheria, 'the killing disease of childhood'. Immunisation was encouraged by the Ministry of Health and progressive local authorities. At the end of 1940, the Ministry undertook the free provision of prophylactics; previously, the cost had been borne by local authorities and this new provision undoubtedly aided the campaign for systematic mass immunisation which under the stimulus of war was vigorously pressed. Attention was drawn to the risk of diphtheria becoming epidemic through the evacuation of large numbers of children from towns where the disease was endemic to rural areas where it was comparatively rare. Over-crowding through the destruction of houses, shelter life and the absence of light and ventilation on account of 'blackout' regulations, were potential aggravating circumstances. Education of parents on the subject by posters, broadcasts, advertisements and health films was instituted. These intensive efforts advanced the practice of prophylaxis, for all local authorities have now the necessary arrangements. It was roughly estimated that between 55 and 60 per cent. of the child population of England and Wales by December 31, 1944 had been immunised.

There was a notable decline alike in the incidence and mortality of diphtheria during the war years. In 1940, when systematic immunisation began, there were 46,281 notified cases with 2,480 deaths; in 1944 there were 29,949 cases with 934 deaths. The decline in the number of deaths has been most marked at those ages at which immunisation has been done. Diphtheria is a preventable disease and steady continuous effort is needed to raise the general percentage of immunised children to at least 75, especially in the pre-school groups, and to maintain by re-inoculation at suitable intervals the state of resistance of children who have received primary immunisation.

Typhus Fever

From immemorial times typhus fever has been favoured by war conditions. Famine, overcrowding, defective hygiene, exhaustion and mental depression pave the way for infection, and the disease is particularly associated with movements of population. Hence, while typhus only rarely occurs in England and then sporadically, for the above reasons the Medical Department of the Ministry of Health in 1942 took special precautions against the risk of introduction of the disease into this country. These precautions comprised:

(a) The establishment of a panel of experienced consultants throughout the country.

(b) The designation of specified isolation hospitals as centres for the reception, disinfestation and treatment of patients.

(c) Local arrangements for the disinfestation of the homes and of the contacts of patients at specified centres.

(d) Formation by local authorities of sanitary teams to deal with the transport of patients and contacts and disinfestation.

(e) Immunisation against typhus fever of the sanitary teams and hospital staffs assigned for typhus work. The Ministry also issued a memorandum on louse-borne typhus fever, giving an account of the clinical features of the disease and suggestions as to the materials and design of protective clothing to be worn by all persons concerned in the work.

(f) Supplies of anti-typhus vaccines were provided and arrangements were made for inoculation of civilians proceeding abroad at any military hospital and at every emergency public health laboratory.

During the war only two suspected cases of typhus fever were reported. After the war 21 cases were detected; all were infected abroad; 14 were ex-prisoners-of-war and seven were medical students who returned from voluntary duty in the infamous Belsen Concentration Camp. All the patients recovered and there were no secondary cases.

During the war medical research greatly advanced the knowledge of typhus, its prevention and treatment. Means for prevention and treatment are now available. The principal method of checking an epidemic is effective delousing of the population at risk; this puts a stop to the activities of the vector of the disease. 'No lice, no typhus', remains the guiding rule. The synthetic compound 'D.D.T.' (dichloro-diphenyl-trichlorethane) has a toxic effect on lice and other pest insects such as mosquitoes (the transmitters of malaria, yellow fever and sleeping sickness) and flies. In powder mixed with kaolin or pyrophyllite and rubbed into underclothes it will protect from lice for two to three weeks. By its use a serious typhus epidemic among the Italian population in Naples and Southern Italy in 1943 was speedily checked. The Americans working under General Leon Fox in Naples blew the powder up the sleeves or down the necks of clothed people and found it effective in delousing as many as 73,000 persons in one day.

The use of D.D.T. requires effective organisation by relief teams. Delousing and vaccine therapy can now speedily control an outbreak of typhus fever. The control of this dire disease was one of the outstanding triumphs of the war period.

Cerebro-Spinal Fever

It is well established that war favours epidemics of cerebro-spinal fever. This is explicable by overcrowding and lack of adequate ventilation in camps and billets, which assist droplet infection, and by movements of troops, which lead to the introduction of fresh and virulent strains of the meningococcus. From the end of 1914 to 1918, cerebro-spinal meningitis was epidemic on an unprecedented scale in this country, the case-mortality-rate averaging about 72 per cent. Previously to the Second World War, the stage had been already set for an epidemic. In 1938 the Annual Report to the Minister of Health drew attention to the fact that as the annual numbers of notifications had not fallen since the epidemic prevalence of cerebro-spinal fever in 1931–33 to so low a level as after the 1914–18 epidemic, and as the number of Group 1 meningococcal infections appeared to be increasing, it was probable that we were approaching another period of epidemic prevalence. That forecast was unhappily fulfilled. In 1939 the number of notifications was higher and in January 1940, four months after the outbreak of war, the disease began rapidly to increase. This increase, with slight remissions, continued into 1941. The total of notifications in 1940 was nearly four-fold that of our previous worst experience in the year 1915. During 1942, 1943 and 1944 the incidence and case-mortality gradually declined. In character the disease displayed its usual severity, and in distribution it prevailed widely. No county in England and Wales escaped. The proportion of non-civilian to civilian cases was not so high as in 1915.

There was, however, balm in Gilead. The use of the sulphonamide drugs and later that of penicillin in treatment achieved the lowest fatality-rate on record; in some outbreaks the fatality-rate was as low as 4 per cent. In chemotherapy, medicine possesses another powerful weapon against a deadly disease.

Malaria

The anti-malaria work of the Ministry of Health in collaboration with other Departments, especially the War Office, the Colonial Office, the Ministry of Shipping, the Ministry of War Transport and the Medical Research Council, was another triumph of preventive medicine. The risks of infection and of the introduction of malaria into Great Britain were great; the administrative precautions under skilled scientific direction were comprehensive, detailed and world-wide. That these precautions achieved their aim is evident from the insignificant number of cases of indigenous malaria that occurred.

After the War of 1914–18, the Ministry of Health had set up an anti-malaria organisation to safeguard the population. This organisation fortunately remained in being in the years between the two World Wars and was further strengthened by the Ministry of Health's laboratory at Epsom. Consequently, when war risks of malaria infection again became imminent, the Ministry of Health had an efficient organisation to hand and an expert staff conversant with the problems that were likely to arise. The anti-malaria work done in Great Britain during the war was blessed by foresight, endowed with scientific direction, comprehensive in character and crowned with success.

The outlook for the conquest of malaria is promising. There are new and potent drugs (mepacrine and paludrine) for the prophylaxis and treatment of the disease; the employment of suppressive mepacrine in highly malarious regions was effective in maintaining our Forces in these areas in a fit condition to fight and defeat the enemy. The onslaught of the infective agent, the *anopheles* mosquito, can be repelled by D.D.T., which destroys both mosquitoes and larvae.

Jaundice

This condition, more accurately described as 'Acute Infective Hepatitis', has given rise to small epidemics in Great Britain from time to time and caused extensive outbreaks among the Forces and civilian populations in Europe and North Africa. The Medical Research Council, at the instance of the Ministry of Health and Army Council, appointed a Jaundice Committee to investigate the disease; and to facilitate the Committee's work, which was conducted from Cambridge, the Minister of Health in 1943 made 'jaundice' compulsorily notifiable in East Anglia. It is now known that the condition is due to a direct parenchymatous hepatitis, and that it is a disease of which the cause is present in the nasal secretion, faeces, urine and blood of patients, more particularly during the pre-icteric stage, and which has certain of the characteristics of a heat resistant virus. Our knowledge of the epidemiology has not yet advanced to permit of the formulation of effective preventive measures.

The infectious diseases which have been considered were those to which special attention was paid during the war and, as has been seen, considerable advances were made in combating them. There was also a considerable amount of dysentery. It was usually mild and of the Sonne type. In July 1941, for the first time a distinction was made between typhoid and paratyphoid fevers for purposes of notification.

Scabies

Scabies, always a disease of war, increased greatly during the War of 1914–18 among both the troops and the civil population. After 1919 there was a rapid decrease and by 1926 it was almost a rare disease, especially in the South of England. About 1930 a rise began, probably of periodic character, and by 1938, judging by the medical examination of school children, the incidence was as high as in 1919 and was rising. This increase was augmented when war began, first by evacuation and mobilisation and later by overcrowding, industrial shifting of population and shortage of laundry facilities, soap, towels, underclothing and bedding, leading to a severe and widespread epidemic of scabies. The Ministry of Health issued a Memorandum on Scabies in 1940, and in 1941 a Scabies Order was made under the Defence Regulations which gave local authorities additional powers to deal with scabies and with verminous conditions generally. An Advisory Committee on Scabies was set up. Many authorities took vigorous action and established efficient scabies treatment centres. In some cases, for instance London, the Minister allowed authorities to make scabies notifiable. Benzyl benzoate treatment proved to be the most efficacious application. The investigations of Dr. Kenneth Mellanby and others showed that efficient prophylaxis mainly depends on the following up of the family contacts and their simultaneous treatment. Disinfestation of clothing and bedding is usually now considered unnecessary.

Tuberculosis

In the War of 1914–18 there was a general rise in mortality from tuberculosis in this country. In some cases there may have been inadequate nutrition, but the main causes of the increase were contact infection, overcrowding and breaking down of bodily resistance to infection through prolonged physical or mental strain. These are difficult things to prevent in war-time. In 1939 the deaths from tuberculosis were 25,623 (war conditions only prevailed in a little over three months of that year); in 1940 they were 28,144; and in 1941 they had risen to 28,670. The figures for the two complete war years do not include Servicemen, but there was evidence indicating a certain increase of the disease among the Fighting Services. There was also an increase in mortality in mental hospitals and mental deficiency institutions.

The figures of deaths for 1942, 1943 and 1944 showed a decline, being 25,549; 25,649; and 24,163 respectively. The most disquieting feature was that deaths from pulmonary tuberculosis and tuberculous meningitis in children increased substantially during the war. The appreciable general decline was maintained. Fortunately, there was no severe epidemic of influenza, which in addition to its own mortality favours death in tuberculous persons. Nevertheless, war conditions inevitably promote tuberculosis, and the effects in so chronic a disease may appear later. A proportion of the deaths in the non-respiratory form are due to persons drinking infected milk. If all milk consumed were either pasteurised or boiled, much disease and crippling from tuberculosis would be eliminated.

At the outbreak of war there was a temporary dislocation of the tuberculosis services in some areas, but excellent work was afterwards done in spite of many difficulties. Evacuation, air raids, shortage of medical officers, health visitors, nurses and of bed accommodation all affected the normal service. The scale of rationing was regarded as adequate for the tuberculous if carefully planned, as in sanatoria and hospitals.

On the problems of tuberculosis in relation to war, the National Association for the Prevention of Tuberculosis, the Joint Tuberculosis Council and the Tuberculosis Association set up an advisory committee at the invitation of the Minister of Health on which the Ministry of Health, the London County Council and the Society of Medical Officers of Health were all represented. The Ministry of Health not only helped to maintain the tuberculosis services, but gave special attention to the question of after care. The Medical Research Council established a committee under the chairmanship of the late Lord Dawson of Penn to assist in promoting an investigation of the extent and causes of the war-time increase in tuberculosis, particularly among young women, and also to advise the Council on possible preventive measures. This committee issued a valuable report in 1942, some of the recommendations of which were rapidly implemented by the Ministry of Health. (See *C.H. & M.S.* Vol. I. pp. 93–95 and *Medical Research.* p. 140.)

The recommendations of the Committee concerning the controlled use of mass radiography among the civilian population were accepted by H.M. Government. Miniature or mass radiography was consequently greatly developed during the war and has proved an important aid to early diagnosis. It reinforces, but does not, of course, supplant clinical examination and pathological tests. (See *C.H. & M.S.* Vol. I. pp. 105–108).

During the war attention was turned to the group of synthetic chemical compounds known as sulphones. Promin was the first of these to be used clinically. Though the results of sulphones in human tuberculosis were then inconclusive the work was of great value for it demonstrated at long last that the disease produced by the tubercle bacillus proved to some extent vulnerable to chemotherapy.

The possibility of obtaining an antibiotic agent active against the tubercle bacillus had been recognised for many years and during the war the search for such an agent was greatly accelerated.

Work on penicillin during the war stimulated research on various moulds and allied organisms directed towards their inhibitive or destructive action on tubercle bacilli, and in January 1944 the important discovery of streptomycin was announced.

Clinical trials of streptomycin were made by a number of investigators in the United States and at certain approved centres in Great Britain under the auspices of the Medical Research Council.

Such war-time work laid the foundation for many post-war advances.

Venereal Diseases

War circumstances, as is well known, favour the spread of venereal diseases. The general state of heightened nervous tension and excitement in persons lacking in self-control, the shifting of large numbers of people, for instance in military camps, in the neighbourhood of munition works, or through evacuation to areas hitherto sparsely populated, may be associated with outbreaks of venereal disease in places unprovided with treatment centres. The War of 1939–45 was no exception to this rule. The following table shows the number of cases of syphilis and gonorrhoea (in all stages) in males and females dealt with for the first time at treatment centres in England and Wales. The figures for 1938 are given for comparison.

| Year | SYPHILIS | | | GONORRHOEA | | | Total Cases |
	Males	Females	Totals	Males	Females	Totals	
1938 .	7,832	4,986	12,818	27,947	7,746	35,693	48,511
1939 .	7,273	4,605	11,878	24,811	6,489	31,300	43,178
1940 .	7,093	4,226	11,319	21,057	5,882	26,939	38,258
1941 .	7,790	4,972	12,762	20,572	7,314	27,886	40,648
1942 .	8,529	6,542	15,071	17,956	8,413	26,369	41,440
1943 .	8,790	7,960	16,750	18,215	10,043	28,258	45,008
1944 .	7,667	8,251	15,918	16,629	10,646	27,275	43,193
1945 .	8,134	8,508	16,642	21,280	11,603	32,883	49,525
Totals	63,108	50,050	113,158	168,467	68,136	236,603	349,761

As regards syphilis it is believed that the majority of civilian cases coming under medical care within a year of infection were dealt with at the treatment centres. These figures do not represent the true incidence, for they were affected by the large numbers of young people, particularly males, who had been drafted into the various Forces of the Crown, as well as by the numbers of these who were sent overseas. By 1939 the incidence of early syphilis had reached the lowest point on record, the number (4,986) being over 45 per cent. less than the corresponding figure for 1931. After 1939, the numbers rose only slightly in 1940 and then more rapidly, to reach a peak of 9,642 in 1943, the number falling in 1944 to 9,318. The trends were apparently different in the two sexes. The figure for males reached its peak of 5,472 in 1942 and then began to decline, being 4,384 (about 53 per cent. more than in 1939) in 1944. The figure for females, on the other hand, rose steadily from 1,412 in 1939 to 4,934 in 1944, an increase of over 249 per cent. over the figure for 1939. This great increase in female syphilitic infections is reflected to some extent in the increase in congenital syphilis in infants under the age of one year that came to the treatment centres. From 1939 to 1944 the number increased from 217 to 346 or by over 59 per cent. In gonorrhoea there was in males a decline from 24,811 cases in 1939 to 16,629 in 1944, but in females an increase from 6,489 to 10,646. The figures are probably not representative, for in this disease there is a greater tendency to seek private treatment, especially since the introduction of treatment by sulphonamides. Venereal diseases increased more rapidly in the ports than in the inland towns.

The Ministry of Health in 1940 encouraged the expansion of diagnostic and treatment facilities and established a new service for rural areas in which private practitioners with approved special experience treated patients at their own surgeries. These expansions were aided by the Ministry making a grant to local authorities of 75 per cent. of the cost. In addition, the campaign for education of the general public in the facts about venereal disease was intensified. In 1942 the Minister of Health issued a regulation (Regulation 33B), which enabled a medical officer of health, on certain conditions, to arrange for the compulsory treatment of persons known to be a source of venereal infection. The existence of this regulation was of value in persuading persons to submit themselves to treatment, in tracing contact infection and encouraged the employment of social workers by local authorities.

Great advances were made during the war in the treatment of venereal diseases. Sulphathiazole was at first found to be the most efficacious treatment for gonorrhoea, but with the advent of penicillin more striking success was achieved. Penicillin cures ophthalmia neonatorum of infants in twelve hours and so diminishes the incidence of blindness and impaired vision in children. It has reduced the time required for the treatment of gonorrhoea to a few days and that for syphilis from a year to approximately ten weeks, though in both these diseases 'following-up' is essential.

It can be said then that the war years not only increased the magnitude of the problem of venereal disease but also witnessed great advances in overcoming the effects of the disease.

Development of Resistance in Organisms

It seems to be the case that when an organism of disease is assailed successfully by some new preparation or drug sooner or later it develops powers of resistance to the remedy. Thus it was the experience of the war that bacteria whose disease activities were inhibited at first by sulphonamide preparations or penicillin later developed resistant properties against these remedies. Fortunately, the discovery of new antibiotics has enabled one of these to act successfully, as a rule, in bacterial infections which have proved resistant, for example, to penicillin. The giving of penicillin in cases where other remedies are available, as for instance, in mild catarrhs and throat infections, is to be deprecated, as its administration may give rise to resistance in more serious infections subsequently, which otherwise would have benefited by penicillin treatment. Again, in the case of a virus infection like influenza, a vaccine at first potent against one strain of the virus may prove ineffectual against a new strain which initiates an epidemic of the disease.

Experience has also shown that disease-bearing insects are developing resistance to D.D.T. and other new insecticides. In 32 countries various types of malaria-bearing mosquito, the body lice which spread typhus, fleas responsible for plague and a strain of mosquito from Trinidad which spreads yellow fever, have all shown themselves to be extremely resistant to insecticides. Should the degree of resistance in such vectors of disease make control by available insecticides no longer possible, disastrous results would occur in many parts of the world. The executive board of the World Health Organisation on January 31, 1956 adopted a resolution that the world must assume responsibility for co-ordinating and stimulating research to combat this new danger.

Hence, in applying preventive and therapeutic measures against disease the possibility that resistance to them may develop has to be remembered.

MATERNITY AND CHILD WELFARE

Throughout the war attention was rightly directed to improving as well as maintaining the health of mothers and young children. The task was rendered the more difficult by the evacuation scheme, which transferred children and expectant mothers from areas generally well supplied with hospital and maternity and child welfare provision, to the more rural and less populated reception areas with less such facilities. In the reception areas the existing health services had to be expanded, maternity homes were improvised, sick bays were set up for minor ailments, residential nurseries for healthy children and hostels for many purposes in connexion with billeting were provided. At the same time, apart from some initial disorganisation at the outbreak of war, the existing maternity and child welfare services were well maintained.

The nutrition of expectant mothers and young children was safe-guarded by priority allowances of milk, cod liver oil, vitamin supplements such as fruit juices, and tablets of ferrous sulphate. The National Milk Scheme was introduced in 1940 by the Ministry of Food, in consultation with the Ministry of Health, to supply liquid milk free, or at a reduced price, to expectant mothers and children.

All this work and provision saw their rewards in the remarkable reduction of the maternal and infant mortality rates in war-time. (See *C.H. & M.S.* Vol. I. Chap. 4.)

INDUSTRIAL HEALTH (See *C.H. & M.S.* Vol. I. pp. 305-346)

Safety and health in factories were promoted by the Factory Department of the Ministry of Labour, which in 1940 took over the functions previously exercised by the Home Office in this matter, and by the statutory arrangements for the detection of scheduled industrial diseases. Research into the hazards of industry and their prevention has been conducted for many years by the Home Office, the Ministry of Health, the Medical Research Council and the Industrial Health Research Council, and the results of these researches have been practically applied to the protection of the worker. During the war the problems of the effects of long working hours at continuous high pressure and of exposure to dangerous substances again demanded consideration. The Ministry of Labour and National Service, by the Factories (Medical and Welfare Services) Order, 1940, required occupiers of armament and munition factories to appoint, if requested by an Inspector of Factories, whole-time or part-time medical practition-ers, nurses and welfare supervisory officers. The Ministry of Supply also appointed full-time medical officers to give medical supervision to workers in certain factories whose health was specially liable to be affected by exposure to dangerous substances. The Ministry of Fuel and Power is concerned with the health of coal miners and has a medical department of its own.

In various ways the health of the industrial worker is safeguarded, but there is still need for the more comprehensive development of indus-trial health services. The Report of a Committee of the British Medical Association points out that medical supervision of the workers in a factory has a wide meaning.

'Such supervision implies the care of the individual worker in industrial environment; the prevention of physical and mental illness; the initial treatment of injury and sickness; and a medical liaison between the factory and outside medical services. It should aim at reducing the general sickness rate as well as the accident rate.'

LABORATORY SERVICES

Prior to the outbreak of war, an increasing amount of laboratory provision was being made by certain local authorities, but this had to be greatly augmented to assist in the prevention of epidemic diseases and to meet the requirements of the emergency hospitals. To provide a new service where needed and to strengthen existing services, the Emergency Public Health Laboratory Service was established by the Medical Research Council in collaboration with the Ministry of Health. By offering greatly improved diagnostic facilities and by co-operating closely with University laboratories, the service has associated medical officers of health, general practitioners and bacteriologists in the public health service. It soon proved its permanent value and has become an integral part of the public health service of the country. Reference must also be made to the hospital unit and epidemiological laboratory under Colonel John Gordon, which was generously provided by Harvard University, the American Red Cross and certain other American Foundations. This was of much help at a critical time of the war.

The Hospital Laboratory Service set up by the Emergency Medical Services under the guidance of Sir Philip Panton, promoted and extended pathological facilities to hospitals throughout the country and was associated with the Emergency Public Health Laboratory Service.

All this progress in the passage of time has implemented the work of Sir John Simon, who as Medical Officer of the Privy Council first called in pathologists to aid in the prevention of disease and first established the principle that the State was responsible for medical research in the national interests.

Of allied interest to laboratory services was the *Blood Transfusion Service*. The Ministry of Health administered the service in England and Wales, except in London and the adjoining sectors of the Emergency Hospital Scheme, which the Medical Research Council controlled. There was close co-ordination with the medical branches of the Fighting Services and many lives of civilians and soldiers were saved by blood transfusion. Without this service the air-raid lists of fatal casualties would have been much heavier. The service is now retained as a function of the Ministry of Health in association with research by the Medical Research Council and the Lister Institute. (See *E.M.S.* Vol. I. Chap.11.)

NUTRITION

It was appreciated that one of the enemy's military objectives would be, as in the previous war, the starvation of the British Isles. The Government long before the war studied the food position and at the outbreak of war the Ministry of Food was set up with wide executive powers for the distribution and rationing of food and for the purchase of food from abroad on a vast scale. The Ministry of Health was made responsible for advising the Government on nutritional policy from the scientific standpoint, and advised other Government Departments on nutritional matters.

The essentials of the food policy were first, to minimise calls on shipping in order to free as many ships as possible for the transport of men and munitions; secondly, to arrange for the equitable distribution of such food as was available in quantities sufficient to ensure an adequate diet for all persons, whatever their income might be; and thirdly, to pay special attention to those on whom the future of the nation depended.

Rationing was introduced on January 1, 1940, and was based on the principle that all the essential foods should be equally available to everyone at controlled prices, to an extent necessary to maintain health. For this purpose, certain foods were rationed and most articles which were not in short supply became subject to price control. Sufficient was known of the general principles of nutrition and of food value to make it possible to arrange a balanced diet for all. During the war a continuous watch was kept on the nutritional state of the people. There were dietary surveys and clinical surveys, while the Oxford Nutritional Survey, under Dr. Sinclair and Dr. Meiklejohn, in association with the Ministry of Health and the Medical Research Council, investigated nutritional problems and added to scientific knowledge.

In this way the average diet of all classes became physiologically a better diet and was more evenly distributed. Rationing, unfortunately, had to continue after the war years owing to a world shortage of food and deficiencies in transport. Certain members of the community found difficulties in the restriction of proteins and fats. This was felt especially by hard manual workers and was recognised by an increase in their meat ration. There was also an increase in minor ailments, some of which, like anaemia and slight forms of peripheral neuritis, were ascribed to dietetic deficiencies. But on the whole, national rationing worked well in an unprecedented time of great difficulty and made an important contribution to the maintenance of good health, especially that of expectant mothers and children for whom special supplements were made available.

CONCLUSION

This satisfactory record of national health during six years of unprecedented strain alike upon the nation and upon the public health and medical resources of this realm is one that evokes pardonable pride. It was a great contribution to national defence, for many wars have been lost by disease and pestilence.

Let us briefly sum up the conditions, under Providence, which helped to secure so excellent a result. First of all can be put the work of organised public health, environmental hygiene and the health services, which, built up during a hundred years, have secured for Great Britain a reputation in preventive medicine second to none.

Next comes the important subject of nutrition. Rationing was ably carried out by the Ministry of Food with expert medical advice and the advances made in recent years of knowledge of the principles of adequate nutrition were well utilised.

A third factor in the maintenance of the nation's health was the special arrangements for war emergencies—air-raid precautions, the Emergency Medical Services, evacuation, the comprehensive laboratory organisation, the blood transfusion service and other triumphs of administrative and scientific organisation, including increased provision for maintaining industrial health and for rehabilitation.

Finally, the years of the war and those immediately preceding it saw great advances in medical science, especially in chemotherapy. For example, the sulphonamide drugs cure many diseases formerly fatal. Sir Alexander Fleming's discovery of the therapeutic value of penicillin and the subsequent work of Sir Howard Florey and Dr. Chain have made this drug another powerful medical weapon. It helps to inhibit the germs of pneumonia, gonorrhoea, syphilis, diphtheria, tetanus and anthrax, and can combat those which infect wounds, cause blood-poisoning and give rise to skin diseases. Malignant endocarditis was formerly a fatal disease; with penicillin 70 per cent. of patients recover. In D.D.T. we possess a most valuable insecticide which assists in the prevention of typhus, malaria and fly-borne diseases. In the application of these drugs, preparations and insecticides the possibility of the development of resistance to them has to be remembered and overcome. New and powerful drugs have been discovered for malaria and affections of the thyroid and adrenal glands. Cancer is still a deadly disease, but surgery, radium and deep X-ray therapy can often abolish it in its early stages. The new physics has not only given a weapon of destruction in the atomic bomb, but through its application in a machine termed the cyclotron, certain ordinary salts can be made radio-active for a time at low cost. This is an aid in the treatment of cancer by radiation.

It was realised that all these developments designed primarily for war must not be lost to peace. To this end a National Health Service was planned in the fifth year of war for all classes of the community and Parliament in 1946 passed an Act for a comprehensive National Health Service which was established in 1948.

PUBLIC HEALTH IN SCOTLAND

The state of the health of the people of Scotland just before the outbreak of war was probably better than it had ever been previously. There was reasonable freedom from major epidemics, but certain preventable zymotic diseases were still too high in incidence. The position as regards tuberculosis was not too satisfactory, and there was room for improvement in the infant mortality-rate. The general medical services covered a large proportion of the working population, although hospital services and treatment and care for chronic conditions were inadequate. There was not yet a real integration of the health services of the country as a whole and laboratory services were not so generally available as was desirable. Expansion of social services and a rising standard of living were contributing to health improvement.

PORT SANITATION

The immediate emergence of submarine warfare led to the virtual closure, for ordinary purposes, of the majority of Scottish ports and to the concentration of all the overseas shipping in the narrow waters of the Clyde Estuary. The bulk of all shipping coming to Great Britain had, for reasons of security, to be diverted to the Clyde. For the Civil Defence arrangements to deal with this concentration of shipping, see *The Emergency Medical Services*. Vol. II. Part I. Chap. 4 in this series. The limits of jurisdiction of the Port of Glasgow were extended to cover an emergency establishment known as the Clyde Emergency Port, and in 1940 an Emergency Port Health Administration assumed responsibility for the enlarged area, the work of which was undertaken by the Port Health Authority of the Corporation of Glasgow. The other constituent riparian authorities co-operated in surrendering their own statutory rights, as a temporary measure. The close liaison which evolved was of material value in the prosecution of the war at sea. The Department of Health acted as the agency through which the details of the scheme, operational and financial, were adjusted. The great increase in the work of port sanitation necessitated by the scheme demanded an increase in the boarding medical staff of the Glasgow Port Local Authority and additional sea transport. Close contact was maintained between the Port Health Office provided at Greenock, the Admiralty and other Service agencies, the various Medical Officers of Health whose duties were delegated to the Port Boarding Medical Officer and the District Hospital Officers of the Department of Health. The ordinary duties of the boarding medical officers covered the whole range of activities relating to sanitation and the infectious diseases, together with co-operation with the Immigration Officers as regards aliens. Food inspection, de-ratisation and the like for ordinary sanitary purposes remained the responsibility of the appropriate local authority.

For the arrangements made for the medical supervision of naval and military personnel—British, Dominion, Allied and United States, see *C.H. & M.S.* Vol. II. pp. 243–245. Close co-operation on an international plane was successfully fostered at the Anchorages. Arrangements were also made for the welfare of refugees and repatriates and of merchant seamen.

AIR PORTS

After an initial period of uncertainty it was arranged at a series of meetings between the local authorities, the Air Ministry and the Department of Health that, for the duration of the war, the medical and sanitary control of the airfields should be the concern of the Medical Branch of the Royal Air Force. In the interests of security and of economy in medical man-power, the arrangement was right and proper and operated well.

EVACUATION AND CARE OF THE HOMELESS

Evacuation in Scotland fell into two distinct phases, the first associated with the Official Evacuation Scheme, the second that which followed the intensive air raiding of the Clydeside areas in 1941. Inasmuch as dispersal of the population is likely to be an important feature of any future war both phases may provide lessons from experience.

The arrangements made for the Official Evacuation Scheme were in line with those planned by the Ministry of Health and the Board of Education for England and Wales, but were naturally modified to serve Scotland's special needs and circumstances. Early in 1939 the local authorities of the reception areas were requested to make a survey of accommodation so as to provide a basis on which the operation could be planned. At the same time the Department of Health, in association with the Scottish Education Department, made a detailed classification of the reception areas and considered the selection of priority classes for the scheme. Three types of area were designated, namely, the sending, the reception and the neutral, the last-mentioned being areas which, while not themselves to be evacuated, were not to be regarded as suitable for reception. They included such populous districts as the City of Aberdeen, the Burgh of Dumbarton and the industrial belts of the Counties of Lanark and Renfrew. The initial sending areas were Glasgow, Edinburgh and Rosyth, Dundee and Clydebank. Later the towns of Inverkeithing and North and South Queensferry were added. The standard of accommodation, applicable alike to existing occupants and evacuees, was one habitable room per adult person, each child under 14 years of age being reckoned as half an adult. Children of school and pre-school age, the latter to be accompanied, if necessary by parents or guardians, formed the evacuation class of first priority. Other classes considered for evacuation after completion of the general child evacuation included expectant mothers and the blind. The Chief Evacuation Officers in the sending areas and the Chief Reception Officers in the reception districts and all those specially concerned were made aware of what was required of them. The Department of Health made comprehensive transport arrangements in consultation with the two railway companies and the road transport authorities.

THE SUPPLEMENTARY EVACUATION

During the six months following the evacuation in mass, a scheme for supplementary evacuation, which comprised registration of children to ensure adequate medical examination etc. before transfers to reception areas, was in force but met with little response.

THE DRIFT BACK

A progressive fall took place in the numbers of those evacuated, for there was a drift back of evacuees to their homes from the outset of the scheme. In theory, Scottish evacuees did not cross the Border and English evacuees were not accepted under the Scottish scheme. But there was a good deal of unofficial evacuation from England in 1940, and certain of these people whose homes were destroyed by enemy action were placed in billets under Government auspices.

THE REVISED SCHEME

In February 1940 a revised scheme was instituted for the evacuation of school children only, designed to eliminate many of the difficulties as to infestation etc. which had arisen in Scotland, as in England and Wales, under the original scheme. Advance registration, full exchange of information between sending and reception areas, cleansing stations in the sending areas, medical inspection and treatment were included. Billet accommodation was supplemented by hostels and five camps were established. Medical and hospital care, clinics and day nurseries were provided. The response of the public was poor, and it was not until after the massive attacks on Clydeside that any further evacuation of moment took place. But soon again the drift back lowered the numbers in the evacuation areas.

COMMENTARY

Except on grounds of security, the evacuation scheme was not advanced by any responsible authority as a desirable thing in itself. Owing to the great extent of the drift back and the readiness of many mothers to terminate the experiment on the first experience of discomfort, the scheme as a whole was a failure in Scotland. It presented few medical problems but revealed unsatisfactory and in some cases deplorable social conditions, whose ultimate solution lies in education in hygienic habits and in improvement of housing. The Scottish experience also emphasises the lesson of the English experience that in time of war evacuation can only be successful if persons accepting evacuation are prepared to sacrifice their personal liberties for the good of their country and their personal protection.

CARE OF THE HOMELESS

In the year preceding the outbreak of war the Emergency Relief Organisation was established. Its three main functions were: (1) the provision in Rest Centres of food and temporary shelter for the homeless; (2) the supply of information and assistance for people in difficulties by reason of enemy attack; (3) the provision of accommodation in billets or unoccupied buildings for people whose homes were destroyed or rendered uninhabitable by enemy action. The Public Assistance Departments, in the main, operated the scheme. The Rest Centres were inspected as to hygienic needs by the medical officers of health, and medical supervision and, if required, nursing care, provided. Information Centres were set up by local authorities of all large burghs and smaller units were established in small burghs and other populous areas in country districts. In each centre a central index was maintained and records kept of the homeless and the casualties. Despite initial drawbacks, the organisation afforded material assistance and relief to the population in times of crisis.

INFECTIOUS DISEASES

No major epidemic occurred. The incidence of cerebro-spinal fever rose sharply in 1940, but mortality was reduced by the use of sulphonamides and penicillin. There were four importations of smallpox during the war, two in the Clyde anchorages, but in only one was there a limited spread to the general public.

Tuberculosis reacted unfavourably under war conditions. The number of new cases rose and so did the deaths. This was a common experience in other countries, but the higher incidence and death-rates continued in Scotland in the years immediately succeding the war. Tuberculosis was the outstanding exception to the general improvement in health.

MATERNITY AND CHILD WELFARE

The services were maintained and after 1942 both the maternal death-rate and the infant mortality-rate declined to new low records.

GENERAL MEDICAL SERVICES

These were maintained as far as possible under war conditions including, in spite of prevailing difficulties, the Highlands and Islands Medical Service.

NUTRITION AND REHABILITATION

These services were planned on similar lines to those in England and Wales. The Bridge of Earn Residential Fitness Centre was an important development in rehabilitation.

MENTAL HEALTH SERVICES

There was an increasing integration of the medical services as a whole including the Mental Health Services. Closer co-operation became possible between the general hospital and the mental hospital. Increasing use was made of new physical methods of treatment in psychiatry, such as electro-therapy, insulin-therapy and leucotomy. Occupational therapy was increasingly developed in various hospitals. In 1944 the After-care Organisation for the treatment and after-care of ex-Service psychiatric casualties was set up by the General Board of Control for Scotland. The foundations of many improvements in the Mental Health Services were laid for development in the post-war years. (See *C.H. & M.S.* Vol. II. pp. 227–326.)

CONCLUSION

While Public Health in Scotland during the war preserved certain independent features, the Department of Health in Scotland worked on similar lines to, and in close co-operation with, the Ministry of Health. High standards of public health administration and work were maintained, and the health of the inhabitants not only remained satisfactory but improved. Plans were made for extensions and improvement in the contemplated National Health Service.

PUBLIC HEALTH IN NORTHERN IRELAND

In Northern Ireland before the outbreak of war there was an increasing appreciation of the value of active immunisation against diphtheria, school medical services, child welfare clinics and efficient maternity services, including adequate ante-natal and post-natal care. Need was felt for the early diagnosis and treatment of disease and the availability of good, well equipped and properly staffed hospitals. No measure had been introduced corresponding to the English Midwives Act (1936). Hospital accommodation for tuberculosis patients was inadequate. The Dispensary Service was still associated with the Poor Law, and about half the population had to make private arrangements for General Practitioner Medical Services. Specialist medical services, except for dispensary patients, were obtainable only in hospitals or by private arrangement.

PUBLIC HEALTH DURING THE WAR

The war proved a stimulus to public health reform. An Emergency Medical Service on similar lines to that in England was established together with a Blood Transfusion Service. Evacuation chiefly concerned Belfast. It was not widespread and had little disruptive effect in Northern Ireland. There were no major epidemics of serious disease. In 1944 the Ministry of Health and Local Government was established and assumed responsibility for the general supervision of the health services. Legislation was passed to provide for the unification and expansion of tuberculosis services with the transfer of tuberculosis hospitals and sanatoria to the new Northern Ireland Tuberculosis Authority. An Act passed in 1946 made provision for the setting up of County and County Borough Health and Welfare Authorities and abolished Boards of Guardians. Amid the stress and peril of war, Northern Ireland took active steps to survey and advance the efficiency of its public health organisation and hospital services. (See C.H. & M.S. Vol. II. pp. 327–402.)

THE CHANNEL ISLANDS

The Medical History of the Channel Islands (Jersey and Guernsey) during the war describes how the medical services were maintained during the German occupation, and narrates the effects of the deprivations on the health of the people. Compared with the occupied areas in the then Colonial Empire, the Channel Islands suffered much less. The experience of the inhabitants of Jersey compared very favourably with those of Guernsey, chiefly owing to an abundance of milk and home-grown wheat, potatoes and vegetables. They were at times short of food, at times many felt hungry and many lost weight, but actual starvation was practically unknown. The Ministry of Health made an inspection of the Channel Islands after the liberation and the food supply, the nutritional state of the population, the state of the public health and other medical matters were investigated. (See C.H. & M.S. Vol. I. Part II. Chap. 5. pp. 418–436.)

PROBLEMS OF DISPERSAL OF POPULATION

In 1938 the storm clouds of international disagreement grew blacker over Europe. Conditions had altered considerably from the warfare of the past, and in preparing for the event of war the Government found it necessary to make special arrangements for the protection of school children and certain sections of the civilian population.

With these considerations in mind, the Ministry of Health and the Board of Education were engaged during 1938 in planning the evacuation from towns and cities and other vulnerable centres of certain 'priority' classes of the population, such as school children, younger children accompanied by their mothers, expectant mothers, and others such as the blind and crippled. Hardly had the scheme been formulated when the September crisis of 1938 almost forced an unprepared rehearsal. Indeed, a number of young children were evacuated from London in the early days of the crisis and were received with much kindness and hospitality. The general application of the scheme took place with the outbreak of war in 1939.

THE SCHEME IN OPERATION

Plans were made in England and Wales for the voluntary evacuation of some three million persons. Some 1,270,000 persons took advantage of the official scheme. Of these 734,883 were school children 'unaccompanied'; 260,300 were young children 'accompanied' by 166,200 mothers or other adults; 12,291 were expectant mothers and some 5,000 blind or crippled persons; the remainder were teachers and helpers. The movement began on September 1 and ended on September 4. The evacuees came from 81 evacuation areas, selected after taking into account size, density and vulnerability, and they were distributed to 1,100 reception areas, mainly small towns or rural areas. There were also large neutral areas neither sending nor receiving evacuees. School children evacuated from London numbered 366,800. From this area some 80,000 persons travelled by motor omnibus, 23,000 by steamboat and the remainder by train from many emergency railheads to avoid congestion at termini. The Ministries of Health, Transport and Education were responsible for organisation, and transport authorities, local authorities, education authorities, medical officers, health visitors, sanitary inspectors, school teachers and school nurses and the general public co-operated.

With the influx of a large population in rural and comparatively isolated parts of the country, local authorities had, in many cases, to extend water supplies, sewerage and drainage, to increase hospital accommodation for maternity and infectious disease, and to obtain many more midwives. Expansions of the local health services, school medical and nursing services were required. Sick bays were established in many areas, and a medical service, chiefly of local medical practitioners, with advice from regional medical officers of the Ministry of Health, provided for unaccompanied children in billets. Concern was expressed at the low standards of cleanliness and behaviour found in many of the evacuees. For their infestation, nocturnal enuresis and bad habits the School Medical Service was unjustly blamed. The fault lay in the low standards of living which persisted in the home of the child. The acuteness of the emergency prevented the children being thoroughly inspected and cleansed before departure. In later evacuations these measures were carried out, so that there were fewer complaints of verminous or contagious conditions. Hutted camps were provided for some evacuated school children.

THE EBB AND FLOW

Owing to the intermissions in enemy activity and air attacks, there was a continual ebb and flow of evacuated persons. On account of the initial lull in the war, large numbers of mothers and children and other evacuees returned to their homes. By January 1940 there were estimated to be only some 520,000 persons in the reception areas. In May 1940, when France and the Low Countries were invaded, voluntary migration of non-essential inhabitants from certain towns on the East and South-East Coasts began. In June and July 1940 there was a second large evacuation from the original evacuation areas which included nearly 134,000 children. In September 1940 heavy bombing of London began and by the end of that year 105,000 mothers and children were evacuated. Later, the numbers of migrants fell with the lessening of air raids on London, but evacuation was begun from other heavily attacked cities, such as Birmingham, Coventry, Manchester, Liverpool and Bristol. Some 123,000 children and 10,000 mothers with children were evacuated. The resumption of bombing of London in February 1944 caused a further flow of evacuation, and the arrival of the flying bombs in June 1944 was responsible for the fourth wave of evacuation.

Some million and a quarter left the now dangerous areas in the July–September quarter. From the Metropolitan evacuation area 285,000 mothers and children, including 101,000 unaccompanied children, were evacuated, as many as 36,750 going in organised parties in a single day. On September 30th, 1944 the evacuees officially billeted numbered 1,012,700, including 284,000 unaccompanied children.

As the Allied Armies advanced northward on the Continent, the bombing menace decreased and in September 1944 arrangements began to be made for evacuated persons to return home. Many were unable, for various reasons, to return and for the time being remained billeted. This number included over 10,000 children whose parents were dead, untraced, or not available to resume the care of their children. Other reasons were that owing to bomb damage there was no home, or room at home, or home conditions were unsatisfactory.

The Government had also to make arrangements for the accommodation and care of refugees. These included foreign refugees from Poland, Holland, France, Belgium and Norway, evacuees from Gibraltar and refugees from the Channel Islands (see *C.H. & M.S.* Vol. I. pp. 218–223). Similar arrangements to those in England and Wales were made for evacuation in Scotland and Northern Ireland. The evacuation scheme in Scotland, as a whole, was a failure, owing to the great extent of the drift back of evacuated persons. In Northern Ireland evacuation was not widespread and chiefly concerned Belfast.

DISPERSAL OF THE POPULATION IN A FUTURE WAR

During the Second World War and subsequently, science put further new and terrible weapons of destruction in the hands of mankind. Atomic warfare would not only destroy fleets and armies and wipe out cities and their populations, but it would leave an aftermath of suffering. There were about 76,000 houses in Hiroshima before the atomic bombing in 1945; 26,000 were left standing. It was the seventh largest city in Japan with some 400,000 inhabitants. The bomb killed about 200,000, including those who died of injuries afterwards. Eleven years later some 6,000 people needed constant treatment as a result of the wounds they received in the atomic explosion. Another 98,000 required regular clinical examination. Fifteen died from delayed after-effects in 1955. The effects of atomic bombing to-day would be greater and more widespread.

The body of man is adaptive, and it is possible that science in the future may discover some effective defence to atomic warfare. Already, research workers are studying the possibility of preventing or alleviating the blood diseases and other ills caused by atomic bombing. But, at the present time the only possible safeguards are evacuation—or to use a better word—dispersal of the population and the provision of deep shelters, together with other precautions, such as decontamination, change of clothing etc.

The most urgent demand will be for dispersal of the population, and in the organisation and planning of a scheme to this end some of the lessons of evacuation in the Second World War should be of service. They can be summarised as follows:

1. In any future war the time for preparation will be short or even non-existent. Atomic warfare may come 'as a bolt from the blue.' It is therefore of the utmost importance that the schemes of dispersal should be planned so that they can be put into force at the earliest possible moment when there are threatenings of enemy hostility.

2. The scheme should have central government direction and control and be sufficiently flexible to provide for autonomous control should communications with central authority be cut off. The country should be divided into evacuation, reception and neutral areas. For the working of the scheme the co-operation of transport authorities, local authorities, education authorities, medical officers, health visitors, health inspectors, school teachers, school nurses, Regional Hospital Boards and Hospital Management Committees should be secured.

3. Local authorities, if necessary, should extend water supplies,

sewerage and drainage and expand their local health services to meet the influx of a large population. Regional Hospital Boards should provide for increased hospital accommodation to serve the needs of isolated areas.

4. Medical arrangements in the reception areas should be on the lines of those developed in the Second World War.

5. Arrangements should be made in the reception areas for medical examination and disinfestation of dispersed persons where necessary, especially school children, before assignment to billets. The ideal procedure would be to arrange for these measures to be done before dispersal, but verminous school children are often reinfested in the home after cleansing, so that arrangements are necessary in the reception areas.

6. As in the Second World War, special arrangements will have to be made for the institutional care of mental defectives, cripples, the blind, 'difficult children' and cases of infectious disease.

7. The chief lesson of evacuation in England, Wales and Scotland in the Second World War is that in time of war dispersal of the population can only be completely successful if persons accepting evacuation sacrifice their personal liberties for the good of their country and their own protection. The possibility of compulsory dispersal of the population under the threat of atomic warfare calls for consideration.

8. Every endeavour should be made to maintain family association. Children should not be separated from their parents, if it is in any way possible. Location of dispersal should be such that the father can visit the mother and children now and then. There was general agreement that the break-up of families was the worst and most lasting evil attributable to evacuation.

9. Another point for consideration in preparing for dispersal in the event of atomic warfare is the preservation of the nation. To leave men within the target area to be differentially killed as against the women would be fatal to any hope of re-emergence as a potentially powerful nation. To meet this, it might prove possible to move out families from the target area to such a distance that men would be enabled to go into the target area to work in relays.

These suggestions which are made from the experience of evacuation in the Second World War are only put forward here for consideration. Obviously, they would need adaptation, alteration and re-planning in regard to policy and new circumstances which might arise in the future.

INDUSTRIAL HEALTH DURING THE WAR

During the war there was a great expansion of industry for the needs of
offence and defence, especially in regard to the provision of munitions
and armaments. In war as in peace it is important to maintain the
health and nutrition of industrial workers as well as hygienic conditions
in the factories. In addition, new processes demand research into the
industrial hazards which they may entail.

Before the outbreak of war the Civil Defence Act of 1938 laid
exceptional duties upon the inspectorate of the Factory Department of
the Home Office in regard to the provision of air-raid shelter in those
factory premises and commercial buildings in certain 'specified areas',
in which more than fifty persons were employed. In 1940 the original
programme of shelter construction in factory premises was completed
and a total number of 13,000 schemes was dealt with by the inspectorate.

With the course of the war and the occupation of France and the Low
Countries by the enemy the conception of 'vulnerable areas' disappeared
and by the end of 1940 the shelter scheme was extended throughout the
country to all factories with over fifty persons employed. The factory
inspectorate were concerned also in training A.R.P. personnel in factories
employing over thirty persons. This included measures for receiving
air-raid warnings, directing workers to shelters, training and equipping
first-aid, fire-fighting and anti-gas squads.

TRANSFERENCE TO MINISTRY OF LABOUR

An Order in Council made in June 1940 transferred the functions of
the Secretary of State under the Factories Act, 1937, etc., to the
Minister of Labour and National Service for the period of the war, and
the factory inspectorate was seconded or transferred to the latter
department. A Factory and Welfare Department was established in the
Ministry and the factory inspectorate was attached to it to continue
work for safety, health and welfare in factories, which had increased in
numbers, productivity and output.

LIGHTING, VENTILATION AND TEMPERATURE

The blackout, prescribed by the Defence Regulations, in many cases
was done without sufficient regard to the resultant interference with
natural lighting and ventilation. It was found that working in artificial
light during day-time affected workers and caused loss of output.
The lighting defects were investigated and largely overcome by application of the Factories (Standards of Lighting) Regulations, 1941. Ventilation was also improved. Attention was also paid to the maintenance
of proper temperatures for workers. In the event of a future war these
problems will recur, especially the lighting problem and the experience

gained in dealing with these matters in the Second World War will be of the utmost value. (See *C.H. & M.S.* Vol. I. pp. 307–310.)

HOURS OF WORK

In the early days of the war the patriotic spirit of industrial workers and the need for increased output of munitions of war led many workers to toil seven days a week without a break. The experience of munition factories in the First World War and the investigations of the Health of Munition Workers Research Committee and its ultimate successor, the Industrial Health Research Board (Medical Research Council), had conclusively shown that this excess of zeal defeated its own object. It was not only prejudicial to the health of workers, causing breakdowns and sickness, but output diminished in fatigued workers as compared with those who worked with a one day break a week. This experience was ignored or forgotten although the Chief Medical Officer of the Ministry of Health early in the war drew attention to the findings of the Industrial Fatigue Board on this question of prolonged hours. When it was seen that prolonged work again resulted in a high sickness rate and diminished output, suitable working hours were resumed with consequent benefit.

MEDICAL WELFARE AND SUPERVISION

The Factories (Medical and Welfare Services) Order, 1940 enabled the Chief Inspector of Factories, on behalf of the Minister, to give directions to the occupier of a factory, in which was carried on the manufacture or repairs of munitions of war or any work on behalf of the Crown, requiring him to make arrangements for one or more of the following services: (*a*) medical supervision of persons employed in the factory; (*b*) nursing and first-aid services; (*c*) supervision of the welfare of persons employed. (For details see *C.H. & M.S.* Vol. I. pp. 311–315.)

CANTEENS FOR WORKERS

One of the more important contributions to the health of industrial workers during the war was the widespread development of factory canteens and other arrangements to enable workers to get hot mid-day meals and other catering services, including meals for night shifts. This provided food over and above the domestic rations and helped to counteract factors prejudicial to health, such as long and tiring journeys to and from work, work at inconvenient times and other war-time conditions. Considerable attention was paid to the nutritional needs of young people under 18.

INDUSTRIAL DISEASES AND POISONINGS

The prevention of industrial diseases, accidents and poisonings occupies a large part of the factory inspectorate's duties in peace-time.

War-time increased these tasks in many directions—an old risk arose in a new guise, a substitute material was found to be poisonous, or a new material introduced new hazards. The use of radio-active substances in industry and the effects on the workers were studied and protective measures devised. Toxic jaundice from tri-nitro-toluene (T.N.T.) poisoning, which was a serious cause of death and illness among munition workers in the First World War until protective measures were instituted, was greatly diminished. (For details of industrial diseases, accidents and poisonings see *C.H. & M.S.* Vol. I. pp. 317-344.)

CIVILIAN MEDICAL RECRUITING BOARDS

After the Military Training Act came into force in May 1939, medical officers of the Ministry of Health were responsible for the supervision of Civilian Medical Recruiting Boards and for advising the Ministry of Labour and National Service on all medical matters connected with the examination of men and women by these Boards; and from June 1940 to April 1945, one senior medical officer, three divisional medical officers and seven regional medical officers were seconded to the Ministry of Labour and National Service for these purposes. These officers also advised the Ministry on all medical questions which arose out of compulsory service in industry, for instance, under the Essential Work Orders. The Medical Boards performed their work well and satisfactorily, and a study of their organisation and duties should be of value in connexion with similar arrangements which war in the future may demand—(for details see *C.H. & M.S.* Vol. I. pp. 346-366).

MEDICAL SERVICES OF THE MINISTRY OF SUPPLY

The Ministry of Supply was formed in 1939. It assumed direct control of the State munition factories known as the Royal Ordnance Factories and acted as adviser to a number of agency factories supplying munitions, the administration of which continued under private ownership.

In October 1940 a Chief Medical Officer was appointed. His primary function was to supervise and co-ordinate medical matters arising at the Royal Ordnance factories and other out-station establishments of the Ministry with the Factory and Welfare Department of the Ministry of Labour and National Service and the Industrial Health Board of the Medical Research Council. This led to the formation of the Ministry of Supply's Medical and Nursing Service. This Service, in organisation and work, naturally resembled that already described for the Factory Inspectorate of the Ministry of Labour and National Service. It had, however, its special problems and features as set forth in *C.H. & M.S.* Vol. I. pp. 367-395, which are of importance in future warfare.

COMMENTARY

The chief lessons concerning industrial health in the Second World War can be summarised as follows:

1. The transfer of the Factory Inspectorate from the Home Office to the Ministry of Labour and National Service and the setting up of a Factory and Welfare Department made for efficiency.

2. The Ministry of Supply established an efficient Medical and Nursing Service co-ordinated with the Factory and Welfare Department of the Ministry of Labour and National Service and the Industrial Health Board of the Medical Research Council. This co-ordination should be fully maintained in a future war.

3. The Ministry of Labour and the Ministry of Supply should be fully acquainted with the value of incorporating their medical branch as an effective member of the team which concerns itself with the human factor in all its aspects alike in peace-time and in war-time. The valuable records of medical experience, of organisation and methods, and above all of the place taken by the medical services in relation to those concerned with labour management, production and research should be available if needed.

4. Of special importance is the maintenance of the full co-ordination established between the Industrial Health Board and the Ministries of Labour and Supply. The scientific experience which the Board possesses of industrial fatigue, maintenance of health in industry, etc., should continue to be applied in workshops and factories, and be available in war-time when factories are expanded and new ones set up.

5. It is of great importance in war-time activities, when patriotic fervour and the need for munitions of war urge the working of long hours to speed up production, to remember that working overtime for long periods and for seven days a week slows production instead of accelerating it owing to the fatigue of workers.

6. War-time canteens to maintain the nutrition of workers and special facilities for welfare, rest and recreation proved their value and necessity.

7. The prevention of industrial diseases, accidents and poisonings is equally important in war-time as in peace-time. War increases these industrial hazards.

8. The use of radio-active substances in industry, their effect upon the workers, and the devising of protective measures demands continued investigation by the medical services of the Ministries.

9. The experience and work of the Civilian Medical Recruiting Boards may serve as a guide to the establishment and organisation of a similar body in a future war.

These suggestions call for consideration, but will naturally be adapted to, and employed for, the needs of any future war under those altered conditions and circumstances, at present unforeseen, which may then prevail.

THE MEDICAL SERVICES OF THE MERCHANT NAVY

The mainspring of victory in the Second World War was sea power, and to this the Merchant Navy made a most essential contribution. Had it not been for this Service Great Britain could not have received food, supplies and reinforcements. Again, all the main operations of the war, for example, the Dunkirk and Crete evacuations, the North African and Italian landings, the invasion of France and the subjection of the Japanese island garrisons, were made practicable through the large resources of British and Allied shipping and, it may be added, through experience down the centuries of seamanship, especially in the First World War.

Here too the Medical Services of the Merchant Navy were of the utmost value in maintaining the health and efficiency of merchant seamen.

SERVICE IN PEACE-TIME

Merchant seamen in peace-time were not under Government control as men are in the Fighting Services, but many of the conditions of service are governed by the Merchant Shipping Acts. These Acts provide for instance that (a) ships must carry medicine chests containing medicines and medical stores in accordance with approved scales; (b) seamen must receive provisions in accordance with an approved scale; (c) shipowners are liable for seamen who are left behind abroad sick. No provision was made for the compulsory medical examination of new entrants or for the periodic examination of those serving, except in the case of young people and the crews of emigrant ships.

Every foreign-going ship having 100 persons or upwards on board must carry, as part of her complement, a duly qualified medical practitioner. On ships carrying less than 100 persons the treatment of any sick members of the crew devolves upon the Master.

SERVICE IN THE WAR

The risks of injury and illness were increased by enemy action, in the air, on the sea and under the sea, by sailing in convoy, carriage of dangerous cargo and blackout on board. There was consequently a substantial increase in the number of seamen requiring medical treatment abroad. Consuls and Shipping Masters dealt with all such cases with sympathy, efficiency and dispatch. While the liability for treatment of sick and injured seamen abroad remained on the shipowners concerned, H.M. Government in the United Kingdom reimbursed them for the treatment of seamen with injuries or illness arising from hostilities or warlike operations. The Ministry of War Transport took over the responsibilities of the Board of Trade for merchant seamen during the war.

WAR-TIME MEDICAL WORK

During the war changes in the recommended treatment of specific diseases and alterations in the medical scales were promulgated by means of notices issued by the Ministry of War Transport. The main changes dealt with the prevention and treatment of malaria, typhoid fever, venereal diseases, tuberculosis, supply of blood products for transfusion, heat exhaustion, heat stroke and heat cramp, immersion foot and frost bite and scabies. (See *C.H. & M.S.* Vol. I. pp. 399–403.)

JOINT ADVISORY COMMITTEE

There was a Joint Advisory Committee on the health of the Mercantile Marine which had been appointed in 1928: 'To consider and advise on any questions affecting the health of the Mercantile Marine which the Board of Trade or the Ministry of Health may from time to time, refer to them'. As originally constituted, the committee was composed of four members representing the Ministry of Health and three members representing the Board of Trade. The Medical Secretary was appointed by the Ministry of Health and the Clerical Secretary by the Board of Trade. During the war two representatives of the Ministry of Labour and National Service were added to the Committee. Questions on the health of merchant seamen were referred to the Committee and its recommendations were implemented by the Ministry of War Transport.

THE EMERGENCY MEDICAL SERVICES PROVISION

Under the Emergency Medical Services Scheme special provision was made for the free hospital treatment and care of officers and seamen of all nationalities who were injured in the course of duty or were suffering as a result of exposure on duty.

HYGIENE, FOOD AND CLOTHING

Special attention was given to the living conditions of seamen, the ventilation of ships, the chlorination of drinking water, food and clothing.

STATISTICS OF MORTALITY AND SICKNESS

These were difficult to procure, but a certain amount of statistical information concerning the mortality and sickness incidence among merchant seamen was obtained. Merchant Navy casualties from September 3, 1939 to August 14, 1945 were given by the Prime Minister to the House of Commons as follows:

Deaths	30,189
Missing	5,264
Wounded	4,402
Internees	5,556

The figures for deaths excluded deaths from natural causes.

WAR-TIME WELFARE WORK

Much valuable work was done under this heading at ports in this country and overseas. Rest and rehabilitation centres were set up and provision was made for training and resettlement.

COMMENTARY

How far all this important and valuable work for the medical care of members of the Mercantile Marine can be repeated, amplified and extended in a future war, it is difficult to say. But the experience gained and the lessons learned should certainly be studied and borne in mind. (See *C.H. & M.S.* Vol. I. pp. 396–417.)

THE MINISTRY OF PENSIONS IN WAR-TIME

The Ministry was established by the Ministry of Pensions Act, 1916 to unify the administration of pensions, grants and allowances awarded on account of disablement or death through service in the Armed Forces. As from February 15, 1917 the Act provided for the transfer to the Minister of Pensions of the powers and duties of the Service Departments in these matters. In 1921 these powers and duties in regard to peace-time claims were retransferred to the Service Departments, but the Ministry's responsibilities in connexion with claims arising out of the War of 1914–18 and earlier wars remained unchanged.

On the outbreak of the War of 1939–45, an Act was passed, giving the Minister of Pensions the same powers in relation to the Armed Forces as he had for the War of 1914–18, and also power to make pensions schemes for the Mercantile Marine. A further Act gave him a new power to award compensation to Civil Defence personnel and civilians. A new Royal Warrant was drawn up for the Forces and pension schemes for the Mercantile Marine and Naval Auxiliary personnel and for the Civil Defence Service and Civilians.

ESTABLISHMENT OF MEDICAL SERVICES

In December 1917 the Ministry formed its own Medical Services Division under a Director-General with a whole-time medical staff. Its main functions were:

1. To advise on the medical aspects of entitlement, to determine the assessment of disablement and to arrange and conduct the necessary medical examinations and boards.

2. To ensure that the medical and surgical treatments and necessary appliances required for war disablement were provided either by the Ministry, or by other agencies, and to provide for the medical administration involved.

3. To provide the organisation and specially trained medical staff required for the skilled provision, fitting and supervision of artificial limbs.

These functions were efficiently carried out by the Medical Services Division. At headquarters this Division was divided into branches to deal with:

1. Medical Boards and the selection and appointment of medical personnel.

2. Provision of medical and surgical treatment including the management of Ministry hospitals and clinics.

3. Provision of treatment concurrently with training and the establishment of special institutions for the purpose.

4. Provision of medical supplies and equipment, artificial limbs and appliances.

5. The Nursing Service.

Between the two world wars awards of pension, or gratuity, were made to nearly a million and three-quarter persons. Of these over 400,000 were still receiving pensions in September 1939.

For the technical meaning in Ministry of Pensions' practice of the terms 'Disability, Disablement, Entitlement and Assessment' see *C.H. & M.S.* Vol. II. pp. 139, 140.

THE SECOND WORLD WAR

As already stated, the outbreak of the Second World War renewed the duties and responsibilities which the Ministry of Pensions exercised in the First World War and enabled them to include provision for members of the Mercantile Marine and Fishing Fleet as well as for the regular Services and their auxiliaries. The Ministry was also made responsible for the compensation of civilians in respect of death or disablement by war injuries and joined with the Emergency Medical Services in providing treatment. The main condition governing entitlement to pension, stated briefly, was that the disablement should have been attributable to or aggravated by war service, or death should have been attributable to or hastened by such service.

The new responsibilities of the Ministry were provided for in the Pensions (Navy, Army, Air Force and Mercantile Marine) Act, 1939 and as regards civilians in the Personal Injuries (Emergency Provisions) Act, 1939. (See *C.H. & M.S.* Vol. II. pp. 152, 153.)

EVACUATION OF H.Q. FROM LONDON

In 1938 preparations were made for the evacuation of the bulk of the Ministry's London Headquarters to Rossall School, near Liverpool. This was started on September 3, 1939. In October 1940, the increased bombing led to almost complete evacuation of London H.Q., only the D.G.M.S. and his personal staff remaining in London. The accommodation at Rossall then became inadequate and Ministry H.Q. had to be moved to hutted accommodation specially built at Norcross, near Cleveleys and St. Annes, Blackpool.

LIAISON WITH OTHER GOVERNMENT DEPARTMENTS

There was close liaison with the following:

1. *The Emergency Medical Services*
   Particularly in connexion with the provision of hospital accommodation.

2. *The Service Departments*
   Especially as regards the keeping of medical records during service and the continuity of medical treatment for invalided members of the Forces without waiting for and without prejudice to the Ministry's decision on entitlement to pension.

3. *The Ministry of Labour and National Service*
   The Ministry of Pensions was particularly interested in the medical boarding of recruits which was the responsibility of the Ministry of Labour and National Service (*see* p. 350). Effect was given to this concern by the appointment of a Ministry of Pensions representative on the Medical Advisory Committee set up by the Minister of Labour and National Service in order to advise him on the medical aspects of recruitment. There was close liaison between the Ministry of Labour and Local Education Committees in the scheme for the education, training and resettlement of disabled persons.

WAR NEUROSIS

The experience of the First World War indicated that in any subsequent war the Ministry of Pensions would undoubtedly again be faced with the prolonged and complex problems inherent in war neurosis. In 1938 the Minister appointed a Committee which included Service representatives and leading neurologists to advise him on the policy to be adopted towards neurosis in the light of current experience. The Committee endorsed the findings of the 1920 'Shell Shock' Committee; they agreed that the First World War produced no unforeseen neuroses, and that those which occurred had previously been recognised in civil medical practice (see C.H. & M.S. Vol. II. pp. 158, 159).

DETAILS OF WORK DURING THE WAR

For details of the Ministry of Pensions' work during the war on regional organisation, expansion and duties of medical personnel, appointment of Matron-in-Chief and expansion of the Nursing Services, increase of hospital provision, air-raid damage and casualties, limb fitting service, incidence of disabilities and other noteworthy developments, see C.H. & M.S. Vol. II. pp. 160–226.

CONCLUSION

The Ministry of Pensions was set up in the First World War and came of age just before the Second World War. Here again, fresh problems had to be faced and solved. New administrative and financial arrangements were needed and on the medical side hospital and other forms of treatment had to be provided, and schemes of rehabilitation elaborated. It was fortunate that medical administrators were still available in the Ministry to apply the knowledge and experience gained in the First World War to the needs of the Second. It was remembered also that peace would bring its problems no less than war and provision was made well in advance for problems which demobilisation would inevitably cause. The record of the Ministry of Pensions in war-time was an admirable one of administrative efficiency and skilled application of medical knowledge and treatment, while in the assessment of entitlement to pension strict justice was often tempered by compassionate consideration.

TRANSFER OF FUNCTIONS OF THE MINISTRY OF
PENSIONS

Following the precedent of 1921, after the Second World War the powers and duties of the Ministry of Pensions in regard to peace-time claims were again retransferred to the Service Departments. Later, a more radical change was made. On August 31, 1953 the Transfer of Functions (Ministry of Pensions) Order, 1953 came into operation.

By that Order the functions of the Minister of Pensions were transferred to the Minister of Health 'so far as they relate to medical and surgical treatment and the provision of vehicles in England, Wales, the Channel Islands, the Isle of Man and the Republic of Ireland, and matters incidental thereto'. With the functions were also transferred 'all property rights and liabilities held or enjoyed by or incumbent on the Minister of Pensions in connection with these functions respectively'. For instance, the Ministry of Pensions' hospitals became hospitals of the National Health Service. The other functions of the Ministry of Pensions, including assessment by Medical Boards, were transferred to the Ministry of National Insurance.

COMMENTARY

In the event of a future war the wealth of experience gained in the two world wars will be of immeasurable value for the administration of pensions, grants and allowances awarded on account of disablement or death through service in the Armed Forces of the Crown, in the Mercantile Marine and Naval Auxiliary personnel and for the Civil Defence Service and Civilians.

In this connexion the following suggestions are put forward for consideration:

1. Having regard to the magnitude and responsibilities of the work in a future war, the question will arise as to whether the peace-time arrangements are capable of expansion or whether the Ministry of Pensions should be reconstituted on lines similar to those planned in the Second World War? A further consideration in favour of the second alternative is that in a future war it will once more be necessary for the powers and duties of the Service Departments as regards pensions matters to be referred to a comprehensive Pensions Authority, such as was the Ministry of Pensions in two world wars.

2. In any case administrative headquarters should be evacuated from London and a regional organisation set up. This will probably entail the provision of new hutted accommodation.

3. Additional medical personnel will be required.

4. The main treatment of pensioners and claimants for pension will be in National Health Service Hospitals. The provision of Pensions Hospitals should also be considered.

5. Substitution of other accommodation for air-raid damaged hospitals requires consideration.

6. There should be full liaison with other government departments, especially the Ministry of Labour and National Service, as in the Second World War.

7. In view of the possibility of atomic warfare the assessment of pensions for casualties, including after-effects arising from this cause, should be worked out.

8. The Limb fitting service will require expansion.

9. Attention should be given to schemes of rehabilitation.

It will be appreciated that conditions in any future war are likely to be unprecedented and that many fresh difficulties and new problems will be encountered. It is hoped, however, that these suggestions may be helpful in constructive planning.

II—THE COLONIES

GENERAL MEASURES

Formerly, the function of the medical services in the Colonies mainly concerned the care of the health of Government officials. But during the thirty or forty years which preceded the Second World War the Medical Departments developed into organised State Public Health Services for the prevention and cure of disease and the preservation of health among the general populations of the Colonies.

When the war broke out every Colonial Government possessed a separate medical department presided over by a senior medical officer, styled in most Colonies the Director of Medical Services. Every medical department included an establishment of District Medical Officers to serve a number of administrative areas, and many departments employed a considerable staff of specialists. These various medical services were unified into a single Colonial Medical Service in 1934.

At the Colonial Office in London the Secretary of State was advised by a Chief Medical Adviser (with an Assistant) and by the Colonial Advisory Medical Committee which contained a number of medical specialists in tropical medicine. The Colonial Office was also in close touch with other bodies investigating tropical diseases, such as the Medical Research Council, the Tropical Research Committee, the Bureau of Hygiene and Tropical Diseases, the Imperial Institute of Entomology and the London, Liverpool and Edinburgh Schools of Tropical Medicine.

At the beginning of the war, or soon afterwards, many officers in the Colonial Medical Service were seconded or released for military service. The depleted Colonial medical staff were chiefly occupied with routine duties, but it was found possible to pursue certain investigations, especially those to meet a number of urgent problems; for instance, from 1939 the occurrence and control of sleeping sickness in Sierra Leone, and the incidence of tuberculosis in the gold mines of the Gold Coast Colony. An investigation of the possible production of a protective vaccine against tropical or scrub typhus was begun at the Institute of Medical Research at Kuala Lumpur in the Federated Malay States and continued, after the Japanese invasion, with the assistance of the Australian Authorities at the Commonwealth Serum Laboratory at Melbourne. Progress was made in several fields of research in the West Indies. The Colonial Development and Welfare Act, 1940 benefited the Medical and Health Services, large grants being made to Colonies in East and West Africa and the Pacific Ocean. These grants were used for the control of malaria, yellow fever and leprosy, to establish health units and health centres, to expand and improve hospital accommodation, to provide better facilities for medical training in local schools and colleges and for many other activities.

PARTICULAR DISEASES

The Colonial Office, with the close collaboration of the military authorities, devoted special attention to the control of diseases prevalent in the Tropics, and of venereal diseases in areas in which troops were concentrated, such as West Africa, East Africa, Palestine, Ceylon and Malaya.

MALARIA

Owing to attacks by enemy submarines and from the air the Mediterranean route to Egypt and the Far East became unsafe for convoys bringing munitions and personnel to the Forces and the Cape route had to be substituted. Freetown harbour in West Africa was constantly full of all classes of ships and in 1940 there was an increase of malaria among the crews of ships calling there and at other ports. A special mission under Professor D. B. Blacklock of the Liverpool School of Tropical Medicine was sent to West Africa. In addition to anti-mosquito measures, prophylactic doses of mepacrine were issued to all personnel in ships from the time of their arrival in Freetown until several days after their departure. Suppressive treatment was also given to all personnel in the shore establishments and also to most of the school children in Freetown. As a result of these measures the incidence of malaria was greatly reduced. Research work was done by others on the breeding of *Anopheles melas* and its control.

In East Africa research units established by the Governments had been engaged from 1930–39 in studies of malaria. On the outbreak of war the experience of malariologists and entomologists engaged in these investigations was used either through their being seconded to the Army for controlling malaria in the field or as consultants in their civil posts. As a result, sickness rates due to malaria were kept at exceptionally low levels during the Abyssinia, Somaliland, Eritrea and Madagascar campaigns. In North Borneo research work was done on *A. leucosphyrus*, a shade-haunting mosquito; it was found that control could be secured by opening up the breeding grounds to sunlight. D.D.T. was used with spectacular results to destroy mosquitoes in malarious areas by the British and Indian Armies in Burma and by the American and Australian Armies in the South West Pacific Campaigns. Experimental supplies of D.D.T. were sent by the Colonial Office to the medical departments of a large number of Colonies. Large scale trials were first carried out with good results in British Guiana for the control of malaria. Ceylon reported that D.D.T. had effected a marked reduction in the malaria infection rates in labour camps.

YELLOW FEVER

The work done on the control of yellow fever was of marked value and prevented spread of the disease in Africa, a danger increased by the extensive movement of Service aircraft. An investigation by the Rockefeller Yellow Fever Institute at Entebbe showed that yellow fever had occurred in the Belgian Congo, Uganda, Anglo-Egyptian Sudan, Eritrea, Somaliland, Kenya and Northern Rhodesia. It had occurred as far east as the Red Sea coast of Eritrea and as far south as Balovale in Northern Rhodesia. When Italian Somaliland and Eritrea were occupied surveys and control were undertaken at once. The incidence of yellow fever in these countries and also in Kenya and Uganda, was greatly reduced by mass vaccination. In Uganda researches incriminated new vectors of disease and proved that monkeys were its hosts. On the advice of entomologists and others in the Colonial Medical Service, elaborate arrangements were made for safe-guarding aerodromes from insect-borne infection.

VENEREAL DISEASES

Special measures were taken to meet the large increase in venereal disease. This increase was most marked at ports and affected not only the transitory population but also the indigenous inhabitants. The problem especially affected the West Indies.

NUTRITION

The effects of the war on nutrition were less serious than had been expected. The supply of rice, the staple diet of many colonial peoples, was gravely affected when Burma and other Far Eastern territories fell into enemy hands. This deficiency was made up by importing wheat. A fuller and more balanced diet introduced through military service and war conditions, if it becomes permanent, is calculated to improve the general standard of nutrition among colonial peoples.

ADDITIONAL WAR SERVICES

The Medical Departments in East Africa rendered the following additional services in the War:

1. Each medical department organised, equipped and mobilised medical units of all races, recruited from members of the department. These formed the nucleus of the East African Army Medical Corps (E.A.A.M.C.) for the East African and Burma campaigns.

2. Medical Examination of Recruits.

3. Hospital facilities for the Armed Forces.

4. Co-operation with Medical Authorities of the Forces.

5. Civil Defence.

6. Housing and health and the hygiene of camps for prisoners-of-war and interned persons.

7. Provision of camps and medical facilities for Polish and Greek refugees coming from the Middle East to East Africa.

8. Supplies of medical stores, especially drugs, comforts and dressings.

9. Training of Africans as hospital assistants, sanitary inspectors, orderlies, nurses and laboratory assistants.

10. Training by Government departments and voluntary bodies of persons of all races in first aid, home nursing and civil defence work.

In many respects these services were also freely made available to the Military Authorities in the West African Colonies.

After this review of the general war-time measures adopted by the Colonial Services, the important experience of the war in certain British Colonies will now be described.

MALTA G.C.

Professor A. V. Bernard, c.m.g., c.b.e., m.d., who was Chief Medical Officer of the Government of Malta throughout the whole period of hostilities, has recorded the impact of the war on the civil population of Malta in *C.H. & M.S.* Vol. II. pp. 16–44. He was chiefly responsible for the organisation and administration of the medical and sanitary services to enable them to cope with war casualties and the increased morbidity and mortality among the civil population due to malnutrition and disruption of the normal way of life.

Experience of protection against the effects of air raids revealed that deep underground shelters tunnelled within the soft limestone rock were the only effective shelters against high explosive shells. A number of these deep shelters were ready by the time of the intensive bombing of 1942. The sanitation of the shelters and refugee centres was effectively dealt with.

The hospitals of the island were organised into casualty hospitals and base hospitals and a scheme for establishment of Emergency Medical Services worked well. A Blood Transfusion Service was provided. Several hospitals were damaged in the air raids.

Infant mortality rose concurrently with general mortality and the maternal and infants health services were expanded to meet the situation that arose. It is noteworthy that the factor that appears to have contributed most to the high infant and child mortality was the lack of proper food. A spectacular decline in this mortality took place in 1943, when the food situation had been eased after the partial raising of the siege at the end of 1942. There had been no improvements in environmental conditions. Rationing of food began soon after the war began and as the siege continued the rations became more and more meagre. By June 1942 the position had become very precarious for the caloric value of the diet was dangerously low. By February 1943 conditions were eased; the caloric value of the diet rose and a rapid and sustained improvement in the health of the people followed.

The picture of war diseases during the siege was as follows:

TUBERCULOSIS

There was an increase both in respiratory and other forms. Rapid improvement set in after 1942 with better supplies of food.

ENTERIC FEVER

A sharp outbreak of enteric fever occurred in 1942. There was a more serious and explosive outbreak in the summer of 1943 due to the contamination by sewage of one of the main water reservoirs situated in close proximity to an aerodrome. The total incidence for the year was 1,566 cases and 202 deaths. A large percentage of the whole population had been inoculated against enteric fever by the end of 1944. The value of this measure seems reflected in the low morbidity from the disease that was noted in this and the following years.

UNDULANT FEVER

Raw goats' milk is chiefly responsible for conveying *Brucella melitensis* infection in Malta. During the siege more use was made of pasteurised milk supplied by the Government and of tinned milk and the supply of goats' milk diminished as the animals were slaughtered for food. In 1943 and 1944 the Government bought up all the milk of the surviving goats and only allowed it to be sold after pasteurisation. There was a negligible incidence of undulant fever in these years. With the relaxation of these desirable measures after 1944 and the rapid multiplication of goats that ensued the prevalence of the disease rose again. In the neighbouring island of Gozo, where pasteurised milk was not in supply, the incidence of undulant fever only fell when many goats had been killed and rose again when the goats re-multiplied. In Malta, as formerly in Great Britain, the value of pasteurisation, in spite of this striking object lesson, was not appreciated.

ACUTE ANTERIOR POLIOMYELITIS

This disease had occurred sporadically in the Maltese islands, but it was not until 1942 that it appeared in epidemic form. From the onset in November 1942 until the end of January 1943 there were 366 cases and 14 deaths in Malta and 40 cases with no deaths in Gozo. The 1–5 years age group was principally affected with a preponderance of male cases. Another, but milder outbreak of the disease occurred between November 1945 and April 1946. The virus appears to have been disseminated by contact (droplet) infection rather than by water or food.

OTHER DISEASES

In spite of conditions favourable to spread (overcrowding, blackout, bad ventilation), cerebro-spinal fever did not give much trouble. Scarlet fever, diphtheria, measles and whooping cough were not affected by war conditions. There were 2,066 cases of influenza in 1943, with only three deaths. The rat population increased enormously during the war and murine typhus appeared in 1944 and became endemic. Gassing with sulphurs and hydrocyanic acid, as well as baiting and trapping were tried, but the rats had their cover and breeding places so deep down under the heavy stones that these methods were not very successful. Rat poisons were scarce. Bubonic plague was prevalent all along the eastern and southern shores of the Mediterranean and was introduced into Malta in June 1945. The large rat population facilitated its spread. The outbreak ceased in June 1946. There were 80 cases with 22 deaths. Scabies was prevalent. Of the deficiency diseases pellagra took the greatest toll of life.

CONCLUSION

The peaceful people of Malta were suddenly confronted with ferocious bombardments and unforeseen dangers and ordeals, and faced them calmly and courageously. Their hardest time was from 1940 to 1942. In 1942, in trying to succour Malta, the British lost three cruisers, nine destroyers and two aircraft carriers, as well as merchant ships. El Alamein, followed by the victorious advance and the Anglo-American landings in North Africa changed the situation. By the end of 1942 the Navy had replenished Malta's stocks of foods and stores and the worst of her ordeal was over. The gallant defence of Malta and the admirable organisation for the prevention and treatment of disease, the hospital organisation and rationing of food make this siege of an island a classic example of the courage and adaptability of human beings. It is indeed an epic story and H.M. King George VI marked its fame by awarding the George Cross to Malta on April 16, 1942 when the inhabitants were at the height of their ordeal.

(*Note*. For a full account of the medical lessons revealed in the siege of Malta see *Civilian Health and Medical Services*. Vol. II. Chap. 2. See also *Royal Naval Medical Services*. Vol. I—Administration, pp. 397–398. Vol. II—Operations, pp. 390–391; *Army Medical Services, Campaigns*. Vol. I. pp. 613–632; *R.A.F. Medical Services*. Vol. III. *Campaigns*. pp. 251–288.)

HONG KONG

Sir Selwyn Selwyn-Clarke, formerly Director of Medical Services, Hong Kong has recorded the tragic story of the occupation of Hong Kong by the Japanese. The deaths from war injuries during the actual period of hostilities in December 1941 were appreciable (1,400 Service personnel and over 2,000 civilians), but in the period of occupation from January 1942 to August 1945 the deaths from violence and starvation, particularly in 1942, rose to appalling heights. The invading forces announced that they intended to reduce the population from one and a half millions to about half a million. They achieved their aim through repatriation (mostly forced), wholesale shootings and starvation. Many dwellings were destroyed by bomb, shell and fire during hostilities in 1941 and many valuable educational institutions, including the University of Hong Kong, were irreparably damaged by looters. The sanitary services, including water purification plants, suffered marked deterioration during the occupation. The community was deprived of most of its medical and health services; its chief hospitals were taken for Japanese troops, its maternal, child welfare and social clinics closed, and vital preventive work against malaria neglected.

As in the United Kingdom the estimate of potential casualties from enemy air action was grossly exaggerated, and similarly the Medical Defence Committee worked on the basis of arranging as many beds for casualties as buildings, staff and equipment permitted. The provision of beds proved adequate, but delay occurred at times in bearing seriously wounded to first-aid posts or mobile first-aid units and to the casualty clearing hospitals, owing to lack of sufficient reliable St. John Ambulance stretcher bearers. Otherwise, the civil defence medical services worked well.

A plan was devised for dispersal of the population to camps in the surrounding hills. Many of the Chinese proved unwilling to join the dispersal and a number of the camps were never occupied.

It had never been contemplated that Hong Kong would be compelled to surrender unconditionally after eighteen days' fighting and no general principles had been laid down for the guidance of Government officers or heads of the essential services should the enemy prevail. Clear directives might have been given to heads of departments and of essential services before the outbreak of hostilities to meet this contingency.

The Director of Medical Services succeeded in maintaining a staff in the hospitals to prevent them from being looted and destroyed, to serve the general community and to prevent the health conditions in the town from deteriorating and bringing in their train epidemics of cholera etc. He was also enabled to assist the prisoner-of-war and civilian camps with food, drugs, instruments and other essentials until arrested and imprisoned by the Japanese sixteen months later, charged with espionage and later sentenced to death. From this fate he was rescued by the end of hostilities.

Most of the members of the medical and ancillary services in Hong Kong were ill-fed, ill-housed and ill-clothed, subjected to frequent humiliations and sometimes to ill-treatment, imprisonment and even death. Yet is is a source of justifiable pride that they maintained the high tradition of the profession under conditions of exceptional stress.

(For a full account see *Civilian Health and Medical Services.* Vol. II. pp. 45-76; *Royal Naval Medical Services.* Vol. II. pp. 256-282; *Army Medical Services, Campaigns.* Vol. II. pp. 1-40.)

MALAYA

R. B. MacGregor, C.M.G., M.R.C.P., M.B., formerly Director of Medical Services, Federation of Malaya, has given an account of conditions in the Malay Peninsula and the island of Singapore from 1939 until the surrender of the Japanese in August 1945. It is written from the civilian point of view, although during the campaign military and civilian medical services were often working together in the same hospitals and first-aid posts.

PREPARATIONS FOR WAR

The Hospital Services were well developed. Excluding mental hospitals and special institutions for lepers, Government Hospitals on the Peninsula contained over 10,000 beds. In Singapore there was the General Hospital with 850 beds, a maternity hospital of 200 beds and a pauper hospital with 800 beds. Additional equipment and beds were supplied for all the larger hospitals. The increase in capacity was about 50 per cent. Throughout the Peninsula arrangements were made for the transfer of convalescent and chronic patients from Government hospitals to estate hospitals, thus permitting the clearance of accommodation for casualties. Subsidiary hospitals were improvised in the larger towns in any suitable buildings, usually schools. Five such hospitals were set up in Singapore with a total of 1,000 beds. The protection of buildings against blast and the provision of air-raid shelters were carried out on a very limited scale. Throughout most of Singapore there were no substantial air-raid shelters; this, undoubtedly, increased the number of casualties. Other preparations included accumulation of medical stores, training of medical personnel, the provision of first-aid posts and an ambulance transport service. A Blood Transfusion Service was organised in the College of Medicine, Singapore. It began early in 1939 to provide a store of blood or plasma for war casualties, and by the time of the outbreak of war in Malaya had recruited 4,000 donors. In each case the donor's blood-group was determined together with tests for haemoglobin and Kahn reaction and a physical examination. This service maintained a supply of blood and plasma to the Army and the civilian hospitals up to the last day of the attack on Singapore.

Dispersal camps were provided but as in Hong Kong they were little used. There was no allowance made in these preparations for the country being invaded and overrun. In practice the provision was determined by using to the full such personnel and accommodation as could be made available, rather than by calculation of what the expected need might be.

THE CAMPAIGN

The Japanese attack on Malaya began on December 8, 1941. It was marked by the bombardment and landing on the coast of Kelantan, in the northern extremity of the Peninsula, and the first air raid on Singapore. The progress of the campaign down the Peninsula was a melancholy story of retreat. Hospitals in turn changed from being civilian hospitals to Army clearing stations, field ambulance stations, regimental aid posts, and, as the retreat continued, they passed into the hands of the enemy. Most of the civilian patients needing treatment were evacuated along with the military patients to the next hospital down the line.

In Singapore after the first raid on December 8, there was a period when air attacks were infrequent and slight. The hospitals and aid posts were fully mobilised, and all the arrangements for dealing with casualties worked well. By the beginning of January, raids increased in number and severity and Singapore was in a state of siege. As a result of the Japanese occupation of the Peninsula medical officers and nursing staff from places further north were driven back into Singapore. In February raids became more frequent, the Singapore docks being one of the most heavily bombed areas. On February 9, the Japanese landed on the north side of Singapore. On February 13, instructions were given that women doctors and nursing staff should leave Singapore. About half volunteered to remain. In spite of siege conditions foodstuffs were plentiful in the General Hospital. There was a shortage of water in the last days. Singapore surrendered on February 15.

The recorded number of civilians in Singapore who were killed or died of wounds was about 3,500. During the last week accurate records could not be kept. Another 3,500 probably were killed or died of wounds in the last week of the siege. The total number of wounded admitted to the hospitals was probably 25,000; those treated in the first-aid posts must have numbered over 40,000. On the mainland, casualties were less severe and it is estimated that for the Malay Peninsula and Penang Island the total of civilian deaths during the Japanese invasion were between three and four thousand.

CONDITIONS DURING THE JAPANESE OCCUPATION

Most of the hospitals and the rudiments of a public health service were maintained under Japanese direction. The Japanese gave scant help with supplies or personnel, but they did pay the staff, provided a limited amount of food for patients, and interfered little, except in the larger towns.

EPIDEMICS

After the surrender there was a severe epidemic of bacillary dysentery which lasted for about two months. An extensive campaign of inoculation against cholera and typhoid was carried out. As a result, there was no typhoid or cholera, except a few local cases traced to infection from a ship.

Malaria appeared in 1942 and 1943 in parts of Singapore which had been free from it for many years. On the mainland, malaria assumed epidemic form in 1943. This was due to the breakdown of malaria control in 1942 and social dissolution and chaos from semi-starvation. The Central Mental Hospital for the Malay States had 3,500 patients when the Japanese took control. There were over 1,000 further admissions, by transfer from Sumatra. When the British returned less than 500 patients remained. Nearly 4,000 had died from dysentery and beriberi.

CONCLUSION

The period of Japanese occupation showed that neglect of sanitation and inefficient administration could cause public health to deteriorate rapidly. There was a breakdown of the unobtrusive but constant precautions which are normally taken to preserve a healthy environment. The selfless devotion of medical officers, nurses and health personnel in the internment camps produced a different picture. Under bad environmental conditions, the application of knowledge, skill and hard work kept the rate of survival higher than would have seemed possible. Mental health and morale were maintained; surgery was carried out; dysentery, tropical typhus and malaria were treated; dental care was provided and much ingenuity was shown in making or improvising medicines and surgical instruments from local materials. When there was opportunity to grow accessory food-stuffs, it was possible to provide a substitute for almost everything except the essential energy value of food.

(For a full account see *Civilian Health and Medical Services*. Vol. II. pp. 77–111; *Royal Naval Medical Services*. Vol. I. pp. 407–409; Vol. II. pp. 173–175. *Army Medical Services, Campaigns*. Vol. II. pp. 41–178.)

NORTH BORNEO

The Japanese occupation of North Borneo, which began on January 8, 1942 met with no resistance. There was no loss of life and little damage to property. Medical officers were allowed to continue at work. A retired Japanese doctor with the rank of Colonel took charge of Sandakan Hospital and the Principal Medical Officer's Office, but interfered little with clinical work. Later the efficiency of the hospital service was impaired by the removal and looting of drugs, stores and equipment by Japanese troops. All credit must be given to the medical, nursing and hospital staffs for their work under great difficulties. As regards the population the usual inefficiency and neglect of public health ensued after the enemy occupation. Malnutrition, beriberi, malaria and, later, hunger oedema were widespread. Indolent ulcers of the legs refused to heal; ankylostomiasis and other worm infestations increased. Mental patients and lepers were turned adrift. The lepers were trans-shipped from their settlement to Boaan Peninsula, where many died or became increasingly diseased in the absence of proper care.

When relief came in 1945, medical supplies and food quickly improved those who had suffered from prolonged semi-starvation. Cases of chronic malaria, ankylostomiasis, other helminthiases and chronic dysentery recovered much more slowly. (See *C.H. & M.S.* Vol. II. pp. 111–114.)

BRITISH SOMALILAND

The occupation of British Somaliland by the Italians lasted from August 21, 1940 to March 14, 1941. The occupation was entirely military and such hospitals as were set up in the country were military.

When the British troops returned in 1941, it was found that there was practically no hospital equipment. Everything had either been removed by the Italians or looted by Somalis. Hospitals were re-equipped from Army sources, and, as soon as possible, Army medical officers took charge of the hospitals for both civilian and military patients, as civilian medical officers had left the country. Later, the civil and military organisations were separated. The Civil Medical Department was staffed by Somali dressers, a few Indian assistant surgeons and by military medical officers, assigned whole time to civilian duties. By August 1945 considerable progress had been made in rebuilding the medical service.

EFFECTS OF THE WAR ON PUBLIC HEALTH

Under-nourishment and tuberculosis increased among the Somalis, especially the town-dwellers. There was a marked drift of recruits and labourers to the towns through the attraction of high wages offered by the Army. In the towns there was gross overcrowding. There was a serious famine in 1943, primarily due to a failure of the rains but aggravated by cessation of the importation of foodstuffs. Another feature of the war was a marked increase in prostitution and venereal disease. (See *C.H. & M.S.* pp. 115–199 and *Army Medical Services, Campaigns.* Vol. I. pp. 408, 413, 446.)

PALESTINE

Colonel Sir George W. Heron, formerly Director of Medical Services, Palestine, has recorded the medical history of Palestine during the War in *C.H. & M.S.* Vol. II. pp. 120–124.

CONDITIONS AT THE OUTBREAK OF WAR

The country lived largely on imported products. About half its grain, much of its dairy produce, eggs, poultry, potatoes and nearly all of its textiles, wood, metal and manufactured articles were all imported. Neighbouring countries prohibited exports, so staple food supplies were imported under Government auspices.

The state of health of the civil population was satisfactory.

There was an organised health service; precautionary measures against epidemic disease had long been established and general sanitation in the chief towns, though not ideal, was under constant control. Public establishments and trades and industries dealing with food were supervised. Water supplies, except in villages, were safe, and the dangers of typhoid and dysentery had been reduced to a minimum in municipal areas.

NUTRITION AND PREVENTION OF DISEASE DURING THE WAR

NUTRITION

By the stimulation of local production of food, by loans to farmers and other forms of assistance, the productivity of the country was materially increased and helped to reduce the call on shipping to supply civilian needs. Rationing control, subsidies and increased production maintained the nutrition of the country satisfactorily.

PREVENTION OF DISEASE

Every effort was made to avoid any deterioration of health of the civil population. This was also important from the military aspects to safeguard the troops from civilian infection. Large numbers of susceptible troops arrived in Palestine from the United Kingdom, from Australia and New Zealand and some from America.

Malaria

By close co-operation between the Department of Health and the Military and Air Force Authorities, the incidence of malaria was slight, and, where it occurred, could be ascribed to the overruling or neglect by the combatant officers of the advice given to them by the medical authorities. The successful co-operation of Army and civil health authorities was also evident in other fields of preventive medicine.

Smallpox

Most of the population had been vaccinated. An occasional case or limited outbreak of smallpox occurred, introduced on one occasion by returning Mecca pilgrims and on another by travellers from Syria where a considerable epidemic raged. Beyond the initial infection there was no spread.

Typhus

There was an outbreak of typhus among imported Egyptian labourers at Sarafad. This was speedily brought under control by the health authorities.

Plague

In Jaffa and Haifa there were small outbreaks of bubonic plague. These were speedily controlled. In the port of Haifa a number of supply ships were effectively 'de-ratted' by the Government 'Clayton' installation.

Venereal disease

There was a rise in cases of venereal disease. The only measures permitted to the civil authorities were the setting-up of free treatment centres, while the police were empowered to close brothels. The Army had to adopt special measures to deal with this menace to the health of the troops.

THE CENTRAL LABORATORIES

For the first two years of the war, when the R.A.M.C. had not yet established all their services in Palestine, the central laboratories of the Department of Health conducted for them much of the bacteriological work and chemical analyses of different kinds. Rabies was prevalent in parts of Palestine and soldiers who were bitten by dogs received treatment with anti-rabic vaccine prepared in the laboratories. This vaccine was selected by the War Office for supply to the British Forces for the invasion of France. Vaccine lymph prepared in the Department's Vaccine Institute was supplied to the Army for local use, and also for the Army of the Middle East.

CONCLUSION

The work of the Department of Health in Palestine provides a striking example of how a country exposed to the constant menace of tropical disease can be safeguarded in war-time.

In many campaigns epidemic disease and consequent wastage of man-power has been the deciding factor. In war it is as important to protect the health of the civil population as that of the troops.

CYPRUS

The Director of Medical and Health Services of Cyprus reported that the war had little significant effect on the general health of the population of the island and there were no major outbreaks of epidemic and infectious disease, except one of measles in 1942 and another of whooping cough in 1943.

REFUGEES

During the period 1941–44 the care of refugees from the Greek islands showed what could be done to meet an unexpected emergency in war-time. The Medical Department undertook the care of these people, who travelled in small fishing-boats and caiques and arrived in a dirty and verminous condition, suffering from exhaustion and exposure. They received delousing, cleansing, food, clothing and shelter and were immunised against smallpox and typhoid fever. In 1944 an U.N.R.A.A. representative took administrative control of the refugees, but their medical care remained the task of the department. Owing to the emergency measures adopted not a single case of dangerous infectious disease occurred among the 15,000 refugees. (See *C.H. & M.S.* Vol. II. pp. 124–6.)

GIBRALTAR

PREPARATIONS FOR WAR

During the year 1939 the usual medical activities continued in Gibraltar, but air-raid precautions and measures to cope with the medical needs of war progressively absorbed much of the time and attention of the medical and nursing staffs. The Colonial Hospital (the chief civil hospital) was expanded to accommodate 700 patients and the new hospital for tuberculosis, known as the King George V Chest Hospital, was completed.

CONDITIONS DURING THE WAR

In May 1940 it was decided to evacuate the women and children and sick, aged and redundant males to England. Some 16,000 persons were evacuated in 1940 and 700 in subsequent years. In June 1940 all mental patients were evacuated. (See *C.H. & M.S.* Vol. II. pp. 126–9.)

The civil hospitals were soon busy with air-raid casualties, the reception of refugees from France and the care of torpedoed and injured merchant seamen. The Isolation Hospital was taken over by the Military Authorities. On September 24 and 25 there were two big air raids, but with light casualties. Substantial damage was done to the new King George V Hospital. In October 1940 the Colonial Hospital also became available for the admission of military cases, and R.A.M.C. personnel were provided to overcome the staff shortage. Through goodwill and co-operation this arrangement between the civilian and medical authorities worked well. In November 1940, the King George V Hospital and the Mental Hospital were taken over by the Army. When cases of tuberculosis increased, a ward had to be set aside at the Colonial Hospital for treatment of the disease.

The health of the population remained good. In 1943 there was an outbreak of mild dysentery and a small epidemic of influenza; two cases of smallpox occurred, with one death. In 1944 the repatriation of the women, children and old people, who had been evacuated in 1940, began; a total of 9,158 returned during the year.

COMMENTARY

Gibraltar supplies another instance of how precautionary measures and good public health administration maintained a satisfactory state of health in civilians and troops throughout the war. (See also *Royal Naval Medical Services*. Vol. I. pp. 398–399.)

CEYLON

Before the war it was not expected that Ceylon would be involved in any future world war, except indirectly, and there was provision for only rudimentary schemes of 'passive Air Defence'. The entry of Japan into the war in December 1941 led to the completion of arrangements for fuller hospital organisation, provision of casualty clearing hospitals and base hospitals and efficient provision of medical services in an emergency. On April 5, 1942 Colombo sustained for some fifty minutes an air raid by the Japanese. They attacked the Ratmalana Aerodrome, railway workshops and the Colombo Harbour area in three waves consisting of some 80 planes and were repulsed with the loss of 24 planes brought down and 20 or more damaged. In this raid 84 persons were killed or died of wounds and 77 were injured. The Colombo A.R.P. and Hospital Air Raid Casualty Services functioned efficiently. On April 8, 1942 an air attack on Trincomalee and China Bay areas developed. Bombers, escorted by fighters came in three waves. Some 36 civilians were killed and 96 injured.

The accepted principles for the resuscitation of air-raid casualties were followed, and the value of a blood bank was confirmed. Operations were carried out under general anaesthesia, and mainly consisted of complete excision of damaged tissues (débridement), cleansing of wounds, manipulation of bones, reduction of fractures and fixation and suitable splints. Skeletal traction was applied when necessary. Five amputations were performed. All casualties who had serious injuries received sulphonamide treatment, either orally or by intra-muscular injections. The mortality from abdominal wounds was very low.

CONCLUSION

Ceylon had to organise and extend its rudimentary provision for air-raid casualties after Japan had entered the war in December 1941. It sustained two severe air attacks in April 1942. The measures taken proved their efficiency and, it is considered, would have been equally effective if heavier demands had been made upon them. The public health of the population of the Island was well maintained. (See *Civilian Health and Medical Services*. Vol. II. pp. 129–136; *Royal Naval Medical Services*. Vol. I. pp. 410–426; Vol. II. pp. 400–410; *R.A.F. Medical Services*. Vol. III. Chap. 11.)

COMMENTARY

The review of the general measures adopted by the Colonial Services during the war shows how the public health services were maintained as far as possible with a depleted staff. It also indicates that the civil authorities rendered all possible assistance to the Fighting Services— Navy, Army and Air Force—that they controlled malaria and were able to institute schemes of research into malaria, yellow fever and other diseases. With no similar experience to guide them they met the medical emergencies of totalitarian war as they arose with a remarkable degree of success.

The British Possessions which bore the brunt of war have been described. In the epic siege of Malta the medical services of the Island, assailed and faced with the perils of war, performed their duties nobly and efficiently. In addition to the casualties of the siege there was an epidemic of poliomyelitis. In Hong Kong and Malaya the outcome of the war was tragic and embittered by the rigours of enemy occupation. These narratives teach many medical lessons gained in circumstances of unprecedented difficulty, and reveal how the spirit of man may overcome and assuage the horrors of totalitarian warfare.

Medical Research

By Sir Arthur S. MacNalty, K.C.B., M.A., M.D., F.R.C.P., F.R.C.S.

(95349)

CONTENTS

MEDICAL RESEARCH

The Medical Research Council (then the Medical Research Committee) played an important part in the alleviation of suffering and the application of new methods to the diagnosis and treatment of disease in the First World War. This tradition was ably maintained in the Second World War.

During the war the work of the Council was orientated in new directions to serve the national effort and as a result it was also greatly expanded in volume. First, the attention of the Council's research workers was mainly directed to war problems. Secondly, the Council were called upon more than ever before to give scientific advice and assistance to administrative Government Departments and also to the Defence Services. (See *Third Report from the Select Committee on Estimates, Session* 1946–47. *Expenditure on Research and Development.* H.M.S.O. 1947. (Appendix 3, Annex B.).) Thirdly, the Council undertook the organisation and direction of certain emergency services of a technical nature.

As Sir Edward Mellanby wrote in the Report of the Medical Research Council for the years 1939–45, *Medical Research in War* (p. 14): 'The response of medical science to the challenge of war has three main objectives. First, it must be directed to maintaining the health of the armed forces and of the civilian population, particularly in the prevention of infective diseases and of malnutrition. Second, it must study methods for rapidly restoring the wounded and sick to full health. Third, an object which became very prominent in the late war, it must find the conditions required for the highest possible efficiency, safety and comfort of fighting personnel and of industrial workers in all the circumstances and tasks of war. Obviously, these aims of application must also be those towards which new research under war conditions is directed.'

CONTROL OF INFECTIOUS DISEASES

Outbreaks of infectious disease have always been a special menace in war, and until the present century have often been a decisive factor. Existing knowledge had helped to reduce the peril, and it was determined to apply and extend this knowledge for the control of diseases such as malaria, typhus, typhoid, dysentery, smallpox and yellow fever. These were all infections to which our troops might be exposed in theatres of war overseas. Nor was the Home Front neglected. The full co-ordination between the Medical Research Council and the Ministry of Health facilitated the setting up of the Emergency Public Health Laboratory

Service in England and Wales and the Council's Committees on Tuberculosis in War-time and on Jaundice (infective hepatitis and serum jaundice).

In some cases it was not known how effective methods discovered by medical research would prove in practice. One example was the value of active immunisation by toxoid injections against tetanus—that type of wound infection so fatal to soldiers in the War of 1914–18. The astonishingly low incidence of the disease among troops of the Allied Armies, immunised with toxoid, bore witness to the efficacy of the method.

Most diseases proved controllable in an impressive degree. In some cases control was obtained only after new investigations had been made, as in the case of preventive inoculation by a vaccine against louse-borne typhus fever which reduced the severity of the disease and by delousing with D.D.T., methods which brought the serious epidemic in Naples in 1943–44 to a rapid close. (See *Medical Research*. pp. 164–169.)

War may bring in its train new diseases or help to make some diseases, rare in peace-time, assume epidemic proportions, like the 'sweating sickness' or 'Picardy Sweat' of the sixteenth century; and trench fever, trench nephritis and *encephalitis lethargica* of the First World War; the great pandemic of influenza of 1918–19; and the cerebro-spinal fever outbreaks of both World Wars. Sometimes a disease, epidemic in war-time, is met where no satisfactory control or remedy can be obtained. Such a disease was infective hepatitis which became a serious problem before the Second World War ended. Knowledge of its causation and prevention is still incomplete but much new information was gathered concerning it. (See *Medical Research*. pp. 150–155.)

The greatest practical advance in control of endemic disease during the war was made in respect of malaria, numerically still the most important disease in the world. The infection was kept in check among the Allied troops, even in hyperendemic areas, such as Burma and Assam, where it might have been expected that the disease rather than force of arms would have been decisive. The optimum dosage of the drug 'Atebrin', introduced by the Germans in 1929, was ascertained and its method of administration improved. Since 1940 it has been made in Britain under the non-proprietary name of mepacrine. Another pre-war German drug 'Plasmochin' was made as pamaquin. These effective substitutes for quinine, especially mepacrine, controlled malaria in the Allied Forces. In addition, there were two outstanding developments in malaria prophylaxis and treatment. The first of these was the application of D.D.T., and of new insect repellents in dealing with the mosquito vectors of malaria. The second was the preparation of a series of biguanide compounds as anti-malarial agents of completely new type. One of these compounds, 'Paludrine' (or Proguanil) proved a most efficient anti-malarial drug, since it is both a true causal prophylactic in malignant tertian malaria and a partial prophylactic in benign tertian. It was not available for field trial until nearly the end of hostilities. (See *Medical Research*. pp. 155–164.)

Mite-borne scrub typhus was encountered in the Pacific area and South-East Asia. (See *Medical Research*. pp. 168, 169.) A protective vaccine was prepared, but the end of the war prevented its large-scale trial. The new antibiotics which have done so much to control rickettsial infections were not available until after the war.

NUTRITION

The impact of modern scientific knowledge on the feeding of Service men and women throughout the war was of great importance, and never before had troops been so well fed. They were given the first claim on supplies. From the point of view of the civil population in the United Kingdom, blockade conditions were at least as bad in the Second World War as in 1914–18, but knowledge and organisation to deal with the situation were much more advanced. On the outbreak of war tests were made on a group of volunteers of experimental diets made up of the limited number of foodstuffs which might be available under conditions of close blockade. The Government were thus informed in advance of the types and quantities of available foodstuffs which were compatible with health in young adults. Rationing did not come into force until January 1, 1940, and it was reassuring to be able to make rationing and dietary plans on the basis of the knowledge gained in this experiment. One of the most important failings of our dietary since the industrial revolution had been its deficiency in calcifying qualities. This caused widespread bone disease, especially in children, as well as much subnormal health and growth. To remedy deficiencies in diet the Medical Research Council advocated the provision of additional milk, cod-liver oil and other sources of fat-soluble vitamins to pregnant and nursing mothers, infants and children. They also recommended the addition of vitamins A and D to margarine and of calcium to bread. Following the discovery, made immediately before the war, that phytic acid has a powerful anti-calcifying influence, and that the raising of the extraction rate of flour from 72 per cent. to 85 per cent. greatly increased the phytic acid intake in the diet, calcium carbonate was added to flour. In this way the calcium intake by growing children and by adults was brought up to a level compatible with a higher standard of health. These changes in the nature of the dietary, together with the more equitable distribution of foods throughout the population probably contributed to the continued fall in the maternal and infant mortality-rates and the stillbirth-rate.

The Medical Research Council also advised the Ministry of Food on matters where changes in, or additions to, the normal rations had to be made in individual cases on account of ill-health or for other special reasons. For this purpose the Food Rationing (Special Diets) Advisory Committee was appointed at the request of the Ministry of Food, Ministry of Health, and Department of Health for Scotland. Its studies produced much information of practical importance in medicine. (See *Medical Research*. Chap. 5.)

RESTORATION OF THE WOUNDED AND SICK

The outstanding advances in this field were the development of the blood transfusion services so that resuscitation of the injured with blood or blood products was possible even in the battle zone (see *Medical Research*. pp. 97–100), the use of sulphonamide drugs and later penicillin to prevent or treat wound infection, and widespread recognition of the desirability of dressing wounds or burns as infrequently as possible, and then only with precautions to prevent extraneous infection. The establishment of mobile surgical units near the front line was of great value in facilitating early operative treatment of battle wounds; skin grafting promoted rapid healing in certain cases, especially of extensive burns; and there were numerous technical advances, particularly in plastic surgery and methods of anaesthesia. Additional factors in the improved recovery of the wounded and sick, as compared with previous wars, were the more extensive and enlightened facilities provided for physiological and psychological rehabilitation.

THE SULPHONAMIDE DRUGS

After the first sulphonamide drug was introduced in Germany as a chemotherapeutic agent in 1935, and its life-saving value in the treatment of puerperal fever was conclusively demonstrated in 1936 by Colebrook and his colleagues in this country, much research work was done on the development and therapeutic possibilities of different sulphonamides in Great Britain and elsewhere. During the war the value of these drugs in the treatment of various infective diseases, particularly bacillary dysentery, and cerebro-spinal fever was more accurately defined; they were also used for the first time in the prevention and treatment of infection in battle wounds and in burns. Many new members of the group were introduced and studied, the war providing opportunities for large scale field-trials which accelerated the assessment of their value and place in therapy.

PENICILLIN

In 1928 Sir Alexander Fleming discovered penicillin. In the wards of St. Mary's Hospital he tried the external application of the filtrate on human wounds. The results seemed encouraging, but the active principle appeared to be too unstable then to be capable of isolation. In 1938 Sir Howard Florey, Dr. Ernest Chain and their collaborators at Oxford began work on penicillin, and in 1939 they succeeded in concentrating it as a stable dry powder. They then made an intensive study of the chemical, biological and clinical properties of this preparation. They showed that it had a powerful chemotherapeutic action against certain microbes, notably the gram-positive cocci and the gonococcus, and that unlike the sulphonamides it is fully active in the presence of body fluids. The sulphonamide drugs had already shown their value in the treatment of diseases such as puerperal fever, pneumonia and cerebro-spinal meningitis. Penicillin was found to be even more efficacious in the treatment of the first two diseases as well as of wounds and burns, of septic meningitis and staphylococcal septicaemia; it also could cure infections such as bacterial heart disease which formerly were invariably fatal. The urgent demands of war led to a quicker exploitation of the clinical possibilities of penicillin than would have been likely under normal conditions. Large-scale production was at first carried out chiefly in America. This was a valuable piece of inter-Allied collaboration since it brought penicillin into widespread field use at a crucial period of the war and must have resulted in the saving of thousands of lives. Of special importance under war conditions was its remarkably rapid effect in curing gonorrhoea and in shortening the treatment of syphilis. Indiscriminate use of penicillin has to be guarded against, especially its use for minor injuries. As with the sulphonamides certain patients treated in this way develop resistance to the drug so that it loses its efficacy; moreover, occasional patients show adverse reactions through becoming sensitised to penicillin.

The discovery of penicillin introduced a new epoch in the treatment of disease. It has been followed by the discovery of other 'antibiotics', and a whole range of diseases due to bacterial infections has now been controlled by substances produced chiefly by moulds, among which penicillin still keeps the chief place. Of these powerful drugs may be mentioned streptomycin which has some success against the tubercle bacillus, chloromycetin, aureomycin, etc. Diseases formerly deadly yield to these new drugs, epidemics of infectious disease are checked, and operations are performed successfully on the lungs, heart and internal organs which no surgeon would formerly have dared to undertake for fear of septic complications. With antibiotics the risk of these complications is largely reduced. But they have to be used with caution for in inexperienced hands they may prove a two-edged weapon and while averting one possible complication may pave the way for another.

The development of penicillin as a therapeutic agent was the greatest practical achievement of medical research in Great Britain during the war.

THE CONTROL OF CROSS-INFECTION IN HOSPITALS

In the War of 1914–18 attention was first drawn to the importance of hospital cross-infection of wounds, particularly by haemolytic streptococci. In the inter-war years and during the Second World War research was made into methods of preventing the principal forms of hospital cross-infection by the use of infrequent, occlusive dressings for wounds and burns, and by adopting new methods of air purification and routines of disinfection for surgical dressing-rooms, operating theatres and wards of different types. (See *Medical Research*. pp. 235–236 and *Medicine & Pathology*. pp. 485–496.)

BLOOD TRANSFUSION AND TRAUMATIC SHOCK

In addition to promoting much work on blood transfusion (see *Medical Research*. pp. 97–110) the Medical Research Council supported a wide range of other researches on those physiological reactions of the body to severe injury which are generally grouped under the name of 'traumatic shock'. These researches, while they did not completely solve the problem of 'shock', led to results of interest and promise. (See *Medical Research*. pp. 86–94.)

PERSONNEL RESEARCH

On the outbreak of war intimation was sent to the Royal Navy, Army and Royal Air Force that all the resources of the Medical Research Council were at the disposal of the Services. The R.A.F. was already associated with the Medical Research Council through its Flying Personnel Research Committee, set up in 1939. This Committee was concerned with investigation of all personal and environmental factors for improving the efficiency and safety of the flying man. In 1940 the Army Council sought the help of the Medical Research Council concerning the protection of soldiers in combat, including the design of steel helmets and the possible value of body armour. The Council were asked to set up a Military Personnel Research Committee which did active and effective work for two years. At the request of the Board of Admiralty the Council also set up the Royal Naval Personnel Research Committee.

The research done by these Committees was concerned primarily with the individual combatant and the improvement of conditions, environmental or instrumental, to make him more efficient in his task and to give him greater safety and comfort. The researches covered such diverse questions as the physiological problems of high altitude flying and deep-sea diving; design of improved clothing for aviators, for men serving in the arctic and in the tropics, and for divers in tropical seas; the habitability of warships for tropical service, and the training and acclimatisation of their crews; the peculiar hazards of service in submarines, including those of oxygen poisoning and escape from submerged vessels; and the design of aircraft, guns and armoured fighting vehicles in relation to human capabilities and needs. The Committees also dealt with research problems of personnel selection for special forms of service, with physiological and psychological factors bearing on the optimal design of instrument panels and engine controls, and with numerous more strictly medical matters such as the choice of drugs for the prevention of sea and air sickness.

It was thus realised that in the design and development of instruments, weapons and machinery which have to be controlled and worked by human beings, the main limiting factor in the efficiency of the machine or weapon is usually the human factor. The need to take human physiology and psychology into consideration applies not only to machine design, but to all matters where human effort is needed, whether in the military or in the civil field.

INDUSTRIAL RESEARCH

The Industrial Health Research Board of the Medical Research Council continued its important studies during the war years. The Board (then the Industrial Fatigue Research Board) was established in the War of 1914–18 and by the outbreak of the Second World War had collected much information on industrial health and efficiency. Much was known about the effect of hours of work and of environmental factors such as lighting, heating and ventilation, noise and, in certain industries, dust and toxic products, upon health and output. The working conditions of the operative were studied; for instance, the optimum height of the working bench, the optimum loads to be carried, the adaptation of machines in relation to the economical expenditure of human energy, and the most efficient timing and nature of movements to be performed. Vocational selection and accident proneness were also investigated. Long hours and excessively strenuous working conditions were unfortunately introduced in factories in 1940. These proved incompatible with a large sustained output and a good standard of health among the workpeople and defeated their very object. If employers, industrial leaders and workmen had appreciated the knowledge gained in the First World War by the Industrial Health Research Board and its predecessor, the Health of Munition Workers Committee, this unfortunate mistake might have been avoided.

SCIENTIFIC LIAISON OVERSEAS

During the war arrangements were made for the exchange of scientific information between scientific workers in the United Kingdom and those in other parts of the British Commonwealth and in Allied Countries. Information regarding much of the new work published in Allied and

MEDICAL SERVICES IN WAR

also in enemy countries during the war years was made available through the publication of the *Bulletin of War Medicine*, which the Medical Research Council issued from 1940 to 1946 with the co-operation of the Bureau of Hygiene and Tropical Diseases. A system was also developed for the exchange and, where desirable, the distribution of unpublished documents. This was supplemented by personal contact. On the one hand, liaison officers from the Dominions and from the United States of America stationed in London kept in close touch with the Council and appropriate research centres; they also attended many meetings of scientific committees. On the other, the Medical Research Council were indebted to the British Commonwealth Scientific Office in Washington for much action taken on their behalf in the United States and in Canada. Visits were exchanged between representatives of the Council and research workers overseas, and visits of British and American scientists were made to inform the scientists of the U.S.S.R. of advances made, for instance, penicillin, and to bring back information given to them by Russian scientists. This helpful exchange of information led to closer official touch being maintained by the Medical Research Council with the Commonwealth, the United States and other countries after the war. A jointly appointed Colonial Medical Research Committee advised both the Council and the Colonial Office after 1945 and in that year an Indian Medical Research Committee was appointed by the joint action of the Council and of the Government of India.

CHEMICAL DEFENCE RESEARCH

Medical research on chemical warfare problems was carried out under the supervision of the Chemical Board of the Ministry of Supply with the aid of various sub-committees. Chemical warfare was not used by the enemy, but the various forms of possible attack were studied as far as possible in case it might be initiated by them. Accordingly, intensive research was organised at the Ministry of Supply Experimental Station and at universities on the modes of action of mustard gas and similar vesicants, of phosgene and of cyanogen compounds, on the treatment of mustard gas burns and of phosgene poisoning, and on protective measures such as respirators, anti-gas ointments and protective clothing.

Three important practical advances in this field were:

(1) The development by Peters and his colleagues at Oxford of 2:3 dimercaptopropanol ('B.A.L.' or 'British Anti-Lewisite') as an antidote to lewisite gas. B.A.L. combines with arsenic and a number of heavy metals and has interesting applications, for example, in the treatment of arsenical and mercurial poisoning.

(2) The development by Ing at Oxford of the synthetic mydriatic,

dimethylaminoethylbenzilate ethochloride as a substitute for atropine in the treatment of mustard gas eye injuries.

(3) The use by Wormall and others of radio-active sulphur to study the distribution of mustard gas in the tissues was one of the earlier examples of that effective application of artificial radio-isotope techniques to biological problems, which since the war has shown far reaching developments.

MEDICAL APPLICATIONS OF NUCLEAR PHYSICS

When the atomic bomb was used in 1945 to end the war against Japan, its effects and its pathological sequelae wrote a new and terrible chapter in War History (see *Surgery*. pp. 737–743). Fortunately this increased knowledge of nuclear physics has not been wholly destructive. It has created new possibilities in the application of physical methods to the treatment of disease and to the study of medical and other biological problems. Research in this field became one of the Medical Research Council's most important preoccupations in the immediate post-war period and can be grouped as follows:

1. The further study of radiations in cancer and other diseases.

2. Determination of the toxic and lethal effects of radio-active substances and the devising of methods to protect the body against these effects.

3. The use of radio-active or stable isotopes of various chemical elements as 'tracers'. This is of great value in the elucidation of biological function, and provides new methods for the study of many fundamental problems of physiology and biochemistry.

In these activities the Council has been advised by their Committee on Medical and Biological Applications of Nuclear Physics, with three sub-committees dealing with the respective branches of the subject, as mentioned above.

(*Rep. of the Medical Research Council for the years 1939–45, Cmd. 7335, H.M.S.O. London, 1947.*)

CONCLUSION

Here in brief outline is an account of the ways in which medical research advanced during the Second World War, including the clinical application in preventing, curing and alleviating human suffering. Never before within so short a time had such conquests been won over so many diseases, never had the medical armamentarium been so well supplied. It cannot be doubted that the accelerated *tempo* of practical discovery was due in large measure to the willing co-operation of biologists with clinicians in their joint contribution to the nation's problems under the stress of war.

Medicine

By Sir Arthur S. MacNalty, K.C.B., M.A., M.D., F.R.C.P., F.R.C.S.

CONTENTS

393

MEDICINE

INTRODUCTION

DURING the present century great advances have been made in diagnosis and treatment in medicine. Instruments of precision, such as X-rays, the electro-cardiograph and pathological and biochemical tests have made diagnosis more accurate and scientific and sovereign remedies for diseases have been found. Discoveries by experimental physiologists made in the laboratory have been applied to the treatment of human diseases, for example insulin by Banting and Best for diabetes, vitamins for deficiency diseases, and liver extract in pernicious anaemia. To these boons concurrently came the triumphs of preventive medicine and immunology.

Chemotherapy attained its first practical triumph in 1909 when Paul Ehrlich and his co-workers discovered Salvarsan or '606', the first really effective remedy for syphilis. Organic arsenical compounds were found for the treatment of trypanosomiasis and allied diseases. Organic compounds of antimony were developed for the treatment of leishmaniasis and other tropical diseases. Alexander Fleming in 1928 discovered the therapeutic value of penicillin but though treatment seemed encouraging the active principle could not then be isolated. Succeeding the work of Domagk with the red dye 'prontosil' against streptococcal human infection, sulphonamide therapy was shown by Colebrook in 1936 as valuable in the treatment of septicaemia. Later the sulphanilamide series was developed in the successful treatment of pneumococcal, meningococcal and gonococcal infections. Other sulphonamide derivatives followed.

Following on the discovery by Bayliss and Starling in 1902 of Secretin (the first of the 'hormones'), which was shown to exercise humoral control in the body, further experimental work showed that the pituitary, thyroid, parathyroids, suprarenals, pancreatic islet tissue and gonads influenced growth and metabolism and led to the founding of the science of endocrinology.

In Great Britain all these advances were greatly stimulated and aided by the Medical Research Council during the First World War and before and throughout the Second World War.

This brief review of progress in the vast field of medical science indicates the stage at which medicine had arrived in 1939. There was a new outlook and conception of the subject, new methods and instruments of diagnosis, and advances in therapeutics had provided remedies for the cure of diseases previously regarded as incurable.

It is now proposed to consider the subject of medicine in the Second

World War and to summarise the advances made and the application of new diagnostic, hygienic and therapeutic measures. These are more fully recorded in the first published volume of this *History* entitled *Medicine and Pathology*. As frequent references will be made to this volume, the abbreviation *M. & P.* will be used in indicating it.

GENERAL MEDICINE

MEDICINE IN THE ROYAL NAVY

General medicine in the Navy was similar to general medicine in the civil population. There were diseases of youth (zymotic diseases), diseases of early and middle adult life like peptic ulcer and diseases of older age, including cancer and cardio-vascular degeneration.

Pulmonary tuberculosis had been for many generations a major naval medical problem. Dudley showed (1938) that ever since accurate medical statistics were available at the Admiralty the invaliding rate for this disease remained approximately two per thousand of the entire force per annum. As this occurred despite changes and improvement in naval architecture and the conditions of service in His Majesty's ships and establishments, Dudley considered that the incidence of pulmonary tuberculosis in sailors arose through infection incurred in the course of their service, and adduced epidemiological evidence supporting this view. He further advocated the application of fluorography (the photography of the fluorescent screen image introduced by d'Abreu of Brazil), whereby rapid and efficient examination of the chest could be made and the first such apparatus was installed and began its work at the Royal Naval Barracks, Chatham in 1939. The Medical Director-General thus made the earliest use of mass miniature radiography, not only for new recruits but also for naval ratings temporarily stationed ashore while ships were re-fitting or under repair. The war's exigencies facilitated and encouraged the general adoption of this method by the Army and the Royal Air Force Medical Services and by the Public Health and Civilian Medical Services. The importance of the problem of tuberculosis in the Navy was further recognised by the appointment of a consulting physician for diseases of the chest and particularly pulmonary tuberculosis (*M. & P.* Chap. XIII).

Skin diseases were common, especially scabies and ringworm of the feet ('foot-rot'). Oil dermatitis in the oil-burning ships was a special hazard. The problem of exposure and the concomitant hazards after shipwreck were studied, especially 'immersion foot' and methods of prevention and treatment were developed (*M. & P.* Chap. XI). The provision of Convoy Rescue Ships was an early advance in rescue work. These ships saved thousands of lives. The clinical work done in them included treatment of compound fractures, head injuries, burns and scalds and shock.

In the old days of sail and long voyages away from port deficiency diseases, especially scurvy, assailed seamen. The prevention of deficiency diseases originated in the Navy when Lind in 1753 advised how to prevent scurvy. With modern knowledge of dietetics, the discovery of accessory food factors (vitamins), rapid passages and wireless communication, deficiency diseases in ordinary circumstances do not occur in the modern Navy. Certain problems of possible food deficiencies were studied by naval medical officers. These were:

1. *The problem of night blindness (defective dark adaptation) in relation to Vitamin A.*

This problem is equally important to the Navy for watch-keeping and flying and to the R.A.F. in night-flying, and was the subject of a joint investigation by both Services. It was found that night vision and dark adaptation were uninfluenced by additional supplies of natural or medicinal vitamin A in the normal individual on an adequate diet. In the Navy age was a factor of importance. Well accredited tests were devised whereby ratings with defective dark adaptation were easily and quickly recognised.

2. *The problem of the possibility of some degree of Vitamin C deficiency (so called sub-clinical scurvy), especially in relation to ulceration of the gums (gingivitis), but also in relation to recurrent boils, sores and slow healing of wounds.*

A full scientific inquiry into this problem was made. McNee and Reid in 1942 found that sailors were rather better than civilians employed in an engineering works in their state of vitamin C nutrition. Gingivitis was due to infection with Vincent's fusiform bacilli and spirochaetes and cure was uninfluenced by the addition of any vitamin (including ascorbic acid) to the diet. No evidence was found of riboflavine (vitamin B2 complex) deficiency in the Services.

It was concluded that no deficiency diseases occurred in the Navy round Britain. (*M. & P.* pp. 3–5.)

Salt deficiency was investigated by K. S. MacLean (1943). It was found that the condition termed 'heat exhaustion' in which a rating coming up from a watch below complains of headache, nausea and dizziness, is but the forerunner of the cramping muscular pains described as 'fireman's cramp', and that both conditions are due to a deficiency of sodium chloride. Salt treatment in most cases caused the symptoms to clear rapidly. An increase of salt intake of those exposed to excessive heat prevented the symptoms arising. Stening described and classified the conditions resulting from salt deficiency into sub-clinical and clinical states, but his view that heat hyperpyrexia supervened upon untreated or incorrectly treated states of salt deficiency was not confirmed by those cases of heat-stroke in which the chlorides in the urine were estimated. It was established, however, that heat exhaustion or heat shock, the symptoms usually being those of clinical shock and heat cramps, were associated with a deficiency of sodium chloride secretion in the urine. Both conditions were remedied by correction of the deficiency of sodium chloride in the body fluids. These investigations have an important bearing for people working in the Tropics. (*M. & P.* pp. 5–7.)

Numerous incidents occurred during the war where men lost their lives through the action of poisonous gases, generated by explosions or fire, by damage to, or misuse of, refrigeration machinery or fire extinguishers containing volatile chemicals or from gases generated by internal combustion engines. The crews of warships were probably more exposed to these dangers than the land forces. Attention was drawn to the considerable frequency of these incidents in war-time and methods of prevention were considered and described (*M. & P.* Chap. XII).

Peptic ulcer (commoner form being duodenal) and functional gastric disorders were as frequent in the Navy as in the other Services, and formed roughly about 10 per cent. of medical admissions to the large naval hospitals. Anxiety neurosis was less common in the Navy than in the other Services. Hypertension and some of its sequelae were often met with and sometimes at a comparatively early age. (*M. & P.* pp. 7–8.)

MEDICINE IN THE ARMY

The impact of the war on medicine accelerated the rate of progress, bringing much of permanent benefit to mankind. The control of malaria, the reduction of dysentery, the influence of protective inoculation on the liability of infection to the enteric group of fevers and the much lower case-mortality of men in the Army to typhoid fever are noteworthy examples. Much was done also in hygiene and sanitation to protect men from food and water-borne diseases. To this Wenyon and others tend to ascribe the low incidence of these diseases rather than to protective inoculations alone. Possibly both played their part. The figures available show no more than that the control of the enteric group of fevers achieved in the First World War was maintained in the Second. (*M. & P.* p. 34.)

The prevention of disease due to uncleanliness and verminous infestation in our armies during the First World War was well maintained in the Second. The troops were exposed to contact with typhus infection in various theatres of war; in Egypt during an epidemic of unusual severity in 1943 on account of the need to employ native labour; through the harbouring of starved and half-clad Polish troops and refugees evacuated from typhus-stricken concentration camps in Russia *via* Persia in 1942–43; in the occupation of North Africa and Naples

under conditions of typhus incidence; and, finally, in 1945 in the
invasion of Western Germany, where the disease had been prevalent
since 1940 and prisoners and refugees were spreading infection. All these
risks failed to overcome to any serious extent the protection afforded by
hygienic control in our Forces. To the measures applied in 1914–18 new
insecticides and prophylactic inoculation were added. A certain number
of troops were infected with louse-borne typhus. In 1943 over 200 cases
occurred among the Middle East Forces. In Persia there were 42
British admissions to hospital and 118 Indian. In Naples only two cases
occurred among the occupying troops. In Germany no exact records of
infections are available, but in Sandbostel Camp, where the infection was
particularly virulent, and in Belsen where there were 60,000 victims of the
disease, the staffs of three British hospitals, immunised, provided with
protective clothing and treated by dusting with D.D.T., worked
unscathed. There were 21 non-fatal cases in the immunised personnel
of a field ambulance. The experience of the Second World War is that
an army can live and work in contact with typhus infection and suffer
only insignificant casualties.

Cerebro-spinal fever has an intimate association with war. In the
Second World War the incidence of the disease began to rise in December
1939 and it rapidly assumed proportions never previously experienced in
Great Britain, while among the troops in France there was an equivalent
rate at approximately the same time. In other overseas commands the
incidence of the disease was negligible. Modern chemotherapy reduced
the case mortality in France to 3 per cent. in contrast with a rate of 40
per cent. in 1918. The severity of the disease was controlled so that
patients could be sent to convalescent depots and rehabilitated for
return to duty. (*M. & P.* pp. 36, 37.)

As regards diseases due to climate, the measures for the prevention
of heat-stroke were acclimatisation, adequate rest and sleep at night,
adequate water and salt-intake, instruction to men on the care of their
health in hot climates, responsibility of commanders in man-management and preventive measures, mobile anti-heat installations, and the
training of officers in the rational treatment of hyperpyrexia, dehydration
and salt depletion. Acclimatisation was so effective that British troops
soon became able to work all day in the open in the hottest weather,
unencumbered by clothing and sun helmets. (See *M. & P.* pp. 37, 38
and 278–280.)

At the other extreme of temperature 'trench foot' which was a cause
of disability in the Army in France and Flanders during the First World
War and investigated then by the Medical Research Committee, was
seen in the Army in Italy during the winter of 1944–45. It is the same
condition as 'immersion foot'. It was again shown that the condition
should not arise in well-disciplined units if the necessary supplies of

suitable footwear are available and the rules for care of the feet, drawn up in the First World War, are observed. (*M. & P.* pp. 38 and 295–303.)

Deficiency diseases were few and of minor significance. The importance of sprue as a factor in wastage of man-power stimulated further research into fat absorption and its mechanism, but the aetiology is still obscure.

Anaemia was common among Indian troops engaged in the operations in South-East Asia. There was reason to believe that this was due to lack of haemapoietic tissue reserves in patients subjected to red-cell destruction or loss, and was related causally to lack of meat in the diet. Milk was introduced into the ration until difficulties in the supply of meat could be overcome. (*M. & P.* pp. 39, 40.)

There was a high relative casualty-rate of skin disease in the armies during the war. This arose from the fact that a minor degree of personal disability may incapacitate a man for the full performance of military duty. Hence the collective results of skin diseases constitute a serious amount of wastage.

Scabies was highly endemic in Europe and Asia during the war, although its incidence in the Army in North-West Europe in 1944–45 was only about 12 per 1,000 per year. At the end of hostilities the rate increased through contact with civilian sources of infection. In the Middle East the so-called 'desert sore' occurred in considerable numbers and proved intractable to treatment. In operations in the jungles of South-East Asia there was a heavy incidence of fungus infections.

Generally throughout the war military dermatological practice hastened cures by new methods of treatment. In the records of campaigns in which statistics of actual incidence were available they showed a lessening rate. Many of these conditions are of a minor nature and Marriott in South-East Asia stated that 95 per cent. of the cases which had to be admitted to hospital might never have become serious if they had been treated efficiently at onset. This emphasises the need for regular inspections of the men and adequate supervision of early treatment by the unit medical officers. (*M. & P.* pp. 40, 41.)

As regards venereal diseases modern chemotherapeutic methods of treatment of gonorrhoea reduced the wastage considerably. There were concurrent advances in the treatment of syphilis, but the policy of retaining a patient in hospital until the primary sore is healed precluded a dramatic change in wastage from this disease, though a considerable reduction took place. (*M. & P.* pp. 42, 43.)

Diseases with jaundice as the prominent symptom were widely prevalent. They included infective hepatitis, leptospirosis (Weil's disease) and jaundice associated with the treatment of syphilis and the parenteral administration of human blood and some of its products.

Infective hepatitis was one of the scourges of the two World Wars, particularly in the Mediterranean theatre of operations.

Weil's disease occurred sporadically among soldiers, as among civilians, in Great Britain from 1939 onwards. In the invasion of Normandy 39 definite cases and 100 less certainly diagnosed cases were reported, with only three deaths. The war saw the first application of penicillin in the treatment of leptospirosis. (*M. & P.* pp. 537, 538.)

A system of rehabilitation was found to be of great value. Specialists in physical medicine supervised rehabilitation, and in specialised units, with their emphasis on orderly controlled remedial exercises, graded physical training in an atmosphere of military discipline; reacting tendencies were controlled, and much was contributed to maintenance of the man-power for which the need was so vital. Army specialists in physical medicine also by physical training improved the physique and stamina of recruits. Over 70 per cent. of the cases sent to these centres attained standards which enabled them to serve in the Army after a period of graduated training averaging six weeks. 'The success of the work points to the advantages which could be expected to accrue to the nation by its wider application in our health service.' (*M. & P.* pp. 44, 45.)

MEDICINE IN THE ROYAL AIR FORCE

The many and varied medical problems in the Royal Air Force required an administrative as well as a clinical solution.

In regard to cardiovascular problems there was a virtual absence of effort syndrome which was so common a diagnosis in the First World War. Conybeare considers that the absence of these cases was due primarily to the employment of other diagnoses to describe them. He is also of opinion that in the previous war the mere term 'disordered action of the heart' used to describe these cases stimulated the production of neuroses which were primarily cardiac in type.

Great importance was attached to blood pressure as a decisive factor in assessing fitness for flying duties. It was laid down that candidates for aircrew with a diastolic pressure persistently over 100 mm. of mercury should be rejected and that those with a pressure persistently over 90, who had more than a faint trace of albumen in the urine, should also be rejected. By 1944 the position regarding hypertension in flying personnel was as follows: all those who showed symptoms such as breathlessness, vertigo, headaches or tinnitus in conjunction with hypertension were grounded, and many were sent to hospital for investigation. Those with symptomless hypertension were usually grounded or given a category allowing them to fly as second pilot only if the systolic pressure was persistently over 160 mm. Hg. and the diastolic over 100 mm.; these limits were often not applied to members of aircrew other than pilots, but the urine in all cases was examined for albumen and microscopically for cells and casts, with reference of the patient to hospital when the findings were abnormal.

In non-flying personnel the problem of hypertension was a much larger one, as many of the officers were older men, some over 50, some even as old as 65, and many accepted for home service only. The Air Ministry, in March 1941, issued an instruction to all principal medical officers both at home and overseas, in which it was pointed out that mild degrees of symptomless hypertension were consistent with efficient service at home and overseas for many years. It was stated that provided the systolic pressure was below 200 mm. Hg. no action need be taken and that symptomless cases need not be transferred to the United Kingdom solely on account of a raised blood pressure. Men with genuine hypertension who complained of symptoms were not retained in the Service. A certain number of cases of coronary occlusion or cardiac decompensation occurred among those retained in the Service.

Some cases of organic valvular disease of the heart were encountered. Though such a lesion, in particular aortic regurgitation, is often consistent with perfect compensation and physical efficiency in ordinary life, the conditions of operational aircrew duty in the air can produce symptoms and men with valvular disease were usually excluded from flying. As regards ground staff in which such disease was found, recruits were usually invalided forthwith. Men who had been trained in a trade, who had no symptoms, and in whom valvular disease was found at routine examination were retained, as a rule. Experience proved this to be justifiable; if symptoms developed later invaliding was advised. Most of the patients gave no history of rheumatic fever.

Cases of acute rheumatism which produced myocarditis, with or without endocarditis or pericarditis, occurred among younger personnel, particularly aircraft apprentices. Patients with acute rheumatism with endocarditis or pericarditis were almost invariably invalided, but it was found that a rheumatic myocarditis was usually transient and that after prolonged rest the patient made a complete recovery. A certain number of cases were diagnosed as myocarditis on very slender evidence. It seems probable that these were of the effort syndrome type of anxiety neurosis.

Coronary disease was found chiefly in the middle-aged. Officers of particular value and experience who had coronary occlusion were often retained in the Service under close medical supervision for at least two years. This policy seemed justified by results. Various forms of cardiac arrhythmia were discovered. They were of no significance, as a rule, unless myocardial damage was present. Some cases presented congenital heart lesions. As a rule, they were regarded as of no pathological significance. Many young men, particularly aircrew, had orthostatic or postural albumenuria of no pathological significance. Occasionally the detection of albumen in the urine led to the discovery of renal disease.

Pilots suffering from renal colic or calculus, provided their progress was normally satisfactory, were regarded as fit for operational duties at home in four months and for full duties at home and abroad in seven months.

Diabetes of any severity was a cause for rejection for service. There was a number of known diabetics, almost all officers, retained in the Service for ground duties. No case of diabetes was found in the Royal Air Force which could be attributed to trauma. (*M. & P.* pp. 51–65.)

MEDICINE IN THE EMERGENCY MEDICAL SERVICES

A special chapter is devoted in this volume to the inception and work of the Emergency Medical Services. The provision was primarily for the casualties of war, but the medical side was well provided for and physicians and resident medical officers were fully occupied with clinical work in the Emergency Medical Hospitals. The patients came from a wider area than the local hospital area. Certain classes of the community were evacuated from urban to rural areas, while the pre-arranged plans of the Ministry of Health and the Board of Education for evacuation concerned school children, younger children with their mothers and some other priority classes of the population. Transference of industrial workers further disturbed normal populations. These evacuated persons brought into the reception areas diseases and ailments which required medical treatment. The Emergency Hospitals also provided treatment for Military and Air Force patients so that physicians occasionally encountered cases of tropical disease. The evacuation of chronic sick from London and the coastal towns into provincial hospitals provided new opportunities of study and teaching. The Ministry of Health effected co-ordination between the municipal and county hospitals. Less well provided hospitals were 'up-graded' to a normal standard, so that physicians throughout the country could diagnose maladies with greater accuracy and treat patients with the full resources of modern medicine. There was a wide distribution of medical specialists, and special treatment centres were established (*M. & P.* pp. 67, 68). Such was the new environment in which hospital physicians dealt with disease during the war.

General Infectious Diseases. These diseases, including epidemic nervous diseases, tuberculosis and venereal diseases, were treated in Emergency Medical Services Hospitals and are considered in *M. & P.* pp. 66–95.

The Chief Fatal Diseases. For tables giving the chief fatal diseases (other than acute infectious diseases) and their percentage contributions to total deaths which occurred in England and Wales, 1939–45, see *M. & P.* pp. 74, 75. As in previous decades the largest proportion of deaths was due to diseases of the heart and circulatory system. Rheumatic fever was less frequently responsible as a cause of heart disease, the majority of these deaths being due to degenerative changes in the heart and blood vessels in adults and old people.

The next killing disease was 'cancer', which included carcinoma, sarcoma, the gliomas and other forms of malignant disease. The number of deaths rose from 67,154 in 1939 to 74,291 in 1945.

Bronchitis, pneumonia (all forms) and other respiratory diseases came next in order. The influence of climate and influenza on mortality from these diseases was noted.

Deaths from diseases of the digestive system rose appreciably in 1940 but thereafter declined.

Diseases of the genito-urinary system, including the various forms of nephritis, were lower after 1940.

The figures of deaths from operations of war were insignificant as compared with the deaths from diseases of the heart and circulatory system and cancer. The Navy and the Air Force protected the British people from the terrors of invasion and from air raids of magnitude, the effects of which would otherwise have been seen not only in a higher rate of bombing casualties but also in deaths from exposure, tuberculosis, deficiency diseases, epidemics and malnutrition.

CHIEF GENERAL DISEASES OF THE WAR PERIOD
DISEASES OF THE HEART AND CIRCULATORY SYSTEM

The numbers of men invalided from cardiovascular causes, organic and functional, in the War of 1939–45 were only one-fiftieth of the large numbers invalided from this cause in the War of 1914–18. (*M. & P.*, pp. 76, 109.) Disordered action of the heart (D.A.H.) or valvular disease of the heart (V.D.H.) were noticeably absent from the casualty lists of the Second World War. This is explained by increased knowledge of cardiovascular disease, largely due to the work of Mackenzie, Lewis, Parkinson and others, the use of the electrocardiograph, X-rays and estimations of blood pressure and the availability of cardiologists for consultative purposes in the Services, the recruiting boards and in the Emergency Medical Services Hospitals. (See *M. & P.* pp. 76, 109–112.) Rheumatic fever, though diminishing, is still responsible for heart disease in an appreciable proportion of cases (P. Stocks) and many recruits were rejected for this reason. Degenerative lesions (arterio-sclerosis, atheroma, chronic myocarditis and endocarditis, occlusion of the coronary arteries and the effects of hypertension) are causes of the greater proportion of cardiovascular disease today. Syphilis plays a much less important part since effective treatment for the disease has been made available. This is shown by the comparative rarity of thoracic aneurysm.

In the treatment of cardiovascular diseases great advances were made during the war. The most striking success was in the treatment of malignant, infective or subacute bacterial endocarditis which, until the advent of penicillin, was almost invariably a fatal disease. Penicillin, in adequate dosage, cured over 60 per cent. of cases. Treatment of cardiac disease and circulatory failure by digitalis and venesection advanced. Coronary thrombosis and angina pectoris were studied and experience showed that in both these conditions, with appropriate treatment, the prognosis was not so grave as was previously believed. Anti-coagulants such as heparin, either alone or in conjunction with dicoumarin, were employed, but modern research shows that their efficacy in the prevention of further attacks of coronary thrombosis is doubtful. In angina pectoris surgical or chemical blocking of the afferent cardiac nervous paths has been tried. Surgical treatment in cardiovascular disease first initiated by H. S. Souttar and by O'Shaughnessy in England was largely in abeyance during the war. Its triumphs are of more recent date.

CANCER

Research into the cause and treatment of cancer was of necessity limited by the war, but the discovery by Professor Sir Charles Dodds that stilboestrol has a beneficial effect on cancer of the prostate was important. At the Imperial Cancer Research Fund laboratories much work was done on Bittner's 'milk factor' in relation to carcinoma of the breast, on the biochemistry of cancer and on the question of a possible cancer virus. The use of the electron microscope in the histological study of cancer was another noteworthy advance.

Advances were made during the war in the study and treatment of cancer of the lung. Clinical experience and hospital and post-mortem records all testify to its increasing prevalence. At the end of the war it was estimated that in England and Wales between four and five thousand people died annually from bronchial carcinoma. The death-rates per million (standardised) during the first decade of this century were 10·2 for males and 7·0 for females, but by 1937 the corresponding figures were 100·9 and 23·2. This increase has continued since the war, especially in males. In England and Wales in 1953 the deaths from cancer of the lung numbered 12,881 in males and 2,251 in females. Lung cancer accounted in the same year for 28 per cent. of all male cancer deaths, giving a record figure of 607 deaths per million living. In females deaths from this site represented 5·4 per cent. of all cancer deaths and 98 deaths per million living.

This increase in male mortality from cancer of the lung is a world-wide phenomenon and is the subject of continued investigation. A statistical correlation between tobacco and cancer of the lung, especially in heavy cigarette smokers, has been shown by Doll and Bradford Hill in this country and Wynder and Graham in the U.S.A. (See also the *Report of the Royal College of Physicians*.)

It was shown in the war that improved methods of diagnosis, including examination of sputum for cancer cells, biopsy, radiography and bronchoscopy, have enabled the condition to be recognised at an earlier stage. Cases of persistent unexplained cough should at once be investigated, since thoracic surgery prolongs life in cases diagnosed as operable with increasing success. Treatment by deep X-ray is now only used in inoperable cases. (*M. & P.* pp. 79, 80.)

For trends of mortality in relation to cancer sites see *M. & P.* p. 95.

RESPIRATORY DISEASES

Pneumonia. In a sample of cases of pneumonia (all forms) admitted to E.M.S. hospitals during the years 1940–5 there was a total case-mortality in 5,930 cases of 0·54 per cent. These were Service cases, for the most part under 30 years of age and with good powers of resistance. The death-rate from acute lobar pneumonia in London hospitals was about 5 per cent. as compared with about 20 per cent. in 1924. These good results were due to the introduction of sulphonamide and penicillin therapy.

There was a number of cases of delayed resolution in pneumonia in patients over 35 years of age. Most cases had been treated with sulphathiazole and about 20 per cent. with penicillin. It seems desirable that no patient suffering from pneumonia should be discharged from medical treatment until a radiograph of the chest shows that complete resolution has taken place. During the war primary atypical pneumonia, a condition believed to be due to virus infection, called for study and attention. (See *M. & P.* pp. 80–85, 509–20.)

PEPTIC ULCER

Deaths from diseases of the digestive system in England and Wales numbered 18,700 in 1939, rose to 19,502 in 1940 and thereafter gradually diminished, being 15,832 in 1945. A proportion of these deaths was due to haemorrhage or perforation from either gastric or duodenal ulceration. War experience revealed a high incidence of peptic (gastric and duodenal) ulceration in the Armed Forces and in the civilian population. This was not a feature of the War of 1914–18, and is due partly to the fact that between the two wars there had been a rise in the occurrence of peptic ulceration, the subjects of which were prone to recurrence of their disease under the stress of war conditions. Before and during the war considerable advances were made in the diagnosis and medical treatment of peptic ulcer with a consequent lowering of mortality. Drip blood transfusions were found beneficial in cases of haemorrhage and lowered the mortality from gastro-duodenal haemorrhage. (*M. & P.* pp. 86–88, 96–108.)

THERAPEUTIC ADVANCES

For a general account of therapeutic advances in the war years see *M. & P.* pp. 88–91.

ACUTE RHEUMATISM

Rheumatic fever is not outstanding as a war disease, but is of importance for it causes a certain proportion of medical casualties and of permanent rejections from the Services.

Its incidence and severity are steadily declining as shown by the fall of admissions to civil and Service hospitals. 'The severest of its clinical features, such as hyperpyrexia, pericarditis and nodes, are nowadays rarities, the age incidence has shifted from the younger adult age-groups to that between 5 and 15 years, while its social incidence is now almost exclusively upon the children of the poor, especially those of great cities'. (*M. & P.* p. 115.)

The inter-war years 1919–39 showed (1) an acceleration of the decline; (2) the inception of systematic preventive effort; (3) the strengthening of the theory that infection by the *streptococcus pyogenes* is the cause of the disease.

The War of 1939–45 showed low rates of incidence (as estimated by admissions to hospital) and mortality from rheumatic fever. This was seen, not only in Great Britain, but also among British troops serving in the original British Expeditionary Force in France (Copeman).

Since the war the decline in mortality from rheumatic fever has continued. In 1944 there were 1,002 deaths from this disease; in 1953 only 310. Good ventilation and avoidance of overcrowding, damp conditions and dust are the chief features of prophylaxis against this disease. Experience with the chemoprophylaxis of streptococcal infection in this country has been largely negative.

CHRONIC RHEUMATISM

A certain proportion of cases in officers and men in the Services occurred in the different theatres as well as in Great Britain during the war; some of these were sent to the spa hospitals for physiotherapy under the Emergency Medical Services of the Ministry of Health. The classification of chronic rheumatism was heterogenous and included such various conditions as sub-acute rheumatism, fibrositis, lumbago, sciatica, rheumatoid arthritis, osteo-arthritis, spondylitis, synovitis, pes planus, gout and other diseases. Of these conditions cases of fibrositis accounted for 52·5 per cent. For an account of chronic rheumatism see *M. & P.* pp. 122–143.

ADVANCES IN TROPICAL MEDICINE

Campaigns ranging from the Mediterranean littoral through the Continents of Africa and Asia to the islands of the South-West Pacific brought the armies of the British Commonwealth into regions where sub-tropical and tropical diseases are endemic. This led to intensive research from which emerged important findings of wide and general application.

MALARIA

Malaria, the greatest source of man-power wastage in regions where it is endemic, was a constant menace in the Middle East, North Africa, Sicily, Italy and in East and West Africa. In Burma it was always a serious problem. Research projects covered the entire range of anti-malaria measures.

Mosquito ecology. Much work was done on the identification of carrier species and on the basis of these observations precise methods of species control were devised and proved effective. For instance, in North Borneo it had been believed that the principal vector was *Anopheles macalatus.* After a prolonged search it was found the responsible vector was *A. leucosphyrus.* Breeding of mosquitoes was controlled with this new knowledge more economically and much more efficiently.

Destruction of larvae and adult mosquitoes. Dichloro-diphenyl-trichlorethane (D.D.T.) proved a valuable aid for the destruction of larvae and adult mosquitoes.

Repellents. Two new repellents, dimethyl-phthalate and dibutyl-phthalate were discovered. The former was more active against mosquitoes. In impregnated fabrics, e.g. head-nets, its value for sleeping men is increased as it is less volatile than when applied to the skin.

Chemotherapeutic control. The soldier must of necessity live in regions where he is exposed to the bite of infected mosquitoes. His only protection is in the use of drugs capable either of destroying the parasites before they can produce an infection (causal prophylactics) or, alternatively, of preventing the appearance of overt symptoms of malaria (suppressants). The entry of Japan into the war and the loss of Java early in 1942 cut off the supply of quinine, which has only a limited suppressive action. Synthetic anti-malarial preparations were studied. Atebrin, manufactured as mepacrine, as a suppressant gave promising results in Malaya, Middle East, North Africa, Sicily and Italy. This and other synthetic preparations were intensively studied at Land Head-quarters Medical Research Unit (A.I.F.) at Cairns, Queensland, from 1943 onwards. Some 850 volunteers were infected with malaria and the action of these various drugs tested under controlled conditions. As a result mepacrine, in doses of 100 mg. daily, was adopted as the standard régimen for malaria suppression. In the Australian Force malaria incidence fell to negligible proportions, and hyper-endemic regions were occupied with impunity. Comparable results were obtained in Burma and Italy.

Treatment. In treatment no new principles were discovered, but it was confirmed that pamaquin (formerly known as plasmoquine), an 8-amino-oxyquinoline, in combination with quinine or atebrin had a powerful action in reducing the relapse rate in *vivax* infection. (See *M. & P.* pp. 195–200.)

BLACKWATER FEVER

Cases of blackwater fever were infrequent. The low incidence is attributed to the use of mepacrine rather than quinine, especially as a suppressant.

VISCERAL LEISHMANIASIS (KALA-AZAR)

Transmission. During the war experiments on transmission of the disease by infecting animals (mice and hamsters) or man by the bite of sandflies seemed definitely to prove that the sandfly is the vector of kala-azar.

Prevention. D.D.T., in the form of residual spray, in huts and dwelling places, was effective in preliminary trials.

Treatment. The variety of kala-azar which occurs in the Sudan is more intractable to antimonial preparations than that found in India or in the Mediterranean area. A new pentavalent antimonial compound, sodium stibogluconate, gave good results in Sudanese cases both as regards immediate cure and lower relapse rate.

Diagnosis. Smears of bone marrow obtained by sternal puncture were used to demonstrate the parasite. The method is safer though less often positive than smears from splenic puncture. A complement-fixation test seemed to be of value.

TRYPANOSOMIASIS IN WEST AND EAST AFRICA

Trypanosomiasis was not a serious menace to the health of the Fighting Forces, but its widespread incidence among native populations from which recruits were drawn made its control important. In mass treatment of sleeping sickness caused by *Trypanosoma gambiense*, in Nigeria, a combined course of antrypol (Bayer 205) and tryparsamide was favoured. Later pentamidine was substituted for antrypol as being less toxic. These drugs have also been used prophylactically. Pentamidine seemed the better and appeared to afford protection for six months. Large numbers of Africans were protected in this way for six months. Progress was also made in tsetse-fly eradication.

AMOEBIASIS

There was little progress to report in amoebiasis. Despite much research no new amoebicides of importance were discovered. In most theatres of war the disease occurred in between 5 and 15 per cent. of all cases showing dysenteric symptoms. Emetine remained the only known drug which exercised a potent action on the trophozoites, especially in metastatic lesions in the liver and elsewhere.

BACILLARY DYSENTERY

Throughout all the theatres of war the dysentery bacilli which were isolated and identified belonged, with few exceptions, to one or other of the recognised types. The *Shiga* infections were, as usual, most severe. Owing to the discovery that certain of the sulphonamide drugs exercise a specific action on dysentery bacilli, it was possible to avert major outbreaks of this disease and to bring about rapid cure in all cases, however severe, which came under early treatment. In the British Army sulphaguanidine was used because of its low toxicity and the negligible danger of renal blockage. Sulphadiazine, being more readily absorbed, was adopted by the U.S. Medical Corps as the standard treatment for bacillary dysentery. The detection of carriers was greatly facilitated by the introduction of desoxycholate medium for the isolation of the dysentery bacillus. It also added appreciably to the number of positive results.

PLAGUE

Apart from a few small outbreaks plague did not occur in the Allied Armies. In India, where the disease was endemic, the mortality rate was appreciably lowered by treatment with sulphathiazole, sulphadiazine and sulphamerazine and the effect was increased when given in combination with anti-serum. Trials of D.D.T. in killing the flea-vector gave encouraging results.

CHOLERA

During the war outbreaks of cholera were reported in prisoner-of-war camps in Thailand and there were epidemics among the civil population in India. A number of small-scale experiments were made with sulphonamide therapy (chiefly sulphaguanidine) which significantly reduced mortality.

RELAPSING FEVER

Several severe outbreaks of louse-borne relapsing fever occurred in native communities in Africa but the armies were never seriously affected. Scattered cases of the tick-borne variety appeared among troops stationed in the endemic areas, particularly throughout the Middle East from Syria to Tripolitania. Both vectors, the louse and tick, are killed by D.D.T. Louse-borne relapsing fever yields to treatment with organic arsenical compounds. The problem of preventing and curing tick-borne relapsing fever was largely unsolved.

SCRUB TYPHUS

Scrub typhus, an acute fever caused by infection with *Rickettsia tsutsugamushi* is conveyed by the bite of larval mites which feed on wild rodents, particularly rats. In peace-time the disease is rare, but in jungle warfare men are exposed to the infected mites. The disease occurred on the Burma front and in the South-West Pacific. In investigation the disease was first identified; the vector was found to be *Trombicula deliensis*, and the bionomics of this mite, with special reference to the infection of man, was worked out in detail. As to methods of prevention, the destruction of rats and other small mammals was found impracticable under jungle conditions. Dibutyl phthalate proved highly effective as a repellent when applied to clothing, the incidence in the Australian Force in New Guinea being reduced to the low figure of 13 in the three months ending December 31, 1943. Tests were made with a protective vaccine, but the end of the war came before definite conclusions could be drawn.

DENGUE AND SANDFLY FEVER

Dengue. Cases of dengue occurred in considerable numbers among Australian troops in New Guinea. The recognised vectors *Aedes aegypti* and *A. albopictus* were absent, and careful research proved *A. scutellaris* to be responsible. By studying this mosquito, attacking its breeding places, protecting troops and especially those suffering from dengue by repellents and nets, the incidence of the disease was controlled. Researches on a protective vaccine against the three dengue viruses were initiated but not completed during the war.

Sandfly Fever. Sandfly fever was relatively common among troops in the Mediterranean area. Natural immunity after an attack may last only a few months, and the same person may suffer from two or even three attacks in one season. No successful vaccine was made. In Malta a 'residual' spray of D.D.T. destroyed the adult fly, and dimethyl phthalate gave good results as a repellent. Thus better control of infection was achieved.

YELLOW FEVER

The control of yellow fever and prevention of outbreaks claimed considerable attention during the war years. As the vector (*Aedes aegypti*) is a common domestic mosquito in most tropical and sub-tropical countries there is a grave danger if either infected mosquitoes or infected human beings are brought into a 'clean' locality. That no such outbreak occurred is a tribute to the efficiency of the preventive measures taken. These comprised anti-mosquito measures in airfields and aeroplanes, and the inoculation with yellow fever vaccine of intending passengers from or through the endemic zone. For those not so protected, rigorous quarantine measures were enforced. The efficacious vaccine universally used was pantropic attenuated virus 17D, developed shortly before the war. The immunity was shown to last at least four years. The vaccine was also successfully used to immunise the population of endemic areas and of troops stationed there. In Uganda and elsewhere in Africa evidence was obtained suggesting that monkeys constitute a reservoir of infection and that the virus of yellow fever is passed on to man by an arboreal mosquito, *Aedes africanus* and a domestic mosquito, *Aedes simpsoni*.

SCHISTOSOMIASIS (BILHARZIA)

By the application of simple precautionary measures based on knowledge gained during the War of 1914–18 there was no repetition of the outbreak which had then occurred in Egypt—a hyperendemic area. In the Eastern theatre, a number of cases, some of considerable severity, occurred among Australian troops who operated in areas where infection with *Schistosoma japonica* was endemic.

FILARIASIS

Filariasis (caused by infection with *Wuchereria bancrofti*) affected United States troops stationed in the Pacific Islands, but not British and Commonwealth troops who were outside the endemic area.

SPRUE

Sprue was of common occurrence in the Burma campaign from 1943 to 1945 when over 3,000 cases were noted. There was defective absorption of both fats and sugar and, in some cases, of salt. In late cases a macrocytic anaemia was common, which arose from a lack of the haemopoietic factor; low absorption of calcium was also present.

A diet rich in protein and relatively poor in carbohydrates and fat was found most satisfactory in treatment. Crude liver extract given parenterally improved the blood condition and lesions in the mouth and tongue.

DEFICIENCY DISEASES

Deficiency diseases were rare, except among troops on the Burma front where difficulty arose from time to time in supplying the authorised rations. Scurvy was practically unknown. The majority of these diseases occurred in prisoner-of-war camps, particularly those under the Japanese. The majority of deficiency diseases were due to a low intake of the components of the vitamin B series. The best treatment was to provide an adequate ration of fresh 'protective foods' with a generous proportion of first-class protein. Yeast extract (Marmite) as a supplement was also beneficial.

In East Africa there were occasional cases of beriberi. When treated with vitamin B (thiamin) and yeast, cure was rapid. Cerebral beriberi, or Wernicke's encephalopathy, was observed in prisoners-of-war in Singapore. A 'spastic syndrome', associated with vitamin B deficiency, was seen in prisoners-of-war in the Far East. (See *M. & P.* pp. 281–294 for 'Nutritional Disorders of the Nervous System'.)

CONCLUSION

The Second World War will be ever memorable in Tropical Medicine for the outstanding advances made in the control of such diseases as malaria, typhus and yellow fever. These triumphs of the pathologist and epidemiologist were great contributions to ultimate victory in safeguarding troops against deadly diseases which for centuries had decimated armies serving in tropical climes. (See *M. & P.* pp. 195–221).

INFECTIVE HEPATITIS

During the War of 1939–45 infective hepatitis appeared among the armies of the world and, as in the War of 1914–18, it made its greatest ravages on the armies massed round the Mediterranean shores. In the six winter months of 1942–43 infective hepatitis cost the British troops in the Middle East over half-a-million man-days in hospital. It was estimated that during epidemics the disease became at least equal to battle casualties in numerical importance and exceeded in importance any other individual cause of temporary loss of man-power.

Investigations. Researches were made by many investigators in the field in all theatres of war, in the hospitals and in the laboratories. At the instance of the Chief Medical Officer of the Ministry of Health, the Medical Research Council set up a team of workers (1943) to investigate the disease and correlate the work of various investigators engaged in studying it.

Pathology. The essential histological picture of infective hepatitis was shown to be one of hepatic cell necrosis and autolysis, associated with leucocytic and histiocytic reaction and infiltration. The centres of the lobules show the first of these changes most markedly and the portal tracts the greatest cellular infiltration. No inflammation was present in the bile canals or ducts. This description was based on aspiration biopsies and necropsies. In fatal cases the post-mortem picture is that of acute or sub-acute necrosis of the liver.

The changes in the liver are related to the severity and duration of the disease.

Aetiology and Transmission Experiments. The disease appears to be due to a virus. It is not transmissible to laboratory animals, but by injections of blood and serum or by urine and dried and filtered faeces obtained from patients in the pyrexial stage, it was possible to infect volunteers with the disease. The causative agent, the virus, seems to be present in the blood and is excreted in the faeces and possibly the urine.

Clinical Picture. The clinical signs and symptoms were carefully noted and described. The disease can be divided into a pre-icteric and a post-icteric phase. A limited number of cases was recognised with clinical or pathological evidence of infective hepatitis which were so mild as not to develop obvious jaundice.

Mortality. The mortality, which appears to increase with age, is about 0·2 per cent. Fatal cases usually die of acute necrosis and cholaemia, often with an associated haemorrhagic state.

Certain observations. The incubation period is about 25 to 35 days. Cases are as a rule infectious for a short period about the time of onset of symptoms. They are only regarded as non-infectious when jaundice is well-established. Contact is the probable mode of spread and chiefly by droplet infection. In England the incidence was highest among children of school age, and, generally, the young are more susceptible than the old. British Army officers in the Middle East and in Italy were affected approximately four and a half times more often than British other ranks. In India the ratio was 2:1. No explanation was found of this predilection.

Much was discovered during the war about infective hepatitis, but the complete picture of the disease, its prevention, treatment and epidemiology, has not yet emerged. (See *M. & P.* pp. 230–267).

Homologous Serum Hepatitis. For an account of this see page 419.

TETANUS

At the beginning of the War of 1914–18 tetanus was a deadly danger to the wounded in France and Flanders. Passive immunisation (prophylactic antitoxin) for all wounded reduced the incidence of tetanus to 0·1 per cent. It also modified the disease and reduced the mortality in those cases which did occur. In 1927 tetanus toxoid was advocated for active immunisation. It was first used to protect Army horses and then to immunise soldiers.

In developing active immunisation against tetanus many problems of technique, including dosage, arose. There was controversy on the advantages of active as compared with passive immunisation. An important discovery was that by combining tetanus toxoid with diphtheria toxoid or T.A.B., its antigenic effect was increased. This enabled large numbers of men to be immunised against both tetanus and typhoid. It was further found that to ensure active immunisation being invariably successful, it is necessary to supplement active immunisation by passive immunisation. In the British Army, active immunisation by the two-dose method, each of 1 c. cm. of plain toxoid, was introduced as a routine in 1939, and about 90 per cent. of those going on active service in that year were so immunised. If a soldier were wounded he was given a single dose of prophylactic antitoxin. If he had previously been actively immunised nothing further was done; if not, he received two further doses of antitoxin at weekly intervals. In 1941 it became a standard practice to give a further dose of 1 c. cm. of toxoid at the end of a year. Before the invasion of Europe the troops in 21 Army Group were practically all inoculated and a third dose was given before going overseas. Any wounded man not actively immunised was given three doses of 3,000 international units of antitoxin at weekly intervals. Actively immunised wounded men received a single dose of 3,000 units as soon as possible. This procedure of continued active and passive protection was adopted in the United Kingdom, Australian, New Zealand and Indian Armies. In South African troops passive immunisation was used alone until 1942.

By the adoption of this procedure the incidence of tetanus among British troops was rendered insignificant. The average per 1,000 wounded (0·12) compares remarkably well with the corresponding figure (1·47) for the Western Front in 1914–18.

AIR-RAID CASUALTIES

In preventing tetanus in air-raid casualties active immunisation of the civil population was impracticable. Reliance had to be placed on the stringent use of passive immunisation. The Chief Medical Officer of the Ministry of Health advised as follows (Ministry of Health, 1942a):

1. A routine prophylactic dose of 3 c. cm. antitoxin equivalent to not less than 3,000 international units to be given by intramuscular or deep subcutaneous injection to every wounded person, however trivial the wound may appear.

2. This dose to be given irrespective of the fact that the patient may have been immunised with tetanus toxoid, and no reduction to be made for children.

3. Two further doses of 3 c. cm. to be given weekly to all patients not previously immunised with tetanus toxoid, and in the case of severe infection this dose to be increased two- or three-fold.

Notification of all cases of tetanus was also instituted.

No rise in the number of deaths occurred in England and Wales from tetanus during the war period; there was a slight decrease in mortality from the disease.

During the first two years of war in a sample of 4,562 civilian air-raid casualties there were only six cases of tetanus, of which two died. None had been actively immunised, but a single prophylactic dose of antitoxin (2,000 to 3,000 units) had been given. Of the patients who died the severity of their wounds probably contributed as much as tetanus to a fatal issue.

TREATMENT

Few cases were available for treatment, but in those that did occur experience emphasised the importance of a large initial dose of antitoxin (200,000 i.u.) given intravenously, as early as possible, followed by thorough surgical treatment of the wound. A further injection of antitoxin was only advised after seven days if the wound was severe. Other treatment was chiefly palliative.

CONCLUSION

The great reduction in the incidence and especially the mortality of tetanus in wounded persons was one of the outstanding achievements in the war.

ADVANCES IN HAEMATOLOGY

This section draws attention to some of the chief advances made in haematology and related subjects during the war.

PHYSIOLOGY

More has been learned about the histiogenesis of haemic cells. The increased frequency of marrow biopsy as a diagnostic procedure has facilitated knowledge of maturation processes in normal and abnormal bone marrow. Terminology is becoming more precise. The term 'megaloblast' for instance, was accepted as referring to the abnormal erythroblast occurring in cases of liver factor deficiency, or in early foetal life, and the main disturbances of the normal process of the development of red cells were described. Physical methods such as micro-spectography and micro-histochemical reactions were applied to the problem of the relationship of morphology to function in haemic cells, and the changes occurring during normal and pathological maturation. This work indicated that the basophilic material of developing red cells is probably ribonucleic acid, and led to the chemical identification of a number of structures. Marrow tissue culture was developed. The life-span of the red cell in the normal circulation and in a variety of pathological states was studied. The function of the lymphocyte was examined and a number of potent enzymes were found to be present. The lymphocyte's regeneration and its part in the formation of antibodies was demonstrated. Improvements were suggested in the estimation of haemoglobin. Important studies were made of normal haematological values, and the normal level of serum iron, an important indicator of iron deficiency, was established.

BLOOD COAGULATION

The war years saw a considerable clinical application of aspects of blood coagulation. Dicoumarin, an anticoagulant, discovered in 1941, was widely used in the treatment and prophylaxis of thrombotic and embolic conditions. Heparin proved valuable in the same conditions and particularly for the prevention of thrombosis during vascular surgery. Fibrin dressings in the form of sheets and 'foam' were used with human thrombin, as haemostatic applications and for filling up cavities in surgery. The theory of blood coagulation was the subject of further study.

OTHER STUDIES

A number of other haematological and associated conditions were studied. Haemoglobin levels in nutrition surveys did not reveal any serious deterioration or severe anaemia in Great Britain during the war years. Further advances were made in pernicious anaemia and related conditions such as the so-called pernicious anaemia of pregnancy, refractory anaemias, the anaemia of sprue, dimorphic anaemia, haemolytic anaemias, toxic haemolytic anaemia, haemolysis associated with cold agglutinations, blackwater fever, sickle-cell anaemia, target-cell anaemia, acholuric jaundice, nocturnal haemoglobinuria, aplastic anaemia and neutropenia, anaemia associated with severe or prolonged infection, glandular fever, leukaemias, the haemorrhagic states, vitamin K deficiency and haemophilia. Each of these studies added something to knowledge of haematology; in some less, in others more. (*M. & P.* pp. 539–550.)

BLOOD TRANSFUSION

From ancient times the value of blood as a life-giving substance has been appreciated and many experimental trials were made from the seventeenth century onwards. Towards the end of the nineteenth century transfusion with physiological saline was adopted for the treatment of anaemia, loss of blood and shock, and blood transfusion fell into disuse. Researches into serology, haematology, haemolysins and prevention of coagulation revived its study, and, especially, Landsteiner's discovery in 1900 that people fall into particular blood groups. In 1914 Agote in Buenos Aires and Lewisohn in New York independently established that 0·2 of sodium citrate acts as an effective anti-coagulant without toxic effects, unless the total amount of citrate administered exceeds 5 g. In 1917 a Canadian medical officer, Oswald H. Robertson, introduced the citrated method of blood transfusion to the Casualty Clearing Stations; it was adopted in our military hospitals in France, and largely developed there by Geoffrey Keynes, who published a standard work on *Blood Transfusion* (Oxford Medical Publications) in 1922. Robertson (1918) stored blood for as long as 21 days and used it with excellent results in the treatment of wound shock on the battlefield. He also showed the advantage of adding glucose to blood. The practice of storing blood was not again used until the Spanish Civil War in 1937–39.

PROGRESS AND RESEARCH

Between 1930 and 1939 much research work in haematology was done by L. Whitby, H. L. Marriott, S. R. M. Bushby, A. Kekwick and Janet Vaughan. In 1935 Marriott and Kekwick introduced the principle of the continuous infusion of large quantities of blood and described their technique. This was a notable advance and all the later modifications of apparatus for giving blood by continuous drip, including the standard apparatus designed by the Medical Research Council and the Army Blood Transfusion Service (Vaughan, 1939; M.R.C. War Memorandum No. 1. 1944), are based upon it.

The risks and complications of blood transfusion were also studied more accurately and prevented by careful technique and scrupulous asepsis. For example, haemolytic reactions for long limited the value and application of blood transfusion. These occur when transfusion of blood, or of a blood derivative, is followed by destruction of the effused transfused erythrocytes at a rate greater than expected, or by an increased rate of destruction of the recipient's erythrocytes. Haemolysis is now a rarity. Accurate blood grouping and the discovery of the rhesus factor (Rh) by Landsteiner and Weiner (1940; 1941) has enabled further precautions to be taken against its occurrence. Simple febrile reactions and circulatory overloading were specially studied by V. H. Riddell (1939).

The transfer of an infective agent from donor to recipient is an obvious risk in blood transfusion; the only safeguard is the careful selection of donors by medical examination. This was realised when the London Blood Transfusion Service (the first voluntary organisation) was founded by the late P. L. Oliver of the Red Cross Society in 1921. Dr. H. F. Brewer, of St. Bartholomew's Hospital, examined the state of health of the donors, including Wassermann test, and estimated their blood groups. The chief disorders of practical importance that may be transmitted were found to be syphilis and malaria. To these a third, hepatitis, must be added. In his report for 1937 as Chief Medical Officer of the Ministry of Health, MacNalty reported the occurrence of cases of acute infective jaundice following inoculation with convalescent measles serum. Out of 109 persons inoculated with serum from a particular batch, 37 developed jaundice, of whom 7 died. Subsequently, a number of other cases were reported after blood transfusion. In 1946, W. H. Bradley of the Ministry of Health reviewed the whole subject of this condition, now known as 'homologous serum jaundice'. Its prophylaxis is a difficult matter.

THE NATIONAL BLOOD TRANSFUSION SERVICE

Before the Second World War the Civilian Blood Transfusion Service was in its infancy. It was a purely local and voluntary organisation and adequate only for the needs of the larger centres of population. The donor was sent for as required for an individual patient, and only fresh 'whole blood' was used.

On the outbreak of war in 1939, the Medical Research Council, in collaboration with the Ministry of Health, set up four centres or 'Blood Banks' in London. These centres were intended to cope with the large number of expected air-raid casualties; to conduct research into the new problem of providing large quantities of blood and the possibility of preserving blood. Subsequent adjustments of the anticoagulant (citrated blood) and, in particular, the addition of dextrose, extended the survival period of the blood. Accuracy of blood grouping was greatly increased by improved technique. Serum, plasma and the dried products were prepared and, in theory, were of equal value with 'whole blood', except in cases requiring haemoglobin. All this valuable organisation was brought into being by admirable co-operation between administrators, pathologists, clinicians and research workers and the patriotic offers of blood donors throughout the country.

The surgical demand for 'whole blood' recurred as the result of clinical experience and had to be met. In the latter half of 1940 a regional blood transfusion service was set up under the Emergency Medical Services by the Ministry of Health. Additional centres were formed at Newcastle, Leeds, Manchester, Liverpool, Birmingham, Nottingham, Oxford, Cambridge and Cardiff, all, except Nottingham, being associated with a university department of pathology. In each centre, as in London, there was a senior whole-time transfusion officer with a staff of assistant medical officers, scientific workers, nurses and technicians, and the necessary transport, maintaining an almost daily link between all the hospitals in England and Wales, was provided. Donors continued to come readily. The total number of donors in the service in England and Wales at December 31, 1944, had reached the large figure of over one million, and the total number of 'blood gifts' up to the same period was nearly two millions. Blood was always available for routine hospital use, for every air-raid emergency and for supplementing the Service (Navy, Army and Air Force) organisations, including those of the United States. Sir Lionel Whitby and Dr. Janet Vaughan rendered conspicuous service in the organisation of the National Blood Transfusion Service throughout the war.

In addition to the E.M.S. Hospitals, all civilian patients were provided for; and a special service, including the provision of rhesus negative blood, was arranged for maternity homes and hospitals. In July 1948, the regional transfusion centres passed from the direct control of the Ministry of Health to the regional hospital boards of the National Health Service.

CONCLUSION

Blood transfusion in the Second World War both in this country and in the campaigns saved the lives of thousands of air-raid and military casualties, who would otherwise have died from haemorrhage or shock. It has now become an indispensable part of ordinary medical practice, not only for cases of injury and shock, but for many medical conditions in which there is a loss or deficiency of blood, such as gastric ulcer, duodenal ulcer and secondary anaemia. Blood transfusion has also helped greatly to reduce the maternal deaths in England and Wales. In 1938 the deaths ascribed to haemorrhage of childbirths and puerperium were 269. In 1948 they were only 122.

Military ambulances in the war were equipped with apparatus so that the wounded might have the immediate benefit of blood transfusion while being conveyed to hospital. This provision helped to save further lives and is now available more generally for civilian casualties.

Blood and blood products in unskilled hands can be highly dangerous and should only be prepared by skilled experts. False grouping, the transmission of infective diseases other than jaundice, neglect to use the proper kinds and proper amounts of transfused fluid and the serious danger of infected material must be overcome successfully by exercising the utmost care.

There is a small risk of transmitting homologous serum jaundice by plasma or serum transfusion. To prevent this risk irradiation of the blood products by ultra-violet light is now being tried. But the benefits of blood transfusion far outweigh the risks, and British haematologists, scientists and clinicians have largely contributed to this valuable therapeutic procedure. The Medical Research Council and the Ministry of Health were responsible for setting up a comprehensive organisation for blood transfusion.

References

1. Blood Transfusion (1949) edited by Geoffrey Keynes. Bristol. (This book contains a copious bibliography of the subject.)

2. Ficarra, Bernard J. (1942): The Evolution of Blood Transfusion. *Annals of Medical History*, New York. Third Series, IV, 302–323.

3. Hirsh, Joseph (1941): The Story of Blood Transfusion: its Civilian and Military History. *The Military Surgeon*, Washington, D.C., 88, 143–158.

4. On the state of the Public Health during Six Years of War. Report of the Chief Medical Officer of the Ministry of Health, 1939–45 (1946). London H.M.S.O., 161–164.

DERMATOLOGY

Skin diseases stand high in the order of incidence of diseases in both civilian and military spheres.

In the Army abroad in war-time dermatologists were given ample facilities in sections of large hospitals devoted entirely to skin and venereal diseases. Dermatological units or centres were established in the Emergency Medical Services and their value was abundantly demonstrated. Unfortunately, there was a shortage of sisters and nurses adequately trained in the nursing of skin diseases, for it was only beginning to be realised that the care of dermatological cases requires specialised knowledge.

SCABIES

Considerable advances in the treatment of scabies were made during the war and were aided by the provision for in-patient treatment. Ultimately, the Ministry of Health recommended as a standard treatment the application of a 25 per cent. emulsion of benzyl benzoate with 2 per cent. lanette wax. This proved to be the most satisfactory method of treatment.

The following points emerged as a result of experience: (*a*) blankets were not a common source of infection; (*b*) the sarcoptes was usually vulnerable; only in a severe epidemic was the disinfestation of bedding and clothing necessary; (*c*) 'silent carriers' were a definite problem; (*d*) in the Army the civilian population was the source of infection; (*e*) there was a seasonal incidence in the United Kingdom, the peak being in the first three months in the year, with an annual fall in the summer; (*f*) with proper therapy men could be treated without having to go off duty; (*g*) accurate diagnoses were not always made by junior medical officers unfamiliar with scabies, the chief error lay in not distinguishing between eczematous eruptions, prurigo, pediculosis and scabies; (*h*) as in the War of 1914–18, ecthyma was a post-scabietic complication, and often developed some days after the scabies was cured; (i) in the average case the patient was not teeming with parasites; (j) the incubation period might be as long as six or eight weeks.

PEDICULOSIS

In air-raid shelters during the war there was not a serious increase of pediculosis among shelterers. Head-lice in town children presented a difficult problem. Pediculosis capitis in entrants to the Women's Services caused much trouble. The introduction of lethane hair oil, a quick, reliable method of treatment, did much to eradicate this infestation.

Pediculosis corporis was not a military problem, except among native civilian labour abroad and prisoners in concentration camps. In the epidemic of typhus in Naples A.L.63 and D.D.T. were of value in disinfesting the population.

Pediculosis pubis in men only occurred in a few military units. The A.T.S. was free from this complaint.

IMPETIGO AND THE PUS-COCCAL SKIN INFECTIONS

The various sulphonamide preparations, especially sulphathiazole (5 to 20 per cent. in a cream or paste) was used extensively in the form of external applications in the treatment of impetigo and other pus-coccal skin infections. Many reports, both from Allied military and civilian sources, showed unfavourable reactions to this treatment. These reactions varied from scarlatiniform, erythema multiform-like, urticarial, purpuric, varicelliform, vesicular, pustular, fixed bullous, exfoliative, and pemphigus foliaceous-like eruptions and might even resemble erythema nodosum or angioneurotic oedema. The skin might be made light-sensitive and the risk of this serious condition was increased in climates where there is much bright light or sunshine. A case of fatal agranulocytosis following sulphathiazole therapy, was reported from Chicago. These unfavourable reactions may render the patient prone to similar reactions if sulphonamides are given even in minute doses. Hence the well-tried remedies should be used for impetigo, folliculitis and other pus-coccal infections, and not the sulphonamides. Penicillin was tried at the end of the war for these conditions but the risk arises also of unfavourable reactions and making the patient resistant to the drug. Aniline dyes (acriflavine, gentian violet and brilliant green) were greatly used in pus-coccal infection, but were discarded for treatment of infections of the face. Ecthymatous sores ('desert sores' and 'jungle sores') were a constant trouble in every theatre of war in hot countries. They caused discomfort, a serious loss of efficiency and some sick-wastage. The use of sulphonamides and later of penicillin helped to obviate sick-wastage, but there was the risk of sensitisation and development of resistance to the drugs.

OTHER CONDITIONS

Ringworm infections were common both among civilians and in the Services. Although many of the industrial processes in war-time entailed contact with skin irritants, the problem of occupational dermatitis was less serious than had been anticipated. Eczema, dermatitis and seborrhoeic dermatitis occurred. Tropical lichenoid dermatitis caused trouble to malariologists and dermatologists. In the Invasion of Normandy and Brittany troops lying in certain fields were severely bitten by harvest bugs. For this benzyl benzoate and di-methyl-phthalate were satisfactory repellents. Severe sunburn was a cause of sick-wastage in North Africa. Adequate sun-tanning was the best prophylactic agent against prickly heat in all hot countries. In old hospital buildings (Netley, Colchester and Harrow Road) sporadic cases of cutaneous diphtheria occurred due to secondary contamination of skin lesions with diphtheria bacilli. It was also a hazard of importance in P.A.I. Force and in M.E.F.

REHABILITATION

This was possibly the most important advance in any dermatological service in the war. An auxiliary hospital (British Red Cross Society and Order of St. John) at Ragley Hall, Warwickshire was used for some three years for the physical and psychological rehabilitation of military skin cases. The results were encouraging—some months after treatment 75 per cent. of those treated were on full duty and 17 per cent. on light duty.

PSYCHOLOGICAL MEDICINE*

Conscription brought into the Services individuals of all mental levels and types. Hence the various forms of psychiatric disorder occurring in the civilian population were found in comparable proportions among the men and women of the Services.

In 1922 the Southborough Committee surveyed the psychiatric problems of the War of 1914–18 in its 'Reports of the War Office Committee on Shell Shock, 1922'. The importance of proper selection procedures in preventing psychiatric illness was emphasised.

In order to cope with the above problems psychiatrists were appointed in the Second World War. Their scope varied considerably from one Service to another. This was due to the different kinds of problems that arose in the respective Services, to the differences in the categories and grades which each Service employed, and to variations in Service organisation and environment.

In the Navy and Air Force, psychiatry and neurology were regarded as two aspects of one subject closely linked with general medicine. In the Army there was a separate Directorate of Psychiatry within the

* See M. & P. pp. 339–407.

Army Medical Department. The Medical Directors-General of the three Services and of the Emergency Medical Services were advised by consultants in psychiatry or neuropsychiatry. The Service psychiatrist worked in a team in collaboration with psychologists, other medical officers and scientists and advised the executive on matters of mental health and adjustment in individual cases.

The Service activities to which psychiatrists contributed were: (1) Selection of Personnel; (2) Training; (3) Morale; (4) Treatment and Disposal; (5) Research and Validation. Psychiatrists diagnosed and recommended placement, treatment or rehabilitation for the following conditions: neurosis, psychopathic personality, psychosis and mental dullness or defect. These conditions might overlap with one another. Special emphasis was laid on early detection of abnormality and on the avoidance of hospitalisation. The longer the delay in treatment the less favourable was the prognosis for return to Service duty. As in civilian life, the treatment and welfare of Service patients was directed to hasten their recovery. The task of readjusting the patient to his environment was a prominent feature. Neurotics often tended to resist treatment designed to fit them again for war duties. In individual therapy, continuous narcosis, insulin treatment, electric-shock therapy and other forms of physical treatment were used together with established methods of psychotherapy. Occupational therapy, remedial training, educational lectures, gymnastics and recreations and group therapy were employed. Social case-work dealt with family problems and vocational guidance, including psychological testing and technical training. Psychiatric treatment played its part in the strengthening and recovery of morale. As in the War of 1914–18, it was found that morale was best near the front line, and the further back towards the Base one went, the worse it became. (For an account of training of Service psychiatrists, instruction of medical officers in psychiatry, see M. & P. pp. 341, 342.)

An important branch of psychiatric work was the selection of personnel. The intellectual resources and personality of individuals were assessed so that each could be directed to the position where he could be of greatest use to the Service. Individuals were no longer liable to be allocated to duties much above or below their capacity, with the result that wastage of training time was much reduced. Introduction of psychiatric selection helped to exclude from the Army many thousands of dullards and defectives; such individuals were formerly a burden to their units, training staffs and medical and disciplinary units. This selection also reduced the intake of individuals with predisposition to psychiatric disorder.

The magnitude of the psychiatric problem in the Services is illustrated by the number of psychiatric patients who had to be discharged. About 118,000 such patients (men and women) were discharged between

September 1939 and June 1944. Between one-third and one-half of all medical invalids (men and women) were discharged from the Services on psychiatric grounds. This ranged from about 4 to 10 per 1,000 of average strength per annum. Of the 118,000 discharged the proportions under four diagnostic heads were as follows:

	Per Cent.
Psychoneurosis and effort syndrome	64·3
Psychoses	21·2
Mental defect	6·4
Psychopathic personality	8·1
	100·0

Surgery

By Sir Zachary Cope, B.A., M.D., M.S., F.R.C.S.

CONTENTS

SURGERY

INTRODUCTION

SURGEONS in the Second World War inherited the physiological outlook that the surgeons of the First World War had to learn for themselves, and they dealt with better human material. They had at their disposal several accessory methods previously unknown or imperfectly developed, e.g., adequate means of intravenous blood or plasma transfusion, gastric or intestinal evacuation by continuous suction, careful salt-balance, and chemotherapy.

In the first two years of the war the importance of immobilisation of the wounded part in transit was realised, the value of the sulphon-amides in controlling general sepsis was appreciated, and the dangers following the application of a completely closed plaster were brought to notice. The second two-year period was noteworthy for the development of mobility, both of the surgical teams who treated the patients and of the wounded themselves. The field surgical unit and the mobile casualty clearing station led to the formation of basic forward medical units. Then (in 1942) came evacuation of the wounded by air and the advent of penicillin. The final two years witnessed a unified and comprehensive treatment of the wound from the moment of its infliction until the patient was rehabilitated and fit again for duty.

The majority of flesh wounds were due to fragmentation-missiles, often of small size. A minute fragment projected at a high velocity often did extensive damage, especially when it struck one of the bones and broke it into fragments. Every wounded patient was thoroughly examined for multiple injuries, fluid loss was made good by plasma or blood transfusion, pain was relieved by morphine (often given intravenously) and every effort was made to raise the systolic blood-pressure to 100 m.m. Hg., before any necessary operation was done. Réchauffement was not utilised to the extent that it was in the First World War.

Pre-operative radiography was done whenever possible. Intravenous anaesthesia (pentothal) was commonly used. The forward operative treatment of wounds consisted of the removal of a minimal paring of skin margin, wider excision of subcutaneous fat, incision of the deep fascia to equal the length of skin incision, and removal of all damaged and devitalised tissue. Time was not spent in trying to remove a poorly localised foreign body. It was found that bone-fragments could often be left *in situ* with advantage. Adequate drainage was essential. Exposed surfaces were dusted with a powder containing 5,000 units of penicillin per gramme. (Sulphonamide was sometimes added.) The wound was dressed with plain or vaselined gauze inserted gently into the depth of

431

the wound; over this was put wool kept in position by bandage or strapping, carefully avoiding any circular constriction of the limb. A split and well-padded plaster splint immobilised the limb. Penicillin was given parenterally. At the base hospital delayed primary suture was done at a favourable time during the next week or ten days. If the wound was frankly infected, secondary suture was performed later.

Field conditions were different from those in the War of 1914-18, when the casualty clearing station and the base hospital fulfilled the needs of prolonged trench-warfare. In the War of 1939-45 there was much more mobility, and forward operating stations were necessary. At first mobile surgical teams were attached to a C.C.S., but soon two entirely new surgical units were formed—the field surgical unit and the field dressing station. Experience showed that the best formation for forward surgery was a combination of two surgical units with a transfusion unit, situated close to a dressing station. At first attached to a C.C.S., by the time of the Libyan campaign the War Office had made both the field surgical unit and the field dressing station independently mobile and self-supporting with their own establishment. It was agreed that surgical centres ought not to be among or in front of our own heavy guns. The post-operative patient suffered less from longer journeys than from the anxiety incidental to the clang of battle. Ideally there was a common pre-operative ward, in which the transfusion officer could work, near to the operating theatre.

The regular use of air transport for the wounded enabled seriously wounded patients to be treated at base hospitals where every facility was available. At one or other of them there were thoracic, orthopaedic, maxillo-facial or neuro-surgical centres. At a later date special neuro-surgical, thoracic and plastic units were sent to different parts of the theatres of war.

BLOOD AND PLASMA TRANSFUSION

The constant availability of blood for transfusion was an important factor in the more successful treatment of wounds. The Army Trans-fusion Service supplied transfusion fluids and equipment for the whole British Army overseas in every theatre of war. Special transfusion units were trained and sent abroad. The needs of the Army increased until more than a thousand pints were obtained daily from a panel of about 350,000 donors. In the later campaigns, with the exception of the B.L.A., the whole-blood service was provided by base transfusion units; most of the blood taken by the home depot (at Bristol) was then processed to form plasma, which was either dried for export to distant war centres, or supplied in fluid form for use in temperate climates. Dried grouping serum was supplied, the different groups being differen-tially coloured for identification purposes. The whole system, from the central depot to the field transfusion units, worked most efficiently.

Transfusion officers became very expert and were regarded as specialists. Large amounts of blood were often needed in massive limb injuries—five or six pints sometimes being required before operation could be undertaken. Caution was necessary in giving transfusion to any patient with an injury to the chest, or who was suffering from the effects of blast.

About 10 per cent. of the wounded needed transfusion and the average protein requirement was about four pints per patient. During the course of the war 756,046 pints of blood were taken from donors in the United Kingdom and distributed as blood or plasma to the Forces all over the world. The Air Force was mainly supplied with blood from the Army Transfusion Service.

At Divisional level only life-saving transfusion was done, chiefly by plasma, for the policy was to evacuate rapidly. Lack of response was usually an indication that surgery was needed, and, in general, resuscitation went hand in hand with surgery. At Corps level it was found that travelling transfusions were unsatisfactory. Multiple injuries were common and the whole body needed to be examined. Forced heating, as done in the First World War, was not favoured. Transfusion was nearly always required for severe limb wounds, for penetrating abdominal wounds, and for burns. Many, but not all, patients with wounds of the chest also required transfusion, but with them there was the risk of pulmonary oedema. Rigors were common with rapid transfusions but haemolytic reactions and air embolism were exceedingly rare. Morphine was best given intravenously in doses of ¼ grain. Overdoses were common owing to faulty recording. Sodium amytal or paraldehyde, given intra-muscularly, were particularly useful when head injuries complicated other wounds. For extreme hypotension methedrine proved useful.

Transfusions was usually done by needle rather than cannula. For speed of administration both arms were sometimes used simultaneously. The sternal marrow route did not permit a rapid enough flow of fluid.

The system of supply in the field never failed. Blood was not held for more than twenty-four hours by units without refrigeration. These units had to rely chiefly on plasma. The blood survived well and was used up to twenty-eight days from the time of collection.

SHOCK AND RESUSCITATION

In the First World War it was shown that the main feature of traumatic shock was a serious diminution of the volume of blood in effective circulation, which led to an instability of the general circulation. It was found that a rapid pulse was not an invariable accompaniment of shock which was indicated better by a lowering of the pulse pressure than by the lowering of the systolic blood pressure.

When war broke out in September 1939, the Medical Research Council set up a committee to investigate traumatic shock, and in 1940 a pamphlet on the subject was issued. This pointed out that the most important requirement in treatment was to restore the blood volume as speedily and as efficiently as possible. Several clinical investigators showed that the symptoms of shock were variable, that mentally the patients were often alert, and that the pulse rate and blood pressure were sometimes deceptive. Though the estimation of blood volume was of value, the size of the wound and the general clinical condition were usually reliable guides to treatment. There was some evidence to support the belief in neurogenic shock. The danger of overheating the patient in the process of resuscitation was emphasised, for the increased sweating caused further loss of fluid. It was thought safer (Wilson) to warm the chilled patient after, not before, starting transfusion. It was agreed that réchauffement should be carried out in moderation.

The view that histamine played a large part in the causation of shock was not confirmed, but H. N. Green obtained from muscle a substance (adenosine tri-phosphate) which had shock-producing properties. Clinical investigations confirmed the experimental work and showed that trauma led to an increase in the blood plasma of substances which are probably derived from nucleotide breakdown. There is therefore some evidence that adenyl compounds are released from injured tissues and that they may be a factor in the production of shock. Further than this one could not go with certainty.

ABDOMINAL AND ABDOMINO-THORACIC WOUNDS

The recovery-rate of patients suffering from abdominal wounds greatly improved during the War of 1939–45, until in the early summer of 1944 there was a 70 per cent. success among the 5,000 abdominal casualties in the B.L.A. The improvement was not due to any great change in technique, but to efficient resuscitation, readily available transfusion of blood, the benefit of the sulphonamides and penicillin, the use of gastric suction and parenteral feeding, better anaesthesia, and the practice of retaining abdominal casualties in an appropriate environment until fourteen days after operation. The exteriorisation of wounds of the colon, introduced by Sir Heneage Ogilvie, proved a life-saving measure. The removal of the coccyx and the incision of the fascia of Waldeyer in extra-peritoneal wounds of the rectum, and more conservative methods of treatment applied to injuries of the kidney, were other advances in technique.

Most patients with abdominal wounds were given first priority, for they required skilled treatment more urgently than other casualties, with the exception of those with severe haemorrhage or threatened with asphyxia. The prognosis was, to a large extent, influenced by the hazards of evacuation. Distance alone had no significance, but the length of time and the roughness of the journey were the important factors. Results were better with an advancing and successful army than when it was in retreat. Soldiers wounded in the abdomen during airborne operations and commando landings usually suffered badly.

The resuscitation department was close to the operating theatre and was in charge of the field transfusion officer. The patient's boots were usually removed and in quiet times he was undressed and put properly to bed. Clean blankets were provided. Electric cradles were not used but a hot water bottle or two were provided. The mouth might be cleaned with a wet swab. A quarter of a grain of morphine was given intravenously and recorded. As a rule two to three pints of blood were transfused but four or five pints might be needed. Those who were exhausted at the time of wounding were often severely dehydrated and needed not only blood but glucose-saline. Rapid transfusion was very dangerous for patients suffering from blast injuries of the lungs or abdomen; it was essential to find out how far the patient was from the site of explosion, and to proceed cautiously if blast injury seemed likely.

Difficulty in diagnosis of abdominal wounds arose when the entry of the missile was away from the immediate neighbourhood of the abdominal cavity, e.g., in the thigh or perineal regions, or in the thorax. Accompanying head wounds causing unconsciousness also sometimes diverted attention from the abdominal wound.

The clinical picture was the most important guide to the seriousness of the injury, but X-rays sometimes helped. All abdominal patients were catheterised as a routine, and digital rectal examination performed in patients with lower abdominal wounds. With perforation of a viscus, abdominal rigidity was usually slight, and absence of liver-dullness of little help. Absence of peristaltic sounds, confirmed and re-confirmed, was a positive indication for laparotomy.

Posterior retro-peritoneal haematoma, without gut-injury, was often difficult to diagnose correctly. Moderate wounds of the liver were best left alone, but continued evidence of bleeding required exploration. The majority of gun-shot wounds of the kidney could be treated conservatively, but nephrectomy was sometimes needed later.

Spinal wounds sometimes gave rise to tenderness of the abdominal wall and hyperaesthesia together with ileus, but the ileus came on sooner than that due to peritoneal contamination.

Operation. The choice of incision for abdominal wounds varied with each case. Speed and gentleness were essential. Systematic examination was carried out, bleeding stopped, injuries repaired, and the abdominal wall sewn up, particular care being paid to the peritoneum. Drainage of the peritoneal cavity was practised less often as the war progressed. If the operation were performed within ten hours of the injury, even faecal contamination did not necessitate drainage. In late cases the pelvis was drained, and a drain was also put into the muscle-layer. In post-operative treatment, gastric or intestinal suction, fluid and chloride replacement, and chemotherapy greatly helped recovery.

Whereas in the War of 1914–18 the recovery-rate of all wounds of the small intestine was 27 to 30 per cent., in the War of 1939–45 from 42 to 63 per cent. recovered. When the injury was confined to the small gut recovery occurred in 34 per cent. in the First World War, and in 63 to 76 per cent. in the Second World War.

Wounds of the colon and rectum. Wounds of the right side of the colon were often treated by conservative measures—suture and caecostomy—but wounds of the transverse or descending colon were most safely treated by exteriorisation. The recovery-rate of wounds of the large intestine varied from 40 to 72 per cent.

Colostomy was an essential procedure in all wounds of the rectum. Intraperitoneal wounds were sutured when possible. With extra-peritoneal wounds free drainage of the peri-rectal tissues was necessary and a rubber tube was stitched in position in the anal canal. The anorectal muscles did not need to be divided. The mortality of wounds of the rectum was about 50 per cent.

Wounds of the Liver. In most cases of penetrating wounds involving only the liver, surgery was unnecessary. Intestinal peristalsis was never absent when only the liver was injured. Small fragments of missiles might remain innocuous in the substance of the liver, but an abscess of the liver sometimes developed. When, on account of continuing haemorrhage, operation became necessary, there were three techniques possible. (1) Suture by the Grey Turner method, perhaps aided by omental or muscle-graft; this carried a mortality of 50 per cent. (2) Packing with gauze rolls or omentum, or a combination of the two. Later in the war use was made of oxidised cellulose which could be firmly packed and left *in situ*. Packing was accompanied by a 60 per cent. mortality. (3) Simple drainage to allow the escape of effused bile was used in the milder cases and had the low mortality of 20 per cent.

THORACO-ABDOMINAL WOUNDS

The percentage of abdominal wounds that involved both thorax and abdomen varied in the experience of different surgeons from 8 to 39 per cent., but, taking a large series of cases it came to about 19 per cent. The chest and abdomen might be penetrated by separate missiles or by the same missile in a vertical, oblique or transverse direction. The organs involved, in diminishing percentages, were the liver, spleen, stomach, kidney, colon and small intestine. Rarely was the diaphragm alone injured. It was sometimes difficult to determine whether the thorax or abdomen contained the more serious lesion. If there was a fair air-entry into the lungs there was less probability of the main injury being in the thorax. Bilateral and persistent abdominal rigidity pointed to a serious abdominal injury which might be confirmed by noting the absence of peristalsis on auscultation. Diaphragmatic injury was suggested by an almost entirely thoracic type of respiration with a catch at the end of respiration, sometimes with a definite hiccup.

Treatment. In view of the danger of respiratory embarrassment fluid was only needed if there were signs of blood loss; blood was of more value than plasma and had to be given slowly, not more than one pint an hour. Any sucking pneumothorax had to be sealed off immediately by an adequate dressing.

Operative approach varied according to the position and nature of the original wound and the predilection and experience of the surgeon. The abdominal approach was adopted rather more frequently than the thoracic. Late thoracic complications were haemothorax, abscess of the lung, empyema, and subphrenic abscess. Diaphragmatic hernia and pleurobiliary fistula sometimes occurred.

The mortality of patients who had both thoracic and abdominal injuries varied according to the viscera involved, from 26 to 84 per cent.

Summary of Treatment Recommended for Penetrating Thoraco-Abdominal Injuries

1. In many traversing (through-and-through) thoraco-abdominal wounds of the right side produced by a small fragment of high explosive or bullet, no immediate active surgical treatment is required, provided that (*a*) no gross damage has been inflicted upon the thoracic or abdominal wall—fractured ribs, explosive effect, etc.; (*b*) the direction of the track of the missile does not appear to involve the general peritoneal cavity or suggest the desirability of its exploration; (*c*) the signs of abdominal haemorrhage or of injury to a hollow viscus are clearly absent.

2. In cases of right-sided thoraco-abdominal wounds in which a small fragment is retained in an inaccessible position in the substance of the liver, an expectant line of treatment is the correct procedure; accessible fragments, unless of small dimensions, should be sought and removed.

3. When there is an open blowing thoracic wound or a severe wound of the thorax, the *chest injury must of course assume priority of treatment*.

4. If the position of the wounds of entry and exit in a left-sided thoraco-abdominal wound indicates a track implicating the fatal left subphrenic area of the abdomen, or if radiological facilities are available and demonstrate a fragment of metal retained in this region, the thorax should be dealt with first and access to the upper abdomen obtained through the diaphragm.

5. When the thoracic injury appears insignificant, but there is evidence of widespread intraperitoneal damage, especially involvement of hollow viscera, the abdomen should be explored through an appropriately placed laparotomy incision. This instruction applies to wounds of thorax and abdomen produced by the same or by separate missiles.

6. When the thoracic injury seems slight, and when the evidence of a radiograph or the direction of a missile track in a through-and-through wound suggests an extraperitoneal course of a small fragment, such a thoraco-abdominal injury may often be left alone.

If in such cases there is evidence of injury to the kidney, the parietal wound down to the kidney should be excised, the condition of the organ investigated, any foreign body removed, and the wound appropriately treated by penicillin-sulphathiazole powder, etc.

7. If a thoraco-abdominal or abdomino-thoracic injury has been approached from the abdominal aspect, it is important not to waste further time trying to complete a difficult suture of the diaphragm in a critically ill patient, unless the aperture in the midriff is so large that immediate or early herniation of the abdominal contents is certain to occur. The liver almost always prevents diaphragmatic hernia on the right side, and therefore repair of the diaphragm on that side is not a vital step.

8. An abdominal approach is necessary in thoraco-abdominal wounds where the colon is implicated; exteriorisation of the large bowel is only practicable by this route.

Suction of the peritoneal cavity, except the immediate infra-diaphragmatic regions, can only be performed efficiently through an abdominal incision. Gross soiling in wounds of small or large gut therefore render this approach advisable.

9. Trans-thoracic crushing of the phrenic nerve is not only unnecessary but undesirable, and only aggravates the insult already inflicted on the diaphragm.

10. Concomitant serious damage of the kidney and colon is probably best dealt with by nephrectomy, and exteriorisation of the colon.

11. As in pure abdominal wounds, gross haematuria lasting 48 hours or more demands exploration.

ANAESTHESIA

In the Navy. At sea, often with unskilled assistance, the anaesthetist had to adopt a method which was simple, safe and reliable. The use of inflammable vapours was inadvisable. Regional anaesthesia, and preferably intravenous anaesthesia, were the best methods. The intravenous route represented a great advance, and pentothal was the commonest substance used.

In the Army an adviser in anaesthetics was appointed to the War Office in February 1941, and he was able to arrange for a proper supply of apparatus, and at a later date to arrange training courses in anaesthesia. Later, special advisers were appointed in the Middle East, in North Africa, in Italy and in India. For the first time it was officially recognised that the administration of anaesthetics was a highly skilled occupation, and that anaesthetists were specialists.

Pentothal sodium, given intravenously, was of immeasurable value, and was used either as a preliminary anaesthesia or as the sole drug. For operations on the head, neck, thorax and abdomen the great value of endo-tracheal administration was recognised. The excellent qualities of cyclopropane as an inhalation anaesthetic became evident and the benefits of closed circuits in maintaining the body-heat and fluids appreciated.

In the Royal Air Force, the need for specially skilled anaesthetists in dealing with seriously ill patients soon became evident, and when in 1941 a civilian consultant in anaesthetics was appointed (who later accepted a commission in the R.A.F.V.R.) he soon arranged the training of suitable medical officers as anaesthetists, and for the provision of the most efficient apparatus. Occasionally members of the V.A.D., and Service nursing orderlies were trained to play a subordinate rôle in routine work and emergencies. Lectures were given to sisters and orderlies, laying stress on the care of the unconscious patient.

The development of the Oxford vaporiser was a welcome addition to the anaesthetist's apparatus. The choice of anaesthetic was influenced by the experience of the anaesthetist and the preference of the surgeon. In the field pentothal was universally popular.

ORTHOPAEDIC SURGERY

Modern orthopaedic surgery, including the treatment of all types of injuries to the limbs, had its origin in the War of 1914–18 under the inspiring leadership of Sir Robert Jones. The Second World War proved a further period of rapid development of orthopaedic knowledge and organisation. Of great importance were the development of special orthopaedic centres, specially staffed by trained orthopaedic surgeons,

P*

and the introduction of systematic rehabilitation of all injured persons. First-aid measures to combat infection were the early application of the field-service dressing, the injection of anti-tetanic serum and gas gangrene antitoxin, the oral administration of sulphonamide, and (at a later date) penicillin injections. Transfusion by glucose-saline, plasma or blood was often done at a very forward level. Early and well-planned evacuation—often by air, was of great assistance. Limbs were usually immobilised by plaster-of-paris (split down the length) and applied over padding. In the lower extremity the 'Tobruk' splint was often useful; this was a Thomas's splint with fixed skin traction which was enclosed in plaster-of-paris. Padding was placed between the plaster and the splint. One-third of the limb was in front of the bars and two-thirds behind. The knee was flexed through ten degrees over a pad, and the plaster stopped three inches above the malleoli, which were well padded. Two or three field dressings were placed between the trochanter and the ring in order to keep it away from the perineum. The skin-extension straps needed to be tightened occasionally to prevent pain. For buttock wounds the posterior half of the ring of the Thomas's splint was removed and a plaster-of-paris spica applied.

For open fractures the plaster treatment of Winnett-Orr and Trueta was carried out. Closed fractures were generally treated by manipulative reduction and plaster-of-paris or Thomas's splint. Rarely, open reduction and plating were done.

Established infection of a joint called for drainage. Wide excision of joints was not practised, and only rarely was amputation necessary. Gas gangrene was rare when wounds were properly treated, and after penicillin became available. Fat-embolism accounted for five per cent. of deaths in all fractures. The clinical picture of fat-embolism was typical. Within 24 to 36 hours of the injury the patient became feverish, with alternations of consciousness and coma, and was cyanosed; petechial haemorrhages developed round the base of the neck and in the conjunctival sacs. The pulmonary type resembled acute oedema of the lungs and was of fair prognosis; the cerebral type came on more rapidly and was usually fatal.

Injuries of the peripheral nerves were for the most part treated by the orthopaedic surgeons. It was agreed that the best time for suture of divided nerves was not immediately but some three or four weeks after injury. The more distally placed the division of the nerve the better was the prognosis. The treatment of peripheral nerve injuries was considered to be better carried out in special centres.

Amputations of the limbs were much rarer than in the War of 1914–18. Almost the only indication for immediate amputation was irreparable interruption of the main blood vessels of the limbs. This improvement was largely due to the prevention of sepsis by better and earlier treatment of the wound, to the more adequate immobilisation of limbs and to the advent of chemotherapy.

Surgeons experienced in the fitting of artificial limbs condemned some of the classical sites for amputation. In the case of the lower limb they advised that the end-bearing should be discarded in favour of the side-bearing or preferably ischial-bearing stumps, and this policy was adopted in Great Britain throughout the war. Four standard amputation-stumps were recommended—below the knee, $5\frac{1}{2}$ inches of tibia; above the knee, 11 inches measured from the great trochanter; below the elbow, 7 inches measured from the olecranon process; above the elbow, 8 inches measured from the tip of the acromion process. These were the only major amputations advised. The Syme amputation was never advised for a woman, and in men only when there was a good chance of primary healing.

In the hand it was advised that every millimetre of thumb or fingers should be saved. Partial amputation of the foot was often advised and gave good results. When sepsis was present a provisional amputation was sometimes performed as a preliminary to the more formal final operation. Neither the Krukenberg nor the cineplastic amputations were employed to any extent. Flaps were designed to give a transverse rather than an anteroposterior scar and placed terminally in the upper limb but often posteriorly in the lower limb.

Prolapsed intervertebral disc was frequently seen. It was usually diagnosed from the history and clinical features. Myelography was only occasionally performed. Some patients were treated conservatively by recumbency or immobilisation in plaster, others were submitted to operation. The results were often disappointing. Only about half those submitted to operation returned to full duty.

Ankylosing spondylitis. There were many cases of ankylosing spondylitis among the Service patients. The cause was unknown. Deep X-ray therapy often seemed to arrest the disease and was the only treatment which gave sufficient relief to enable men to return to full duty. Recurrent dislocation of the shoulder was seen many times. The Putti-Platt operation gave better results than the Nicola operation.

Fractures of the carpal scaphoid were common. Treatment was by prolonged immobilisation. Bone-grafting gave indifferent results.

Division of the flexor tendons of the palm was treated by improved methods. The new principle was that no suture-line should be placed within the digital sheath, except at its distal extremity. The injured tendon was removed from the mid-palmar level to its insertion into the distal phalanx. The excised tendon was then replaced by a free tendon graft, preferably from a tendon which has an investment of paratenon, such as the palmaris longus. Inert material, e.g., stainless steel wire, was used for suture purposes.

Internal derangement of the knee-joint was treated by removal of the entire injured cartilage with the least possible trauma to the tissues of the joint, followed by adequate physiotherapy and rehabilitation. The patient returned to full duty from eight to twelve weeks after operation. Arthrography was seldom used in diagnosis.

Fractures of the astragalus were more common than in civilian practice. Uncomplicated fractures were treated by simple immobilisation in plaster until union occurred. Complicated fractures sometimes required removal of the astragalus, and in some instances tibio-calcanean fusion was necessary.

Rehabilitation of orthopaedic cases was more extensive and systematic than in the War of 1914–18. Even bed patients were encouraged to exercise the trunk and limbs as early as possible, and to do some form of occupational therapy. For ambulatory patients many forms of active exercise were arranged. Spontaneous exercises, 'resisted' exercises, movements auto-assisted by means of cords and pulleys, were all utilised. Passive treatment was less used. Games calculated to exercise weak muscles were instituted, and all varieties of occupational therapy were employed.

In fracture cases early use of the damaged limb and earlier movements of the joints, and in the case of the leg, earlier weight-bearing were encouraged.

More than a third of all cases referred to the orthopaedic centre were for complaints of the feet. Fatigue was often the cause of the trouble, and the treatment was rest and graduated exercises. Operative treatment was discouraged, for a soldier rarely returned to full duty after operation.

BURNS

Burns were more frequent than in the First World War on account of the increased use of armoured vehicles, tanks, and aircraft. Many burns occured also from the careless way in which the soldiers used petrol for domestic purposes.

The aviator's burn had a characteristic distribution involving the face and hands, and sometimes the legs and thighs. At the beginning of the war picric acid, tannic acid, and gentian violet solutions were chiefly used as local applications, but picric acid was soon discontinued, and so was tannic acid on account of its tendency to cause circular constricting scars on the fingers, and because it sometimes caused serious degenerative lesions in the liver.

The Medical Research Council initiated and supported research on burns, and special centres for burns were set up in different parts of the country. Trained staff and good team work brought better results. Advances were made in several directions.

(1) Relief of pain. Research showed that the inclusion of an analgesic in a local application did not relieve pain either certainly or completely. Morphine was usually necessary.

(2) Local applications. In the Navy a triple dye jelly was often used. It consisted of brilliant green · 1 per cent., euflavine · 1 per cent., gentian violet 1 per cent. A suspension of sulphanilamide in oil or petroleum jelly gave good results. The trend gradually turned towards simpler antiseptic dressings, e.g., simple boric acid ointment, so long as sulphanilamide was given internally. At the Glasgow Burns Unit the first-aid treatment was to apply a sterile cloth, then (in hospital) to swab with 1 per cent. 'cetavlon' and apply a 3 per cent. sulphonamide cream. Towards the end of the war local application of penicillin by compress, cream or powder, came into use. Continuous or intermittent saline baths were recommended by some, but this required special apparatus and trained attendants. The Bunyan-Stannard irrigation envelope was adopted in some places; a solution of electrolytic hypochlorite was used. Pressure dressings were used by some American surgeons; they applied vaseline-gauze strips, then gauze dressings, then fluffed sponges and finally a folded gauze roll. Others dressed the part with gauze impregnated with petroleum jelly and covered the whole with plaster-of-paris. For certain cases in which the whole thickness of skin was destroyed, immediate excision and prompt skin grafting were employed. At the end of the war simplicity of both first-aid and of definitive treatment was found to give the best results.

(3) Prevention and treatment of shock. This was achieved by early and adequate fluid replacement. In every serious burn much fluid is lost from the circulation into the tissues during the first twenty-four hours. Intravenous plasma or blood will make good this loss. Prevention of shock by prophylactic administration of plasma was more efficacious than curing shock when once it had developed. Amounts of plasma varying from two to seven litres were necessary according to the extent and severity of the burn. Roughly 50 c.cm. of plasma for every 1 per cent. of the body surface affected by a blistering burn was advised. The estimation of body surface was done by Berkow's method. Transfusion was necessary in adults in whom 15 per cent. and for children in whom 5 to 10 per cent. of the body surface was affected. The replacement of fluid had to be continued for at least twenty-four hours after the occurrence of the burn. Fluids were also given by mouth if there was no vomiting.

(4) Prevention of sepsis. The surface of the burn was swabbed gently with lint soaked in a detergent antiseptic solution ('cetavlon').

Then various applications were made, but opinion gradually decided in favour of some form of sulphonamide or penicillin dressing. It was of the greatest importance to dress the wound aseptically by the no-touch technique.

Skin-grafting. The final result of a burn was found to be much better in proportion to the rate at which the raw surface was covered by new epithelium. Large raw surfaces were often accompanied by anaemia and constitutional illness. Earlier skin-grafting became possible when raw surfaces were able to be rendered sterile by the local use of sulphonamide or penicillin. The common type of graft was that of split-skin, though whole-thickness grafts were sometimes used on face or hands. Autogenous grafts were always necessary. More rapid healing was sometimes obtained by use of 'postage-stamp' grafts.

Chemical burns. Burns due to strong acids or alkalies were best treated by immediate washing in running water. The correct chemical antidote was then applied. Phosphorus could be detected by its pungent smell, by the emission of fumes or (in the dark) luminosity. It stained muscle a grey colour. The essentials of treatment were to keep the part moist and allow no dry material to touch the wound, and to remove particles of phosphorus by moist gauze held on forceps; then to apply a solution of sodium bicarbonate (two teaspoonfuls to a pint of water). After that some recommended washing the part with a 1 per cent. solution of copper sulphate.

(For treatment of burns by saline baths see *Surgery*. p. 312.)

PLASTIC SURGERY

Plastic surgery developed rapidly during the war. Most of the plastic work was centred round E.M.S. units, but the Ministry of Pensions had a centre at Sidcup, which was later transferred to Roehampton and later still to Stoke Mandeville. The R.A.F. had several centres for maxillo-facial injuries and for burns. Apart from battle casualties, severe burns and frost-bite furnished many cases for the plastic surgeon.

Several new techniques came into use during the war. In 1940 split-skin grafts (aided by insufflation of sulphonamide powder) were used to make good the loss of skin over an open fracture. This gave the best results in dealing with more deeply placed bones; in older fractures the method was sometimes used at the time of the first change of plaster. Another advance was the use of metal pins to control the mobile fragments of a fractured mandible. The pins were driven into the fragments and the protruding portions were rigidly fixed by external nuts and cross-pieces.

In 1941 Mowlem introduced the cancellous-chip bone-graft. Chips of bone (from the iliac crest) of a size 1 by ·5 by ·2 cm. were inserted to fill the gap or defect. In about ten days, even when septic discharge had only recently ceased, the mass was clinically united. This method could be used for gaps in the lower jaw when the ends of the bone were immobilised by dental-cap splints or external bone-pins.

Knowledge of crush-fractures of the facial bones was advanced, and McIndoe urged the necessity of correcting the resulting deformity at the earliest possible moment. At Park Prewett several patients who had lost both lower lip and mandible were successfully treated in stages. Fan-flaps from the cheek made the 'mouth-ring', then the gap below was closed by a mucosal flap on the inner side, and a large rotation-flap from the neck on the outside. The mandible was then bone-grafted, and finally a buccal inlay prepared the way for a lower denture.

The Padgett dermatome simplified the cutting of skin-grafts. The grafting of a raw surface by many small grafts about one-fifth of an inch apart, led to quicker healing. Sano recommended fibrin-glue to attach the graft to its bed. Some used tissue extract or thrombin for the same purpose. Only homografts survived. The difficult deformity resulting from loss of skin (and sometimes tendons) on the back of the hand was remedied by excision of the scar, followed by whole-skin graft and tendon graft (Cuthbert).

In addition to the plastic work done in England and Scotland, there were six Army maxillo-facial units and two Indian Army units which did good service in the different theatres of war. An important administrative step was the formation of forward units which, by early and prompt treatment, often saved the patient many months of stay in hospital. It was found advantageous to associate maxillo-facial units with other specialist units, notably neuro-surgical and ophthalmic. It was agreed that a consultant in plastic surgery should be available to visit units in the field as well as home units, and that nurses experienced in that special kind of work should be provided. One advantage of having a forward maxillo-facial unit was that facial wounds could receive earlier skilful treatment. The greater number of battle-wounds of the face lent themselves well to primary closure. This avoided the sepsis inseparable from the dribbling of saliva over the wound and consequently reduced the number of operations and expedited return of the patient to duty. Tracheotomies were seldom needed, for better air-entry was facilitated by transporting the wounded in the prone position with the head downwards, by external fixation of the middle fragment of the jaw, and by the introduction of a wide bore nasopharyngeal tube when necessary.

The anaesthetic for most patients was induction with pentothal, followed by intubation and continuation of the anaesthetic by inhalation anaesthesia, using the Oxford vaporiser or the Heidbrink apparatus. (For the technical improvements for maxillo-facial injuries *see* Chapter 9, in *Surgery*.)

NEUROSURGERY. THE SKULL AND BRAIN

The War of 1939–45 was the first war in which any military force developed an effective organisation for the segregation of patients with wounds of the head. Special neurosurgical centres were provided by the E.M.S. and by the Scottish Board of Health. In the Army the outstanding feature of the new Head Injury Service was the creation of mobile neurosurgical units. There were eight such units which all proved their worth. The Royal Navy had its own neurosurgical service. The R.A.F. made use of the centres provided outside their Service.

Before the war too often a head injury was followed by a long period of invalidism, mainly because the patient developed a neurosis. It was found that after a head injury persons with an unstable pre-traumatic personality did not adjust themselves well to life in the Fighting Services; they had a better chance of avoiding a neurosis if they were promptly returned to civil life.

Journeys of several hours were well borne by patients suffering from head injury, so that it was usually safe to evacuate them to a neuro-surgical centre. In all campaigns effective segregation of head cases depended largely on air evacuation. The majority were operated on within forty-eight hours of injury. In over 80 per cent. of those who survived the initial brain damage, wounds healed by first intention. In non-penetrating wounds the death-rate was under one per cent., and the mortality from infective penetrating wounds was as low as five per cent.

In 1943 it was found that the adequate local use of penicillin provided a measure of control of the severely-infected head wound never before attained, and in grossly infected wounds and brain-fungus, systemic penicillin proved of great value.

Early excision of the wound, débridement of the injured track in the brain by suction, and primary closure became the rule. In 1944 the use of fibrin-foam was introduced to stop bleeding from brain cavities and venous sinuses. Blood transfusion was often needed. Most neuro-surgeons preferred general anaesthesia for their patients. Pentothal by intravenous drip, or pentothal followed by intra-tracheal gas, oxygen and ether, or by cyclopropane, were the methods of choice.

The late prognosis of penetrating wounds was fair. The patients adapted themselves to their handicaps and after the first year the general health and working capacity greatly improved. Ritchie Russell found that 55 out of 200 patients with penetrating head wounds had not attempted any work eighteen months after the injury.

Dural tears accompanying blunt head injuries were not uncommon, particularly when there was a fracture of the anterior fossa and the air-sinuses. Careful radiological examination was necessary to reveal fractures of the roofs of the ethmoidal sinuses. Compound blunt injuries of the frontal region were treated by débridement of the cranial wound, drainage of the paranasal sinuses into the nose, sealing off the subdural and subarachnoid spaces, and closure of the scalp without drainage.

Missile wounds of the air sinuses and dura might take many forms. Many needed the co-operation of the maxillo-facial, dental and plastic surgeons. The removal of completely loose or contaminated fragments of bone was usually all that was necessary to avoid all complications which might arise from faulty drainage of damaged air sinuses.

Wounds of venous sinuses sometimes bled freely. The bleeding was controlled by finger pressure, and when the tear was exposed, artery forceps were clipped on to the torn margins of the dura and allowed to hang over so as to occlude the sinus. Fibrin-foam or muscle was then applied.

Infection in head wounds was largely controlled by chemotherapy, but various delayed infections occurred. The recognition of cerebral abscess was not always easy. When there was local pain and swelling and the X-ray showed indriven bone chips in the substance of the brain, an abscess could be suspected. Among 354 cases of brain wound there were 23 instances of intra-cranial abscess, with four fatalities. One patient recovered, under treatment by penicillin, though both cavernous and lateral sinuses were thrombosed. Meningitis occurred in ten per cent. of brain wounds; it was more common with trans- or para-ventricular wounds. Late meningitis usually spread from the paranasal sinuses through an overlying dural tear.

Brain-fungus almost always meant infection, ensuing after brain tissue had been destroyed by a shearing stress. Treatment was the administration of sulphadiazine and penicillin systemically, and the application of penicillin-sulphamezathine locally. Sulphathiazole was never to be applied locally to brain tissue.

Chronic abscesses often showed few symptoms. Occasional purulent discharge from an old wound, headache, vomiting, or an epileptic fit, might suggest abscess, and ventriculography might show deformity of the affected part. The best treatment of a chronic abscess was complete excision of the abscess with capsule; infection was kept under control by sulphadiazine and penicillin. Among 354 patients with penetrating wounds of the head, 49 developed major infection, but only 19 died from infection.

The Prevention of head injuries. The experiences of the war proved beyond question that the wearing of crash helmets by motor cyclists greatly reduced the incidence and severity of head injuries. On the recommendation of Sir Hugh Cairns, the Army Council made it compulsory for all motor cyclists in the Army to wear crash helmets.

There is no doubt that the adoption of a crash helmet as standard wear by all civilian motor cyclists has resulted in much saving of life, of working time and of time in hospitals.

Concussion. Views on the nature of concussion developed during the war. Basing his arguments on some remarkable clinical data Jefferson concluded that unconsciousness, or as he preferred to call it, the traumatic stupor of concussion, was produced by a low level lesion— hypothalamic and brain-stem—and he coined a new word 'parasomnia' to indicate the condition. The word parasomnia was defined as a state following injury in which there are no responses to stimuli, verbal or mechanical, except those of a reflex nature. From a study of closed head injuries Jefferson concluded that unconsciousness was in itself the most serious single sign. Rapid death was due to brain-stem contusion.

Treatment of concussion. One of the surprises of the war was the proof that the prognosis of concussion was not so bad as it had previously been thought to be. In treatment dehydration was found to be unnecessary and was abandoned. The 'head-low' position was also given up, and, if the patient was able to swallow well, the head was kept high. The lumbar intrathecal pressure was not regarded as of such importance as had previously been held. Often there was no blood in the cerebral-spinal fluid in cases of concussion.

Headache as a sequel of concussion was regarded as more often due to psychical than physical causes. This naturally led to the policy of systematic rehabilitation beginning as soon as possible after recovery of consciousness.

Intra-cranial and intra-cerebral haematoma. It was recommended (Schorstein) that the dura mater should only be opened in patients who gave evidence of widespread inhibition of cerebral function. Linear incision of the dura was sufficient. With a deep collection of blood the X-rays sometimes showed a circular arrangement of indriven bone-fragments.

Electro-encephalography in head injuries. In the acute stage there were widespread abnormalities which affected all parts of the cortex; later local abnormalities persisted. The irregularities consisted of widespread abnormally slow waves whose frequency varied from less than $\frac{1}{2}$ per second up to 7 a second, a suppression of the normal dominant frequencies of 8 to 12 per second and clear-cut outbursts of high-voltage sine waves of 2 to 3 per second. (Denis Williams).

Late effects. It was found that 50 per cent. of patients who had suffered head injuries had an abnormal E.E.G. It was almost always generalised and of low voltage, 2 to 7 a second slow waves underlying the more rapid dominant waves. The E.E.G. was of assistance in diagnosing subdural haemorrhage.

The rehabilitation of patients who had suffered a head injury was carried out at special centres, specially equipped. The results transformed the prognosis of this serious class of case.

INJURIES OF THE SPINAL CORD

During the Second World War a fundamental change took place in the whole conception of the treatment and prognosis of paraplegic patients. In the First World War and the inter-war period the outlook for those afflicted with injury of the spinal cord was almost hopeless. It was thought little could be done for them, and in fact little was attempted for them. The mortality within three years of the injury was 80 per cent. and those who survived lived a miserable life. Factors which made for better treatment were better facilities for transport, a more conservative attitude towards laminectomy, the advent of blood transfusion, and the introduction of chemotherapy to combat sepsis.

During the course of the War of 1939–45 ten special spinal units were set up in different parts of the country, and adequate technical staff and facilities were provided. Into these centres patients were admitted suffering from cord-lesions due to other causes than gun-shot wounds—e.g., Pott's disease, syringomyelia, amyotrophic lateral sclerosis, etc. The majority of lesions were in the distal parts of the cord and in the cauda equina.

The death rate of spinal casualties in the Second World War was reduced to 9·3 per cent. The major factor in the mortality was not the completeness nor the level of the cord injury, but the degree of care and attention to the prevention and cure of urinary infection and pressure sores.

Patients were admitted at varying dates after injury. Sometimes there had already developed multiple pressure sores and infection of the bladder; occasionally also the condition was complicated by severe contractures or a deteriorated mental state.

Ludwig Guttmann found that the accepted opinion that there was a characteristic reflex pattern for a particular type of cord lesion was not correct. The pattern of spasticity was considerably influenced by the attitudes and posture of the paraplegic in the early stages after injury. Experience also showed that the isolated spinal cord was capable of some re-adaptive change. Under appropriate stimuli local reflex arcs were capable of producing useful static reflexes. Thus by training it was possible to rehabilitate the paraplegic. It was possible to mobilise and utilise certain muscle-groups of the trunk which, by their attachment to the pelvis and spine, could restore the upright position, permit standing, and maintain postural control. By exercising and over-developing the latissimus dorsi, which has attachments to the pelvis, spine, ribs and humerus, a new pattern of postural sensibility was developed, for the muscle is supplied from the brachial plexus above most traumatic spinal lesions.

After a complete lesion of the spinal cord the disturbance of the autonomic nerve-supply led to a failure of regulation of blood-pressure, blood-flow and body temperature, which imposed great limitations on the paraplegic patient. These postural circulatory disturbances could be overcome by systematic exercises. The isolated cord itself played a part in this adaptation.

In high lesions of the cord, deep inspiration elicited vaso-constriction and prevented or delayed the fainting which would otherwise have occurred from any postural hypotension. The paraplegic could be trained to compensate for the paralysis of the intercostals by the over-development of the auxiliary muscles of inspiration.

Guttmann, by using the quinizarin method of testing, showed how the capability of sweating could help to diagnose the level of the cord lesion. He also demonstrated that sweating and other reflex responses of autonomic mechanism could be elicited in the upper part of the body by certain stimuli originating in the paralysed parts of the body, especially by distension of the bladder. In high cord lesions distension of the bladder was accompanied by patchy vaso-dilatation in the face and neck; thus the facial appearance often gave the signal for immediate attention to the bladder.

MANAGEMENT OF PATIENTS WITH INJURY OF THE SPINAL CORD

First aid. The patient was warned not to move. Hard objects were removed from pockets, and pillows or a blanket placed under the calves. Body heat was preserved by covering the patient with blankets. Whether carried in the prone or supine position the patient was always to be moved gently by three or five persons. He was to be 'shifted and moved in such a way as not to be bent either backwards or forwards'. Fluid by the mouth was restricted for 24 hours, and shock was treated by blood transfusion, if necessary. Patients with cord injury had high priority for evacuation by air.

Surgical aspect. The general view was in favour of the non-operative reduction of dislocations and fractures of the spine which were accompanied by complete lesions of the cord. Hyper-extension of the spine in a physiological position was satisfactorily achieved by placing a blanket roll under the sorbo mattress, and gradually increasing the extension. In cervical lesions, skull-traction by Crutchfield tongs was the accepted practice.

Prolonged immobilisation and recumbency were discouraged because they led to stagnation in the renal system with consequent pyelitis and stone-formation. Plaster jackets and beds were considered bad forms of treatment, for they often caused dreadful pressure sores and contractures. They were only sanctioned for purposes of transport.

In open spinal injuries early operation was required to perform débridement and remove foreign bodies. Dural tears were closed and penicillin and streptomycin applied locally. Intact dura was not opened unless there was evidence of subdural haematoma.

With closed spinal injuries accompanied by complete paraplegia immediate laminectomy was not recommended. Even when the paraplegia was incomplete it was wiser to postpone operation.

Early laminectomy was indicated, not only for open spinal injuries but for incomplete lesions in which the neurological signs gradually increased. It might also be required for the rare condition of severe irritation of the spinal roots, or for permanent manometric block without evidence of fracture.

Late laminectomy was recommended for incomplete spinal syndromes with increasing neurological symptoms; it was seldom indicated for complete lesions at any level.

Relief of spasticity was accomplished by diminishing stimuli (constipation or full bladder), placing the limb in correct position, and by passive movements of the paralysed spastic legs. The standing position in parallel bars enabled the patient to overcome exaggerated action of the flexors of the lower limb. The value of drugs was doubtful. Resection of the obturator nerve was sometimes needed for severe adductor spasms. Intrathecal injections of 80 per cent. alcohol proved very effective in relieving severe spasticity, and at the same time relieved pain. Rhizotomy was not called for. A factor which predisposed to pain was a lowered general condition of the patient, due to infection; relief was obtained by improving the general condition and adopting proper psychological measures, e.g., by giving pre-vocational training. Sedatives were reduced to a minimum.

The treatment of the paralysed bladder. If voluntary or reflex micturition had not developed within 24 to 48 hours, continuous drainage of the bladder was needed. Urethral catheterisation, carried out by strict no-touch technique by experienced medical officers, was a satisfactory method favoured by some. (For technique *see* page 465 of *Surgery.*) An alternative method was the open insertion of a small catheter into the upper part of the distended bladder in an oblique downward direction; the closed method of insertion (Riches) was very suitable. The sooner suprapubic drainage was discontinued, the better was the prospect. The patient gradually learnt to appreciate the fullness of the bladder and to induce emptying by certain trick mechanisms. Most paraplegics needed a urinal but incontinence was overcome by training the patient to adjust the frequency of micturition to the amount of fluid taken.

Urinary infection was prevented by avoiding prolonged recumbency and by encouraging active movements; by ensuring that the patient drank about five pints a day (of tea, barley water, or fruit juices); and by regular or intermittent bladder washouts or tidal drainage. The older urinary antiseptics could be used but a new era in the treatment of urinary infection of the paralysed bladder was begun with the discovery of streptomycin, aureomycin and chloromycetin, which were powerful agents against gram-negative organisms. Streptomycin was not so useful when there was obstruction in the urinary tract, or when there were calculi, or undrained abscesses. Calculosis was prevented or diminished by proper drainage, frequent change of posture, restoration of the upright posture, physical activity and acidifying of the urine.

In the early stages of an acute transverse spinal lesion benefit was gained by intramuscular injection of $0 \cdot 5$ to $1 \cdot 0$ mg. of prostigmine every four to seven hours, for this helped to overcome intestinal paralysis. In later stages constipation had to be prevented.

The stimulating effect of prostigmine ($\cdot 3$ mg. intrathecally) on the reproductive organs was used to distinguish varying degrees of reproductive deficiency, and to rehabilitate the sexual function of paraplegic patients.

The skin needed to be kept in good hygienic condition, particularly in those areas likely to be soiled by urine or faeces. The soles and heels were never allowed to become scaly, and toe-nails were carefully trimmed. Hot water bottles were never used; instead, woollen socks were worn in bed. Great care was used to prevent burns from hot water pipes, open fireplaces or electric fires.

Pressure sores. The incidence of pressure sores was very high. They were chiefly found on skeletal prominences and varied from a reddening of the skin to a deep necrosis. Infection, and the loss of protein-containing discharge from these sores was one of the main causes of nutritional deficiency. Acute nutritional deficiency was best countered by blood transfusion, by a special diet rich in protein and vitamins, by the administration of liver extract or B.12 injections, and by iron.

Prevention of sores was attained by cleansing and hardening the skin, by frequent change of posture, and by redistributing the pressure by the use of a rigid bed with an air or sorbo mattress. Pillows placed under the calves prevented sores on the heels.

Cure of pressure-sores necessitated the treatment of anaemia and of the nutritional deficiency. The maintenance of the prone position for several hours at a time was helpful. Sloughs were freely excised and adequate drainage provided. Various local applications were used—flavazole 1 in 2,000, boric acid solution, phenoxetol $2 \cdot 4$ per cent., Milton 5 per cent., streptomycin or penicillin, according to the type of infection and stage of healing. The patient was taught to be pressure-conscious. Excision of the scar with resection of the callous or macerated underlying bone followed by primary suture, gave good results in the case of sacral or trochanteric scars of moderate size. The great majority of sores were healed by conservative means.

Mental condition. Careful psychological handling of the paraplegic was most essential. The creation of a cheerful atmosphere and good morale was striven after.

The Rehabilitation of the paraplegic. The two fundamentals in the physical treatment of the paraplegic were an early start and a continuity of treatment. The paralysed limbs were placed (not fixed) in the correct position and passive movements were carried out several times a day. Daily electrical stimulation of denervated muscles was carried out. Those muscles necessary for the upright position (latissimus dorsi, trapezius, abdominal and long back muscles) were caused to hypertrophy by regular exercises. Restoration of postural sensibility was encouraged by exercises performed in front of a mirror. Vaso-motor control was re-adjusted by frequent change of posture and breathing exercises. The patient was trained to dress himself and even to stand and walk with arm or elbow crutches. Cumbersome appliances were not used but walking calipers were sufficient. Sport was of the greatest assistance—darts, billiards, skittles, punch-ball, netball, and archery. Cultural entertainments were encouraged and useful work often helped to complete the rehabilitation. Quite a number were able to look after themselves at home, or in special residential settlements. (See *Surgery*. pp. 422–516.)

PERIPHERAL NERVE INJURIES

Service patients with peripheral nerve injuries were segregated in special centres specially staffed by medical officers experienced in the diagnosis and treatment of such injuries. Local and general remedial therapy was begun in hospital and continued after discharge from the centre. No elaborate appliances were used in sensory examination or in grading muscular power. Electrically, the ordinary galvanic and faradic apparatus was inadequate; most useful information was obtained from the strength-duration curves. Electro-myography was clinically useful. In 1942 Seddon introduced three new terms. Neurotmesis implied a nerve either divided, or interrupted by scar tissue which prevented regeneration. In axonotmesis complete degeneration resulted but repair took place readily since the endoneural tubes were preserved. With neurapraxia there was a local degeneration of the myelin sheath leading to temporary paralysis and sometimes loss of sensation.

Causalgia was seen less frequently than in the First World War. The pain caused by it, if persistent, was best relieved by upper thoracic ganglionectomy. The most important factor in keeping the limb in a healthy condition while under treatment was the preservation of mobility. Persistent over-stretching of a paralysed muscle was very damaging. If splints were used it was essential to put the paralysed part through a full range of movement at least once daily.

In war wounds primary repair of a nerve was inferior to early secondary suture. At the initial treatment of the wound the nerve-ends were tacked together, and the wound closed. Secondary suture was done three or four weeks later. Of those wounds which arrived at the centres, every case which showed signs of complete loss of conductivity was explored, unless the early notes contra-indicated this. The greatest extent of the gap which could be closed with fair prospect of success was, for the median 7 to 7·5 cm., for the radial 7·5 (with anterior transposition) to 5·3 cm. (without transposition), for the ulnar about 6·0 cm. Any suture requiring more than 90 to 100 degrees of flexion of a joint ran a risk of failure. Autogenous nerve-grafts, cable grafts, and nerve pedicle grafting were sometimes successful. Fibrin-clot was used to glue small nerve stumps together. In suitable cases satisfactory results were obtained in most patients with radial, median and internal popliteal nerve injury. Repair of the ulnar nerve proximal to the elbow was hardly worth attempting, and repair of the lateral popliteal was rarely successful.

VASCULAR INJURIES

The outlook for a patient with a vascular injury was better than in the First World War, but this was largely due to better organisation. Operations for removal of a foreign body from the heart were performed a number of times by the Americans. The great development of cardiac surgery took place after the war.

THORACIC SURGERY

Thoracic surgery had begun to advance towards the end of the First World War; it developed rapidly between the two world wars, and became a robust and efficient specialty during the Second World War. It was greatly helped by the improvement in anaesthesia, the availability of blood transfusion and the introduction of the sulphonamides and penicillin. Special centres for thoracic surgery were organised and numbers of young surgeons were trained in the specialty. Mobile thoracic teams were made available to travel to any region where they were needed. The bombing of industrial towns resulted in many thoracic wounds.

With thoracic wounds several special points needed attention. Paradoxical respiration was controlled by effective strapping. Acute dilatation of the stomach had to be looked for and guarded against.

Bronchial secretions required evacuation by postural treatment, by encouragement of coughing, or by direct intra-bronchial suction. The treatment of haemothorax went through several stages, starting with aspiration and air-replacement, going on to open operation and removal of the clots. It was only in 1942 that decortication became the rule.

Apart from the hastened general evolution of thoracic surgical organisation, the great contribution of the war-time thoracic surgery to civilian work was the advance in the treatment of clotted haemothorax. During the acute phase of haemorrhage and exudation the lung was collapsed, compressed and often grossly distorted. Superadded infection led to the formation of a large chronic empyema, which was perpetuated by rib-resection and drainage. Decortication proved to be the remedy. If, after formal thoracotomy and clearing out the clot, the lung did not expand when inflated by the anaesthetist, decortication was performed. The display of the compressed distorted lung and its immediate conversion after decortication into a freely aerating normal sized organ, was one of the most dramatic sights of surgery. The cortex might be thin and filmy or as much as 0·5 to 1 cm. in thickness. Lung expansion was maintained by closed pleural drainage, and by ensuring that bronchial secretions were removed by suction. Two intercostal tubes were used for pleural drainage, one at the base and one high up in the back. For 12 to 24 hours they were attached to simple underwater seals; after that time suction could be applied if the lung had not fully expanded. Usually the tubes were removed within three to five days. The patient could be out of bed in 2 to 3 days and the wound healed in 10 to 20 days.

Post-operative physical treatment ensured perfect chest expansion. Often the patient returned to his unit with only temporary or slight down-grading. In chronic empyema excellent results were also obtained by similar methods.

In the Field. In the field the surgery of thoracic wounds had two phases. The first phase was carried out at the forward surgical unit, or advanced casualty clearing station; the chief duty here was to aspirate any haemothorax, though when haemorrhage was continuing operation was necessary. Open sucking wounds were formally excised, the haemothorax sucked out and the thorax closed by suture of muscles. The skin was left open for delayed primary suture.

The second phase took place at the chest centre at the base hospital. The members of the chest team consulted together over each patient. Clinical and radiological examinations were made, aspiration done if needed, the bronchi drained or sucked dry, and blood given if required. Delayed primary suture was then carried out when justified, or major operative interference undertaken when indicated. The physiotherapist greatly helped in the re-establishment of full respiration.

The old view that major thoracotomy in the presence of pleural infection was dangerous, was abandoned. The use of penicillin, though not essential, made this procedure safer.

In the Italian theatre of war the tendency was to remove all retained metallic foreign bodies of the size of 1 cm. or more. The results were very satisfactory.

RADIOLOGY

X-ray examinations at advanced surgical centres were only considered necessary when the findings were expected to affect immediate treatment or the disposal of the patient. Routine radiography was out of the question. The radiologist was responsible to the commanding officer.

Most radiological war work concerned injuries of the extremities, and the radiologist had to be acquainted with the special types of fractures incidental to flying, to paratrooping and to marching. In war wounds of the chest Hodson demonstrated three types of missile track in the lung which could be shown radiologically: hollow tracks, solid tracks, and tracks outlined by metallic fragments. In abdominal wounds X-rays might show the site of a foreign body, give evidence of free gas or distended gut, indicate the track of a missile or point to a retroperitoneal haematoma.

Radiography of a lung injured by aerial blast showed areas of mottling in the periphery of the lower lobes and sometimes areas of collapse; the upper parts of the lung were often emphysematous. X-rays also served to help in the diagnosis of haematoma of the lung, mediastinal emphysema, traumatic asphyxia, and sometimes fat embolism. (For details of technique see *Surgery*. Chapter 14.)

OPHTHALMOLOGY

Night vision. Tests were carried out to distinguish those with good from those with defective night vision. Individuals varied greatly in this respect, but there was no relation between the amount of vitamin A in the diet and defective night vision. Night blindness was so easy to simulate and so rare in fact that an official notice was issued to the effect that the Army did not recognise night blindness. From the practical point of view that solved the problem.

Ophthalmic casualties formed 2·5 per cent. of all casualties in battle. They were often grouped, for purposes of treatment, with the neuro-surgical and maxillo-facial patients.

Concussion injuries were common; in the majority of blast injuries a traumatic keratitis developed. Visors were sometimes used to protect the eyes from missiles; superficial and larger particles in the cornea were removed, but persistent efforts to remove more deeply embedded particles did harm. Magnetic metal fragments were often extracted by the aid of a magnet. Deep particles of cordite or quartz did not cause much inconvenience, but retained copper particles caused pathological changes.

The final effect on vision of through-and-through wounds of the globe depended upon the size of the entering fragment. Sepsis was reduced by care in dressing the eye, and by the use of sulphonamides and penicillin. Sympathetic ophthalmia was exceedingly rare.

Disease of the eye due to dietetic deficiencies occurred on an epidemic scale among the British prisoners-of-war held by the Japanese in camps in Asia. It took the form either of a granular keratitis which responded well to the administration of Marmite, or of paracentral or central scotomata due to a demyelination of the optic nerve. The latter was due to the lack of first-class protein and portions of vitamin B complex from the diet.

Localisation of fragments of missiles in the orbit by radiological means was greatly improved. The more exact methods comprised the techniques of Sweet, McGregor and Comberg, and later Bromley and Lyle's 'eye localiser', and the limbus ring and equatorial techniques.

OTO-RHINO-LARYNGOLOGY

In the War of 1939–45 specialists in diseases of the ear, nose and throat were provided in a better manner and more adequate numbers than in any previous war. A consultant with the rank of brigadier was also appointed as adviser to the Army. The Admiralty had a civilian consultant and several specialists. In the R.A.F. there was a regular medical officer who combined specialist knowledge with long experience, and he both organised the service in this department and also supervised research. In the E.M.S. regional consultants in oto-laryngology were appointed.

Chronic otitis media led to the greatest loss of fighting power. Though at home the results of treatment of this condition were most encouraging, it was found that relapse almost invariably occurred when the patient went on active service abroad. A man with chronic otitis media never paid a dividend in fighting efficiency. The condition was an absolute bar to service in submarines, in diving, or in the Fleet Air Arm.

Otitis externa was also troublesome.

Motion sickness was rare in the R.A.F. but was more common among the commando personnel in landing craft. Ruptured tympanic membrane was not an uncommon lesion and was often due to blast, either from bomb or gunfire. Cochlear deafness, either acute or gradual, also often occurred from the effects of gunfire. Rubber ear plugs or cotton wool packing in the external ear served as protection against blast.

Barotrauma. The term barotrauma was introduced to signify that condition accompanied by aural pain and deafness, in which the barometric pressure in the middle ear differed from that in the surrounding atmosphere. It was due to blocking of the eustachian tube which was more likely to occur when there was some naso-pharyngitis.

Barotrauma usually occurred in making rapid descents. Sinus barotrauma was a similar condition due to sinusitis. The symptoms were aural pain, deafness, inability to clear the ears, tinnitus, and sometimes vertigo. It persisted until landing was effected but was immediately relieved by restoration of the intra-tympanic pressure by auto-inflation, catheterisation, or by politzerisation. It was usual to 'ground' those who were suffering from head colds if Valsalva's test were negative. Mild attacks of barotrauma occurred more readily in fatigued persons.

In the Navy trainees for offensive diving were trained to perform Valsalva's test under different conditions and pressures, and were encouraged to clear the ears at an early period when diving. Barotrauma was accompanied by varying degrees of congestion of the membrana tympani.

Treatment of barotrauma was by steam inhalation and occasional politzerisation. Irradiation of the lymphoid tissue in the nasopharynx—a dosage of 1,200 r. spread over 14 days—was beneficial. A better hearing test was introduced and consisted of two parts. The first was designed to give a rough form of pure tone audiogram, and the other to indicate whether an individual was likely to be able to work in a loud noise, and to receive speech signals in such a noise. The former consisted of testing by a series of pure tone signals at a low intensity.

GENITO-URINARY SURGERY

No great advance in genito-urinary surgery took place during the war. Gunshot wounds of the urethra were sometimes treated at special centres. Haemorrhage was stopped, the urine diverted (in any serious wound) by suprapubic cystostomy and the continuity of the urethra restored as soon as possible.

Traumatic uraemia occurred in some severely wounded patients and after some crush injuries, probably due to renal anoxia. The symptoms came on from two to six days after injury; anorexia, hiccup, vomiting and oliguria were early symptoms. The patient became dull and drowsy, and cyanosis and a petechial rash might occur. If recovery were to take place the improvement occurred from the 6th to the 8th day.

In each of the Services there was a marked increase in the incidence of epididymitis for which no particular cause could be found. In an epidemic in Malta there was prodromal fever with headache, backache, and anorexia lasting about five days. After a period of normality of six days there occurred pain in the groin followed by pain and swelling of the testicle. There was a raised sedimentation-rate of the red cells.

THE EFFECTS OF BLAST

In the War of 1939–45 the injurious effects of blast were more serious than ever before. Experimentally the primary effects of blast were only experienced when close to an explosion, e.g., within 20 feet. With aerial blast the chief lesion was haemorrhage into the lungs. There might be local, scattered or confluent areas of haemorrhage, often following the lines of the ribs. Zuckerman thought the internal injuries were mainly caused by the impact of the pressure wave on the body-wall. The actual blast-pressure needed to cause death was estimated at about 400 pounds per square inch.

The clinical symptoms of aerial blast were shock, dyspnoea, cyanosis, pain in the chest and abdomen, haemoptysis, cough and restlessness. The main signs were bulging of the chest wall, poor respiratory excursion, and slight local impairment of the percussion-note, distant breath sounds, and some coarse râles. X-rays showed mottling of the lung fields.

Underwater blast from an exploding mine or a depth charge was often serious and affected chiefly those who were swimming. Those who floated on their back often escaped injury. The maximal injurious range of a charge exploding at depth was about 20 yards. The main lesions in the abdomen were haemorrhages into the wall of the intestine or perforation of the gut. The symptoms of underwater blast were sharp pain in the back or round the waist followed soon after by varying degrees of abdominal pain. Sometimes bleeding from the bowel or haematuria occurred. There might be the classical symptoms of intestinal perforation.

Treatment of blast injuries. Nearly every patient suffering from severe blast injury needed morphine to control restlessness. Great judgment was needed in giving transfusion owing to the injury to the lung. Sulphapyridine was given prophylactically and oxygen administered for the dyspnoea. Definite signs of intestinal perforation demanded operative exploration.

The mortality of underwater blast was high but varied according to the distance of the victim from the explosion, his position in the water at the moment of explosion and the presence or absence of some form of bodily protection.

THE CRUSH SYNDROME

The crush syndrome, under another name, had been described in Germany during the First World War, but it was not noted in Britain until attention was called to it by Bywaters and Beall in 1941. It was a condition which usually followed the prolonged crushing of a limb, in which, some hours after release, severe symptoms resembling shock ensued; ischaemia of the limb developed and death often resulted a few days later from anuria and uraemia. At post-mortem muscle necrosis was found and the microscopical examination of the kidneys showed changes resembling those found after a mis-matched transfusion.

The pathology appeared to be that of an ischaemic necrosis of the muscles; shock was due to the loss of plasma into the tissues. The exact cause of the renal lesion, which in severe cases led to fatal anuria, was not definitely known.

The treatment of established renal damage was difficult; threatened renal damage was treated by giving fluid and alkali bicarbonate by mouth, and lactate by vein along with plasma transfusion.

IMMERSION FOOT

Immersion foot was a term used to signify a condition of peripheral vasoneuropathy which occurred after chilling rather than freezing of the tissues. It was often seen in survivors from shipwreck. Any general debilitating condition or any local constriction of the limb helped to produce the condition. The tissue damage was due to the indirect effects of cold, particularly on the blood vessels which became constricted.

During exposure the limb was numb and swollen. After rescue the foot passed through three stages. For some hours the limb remained cold, pulseless and numb, with a 'stocking' anaesthesia. Then followed a hyperaemic stage accompanied by pain; the foot became hot and reddish-blue and blisters might form. The third stage followed a day or two later; the foot became paler and areas of gangrene might appear. Sensory recovery was slow and was accompanied by radiating pains and by hyperhidrosis. The nerves showed degeneration but slowly recovered.

When rescued the patient was not allowed to walk but was made to lie with the feet elevated and exposed to the air. Direct application of heat to the limb was forbidden. In the second stage pain was relieved by cooling the feet with icebags, or by a fan. 21° Centigrade was the optimum temperature for therapeutic cooling. Sedatives and analgesics were required. A prophylactic injection of anti-tetanic serum was given. The feet were cleansed daily with soap and water followed by spirit, the toes were dusted with sulphanilamide powder and separated by pledgets of sterile gauze. Minor amputations were occasionally required later. Persistent hyperhidrosis and cold-sensitivity were sometimes treated by preganglionic sympathectomy.

AMPUTATIONS

The limb-fitting surgeons of the Ministry of Pensions laid down the ideal lengths (which have been given in the section on orthopaedic surgery) for amputations of both upper and lower limbs. British surgeons did not favour end-bearing amputations such as the Syme and the Stokes-Gritti, though they were used by the Canadian surgeons. Surgeons were advised not to perform a definitive amputation at a site of election unless they were reasonably certain of primary healing. It became the rule to perform a provisional amputation at a low level with a view to a higher definitive amputation later. With the advent of the sulphonamides and penicillin surgeons were often able to perform a primary definitive amputation at the site of election.

Antero-posterior skin flaps were cut, each equal to half the diameter of the limb. The deep fascia was cut through at the same level and the flaps of skin and fascia dissected up to where the bone and muscles were to be divided circularly. Neither nerves nor periosteum received any special attention. Drainage was optional. Neither the Krukenberg nor cineplastic operations were in favour with British surgeons. It was important to see that a patient fitted with an artificial limb was properly trained in its use.

THE REHABILITATION OF THE PATIENT

In the application of the methods of physical medicine there was an outstanding clinical advance during the war. The main feature was the substitution of active movement by the patient for passive movement performed on him by the physiotherapist. Moreover, general bodily activity was found to be almost as important as local activity of the affected part. Some measure of activity was increasingly employed to restore the patient's strength after almost every kind of injury or illness, unless there were some special reason for not doing so. The method was also practised in obstetric work and after almost every type of surgical operation, particularly after operations on the thorax. Active movement had a physical effect in maintaining and restoring normal circulation in the muscles and joints, and it also had a very useful mental effect in keeping up the spirits of the patient. Breathing exercises were practised both before and after operation, and general exercises were gradually undertaken by bed-fast patients as soon after operation as was practicable. As regards physiotherapeutic techniques, it was found that little result could be expected by applying them once or twice weekly; to be efficacious they needed to be applied several times daily.

Diseases and injuries of the chest. Following the lead of Dr. F. S. Cooksey, remedial exercises were found to be of great assistance in conditions affecting the thorax. Breathing exercises constituted the main feature. The value of early, vigorous and progressive breathing exercises together with early ambulation was soon established. Close liaison between the medical and the ancillary staff was essential since it was often necessary to suspend or modify the exercises from day to day. Beginning with individual treatment in bed, patients progressed to group exercises in bed, sitting group exercises in the ward, easy group exercises and games in the gymnasium or out of doors, and finally to advanced exercises and games. At each stage the exercises were increased in strength and duration until they occupied thirty minutes or longer twice or three times a day. The effect of this was seen in the full restoration of respiratory function and physical fitness.

Inspiratory exercises were used in atelectasis, pneumonia, empyema, after the removal of a lobe or lung, and as a prophylactic before and after operations on the upper abdomen. Expiratory exercises were used in asthma and chronic bronchitis, and were found useful when combined with postural drainage in lung abscess, bronchiectasis and post-operative basal congestion. Thoracoplasty for phthisis required breathing exercises for a few days after each stage to prevent atelectasis of the unaffected base, and postural bed-exercises to prevent scoliosis. Massage, electrotherapy and occupational therapy were also found useful and in some thoracic cases it was necessary for the patient to undergo vocational training for a less strenuous occupation. This was facilitated by the passing of the Disabled Persons (Employment) Act of 1944 which made provision for the training and resettlement of all disabled persons.

Foot-Strain. With the strenuous training which recruits had to undergo it was found that foot-strain became common. This sometimes resulted in painful, stiff and often swollen feet, sometimes accompanied by spasm of the extensor longus digitorum muscle. This was treated by complete rest in bed until pain and spasm had gone. Non-weight-bearing exercises were then performed in bed for several days. Then carefully graded remedial exercises were performed in classes until the patients were fit to go to a convalescent depot. Severe spasm of the extensor longus digitorum required special training to strengthen the tibialis anticus muscle.

Medical Electrology made some advances during the war, both in the direction of obtaining quantitative measurements of excitability, and of improving diagnosis and prognosis by a study of the potentials produced in muscles. Bauwens devised an apparatus whereby the amount of denervation of a muscle could be readily estimated, and Weddell, Feinstein and Pottle introduced a technique so delicate that theoretically it would be possible to detect one single motor unit among denervated ones, and a single denervated fibrillating fibre among normal ones at rest.

Occupational Therapy. Occupational therapy had been established as a useful method of therapy as early as 1930 by Dr. Elizabeth Casson. During the war great developments took place, several schools were started and occupational therapy became a very useful method of rehabilitation.

SURGERY IN A PRISONER-OF-WAR CAMP
(*Singapore Island 1942–45*)

One of the most important lessons taught by the war was that good major surgery could be successfully done under the most disadvantageous circumstances, provided that there be in control a skilful surgeon with fertile ideas for improvising, and with the requisite patience and wisdom to train subordinates in the essentials of surgical technique and of nursing. After the capitulation to the Japanese on February 15, 1942, there were 2,500 wounded to be cared for in Singapore but only accommodation for 986 was provided; the remainder had to be treated as out-patients. The Changi 'Hospital' in Roberts' Barracks was overcrowded; 140 patients were packed into a ward meant for only 40 soldiers. There was difficulty in getting water and for several months no electric light was available. Instruments and dressings had been smuggled into the hospital but sterilisers had to be heated by means of paraffin until a mechanism was improvised for obtaining steam pressure. The nursing was done by R.A.M.C. orderlies, and some Assistant Surgeons I.M.D. There was a staff of seven surgeons under the able leadership of Mr. Julian Taylor, one consultant anaesthetist, two radiologists, and several junior medical officers. There was a shortage of bed linen, pillows and mattresses. The diet was chiefly rice with a minute amount of protein furnished by some dried fish. In spite of all these disadvantages nearly all the war wounds had healed before the end of 1942 and there was a rapid return to good function in nearly all the wounded limbs.

Moreover a special fly-proof theatre was made by the Royal Engineers and to this no unhealed wound was admitted. In this theatre clean operations were performed, including nerve-suture, herniorrhaphy, bone-grafting, craniotomy, operations on joints, appendicectomy, cholecystectomy, laminectomy, and even partial gastrectomy. Gastrectomy was called for because there were many instances of severe and extensive duodenal ulceration. Operation was never performed unless the patient was in extreme pain. The operation was carried out on 22 patients, on three occasions for severe haemorrhage which had recurred after blood transfusion. Only two patients died, one from miliary tuberculosis and the other from acute oedema of the lungs. The operations were usually carried out under regional intercostal novocain or under chloroform anaesthesia. Milk powder was difficult to obtain and each patient with duodenal ulcer treated by gastrectomy could only be allowed one gallon of milk during after-treatment. Everyone will agree that 'to offer gastrectomy to a man when there are no sheets, only mattresses and perhaps pillows, shiny and black with dried shed blood, pus and sweat, is not a pleasant duty, eagerly though it was accepted', but the results justified the offer. No wonder, however, that the patients had a stormy passage in many instances, and that in some cases there was some suppuration which could not even be prevented by the sulphonamides.

Great credit was also due to the orderlies who worked in the theatre and did the nursing. The following fact needs no comment. 'From early in 1943 until the end of captivity, i.e., during two and three quarter years, not a single bedsore was seen on the surgical side', and again— 'It is to the credit of the nursing orderlies that in spite of the conditions indicated above, in spite of the malnutrition, the thin stretched skins, the fleshless bony backs, shoulders, buttocks, the muscleless legs, without linen and without rings, with no pillowcases and hardly any

Summary of Results on December 31, 1942
in Soldiers Treated in Changi

Compound fractures	489	Chest—penetrating lung.	25	
Un-united—Tibia	2	Deaths	2	
Humerus	1	Brain	25	
Ulna	1	Deaths	3	
Radius	1	Spinal cord	5	
Secondary haemorrhage	26	Deaths from urinary in-		
Deaths	6	fections	5	
Femur	37	Cauda equina	3	
Deaths	7	Deaths	0	
Hip Joint	3	Peripheral nerves	72	
Deaths	2	Nerves repaired	40	
Knee Joint	26	Aneurysms		
Deaths	8	Excision of aneurysm in 5		
Amputations 18, with sur-		patients, 1 amputation		
vivals	12	through thigh	6	
Artificial limbs—Manufacture		Deaths	0	
proceeding slowly		Abdomen	28	
		Deaths	14	

pillows, large numbers of patients suffering from grave surgical diseases were nursed to recovery'. As for the operating room attendants from the Services, the following testimony from the surgeon in charge speaks volumes—'though they may have had little experience of responsible work in theatres, such as that carried out by theatre nurses and sisters, yet they are easy to teach, are truly reliable, rapidly learn to be extremely good assistants at operations, and acquire impeccable asepsis'. The last mentioned must have been very necessary for we read that 'the theatre roofs were full of rat-droppings through which the wind would blow and the rain would drip'. It was found that with a thorough use of soap and water there was not much need for antiseptics.

A very good idea of the results obtained under the terrible conditions above related can be seen by studying the table of statistics of war wounds treated on p. 464.

PART II

Canada

The Canadian Medical Services

By William R. Feasby, B.A., M.D.

Detailed official accounts of the work of the Canadian Medical Services during the Second World War will be found in the following volumes:*

Vol. I   Organisation and Campaigns ⎫
                                      ⎬ W. R. Feasby
Vol. II   Clinical Subjects   ⎭

---

* Published by Edmond Cloutier, Ottawa, Queen's Printer and Controller of Stationery.

CONTENTS

I—ORGANISATION OF THE MEDICAL SERVICES IN THE ARMY AND THE ROYAL CANADIAN ARMY MEDICAL CORPS

EARLY HISTORY

THE early history of the Medical Corps dates from 1885, the year of the North-west Rebellion, when troops were sent to crush Riel and his followers. It was Lieutenant-Colonel Darby Bergin, a surgeon of Cornwall, Ontario, who directed the first military medical corps. After this brief campaign we see the first dissolution of a medical force as a prelude to a long gap before the next emergency arose, with consequent lack of preparation and orientation of a medical service.

It was not until February 1898 that a Director General of Medical Staff was appointed; in 1899 a Canadian Army Militia Medical Department was created. During the South African War certain units served. In 1904 an Army Medical Staff and the Army Medical Staff Corps were formed with only a small permanent establishment. It was not until Great Britain inaugurated the Royal Army Medical Corps in 1898 that military medicine began to have a proper relationship to the other arms of the Service.

THE FIRST WORLD WAR, 1914–18

It was during this period that the C.A.M.C. faced a great test of organisation. Because of the length of the war and the great demands for men there was a constant increase in the number of active military medical units in the field; and, beginning with less than a hundred personnel, the strength overseas had increased by June 1918 to 15,519 all ranks and the number of units had increased to 68, of which 37 were hospitals of various types. The C.A.M.C. proved equal to the rapid and enormous expansion experienced. There were minor failures and one major investigation but as Sir Andrew MacPhail, the official historian wrote: 'The Canadian Army held the field for four years without any of those failures in the medical service by which so many campaigns have been marred.'* In 1916 a serious controversy over the administration of the corps developed and a bitter dispute arose which led eventually to the resignation of the Minister of Militia and Defence in 1916. Thereafter, the system of controlling the overseas force was reorganised to ensure as nearly as possible the correct division of

---

* MacPhail, Sir Andrew—*Official History of the Canadian Forces in the Great War 1914–1919; The Medical Services.* p. 402.

responsibility between the civil and the military authorities. This dispute represented a fundamental problem which confronts all who manage armed military forces, and its resolution in this instance was never satisfactorily achieved. During the First World War a Military Hospital Commission was formed to take charge of returning casualties, but this civilian organisation, completely independent of the military authorities, eventually assumed control of hospital arrangements for all casualties and for those originating in the units stationed in Canada. This arrangement was not satisfactory and a large number of hospitals operated by the Commission were taken over by the Department of Militia and Defence; all military patients were brought under the control of the Adjutant General until they were discharged to civil life. At this time they became the responsibility of the Department of Soldiers, Civil Re-establishment. These incidents are related to indicate that certain problems recur; these are connected with the provision of medical services for men who enter the armed forces on a temporary basis during war-time.

THE INTER-WAR YEARS, 1919–39

During this period financial economy dominated the pattern of the medical services and the strength of all units was greatly reduced. By 1936 the international situation had reached such a point, with the Japanese invasion of Manchuria in 1931, that the implication in terms of national defence could no longer be ignored. Appropriations for military defence were greatly increased and as a result there were some increases in the number of serving medical officers, but even so on March 31, 1939 the R.C.A.M.C. could muster only 4,169 all ranks. Although it was such a small force this Corps held many responsibilities during the economic depression of the thirties. Among others was the formation of a section to deal with the new air force medical problems, and with the work camps for the unemployed. During this period, also, many units were formed in the Non-Permanent Active Militia, and although these units received the designation of R.C.A.M.C. (N.P.) they were an important factor during the mobilisation period of 1939. Training was seriously hampered during this period by lack of equipment and it is not surprising that the medical corps faced the opening months of war with inadequate personnel, relatively poor training and equipment that was already obsolete.

MOBILISATION PLANS

A general plan of mobilisation had been prepared and was in readiness early in 1939. Unfortunately the Director General of Medical Services was not fully informed of the medical plans and he was frustrated in his efforts to secure an adequate mobilisation document for the medical forces that would be required. There were long delays, up to two years, in the approval of the D.G.M.S.'s plans for the mobilisation of base hospitals in the so-called intermediate zone. At this time Major-General E. C. Ashton (Chief of the General Staff), and himself a physician, expressed complete dissatisfaction with the medical planning and especially with hospital arrangements. He stated: 'Apparently the D.G.M.S. has been earnestly endeavouring to press forward the arrangements in connexion with medical services for some years. He does not appear to have been given the necessary information.'

It was at this stage that a long and distressing argument developed between the Department of National Defence and the Department of Pensions and National Health. The Deputy Minister of the latter department, Dr. R. E. Wodehouse, raised the question before a standing inter-departmental committee on defence co-ordination which had been formed by the Government in May 1938. He put forward the suggestion that the R.C.A.M.C. ought to look after casualties in field units, but that the Department of Pensions and National Health should provide all other tretament for those in military service in Canada. It was implied that the Department of National Defence would only clear casualties from the fields of conflict and that thereafter their care would be the responsibility of the Department of Pensions and National Health. Finally, the offer of the Department of Pensions and National Health was accepted on a provisional basis until the armed forces could provide hospitalisation for the troops under their command. This was only one example of the lack of preparedness in the armed forces. The D.G.M.S. had done his utmost to make the necessary arrangements for hospitalisation of casualties in Canada and at bases outside Canada. He had met with complete lack of co-operation and there was inadequate planning in this field. Similarly, over the medical examination of recruits there were many misunderstandings, which were not cleared up until the issue of the new publication in 1938. Even with this document there had been many delays in securing the necessary definitions of categories. The question of adding a chest X-ray examination and that of enlisting personnel of categories lower than A, for whom remedial measures could be provided, had yet to be decided. Finally, in May 1939, decisions were reached; in addition, new medical records were required and urine analysis was added to the examination procedure. In other ways planning was delayed and inadequate; the provision of mobilisation plans in the districts could not be completed because the district medical officers were to be informed by the D.G.M.S., who himself had no adequate information about mobilisation.

In June and early August of 1939 an Adjutant General's Branch representative was sent hurriedly to all military districts in order to bring about revisions of mobilisation schemes. He recommended the use of civilian practitioners to implement the mobilisation medical plans. A scheme was recommended as a practice exercise for the integration of such personnel, but it was too late by now to put it into operation.

THE FIRST MONTHS OF THE WAR

On August 25 war was apparently inevitable, and orders were despatched to district officers commanding to mobilise certain units. Since the Government had decided on a policy of active defence of the Canadian shores and territorial waters and of adjacent British Possessions, combined with extensive economic assistance to Great Britain and France, only one corps of two divisions with ancillary troops was to be mobilised as part of a Canadian Active Service Force for overseas duty. The R.C.A.M.C. was seriously affected by the limitations placed at various times on mobilisation; it was more serious since the Department of Pensions and National Health made a determined effort to secure permanent control of the treatment and hospitalisation of all military patients in Canada. At the same time problems relating to the examination of recruits occurred. In spite of these difficulties active service units were mobilised quickly and their strength rapidly completed; others, however, were deferred in keeping with the national policy of limiting the forces who were to serve abroad. Matters actually reached a climax when, on September 18 the Adjutant General found himself with a draft Order in Council which relieved the R.C.A.M.C. permanently of all responsibility for the treatment of military patients in Canada. A little later another draft of an Order in Council was to have been submitted by two Ministers, this time proposing that although the military patients were to be treated in Pensions and National Health hospitals, they were to be under the laws of their own Service with officers of the Department of Pensions and National Health being in charge of discipline. At this juncture, Major-General E. C. Ashton was recalled from retirement to undertake the supervision of R.C.A.M.C. hospitalisation plans in Canada. He promptly took a stand supporting the institution of R.C.A.M.C. hospitals, so that proper training and experience would be developed and proper discipline of those being treated in the hospitals could be maintained. As a result of all these discussions an Order in Council (P.C. 3004) was issued on October 5. It was arranged that the control of military patients was firmly in the hands of the R.C.A.M.C.; the remaining difficulties about the number of military hospitals to be established was settled during the next few months, but not without considerable discussion and much pressure from interested civilian authorities. Dr. Wodehouse appears as the central figure throughout this controversy and it was he who pressed for absolute control as soon as possible of the care of soldiers in pension hospitals. His recommendations were rejected by General Ashton and the Department of National Defence eventually settled the problem without further reference to him. A policy statement on military medical arrangements was issued on October 23 and sent out to district officers on the 26th. It pointed out that all military or station hospitals were to continue to operate at full capacity for naval, military, and air force patients and were to employ such staffs as might be required. It also authorised the organisation of treatment hospitals in areas where there were to be large concentrations of troops. The freest possible use, consistent with efficiency, was to be made of the laboratory and technical equipment of the Department of Pensions and National Health. This policy was to apply equally to the Royal Canadian Navy and to the Royal Canadian Air Force. With the members of the three Armed Forces to be dealt with certain problems arose as to the appropriate authority for maintaining discipline; but these were rapidly settled by a new Order (P.C. 3988) in which the Minister of Defence was empowered after November 14 to appoint any officer of the three Services to deal with offences committed by members of the forces who were receiving hospital treatment or other care in the Department of Pensions and National Health hospitals.

The long controversy concerning the control of military patients thus ended with the decision in favour of military authority. This was a fundamental issue; had preparation been adequate and understanding of what had occurred in the First World War sufficient, the long delays and the time wasted in negotiating this matter need never have occurred. It illustrates the great weakness in the planning phases before the Second World War. Sound planning should ward off any technical obstacles to the efficient mobilisation of forces and their medical care.

OVERSEAS MEDICAL COMMITMENT

While these discussions were progressing, units were being mobilised to form a headquarters in the United Kingdom to accompany the first division. Large numbers of recruits had to be medically examined at short notice. On the whole the examinations were satisfactory; a final re-examination before going overseas included urine analysis, colour vision testing, and X-ray examination of the chest. Advance units were despatched to the United Kingdom on November 24, 1939, the main force following in December. Medical arrangements comprised allocation of conducting medical officers, hygiene sections and duties of medical officers on board troop trains, on ships and at embarkation points. These arrangements proved satisfactory.

ADMINISTRATIVE CHANGES

The Directorate of Army Medical Services began the war with four officers and three other ranks, and with many departments dormant. In the autumn of 1942 it was divided into two branches, administrative and professional. The D.G.M.S. remained the chief executive officer with two deputies, each in charge of one of the new divisions. In 1945 the directorate reached its peak strength, with 104 officers and 188 other ranks, a total of 292. The lesson is that at all times the structure and organisation of the medical directorate should be kept under revision and not left dormant and stagnant as this one had been for over 20 years.

By 1942 it was possible to add senior consultants, in all specialties, on a regional basis for Canada. This maintained professional standards, improved medical care and helped younger men brought into the Service before completion of post-graduate medical training.

SOCIAL SCIENCE

Prior to 1943 social welfare in the Armed Forces was a haphazard service. Most of the social welfare was left to the regimental officer; but late in 1942 an unofficial arrangement was adopted in the medical reception centre at Military District 2, whereby local civilian welfare agencies were added to assist the medical board in securing social and health data. This did not solve the welfare problem of the serving soldier and in March 1943 the D.G.M.S. established social workers from the Canadian Women's Army Corps to be employed wherever needed. District welfare officers were appointed in 1944; this provided information on service that might be required by the D.G.M.S., a notable advance, which led to a most interesting development. A directorate of social science was established under the D.G.M.S. for a trial period of six months; this experiment proved successful and the arrangement was continued. It was during this period that Major-General G. B. Chisholm was exploring the possibility of a much broader and quite revolutionary plan for the establishment of a Royal Canadian Army Health Service.

He proposed to incorporate in the R.C.A.M.C. not only social science but psychology, selective service, and even the auxiliary services. He argued that all these services were primarily concerned with the health of the individual. This plan received wide approval from all professional and scientific bodies in Canada and from the district medical officers' conference. A proposal was submitted to the Adjutant General, and later to the Chief of the General Staff; both were of the opinion that the proposal deserved 'careful consideration', but before the plan came up for further discussion its sponsor, General Chisholm, had retired and the end of the war was in sight. Although the plan was never formally completed, its realisation was very close at hand, since social science and personnel selection were closely integrated with the medical services. The amalgamation of personnel selection with the

R.C.A.M.C. was approved in Canada, but since it was not approved in the United Kingdom its implementation proved difficult. The proposals advanced by General Chisholm for a Royal Canadian Army Health Corps, while they seemed to be sound at the time, under his persuasive leadership, were never whole-heartedly accepted by the great majority of serving medical officers. Indeed, they were understood only by a very limited group, and those who had practical experience with the integration of non-medical formations into a medical corps, were distinctly opposed to the plan. The reasons for this are somewhat obscure, but perhaps they lie in the ingrained disciplinary pattern which applies to the medical profession, but which cannot be applied so well to other less homogeneous elements. It may perhaps be significant that the personnel service dealing with the selection of personnel for the Armed Forces has subsequently been removed to its traditional position in the division of the Adjutant General, and no further attempt to form a Royal Canadian Army Health Corps has been made.

HOSPITALISATION IN CANADA

Provision of hospital beds in Canada proved to be one of the major problems of the medical services on the home front. The dispute with the Department of Pensions and National Health, wide dispersal of troops over an enormous area, the problem of co-ordinating hospital activities in three Services, all presented difficulties. After promulgation of Privy Council Order No. 3004 on October 5, 1939, there was still a difference of opinion as to its interpretation, and both the Department of National Defence and the Department of Pensions and National Health began the rapid expansion of hospital services and beds. This expansion had to be placed under strict governmental supervision and the Associate Minister of National Defence found it necessary to recommend a full review of the medical and hospital services. This resulted in the formation of an inter-departmental committee of hospitalisation. It was this committee that established firmly the primary function of each department. The Treatment Branch of the Department of Pensions and National Health was to provide treatment and hospitalisation for veterans of the First World War and all members of the Canadian Active Service Force who were discharged from the Service and still required treatment. The secondary function of this Department was to offer hospitalisation for cases of the Forces that could not be accommodated in the Service establishments, when beds were still available in existing Department of Pensions and National Health institutions. It was further decided that any further expansion of hospitalisation for the present treatment of any overflow of Active Service cases, requiring the taking over of extra buildings not immediately a part of the existing Department of Pensions and National Health institutions, would be the responsibility of the Department of National Defence, and not that of the Department of Pensions and National Health. It was thus the final discussions of this committee which settled the long drawn-out argument between the two departments. All requests for the enlargement of pensions hospitals were referred to the Inter-Departmental Committee but a completely amicable solution was not always effected. In fact, dissension reached the special Parliamentary Committee of War Expenditures and the sub-committee had the duty of arbitrating such divisions of opinion. Having in mind the disastrous effects upon the Government and the Minister of Defence in the First World War, this committee discussed hospitalisation very fully and reached the conclusion that the Defence Department should treat serving men until they were placed in category E, that is until they were no longer considered physically or mentally fit for active service. The Parliamentary Committee based its decision on cost factors since temporary hospitals can be built very much less expensively than permanent Pensions hospitals, and upon the time factor; they believed that temporary hospitals could be built much more quickly. This Parliamentary Committee strongly recommended that regular meetings of the Inter-Departmental Committee on Hospitalisation ought to be held and in order to give direction to such a committee the Deputy Minister of the Department of National Defence was to be appointed as Chairman. This committee was given wide powers, including a survey of existing hospital care, consideration of all new public hospitals to be built in Canada and elsewhere, and in general to study the most efficient and economical use of our hospitals and auxiliary services. This committee's name was changed to the Wartime Committee on Hospitalisation in May 1942, with the Deputy Minister of National Defence (Army) as Chairman and a representative of the Treasury as a member. The work of this committee during the next five years was very important and strenuous. It worked out the categorisation of hospitals and their proper distribution to serve various areas and various arms of the Forces. By 1944, 13,057 hospital beds were in operation, many of them in installations of more than 400 beds; these hospitals were equipped to deal with the most advanced type of surgery, staffed by the best medical and surgical specialists in Canada. The appointment and operation of this committee was a highly significant step forward. It was not arrived at without considerable difficulty. It clearly illustrates the necessity for forethought and planning and for adequate co-ordination between departments concerned with the care of the serving man. It also demonstrates how certain opinions and actions of departmental officials, however well-intentioned, may seriously disrupt the proper chain of events.

CONDITIONING CENTRES

Many men were found to be unfit but to have disabilities which could be improved. Various centres were established in Canada both for the men's and for the women's services. Two were concerned with treating special problems of women in the Fighting Forces. Special treatment centres were also set up, particularly for plastic surgery.

HOSPITAL SHIPS AND TRAINS

In 1943 the first Canadian Hospital Ship appeared; in 1944 a second was added. These ships were of great importance to Canadians serving abroad as there had been long delays in the return of casualties from the United Kingdom to Canada.

Hospital trains were made available early in the war and others were added as required. They were an important link in the administrative arrangements for casualties disembarking at the ports.

TRAINING CENTRES

Training Centres were lacking at the outbreak of war and it was 1940 before a training centre for officers and other ranks in the R.C.A.M.C. could be established. This should, in the future, be remedied by the maintenance of a permanent training centre with adequate teaching staff.

THE R.C.A.M.C. IN BRITAIN, 1940–43

The Canadian Forces spent three years in the United Kingdom in training and in guard duties. The Canadian hospital medical units served as base hospitals, and proved satisfactory. Experience over a long period of training led to a definite pattern of operation. During the winter of 1941–42 each regimental aid post kept five or ten beds available for those who were not expected to need accommodation for more than 24 hours. Each field ambulance maintained 25 to 75 patients, depending on the amount of space. In each division two field ambulances normally looked after the sick while a third participated in training. Casualty clearing stations functioned with 150 or 160 beds for patients requiring three or four days care; for longer periods patients were sent to one or other of the Canadian hospitals that were then active.

REORGANISATION OF FIELD MEDICAL SERVICES

During 1940 and 1941 much attention was given to the reorganisation of field units, and a committee under the chairmanship of Brigadier W. C. Hartgill studied the problems relating to this subject. The Hartgill report stated that a reorganisation of the medical service in the corps and division was long overdue. It concentrated on changes within a division as follows: (1) The field ambulance without its main dressing station was reorganised as a fully mobile collecting and evacuating unit composed of a headquarters and two bearer companies, each of three sections. (2) The corps field ambulance was abolished and in its place a field dressing station was recommended. (3) The casualty clearing station was reduced in size and its equipment somewhat altered. (4) Field surgical and field transfusion units were classed, some as Army and some as G.H.Q. troops. A field surgical unit was sometimes attached to a dressing station to form an advanced surgical centre. (5) The recommendations outlined the flow of casualties under this new system.

The Canadian reaction to the new British organisational plan was at first unfavourable, but a Canadian alternative, when tested, was discouraging and the British scheme was adopted in January 1943.

HOSPITAL POLICY OVERSEAS

From November 1939 it was planned to send two base hospitals to the United Kingdom and to establish them near the concentrations of Canadian troops. One was equipped by the Canadian Red Cross Society, which also provided extra equipment at other hospitals. At Basingstoke a special hospital was set up which served throughout the war as a centre for both neurological and plastic surgery cases. Satisfactory convalescent units were established. Accommodation throughout 1940 and 1941 expanded in the two base hospitals. Hospital units were brought from Canada and integrated with the existing hospitals. By 1943 a group of well-equipped general hospitals was based in England with a competent staff of officers and nursing sisters. It was not until late in 1943 that a reasonably firm estimate of the Canadian quota for a joint British-Canadian Expeditionary Force could be provided, but fortunately hospitals available were adequate to supply the proposed hospitals for the Force without impairing the efficiency of the base hospitals in the United Kingdom; and a constant flow of new hospitals from Canada made up any replacements. Eventually Canadian hospital beds for active treatment numbered 19,600, as well as 2,500 special hospital beds for various purposes, including convalescence.

II CAMPAIGNS

THE DIEPPE RAID

In the Dieppe raid on August 19, 1942, the Canadian medical organisation met its first severe test of the war. A raiding force was mobilised with the utmost secrecy at various ports and medical equipment and stores were limited to what could be carried by the raiding party. Medical officers accompanied the landing units and some of them were taken prisoner along with the fighting troops. Casualties were heavy. One of the lessons recorded is that the senior medical officer of the force should have been on the headquarters ship and not on the reserve headquarters ship because of the difficulty of keeping in touch.

So much secrecy was observed before the raid that the field ambulances concerned first heard about the operation on the morning of the event. Although there was some difficulty in siting the dressing stations that were to evacuate casualties, in general this was carried out in a commendable manner. Mortality rates for these casualties were low, and valuable experience was gained as to flexibility, the necessity for accurate advance information and better means of communication during action.

SICILIAN CAMPAIGN

Medical planning for the Sicilian Campaign was hampered in the beginning by delay in reaching a firm decision as to the operational plan. This was a serious matter for the Canadian units because although the units of the 1st Canadian Division were fully trained and at a peak of efficiency rarely achieved by a fighting force, the units were divorced from centralised direction. Reasonable liaison was maintained in the Middle East Command but the co-ordination of this attack, which was to come from widely scattered points, was a very difficult matter. Medical plans were finally satisfactorily achieved, but the difficulty of providing information to the subordinate formations, including the Canadians, was very great. The division had no medical representative at H.Q. XXX Corps. The problem of physical separation was thus aggravated for the medical staffs. Matters were improved by a visit of the D.D.M.S. British XXX Corps, although by that time it was difficult to change Canadian plans. One serious lack was discovered during these conferences with the D.D.M.S. He found that though everybody was to receive one mepacrine tablet daily at sea for six days prior to D-day, no adequate provision had been made for continuing this treatment ashore, the first follow-up supply of mepacrine being due to arrive on D-day + 3 and to be unloaded an indefinite number of days thereafter. This oversight was speedily rectified. The Canadian medical planners had grave difficulty in securing information to help them in their plans for an anti-malaria campaign. The time for training in anti-malaria routines was limited, the equipment was provided very late, and the specially trained anti-malaria officer from the Middle East failed to reach the division until three days before embarkation. Some of the deficiencies were remedied by the appointment of divisional anti-malaria officers, and late in the day three anti-malaria control units were formed. It took some painful practical experiences of the disease before all ranks became reasonably conversant with the methods and the need for protection and control. Just before the battle was to begin there were many changes in the medical order of battle and this

complicated matters considerably. It was not until very shortly before
the attack that five additional Canadian medical units were added
to the order of battle.

Medical units in the Mediterranean were strengthened by the
addition of general hospitals and field medical units, on the advice of
the Deputy Adjutant General, C.M.H.Q., Brigadier A. W. Beament.
The shipment of two hospitals overseas presented technical difficulties;
the bulk of their field ordnance and medical equipment was assembled
and shipped without the officers of the hospitals ever having seen it;
the results on arrival at the field of operations were chaotic. The units
had limited experience in the erection of hospital canvas and the time
allowed for training was extremely limited. Neither unit had any
opportunity to function under canvas, and with field equipment only.
This was a valuable lesson which was applied in later training exercises
for other hospitals that were proceeding to theatres of war. Each of
the medical units functioned well in the advancing campaign in the
Sicilian countryside. The great problem that faced the Canadian forces
was that of malaria. There was an epidemic of serious proportions
during the latter part of August 1943. It was necessary on August 27
to apply a drastic 'blanket' quinine therapy to the whole division,
and this campaign was instituted on the 28th. The assigned cause of
this outbreak was the laxity in anti-malaria precautions by units and
individuals during the period spent by the division in the vicinity
of Agira and Regalbuto, both situated in the midst of the highly malarious area encompassed by the valleys of the Dittaino and Salso rivers.
It is more likely that the laxity in many instances followed the cessation
of fighting. The majority of the cases occurred during the latter half
of August. From all aspects it would appear that the root cause of the
Canadian malaria epidemic in Sicily was general neglect on the part of
units and individuals to implement the measures laid down, a neglect
induced by inadequacy of training. It is only too evident that as soon as
the division was seriously exposed to malaria, cases developed rapidly
and the disease was most rampant after the stress of battle gave place
to a period of relative relaxation. The monthly rate during the latter
half of August was 42·7 per thousand, if all identified fever cases are
included without being firmly diagnosed as malaria. So serious were the
epidemics of malaria in both the British Army and the Canadian Forces
serving with it, that every effort was made to bring them under control
and to guard against any recurrence. Many Canadian medical officers
were sent to British malaria centres for short courses and the reorganised anti-malaria control units were attached to British units for
training in field work. Canadian casualties in the Sicilian campaign
were evacuated to No. 15 Canadian General Hospital in North Africa.
This hospital was located on a steep slope of an undulating valley six

miles long and four miles wide. It was exposed throughout the day to the direct rays of the tropical sun, and as the soil was clay, poor drainage and deep mud were expected in the rainy season. Malignant malaria was prevalent in the area, and the convalescent and reinforcement depots were too far away. Although the commanding officer made strong recommendations, the unit remained in this unsatisfactory location and no alternative site was ever found. The hospital was housed in tents, water was piped but was grossly inadequate when the unit moved in and began to function with the temperature at 100° F. The engineering work was not efficiently carried out and electricity was not available for some time. The laboratory and X-ray equipment were not in full operation for nearly a month and many engineering projects were long delayed. As a result of these unfortunate events, many Canadian casualties were admitted to British hospitals. A remarkable achievement of this Canadian hospital was its malaria control campaign, which was not only active among the staff and patients but also among the local population. Because of administrative miscalculations medical units are sometimes badly located and equipped; but even in these conditions excellent work can be done with improvisation and hard work.

ITALIAN CAMPAIGN

The opening of the campaign in Southern Italy was an operation known as 'Baytown'. The Eighth Army, with its experience in amphibious warfare, gave a brilliant example of military planning in this operation. The medical requirements in such an amphibious operation had been well understood during the operations in Sicily and the control of medical units was largely decentralised for the assault phase. It was in this operation that the 'beach brick', was introduced, an early term for what later developed into the beach group. The Canadian divisional medical units were reinforced by such a segment during this operation. It was during this campaign that evacuation by air came into more general use, although ships and tank landing craft were to be used to the fullest extent. The problem of malaria came into focus, and the distribution of malaria maps and the very careful administration of precise instructions had a great deal to do with the success of the control programme. Medical authorities recommended that shorts be withdrawn and that long trousers be worn by all ranks at all times.

The rapidity with which the campaign developed in Southern Italy created problems in the maintenance of an efficient system of evacuation. Although battle casualties were light there was always the possibility of a serious engagement and the flow of sick was considerable because of exposure to new types of infection and to malaria. During this phase evacuation from the far-flung forward units to the base field ambulance had to be employed. Distances of more than 100 miles had to be traversed at this period. During this campaign an administrative centre was developed at Campobasso, where there was a considerable concentration of medical units. All Canadian casualties were collected at this point, and this made a valuable contribution to the morale of the forces fighting in Southern Italy.

MEDICAL ARRANGEMENTS BEHIND THE FRONT

No. 5 General Hospital remained in Catania and No. 15 General Hospital in North Africa at El Arrouch. One of the difficulties of this campaign was that these hospitals were at an undesirable distance from the fighting troops, but neither could be moved to Italy until an advance base had been established there; it was not until October that this was achieved. Fortunately two other Canadian hospitals had already arrived direct from the United Kingdom.

WINTER CAMPAIGNING, 1943–44

The long and bitter winter campaign in Italy found the medical units able to cope adequately with the casualties flowing through from the fighting in the mountains. Through the long campaign in the Ortona salient medical arrangements ran smoothly and the deficiencies of equipment were gradually made good.

CANADIAN HOSPITALS, NOVEMBER 1943–MARCH 1944

Nos. 1, 14 and 15 Canadian hospitals located in this theatre were overtaxed in this period, but with the opening of No. 5 General Hospital in February 1944 the burden was somewhat eased. It was at this juncture that it was possible to evacuate Canadian casualties to Canadian hospitals, and an order was issued, 'Canadian battle casualties and sick will in the main be admitted in the first instance to the Andria group of Canadian hospitals.' They were then to be transferred to the Caserta group, which was to be the Canadian base from which evacuation to the United Kingdom was to be undertaken. At the end of February 1944 a careful review of the hospital beds available in the Italian theatre was undertaken. In view of the impending campaigns a critical decision concerning the number of beds to be provided had to be made. It was decided not to increase the number of hospital units in the theatre but to expand existing hospitals to capacity. This was accomplished before the summer campaigns, and although there were some anxious days, the arrangement proved to be adequate.

THE LIRI VALLEY

The development of strong German defence lines in the Liri Valley led to a long drawn-out campaign for the capture of the Gustav Line. Medical plans for the evacuation and treatment of casualties during this phase of the fighting were adequate and successful. It was at this time too that the field medical organisation devised by the Hartgill Committee was fully tested in battle. Apart from the grouping of all field dressing stations under the control of the D.D.M.S. the tactical doctrine evolved by the committee was strictly followed, and an ideal testing ground was provided; at the conclusion of the operation Major-General Hartgill, at this date D.M.S. to Allied Force Headquarters, expressed himself as delighted with the manner in which the field medical organisation he had done so much to shape had been employed by 1st Canadian Corps: 'Never before', he said, 'have casualties reached hospital so quickly and in such good condition.' The functions of the field and the light field ambulance were fully worked out during this period and the new unit, the field dressing station, functioned principally as a nucleus to which were added field surgical and field transfusion units. These were usually established on the down-traffic route and provided a most valuable system of nesting casualties while the advance continued. The consulting surgeon at Canadian Military Headquarters, Brigadier J. A. MacFarlane, stated after a visit to one of these nests: 'The post-operative nursing care at the casualty clearing stations and at the small 200 bed general hospitals was excellent and was assisted by nursing sisters attached to general hospitals. Without this excellent care much of the brilliant surgical work would have been of no avail.' The part of the mobile laboratories in this new system should not be overlooked for they were invaluable in the provision of blood and bacteriological services. The use of the motor ambulance corps and the distant evacuation procedures all went smoothly. It was during this period of evacuation of casualties that the breaking point was reached. No. 14 General Hospital had received about 900 battle casualties and No. 15 slightly more than a thousand, bringing the total on hand in each hospital to approximately 1,600. No. 15 found its resources severely taxed by this time and No. 14 was not in a position to accept further patients. During the night at this point No. 15 had to close for fifteen hours and some casualties were diverted to No. 5 General Hospital at Cancello and No. 1 at Avellino. Furthermore, a surgical team and several medical officers were transferred from No. 1 to assist the staff at No. 15 General Hospital. These measures taken in the emergency proved sufficient to restore the hospital situation to a reasonably satisfactory position. The flow of casualties diminished and a number of long-term cases were cleared from the area by hospital ship. On May 31, only five days after the peak of the casualty flow, each hospital had a substantial reserve of beds. All ended well, but it is very apparent that the margin of safety was small, even bearing in mind that intentionally the facilities of No. 1 and No. 5 were not employed fully. The hospital staffs were strengthened by the provision of auxiliary surgical teams from the field, but these could only be sent to the hospital at the expense of forward surgery. Had the Germans been able to prolong a stubborn defence of the Hitler Line and the Melfa River, the number of Canadian hospital beds in the theatre would probably have proved insufficient. Marginal decisions of this kind must be taken in an active conflict but they should only be taken after adequate advice and consultation with competent medical advisers.

ADVANCE TO THE SENIO

After the battles of the Liri Valley there was a summer interval for the Canadian Forces, during which re-grouping and re-equipping were necessary. New campaigns were soon under way and the hospital units found themselves full of casualties from the bitter fighting for the Gothic Line. Medical arrangements, with what were now very experienced medical forces, functioned smoothly. The flow of casualties was great and the strain on the units was increased because of the long distances. At the end of this summer campaign a medical reorganisation took place. The D.D.M.S. felt that the existing organisation was unbalanced as to its personnel. Some units had too many and some units had too few personnel for the functions they fulfilled. Field ambulances became light field ambulances with a headquarters and four sections each. Some field dressing units were made corps troops and one was made into a field hospital. The field dressing stations were given increased transport and equipment, and the casualty clearing stations were given additional medical officers and staff. Two surgical groups came into more or less permanent existence and each was based on the casualty clearing station. An important change was disbandment of the 2nd Light Field Ambulance. There was a relatively small saving of man-power and divisional resources were reduced to the point where the A.D.M.S. considered them inadequate to meet the normal commitments. Requests for reinforcements, except for a stretcher-bearer officer, were refused. These changes were questionable and it is notable that when the 1st Canadian Corps eventually joined the First Canadian Army in North-West Europe it was ordered to undo all these changes in its medical service. Sometimes individual enthusiasm and judgment, inadequately tempered by wise counsel, can create considerable confusion.

ACROSS THE SAVIO

Intense battles across raging rivers characterised this phase of the Italian campaign. Medical arrangements were swift and satisfactory. A month of rest was arranged for the 1st Canadian Corps during November. Diphtheria made its appearance in the area at this time and provided additional problems for the Canadian troops. They had not been immunised and, although a considerable number of Canadians had been immunised during childhood, there was still sufficient not immunised to permit an epidemic in the Canadian Corps at this time. Special hospital evacuation was arranged and an immunisation programme decided upon, but this had only been started when the corps was again committed to action, completely interrupting the procedure. Venereal disease also created a serious problem at this time, and a special educational exhibit was set up to assist in its prevention. During December the Canadians participated in heavy fighting and the evacuation of casualties was carried out smoothly and satisfactorily. At the end of the year the 1st Canadian Corps found itself firmly established along the Senio and this was virtually the end of Canadian operations in Italy.

Because of the development of the campaign in Italy, the geographical relationship of Canadian hospitals to each other and to the scene of Canadian operational activity in Italy was far from ideal during this period; and so it remained to the end of the Canadian participation in the Italian Campaign. The provision of surgical care for the casualties admitted to No. 14 at Perugia became a serious problem, and it illustrates the point that a more generous provision of hospital beds in the Italian theatre would have been wiser. An even distribution of patients was impossible; sometimes No. 14 was completely filled and at other times it had empty beds because of the severance of road communication. No. 15 could not handle all the patients directed to it, expecially during September and October, with a consequent overflow into British hospitals at Caserta. The fundamental tenet of Canadian medical policy, namely, to treat Canadians in Canadian units, had to be broken; responsibility for this rests, not with medical officers, but with senior administrative officers who made decisions in the planning period that severely limited hospital beds. Early in January 1945 the decision was made to withdraw certain Eighth Army units from the Italian campaign. In accordance with the overall plan the medical units were transferred to the European theatre of operations. At the conclusion of the operations in Italy certain hospitals were evacuated and others were closed down, including No. 14 and No. 15 General Hospitals. The closing and moving of hospitals was under the direction of Allied Force Headquarters and was effected through British channels.

THE INVASION OF NORMANDY, JUNE 1944

Plans for the invasion of Normandy were made from April 1943 onward and the Canadian Forces were involved in these from the outset. All casualties, from D-day until the establishment of adequate hospitalisation in the bridgehead, were to be evacuated to the United Kingdom, with gradual extension of the period for which casualties were to be retained in the European theatre of operation as more hospital beds became available. Most careful estimates of casualties were made and with the landing of 70,000 British and Canadian personnel on D-day, 6,250 were expected to be casualties, 4,495 requiring medical attention. Casualties in the first flights of the assaults were to remain in the craft and to return to the parent ship. On shore, no attempt was to be made to evacuate casualties until the beachhead was secure. At this time the casualties were to be given first-aid treatment and nested in protected areas in the region of regimental aid posts. A beach sub-area was to be formed immediately following the assault with medical components for the treatment of casualties. With the establishment of a casualty evacuation point, casualties were evacuated by naval transportation. Coastal hospitals were to be established and treat urgent cases, which were later moved to base hospitals as quickly as possible. Base hospitals were to take only third priority patients, those who could stand a journey of some distance. There were to be 30 hospital ambulance trains, as well as sea transport. Canadian medical planning for this campaign began actively in May of 1943 so that they were integrated adequately and early into the picture. Since the Canadian Army was actually based in North America it was important that decisions be made early and this complicated the planning. In addition, the desire to have Canadian casualties treated in Canadian hospitals and returned to Canadian units at the earliest possible moment introduced many complicating factors. Thus the evacuation through the Emergency Medical Services' chain might delay their return to units unnecessarily. Through the good offices and intelligent management of Brigadier R. M. Luton, there was close liaison between 21st Army Group and Canadian Military Headquarters in London. Largely due to his initiative there was a minimum of misunderstanding, and Canadian hospitals were integrated into the programme with the minimum of difficulty. The medical corps was to be required to operate on the basis of 22,100 hospital beds. The allocation of hospital units to static and mobile rôles was the first project. It necessitated the arrangement of an additional group of hospital beds and their movement from Canada to the United Kingdom. This led to an extensive mobilisation of hospital units and to their despatch to the United Kingdom, and arrangements were made for their transfer to France when necessary.

The training phase for the 'Second Front' was adequately handled and all field units, including many base hospitals, were given experience in landing in amphibious craft. During the landing and lodgement on 'Juno' beach all medical arrangements went forward satisfactorily. Inevitably with the advances and the events of the first few days, field ambulances operated without any new divisional orders, but each field ambulance commander maintained close liaison with his respective brigade and moved within reach of brigade headquarters at all times. This was one of the most important lessons of the type of warfare being waged at that time, and the close liaison of fighting units with medical service units cannot be over-emphasised. The establishment of an exhaustion centre early in the fighting was an important development which was not fully anticipated, for during the first 25 days of the operation of such a unit in France it cleared 977 casualties through its various installations. The establishment of the beach group with its relevant Canadian components went satisfactorily as did the evacuation of casualties. Evacuation by air began a full week earlier than had been anticipated in the planning. One of the unforeseen difficulties was the provision of facilities for holding casualties near suitable airstrips, and on June 18 the whole evacuation system was centralised under No. 11, Lines of Communication Sub-Area, and a medical liaison officer was attached to 83 Group of the Royal Air Force. Two British hospitals were made the principal collecting centres and R.A.F. casualty air evacuation units began to arrive at this time and assisted in holding these casualties. In the first three weeks of the assault the casualties in the British-Canadian sector were 21,000 approximately, of whom 2,900 were Canadians. This was substantially below the estimated flow of casualties, with the result that not all the facilities were operated at their capacity. An excellent supply of all types of goods and equipment was available at all times.

The reception of casualties in England at the coastal hospitals was eminently satisfactory. The coastal and transit hospitals were able to handle the greater proportion of all casualties evacuated from the Continent. The base hospitals in the scheme of evacuation received fewer casualties than had been anticipated, and their principal function continued to be the hospitalisation of troops remaining in the United Kingdom.

THE NORMANDY BATTLES, JULY 1944

Following the establishment of a bridgehead, the offensive for the capture of Normandy began, and with the attack on Caen medical units became heavily engaged. The medical units functioned smoothly throughout this phase, except for the failure of the D.U.K.W. evacuation route across the Orne and the Caen canal because of perpetual shelling by the enemy. Temporary bridges across the Orne shortened the evacuation route and the divisional casualties flowed smoothly rearwards. During the forward advance from Caen, Canadian casualties were heavy but they were dealt with by the existing medical units. In the early stage of the campaign total exhaustion casualties were comparatively few and were held for 48 hours in a small rest camp attached to one of the field ambulances. Later on, a field dressing station was set up to deal with these cases and, subsequently a corps exhaustion centre had to be established. The movement of Canadian hospitals to the Continent was delayed for a month because of crowding in the bridgehead area but by mid-July three of them had been established.

BREAK-OUT AND PURSUIT

During August First Canadian Army was to break out of the Caen perimeter and to pursue the enemy across Normandy. Medical organisation for this part of the campaign went smoothly, except for some congestion of casualties in the casualty clearing station area. The problem was accentuated during the further extension of this campaign and the D.D.M.S. of First Canadian Army remarked: 'Apparently the limiting factor in a casualty clearing station is not bed capacity but surgical capacity.' A sudden influx of casualties late in the day taxed the surgical capacity of the clearing station and delayed treatment. Various remedies were attempted, including the attachment of additional surgical teams or of field dressing stations to care for the walking wounded. Congestion of ambulance cars resulted and they were eventually sent first to the dressing stations before being passed on to the casualty clearing station. Field dressing stations were later attached to each casualty clearing station to avoid this difficulty. It soon became apparent that this was the ideal system.

The catastrophe which overtook the Germans in the Falaise pocket made resistance very much less, with the result that Canadian medical units were not seriously taxed during this period. A problem encountered was the rapidity with which units had to be moved, and for those who had little or no transport, this was serious. The crossing of the Seine occurred so rapidly that units were in continuous movement. The problem for medical units was complicated by three factors, in addition to congested roadways. Each unit was required to leave a small section behind for the care of casualties, and at one time there were eleven of these nested along the route. They had to continue admitting casualties while the main unit was on the move. A trickle system was devised and No. 6 Canadian Field Dressing Station, for example, moved several times without closing. A third complication was that of communication; keeping in touch with forward units to control the flow of casualties was solved most easily by the use of despatch riders. But they had great difficulty, especially in night moves through congested areas. The assignment of wireless units was of some help, but the Slidex Code did not elaborate certain phrases, resulting in ambiguous messages including 'dispose of diphtheria, dispose of ampoules, dispose of . . .' It was, however, most useful in getting emergency information and saving despatch rider runs in bad weather and at night. It was the first time in this theatre that the necessity for this type of communication

had become evident. Air and sea evacuation had limited the usefulness
of hospitals and convalescent units brought to Normandy. One convalescent unit provided an excellent centre for exhaustion casualties,
a problem which had not been fully appreciated, and which previously
was dealt with in field ambulances. The advance from the River Seine
to the Albert Canal was completed between September 3 and 30, thus
greatly extending the communication lines. The capture of the Channel
ports became imperative in order to shorten lines of evacuation, and
in these hard-fought battles medical units played an important rôle.

The advance of the Canadian divisions after the Seine crossing in
September 1944 was so rapid that some of the corps units were so far
behind the line of advance as to be of little use in the treatment of
casualties. This difficulty was lessened with the decrease in the speed of
advance by the Corps after the middle of September. Similar problems
were faced by the First Canadian Army. The time taken by the ambulance convoys was greatly increased and transport upon which medical
units depended for their moves was engaged in the vital task of supplying
the advancing army. No casualty clearing station was opened north
of the Seine before September 10, so that evacuation was from advanced
surgical centres direct to general hospitals. The load on ambulance
car companies was tremendous, and the employment of advanced
surgical centres helped greatly to relieve it.

During this period an acute shortage of hospital beds was experienced.
The quarterly medical report of First Canadian Army sums up the
situation at this time: 'On the night of September 11, every available
hospital bed was full, every ambulance car on the road, no air evacuation
had taken place in the previous ninety hours. It was then a miracle
happened. A flight of nine Dakota aircraft dropped in at B/31 airstrip
on their way back to England. A R.A.F. officer was able to persuade
this group to take back 195 casualties the following morning.

At the end of September, the rapid advance having ceased, the
medical situation was eased. *The Official History of the Canadian
Medical Services*. Vol. I. p. 253, summarises the work of the
Canadian Medical Services during the Normandy Campaign, as follows:

'Medical plans during the period prior to the capture of Falaise worked
admirably despite the difficulties encountered. Casualties were given
every possible attention; rapid collection, early surgery, and speedy
evacuation were always provided. Medical units were greatly assisted
in their task by the fact that the distance from the front line to the
hospital area at Bayeux was never great. Most of the early surgery was
done at casualty clearing stations. Field dressing stations were, for the
most part, not called upon to form advanced surgical centres but worked
in conjunction with casualty clearing stations, doing triage and assisting
in evacuation. Transport facilities by land, sea and air were excellent

for the greater part of this period and evacuation did not present a problem. Evacuation by sea to base hospitals in England was under way almost immediately after the campaign began and air evacuation commenced as early as June 13.

'After the Falaise gap had been closed the period of almost static warfare gave way to one of rapid movement. The advance to the Seine, though swift, was not without bitter fighting and the First Canadian Army suffered many casualties. Lines of evacuation had as yet not been extended to impose great difficulties on medical services. After the Seine was crossed, the advance was greatly accelerated and the Canadians swept across France and into Belgium. This new situation severely strained the resources of the medical as well as those of other services, especially during the first two weeks of September.

'Medical plans for this phase consisted of evacuation of casualties from Dieppe to the United Kingdom, rail evacuation to Bayeux, air evacuation either to Bayeux or the United Kingdom, and the establish- ment of an advanced hospital area north of the Seine pending the establishment of a new hospital base in the Antwerp–Rotterdam area. These plans were essentially sound, but difficulties were immediately encountered. The port of Dieppe was not used for casualty evacuation until September 16. The railhead, although operating as early as the 6th, extended only to Mézidon. An air evacuation strip north of the Seine which was essential for the direct transport of casualties to England, was prepared by September 6 but did not begin to operate for another five days due to bad flying conditions. Casualty evacuation during this period depended almost entirely on ambulance car companies which, to make matters worse, were forced to haul their own fuel. As a result there was a serious overcrowding in forward medical installations which was not improved by an influx of prisoner-of-war casualties from captured enemy hospitals. Lack of transport vehicles, which had to be used to bring forward supplies of fuel, food, and ammunition over the now vastly lengthened lines of communication stretching back to Bayeux, and unprecedented congestion on the roads, delayed the establishment of the advanced hospital area north of the Seine.

'These difficulties might not have proved so serious had there been sufficient holding capacity farther forward. The same reasons delaying the establishment of hospitals were partly responsible for preventing the movement of casualty clearing stations. There seems to have been some timidity in pushing these units forward when transport was available, and there were delays in opening them when they were vitally needed which the records do not explain.

'The bulk of forward surgery was ably handled by advanced surgical centres, formed for the most part by corps field dressing stations, but due to the rapidity of the advance even these units were often far behind the fighting troops. Many casualties took as long as 18 to 24 hours to reach a surgical centre. It was reported that not only time but distance travelled affected the mortality rate. It was suggested at the time that an advanced surgical centre should be located much closer to the actual fighting and that a divisional field dressing station be used for this purpose.

'For the greater part of September divisional medical units evacuated all types of casualties to the nearest advanced surgical centre. This practice was carried over from the period of fighting in Normandy when casualty clearing stations did advanced surgery and the field dressing station did triage. With the field dressing stations operating as advanced surgical centres it was apparent that triage should be done farther forward; failure to do so was resulting in additional and unnecessary burdens for them and occasioning delays in giving surgical treatment to serious cases. When triage was carried out in forward areas it was often possible to evacuate the less seriously wounded by taking them to casualty clearing stations or general hospitals. Toward the end of the month this difficulty was overcome. On September 25 the army's surgical adviser reported that triage forward was much improved and that only the more serious cases were arriving at the advanced surgical centres which he visited.

'During the month of September the problems confronting the medical service were enormous. The pursuit of the fleeing German Armies has been described as one of the most spectacular in the history of warfare. Every energy was directed towards maintaining the momentum of the advance, and whole divisions were "grounded" so that their transport could be used to support those leading the pursuit. The fighting units and the services intimately concerned with the supply of these units had first priority, not only in transport but in roads. In these conditions the medical services' problem of keeping pace with the advance, complicated as it was by a rapidly extending left flank stretching from Dieppe to the Dutch border, a distance of over 200 miles, almost defied solution. Medical units fortunate enough to have their own transport were able, by heroic efforts, to keep pace with the advancing troops. Casualty clearing stations and general hospitals, dependent as they were on borrowed transport, soon found themselves far behind the battle line. Air evacuation, always at the mercy of the weather, rendered vital assistance at a time when other methods of evacuation were being extended almost to the breaking point. Great praise is due to the ambulance car companies, confronted as they were by almost insurmountable obstacles. They continued, both by day and by night, to maintain a constant service from forward units to base hospital. Any criticism of the medical service during this period should be weighed against the colossal difficulties that confronted it.'

OPENING THE PORT OF ANTWERP AND THE WINTER ON THE MAAS

The clearing of the Scheldt Estuary was now to begin and was to be accomplished in the face of the most difficult conditions of ground, weather and enemy resistance. The troops assigned were experienced veterans, but the task was a very difficult one. During October and the early part of November the Canadian Forces were engaged in heavy fighting in the area of Belgium and the Netherlands close to the Scheldt, and medical units were active. Medical operations throughout these activities went smoothly.

A most spectacular and difficult operation was the capture of Walcheren Island. A period of intensive training was undergone and it was on November 1, that a flotilla of landing craft sailed out of Ostend harbour bound on this dangerous mission. The night was cold and for some hours the convoy made a circuitous sweep in order to begin the assault at daylight. Five minutes before the two landing ships, prepared as hospital ships, were due to arrive, they were sunk by mines. The German shore batteries opened up and whole ships began to disappear. Medical units landed in close support of the assault troops; all casualties had to be held at a field dressing station in Ostend after being evacuated during the night by landing craft. Casualties were high, and although the operation was carried out by a British brigade, medical services were provided by the R.C.A.M.C.

MOVEMENT OF CASUALTIES

The movement of casualties during the autumn and winter was relatively easy because the units were not so far apart and it was possible, especially after the number of casualties was reduced, to increase the holding period in the theatres to 30 days. At the end of the month eight Canadian general hospitals were north of the Seine.

Cold weather medical problems included provision of sufficient hospital units in the forward area with adequate covered accommodation. The weather was consistently wet with temperatures from 40 to 50 degrees F.; the siting of some units well forward greatly increased the difficulties. The use of V-2 weapons during this period also caused some casualties and disruption of the medical services.

A long wait on the bank of the Maas was now to begin; because it was the first natural barrier following the break-through in Normandy, the German forces determined to make a firm stand at this point. This led to much re-grouping and re-deploying of the units during this period, both in the division and corps, as well as in army medical units. The movement of hospitals at this time was reduced to a minimum because of the difficulties of obtaining undamaged buildings in the forward area. The work done in the 1,200-bed hospitals varied considerably. It was actually demonstrated that if all Canadian sick and wounded had been concentrated in Canadian hospitals not more than 41 per cent. of the authorised number of beds would have been occupied at any one time. Some of the hospitals operated at their full capacity, but during November the admission rate dropped rapidly. This was not quite so true of the 600-bed units because of the speed with which they could be opened and the greater ease in moving them as the situation warranted. They operated at a higher rate of bed capacity than larger units and were at various times used as casualty clearing stations.

THE RHINELAND OFFENSIVE

From early in November 1944 until early in February 1945 the First Canadian Army held the line of the Maas and the Nijmegen salient. Before long it was to join a mighty offensive which took the war into the heart of Germany. In this enormous operation the Canadian Army medical plan was carefully drawn up, with a proper system of evacuation in the usual pattern. Siting of the units and locations began and much use was made of jeep ambulances in the brigade areas. From February 8–26, the operation went forward to face some of the most severe fighting of the war. The Canadians next took part in the battle for the Hochwald, and the general pattern of medical evacuation was the same as in previous battles. The terrific air and artillery bombardment preceding this attack had destroyed so many buildings in the forward areas that units were required for the first time since the early battles to operate under canvas.

THE FINAL PHASE AND THE OCCUPATION

When operation 'Veritable' was completed First Canadian Army undertook the holding of the front, while forces were re-grouped for the Rhine crossing; the line of defence ran from Emmerich to the sea. When it was agreed that casualties were to be cared for by Canadians, arrangements were made to have them returned from the divisional medical units across the Rhine *via* the casualty clearing station at Bedburg and thence to Nijmegen and its group of hospitals whence they would be evacuated by air, rail or road to hospitals on the Continent or in the United Kingdom. With the beginning of the operation to cross the Rhine on March 23. Canadian Forces were involved. A most successful airborne operation was conducted during this phase by the 6th Airborne Division, and it was during this battle that Corporal F. G. Topham received the Victoria Cross 'for sustained gallantry of the highest order for six hours, most of the time in great pain.' There was much movement of units following the crossing of the Rhine, and with the liberation of Holland in April 1945 Canadian participation was almost at an end. One of the most difficult problems during this period was the supply of medical equipment, but this gradually disappeared with the opening up of rail and road traffic. On April 28, what amounted to a truce came into effect on the 1st Canadian Corps' front, and with the end of hostilities on May 8, the 1st Canadian Infantry Division was employed mainly in containing the German movements in Western Holland. During this period the rapidity of the Canadian advance had called for reorganisation of the forward evacuation system, and a new medical operation instruction was issued on April 24. At the close of hostilities plans were made for the disposition of hospitals in the occupation zone when a new rôle for Canadian medical personnel made itself apparent. Valuable experience gained in earlier stages of the campaign was applied during this period and the medical units, in addition to caring for the troops in the occupation area, were called upon to supervise and control medical administration of the German Army, Navy and Air Force. They shared in the task of controlling all medical stores of the German forces and maintaining close liaison with the public health section of the Military Government Branch over joint problems affecting military and civil requirements.

One of the first medical problems to be dealt with was the provision of attention for liberated prisoners-of-war in camps which had been overrun prior to the cessation of hostilities. Medical conditions in these camps were bad because of overcrowding and inadequacy of treatment of the sick. Another duty was the taking over of German military hospitals which, in contrast with those for prisoners-of-war, were well housed, staffed and equipped. British or American prisoners in these hospitals were rapidly passed into Allied hospitals. Nationalities were re-grouped in hospitals in various cities, and the removal of German medical equipment began. The provision of the care of German troops on the move back to Germany also required much attention from medical units of the Canadian Army. The gradual disbandment of certain units began to take place at this time, and many personnel began to move toward the concentration areas for disbandment and return to Canada.

Medical units were part of the Canadian Army Occupation Force, which was to consist of one division of approximately 25,000 men. On July 11, 1945 this division took over its new duties. Each regimental medical officer had a sick-bay of ten beds, and each field dressing station had 40 beds and held patients up to 14 days. General hospitals held cases likely to recover in six weeks, discharging patients to the 3rd Canadian Infantry Division reception centre or directly to the soldier's previous unit. During this period the A.D.M.S. was medical adviser to the G.O.C. who was the military governor of the area, and a great responsibility fell on him for the restoration of normal health to the people dwelling in that vicinity. By May 15, 1946, all medical units had been closed and a British force took over. It was six years and nine months after Canada had declared war and almost two years after the opening of the great offensive to capture Europe from the Germans.

HONG KONG

On October 27, 1941 Canadian forces left Vancouver for Hong Kong. The medical arrangements were found to be those of a normal British

501

command, with two military hospitals and a naval hospital. Some of the Canadian medical officers and nursing sisters were posted to the British military hospitals and other medical officers remained with their battalions in the Kowloon Peninsula. Separate records were maintained for Canadians admitted to the British hospitals. The only serious problem during this period was the incidence of venereal disease which had become a marked problem by the first week in December, threatening to impair the fighting efficiency of the force. At approximately eight a.m. on December 8, the Japanese opened their attack on the Colony by bombing various targets on the Kowloon Peninsula. During the first bombing of Kowloon the personnel of the medical inspection room at Sham Shui Po Camp transferred their equipment and medical supplies to Wan Chai Gap, the Island headquarters of the Grenadiers. Casualties from the mainland were evacuated to the Combined Military Hospital in Kowloon and later moved to St. Albert's Convent on the Island. Subsequently casualties were evacuated to the Bowen Road Hospital. During this period ambulance cars with large red crosses were frequently attacked by Japanese aircraft. When Hong Kong surrendered there began for the survivors a long period of dreary captivity in conditions that are almost indescribable. For four years they were herded together like cattle in prison camps, kept on a near-starvation diet, and compelled to perform hard manual labour. The Japanese, with a few exceptions, were largely indifferent to the needs of the sick and wounded, and they made no effort to provide adequate medical facilities. When they began to pay Canadian officers it was possible for these men to purchase some medical supplies. At Sham Shui Po Camp there was a dysentery epidemic following a shortage of cooking utensils; there were few medical instruments and only chloroform was available as an anaesthetic. At the end of January 1942 the Canadians were evacuated to North Point Camp where conditions gradually improved and liaison was permitted with the Bowen Road Hospital. During August a diphtheria epidemic occurred. Antitoxin was not available, except in very small quantities by private purchase. In January 1943, 650 Canadians were sent to Japan to work in various industries. The medical officer, who was chosen by lot, acted also as commanding officer. The measure of his success in dealing with the Japanese, and in persuading his fellow prisoners to make the best of things, is that only 25 of this group died. Although it was the largest group of Canadians in Japan it had the smallest number of deaths. Three further batches were sent, making a total of one medical officer and 1,183 other ranks. Two nursing sisters continued to work at the Bowen Road Hospital after the Japanese occupation. Despite many hazards they survived and were returned, after being interned with civilians at Stanley Camp. It was through them that the first news of the events in Hong Kong reached the Allied Forces.

Japan was not a Signatory of the Geneva Convention. Had it been so, its treatment of prisoners-of-war would have violated the Convention incessantly. For example, at one point during the fighting a medical aid post was overrun by the Japanese and the personnel were killed. The medical officer's life was spared only after he had been barbarically treated by his captors.

III. ARMY ANCILLARY MEDICAL SERVICES
NURSING SERVICE

During the Second World War the nursing sister attained the status of a fully commissioned officer for the first time in history. Preparations for war were made by the nursing profession and a list of those who were willing to serve was maintained by nurses in their own areas. This list proved invaluable. It was during the Second World War too that nurses served in forward areas with the Canadian Forces, going as far forward as field dressing stations. The experience with this method of distributing nursing sisters was entirely satisfactory and they all conducted themselves in a highly efficient manner. It was also during this type of warfare and during the active and rapid movement of the campaign in Europe that the battledress uniform was adopted with great success for nursing sisters.

DIETITIANS

The appointment of dietitians to the R.C.A.M.C. was an advance during the Second World War. They made a valuable contribution to the smooth and efficient operation of Canadian military hospitals. The appointment of a chief consultant in nutrition at N.D.H.Q. was of significant value.

PHYSIOTHERAPY

The enrolment of physiotherapists in the R.C.A.M.C. was another innovation during the Second World War, and the appointment of a chief physiotherapist was also made for the first time. Their work became an integral part of the programme of rehabilitation which included in its scope many fields of curative effort. Physiotherapists began their work at the bedside of the patient and continued until the soldier had been returned to his unit or to civilian life.

OCCUPATIONAL THERAPY

The formation of the occupational therapy branch of the R.C.A.M.C. was also an innovation in the Second World War, as was the appointment of a consultant in this field. Recruitment of personnel was carried out by a special committee under the direction of the Canadian Occupational Therapy Association. The Red Cross assisted in this sphere until the occupational therapists became fully organised and integrated into general hospitals.

HOME SISTERS

A new branch of the Nursing Service, R.C.A.M.C.—'Home Sisters' was created during the war. 'Home Sisters' were responsible for the care and household management of the nurses' residences. They served in all types of accommodation from permanent hospitals in Canada to tents in Sicily.

RULES AND REGULATIONS

Dietitians, physiotherapists, occupational therapists and home sisters, on appointment, were carried on the Nursing Service, General List R.C.A.M.C., and were referred to as members of the Nursing Service. There was little distinction between the various branches with respect to rules and regulations. During the long and colourful history of the nursing service members were granted the relative rank of officers, but they did not possess the status of officers because it did not carry with it the power of command exercisable by a commissioned officer of corresponding rank. In 1942 P.C. 4059 was passed, giving authority to grant commissions and the power of command to members of the nursing service selected to serve as officers. Their powers of command were restricted to such personnel as were placed under their command and they did not have individual powers of punishment. They were eligible to sit as members of courts-martial at trials of members of their own service but were not permitted to be appointed as presidents. The granting of commissioned rank to members of the nursing service marked a very definite turning point in their army career. They were put on an equal footing with all other commissioned officers and they were proud of this honour. A regulation which caused considerable difficulty was that concerning marriage. A pre-war regulation compelled a member to relinquish her appointment on becoming married. This was not a great deterrent and many personnel were married in the United Kingdom. This caused some concern among those who felt there was a wastage of public funds in training and transportation and an amendment of the attestation form required all members of the nursing service to sign an undertaking not to seek permission to marry until they had given at least one year's service. It was not very helpful. Soon steps were to be taken to permit the retention of those who were married in the service if they had been given permission to marry. In February 1943, G.O. 49 authorised the retention in the service of a married member of the nursing service until she was physically disqualified for active military duties. She was then retired on compassionate grounds but could be reappointed on the recommendation of the D.G.M.S., or the D.M.S. (overseas).

CANADIAN NURSES IN SOUTH AFRICA

The serious shortage of nurses in the Union brought about the despatch of 300 nurses to South Africa for service in the military hospitals which were to be used for the evacuation of casualties from the Middle East. The rates of pay and allowance were those of the South African Military Nursing Service, and this created some difficulty; nearly 100 sisters returned at the end of a year's service. Towards the end of the war nurses who served in the South African Military Nursing Service were granted the same re-establishment benefits as other members of the Canadian Forces.

IV. THE MEDICAL BRANCH OF THE ROYAL CANADIAN NAVY

The naval force of Canada between the wars was small, comprising only six small destroyers and 1,700 officers and men. There were no permanent medical officers with the force, the last having left in 1924. From that time until the beginning of the war, the requirements of the Canadian Navy were met as part of the normal duties of medical officers of the Canadian Army. Personnel of the ships were attended at the naval dockyard or at military sick parades. When ships were on manoeuvres, a military medical officer was detailed for duty afloat. Six of the 20 divisions of the Royal Canadian Naval Volunteer Reserve were distributed in 20 Canadian cities and received care from practising physicians.

RECRUITING

The work of medical officers at recruiting centres was of a high order. This is shown by the fact that of 105,000 recruits examined only 10·1 per cent. were rejected on medical grounds and of those accepted only 3·5 per cent. were later eliminated for medical reasons. Since the wear and tear of Service life in six years of war would give cause for more than half of these discharges, it will be seen that the error of recruiting medical officers was little more than 1 per cent. including the recruits who did not admit to serious organic disease. It was the policy of the Canadian Navy to require service at sea of all its medical officers, after they had first become acquainted with naval life and ship's procedures at an inland centre. In this way the service was less of a mystery to the newcomer when he reported for duty at a large naval base.

ROTATION OF DUTY

One of the remarkable features of service for medical officers in the Royal Canadian Navy was the rotation of duty. An officer was seldom left for six months at a recruiting centre, or more than six months at sea. He was also never left for more than one year at any naval base, thus avoiding any suggestion of an officer becoming a forgotten man. This prevented boredom, distributed appointments equitably and enlarged each medical officer's experience throughout the whole naval service. Even the most experienced consultants at naval base hospitals spent time at sea and shared the dangers and hazards afloat of crews in war-time.

NAVAL HOSPITALS

When war broke out there were no naval hospitals, not even a bed! Ultimately, temporary hospitals were erected at Halifax and Esquimalt, to be followed by the addition of some permanent structures there as the Service needs developed. A hospital was established in H.M.C.S. *Niobe* at Greenock and was of value to those employed on the convoy routes. This hospital maintained close liaison with the R.C.A.M.C. in the United Kingdom and frequently benefited by advice and counsel from the visiting army consultants.

HEADQUARTERS

When the Second World War began, medical problems were referred to the Director General of Medical Services of the Army. A D.N.M.S. was subsequently appointed. He later became Medical Director General of the Royal Canadian Navy. Every naval base had a competent staff, so reference on clinical matters to headquarters for advice was infrequent. Central medical stores met all naval needs; problems of mutual concern were discussed with members of the other Forces. Primarily the office of the Medical Director General acted as adviser to naval headquarters on medical policy, and with the continued growth of the navy the medical officer strength at the office of the Medical Director General rose from a single officer in 1940 to ten by the end of the war. The rotation of duty also applied to medical officers serving in this office in order to broaden their experience.

NURSING SERVICE

Registered nurses were recruited for naval nursing, and eventually numbered 323. They had the status of other officers of equal rank in the naval service and the registered nurse wore the maroon distinction cloth already used by wardmasters of the sick-berth branch. Other members of the nursing branch including dietitians and physiotherapists, wore the green distinction cloth. The style of the uniform closely followed that already in use by nurses of the R.C.A.M.C. and made easy the recognition of a nursing officer of the Canadian Armed Forces in whatever country she might be. Though the Medical Director General was responsible for the nursing branch, detailed administration was by a matron-in-chief who later became the Director of Nursing Service at M.D.G. Headquarters.

SICK-BERTH BRANCH

This branch expanded from 20 men to over 1,200 before the end of the war; to this were added 350 women of the Women's Royal Canadian Naval Service. They were suitably trained and rendered good service at sea and on shore.

MEDICAL INTELLIGENCE

A special branch effectively provided the latest medical information to the members of the medical service in the Royal Canadian Navy.

LOAN OF MEDICAL OFFICERS TO BRITAIN

Forty junior medical officers were loaned to the Royal Navy during the early period of the war. They served for two years. As volunteers for this duty were numerous it was always possible to send a replacement when an officer returned at the expiration of his two-year tour of duty. The original 40 had been replaced two and a half times, so that approximately 100, or nearly one-quarter of all medical officers who entered the Canadian Navy, saw service in the Royal Navy.

PROFESSIONAL TRAINING

One of the difficulties for serving medical officers in any armed force is loss of contact with academic pursuits. The Navy was quick to appreciate this difficulty and organised a series of courses to replace the limited clinical experience that the officer would have had during his service at sea. At every naval base there was a hospital with specialists who needed assistants, and medical officers who showed aptitude in a specialty were selected for further training before assignment to duty in these locations. When they had demonstrated their abilities they were placed for further training in teaching hospitals. There was a special group of officers sent for courses in tropical medicine, and some took a diploma in public health. At the close of the war almost 200, or nearly half the total strength of medical officers, had received some form of refresher or post-graduate work, spread over 26 hospitals in Canada, the United States and the United Kingdom. In the case of those who returned to civilian life the additional training in the Navy helped towards specialist certification and proved useful in the resettlement of these officers.

The quality of leadership in the Royal Canadian Navy Medical Service during the Second World War was of a high order. It illustrated one of the most important lessons of war, that the prime requisites for those who are destined to command are leadership, imagination, judgment and a spirit of friendliness and goodwill—qualities which permeate to all levels of their commands.

V. THE ROYAL CANADIAN AIR FORCE MEDICAL BRANCH

At the beginning of the Second World War the medical care of those serving in the Royal Canadian Air Force was provided by medical officers drawn from the R.C.M.A.C., their activities being co-ordinated by District Officers and the staff at National Defence Headquarters. The need for the creation of a separate medical service was represented to the Minister of Defence and after considerable discussion this Service was established in September 1940. A Principal Medical Officer was appointed in each area with direct access, on professional matters only, to the national headquarters in Ottawa.

HOSPITALS

The principal R.C.A.F. units were provided with hospitals. Most of these were on new stations and were standard hospitals of good size and construction, built under the authority of the war-time committee on hospitalisation. Eventually there were 100 of these hospitals, with a total bed capacity of 5,383. The largest of these was at St. Thomas at the Technical Training School, which was capable of looking after 700 patients. In October 1943 arrangements were made for the use of certain beds by the R.C.A.F. in Department of Pensions and National Health hospitals throughout Canada. Eventually these units became known as Regional Medical Board Hospitals. In 1943 also a number of convalescent hospitals were provided.

This interesting development and utilisation of Department of Pensions and National Health beds was the end of the long effort on the part of the departmental officials to have more active participation in the treatment of war patients. The R.C.A.F. were, in effect, in control and at least the departmental beds were being used. Difficulties of control were circumvented by the administrative arrangements. On the other hand, these arrangements suited the R.C.A.F. because it removed the necessity of creating entirely new hospital units in order to give the service the autonomy required to make it function efficiently.

THE MEDICAL BRANCH IN THE WOMEN'S DIVISION

The Royal Canadian Air Force (Women's Division) was created in February 1941. This innovation brought special problems including, for example, the alteration of existing hospital facilities. Two station hospitals were specially built for women, and staffed and administered by women doctors. Women who entered the medical trades were trained by women doctors. Special difficulties arose, for example concerning the shoe, which had a rigid toe-cap similar to that worn by men. Because of the thin stockings worn by women the toe-cap frequently caused sores, and the type of shoe had to be abandoned in favour of one more suitable for women. Special uniforms and clothing had to be designed. Some doctors trained in gynaecology were appointed and the Department of Pensions and National Health appointed gynaecological consultants for the women's division. Venereal disease was not a serious problem, and personnel affected were not discharged from the Service unless there were other indications to make it advisable. An effort was made to maintain confidential records and posting to another station was carried out if the medical officer in charge felt it was necessary to help re-establish the airwoman in the Service.

Pregnancy was a more important problem but its incidence was not unduly high. Social implications, however, added to its significance. Special regulations were devised, diagnostic facilities developed, and proper care was provided until the women concerned were re-established in civil life. Senior officers of the medical branch were of the opinion that the frequency of illegitimate pregnancy among Service women during the war was no greater than that among the civilian female population of the same age group.

DIRECTORATE OF MEDICAL SERVICES (AIR)

Gradually a pattern of administration was evolved similar to that of the Army. The various sub-directorates dealt with administration, professional matters, aviation research and nursing. A board of honorary consultants formed an advisory consultant body on professional matters which was directly responsible to the D.M.S.

MEDICAL ARRANGEMENTS OVERSEAS

In the United Kingdom Canadian squadrons had their own Canadian medical officers. Initially, medical care had been an army responsibility and air force personnel were hospitalised in army hospitals. During the later stages of the war the R.C.A.F. was closely integrated with the R.A.F., and many of the medical arrangements were made through R.A.F. formations. This led to some difficulty, since the standards of British medical care in Service hospitals differed from those in Canadian hospitals. Partial solution of the difficulty was effected by referring air force patients to Canadian Army general hospitals.

Function of the small medical headquarters in London was restricted by the close integration mentioned above. Medical documentation and statistics became an important function of this headquarters. It was necessary to adopt the R.A.F. system of records which was the only workable arrangement at the time. In view of the varying requirements of pension boards this information was not always suitably correlated and it would have been better if a system of Canadian medical records had been available to the R.C.A.F.

Because of the widespread distribution of R.C.A.F. units in the United Kingdom the provision of special R.C.A.F. hospitals was not practicable. There were small station hospitals but serious cases from R.C.A.F. squadrons were sent to E.M.S., R.A.F., R.A.M.C., and R.C.A.M.C. hospitals. Though the question of a separate R.C.A.F. hospital was seriously considered from time to time this was never brought about. In 1944 a hospital at Northallerton was offered to the R.C.A.F., but they were no longer interested. Canadian medical officers and nurses were posted to this hospital to assist in caring for the large number of Canadian casualties going through that area.

A large sick quarters was maintained at the repatriation depot at Warrington in Lancashire. It was opened in 1942. Subsequently it moved to Torquay. Boarding facilities expedited the arrangements for repatriation.

Air force casualties needing plastic surgery were treated from 1942 in the plastic surgery unit at East Grinstead where much successful and pioneer work was done.

R.C.A.F. MEDICAL BOARD IN LONDON

This was opened on May 1, 1944. The Board acted mainly as the instrument of R.C.A.F. repatriation policy. Liaison was maintained with R.A.F. consultants and specialists and members of the board attended R.A.F. medical committees. The creation of an all Canadian Board proved justifiable as Canadian medical officers knew the men's personal difficulties. It was not possible for the specialists employed to keep their colleagues at home fully informed owing to the pressure of board work but valuable information was sent to Canada from time to time. More opportunity might have been afforded for specialists to visit units and study station conditions; this was of particular importance to the psychiatrist who needed to be familiar with the stresses to which aircrew and ground crew were exposed. In psychiatry the board did valuable work.

It may be observed that Canadian psychiatrists took a more lenient view of a man's nervous breakdown and refusal to fly than did those in the R.A.F.

MEDICAL ARRANGEMENTS IN OTHER THEATRES

One squadron of the R.C.A.F., No. 417, served in Egypt in 1942 and, subsequently, in the Western Desert, Tunisia, Sicily and Italy. A Canadian medical officer was responsible to the R.A.F. formation and patients were treated in non-Canadian units. Similarly other squadrons served in the Kairouan area of Tunisia in 1943 and three squadrons operated in Asia.

No. 52 (R.C.A.F.) MOBILE FIELD HOSPITAL

This self-contained mobile unit equipped with trucks, trailers and tenders to carry its staff and equipment, had a number of ambulances attached for moving patients, and served during the North-West European campaign. It functioned well in air evacuation in 1944 and 1945. From D-day to the end of June 1945, 16,531 Canadian casualties were evacuated by the R.A.F. and R.C.A.F. to England without a single aircraft accident or death.

In Canada, from 1943, special aircraft were held at each command for the transport of cases to command hospitals difficult of access by road or rail, where specialists in various fields of medicine were available. Patients were also transported by air from Labrador and Newfoundland. Some of the early problems included the development of a suitable stretcher, and this was supplemented by a casualty bag with zip openings to permit access to different parts of the patient. In severe cold these were of great value but in temperate weather blankets were a more satisfactory means of controlling the temperature of the patient.

VI. MEDICAL ARRANGEMENTS FOR THE BRITISH COMMONWEALTH AIR TRAINING PLAN

The development of schools in Canada for the training of aircrew drawn from various parts of the British Commonwealth placed a great burden on the R.C.A.F. which at the time of the agreement to this plan was a small force with a strength of 8,000. Four training commands were developed and a large number of stations opened. Early in 1942 much progress had been made with the training of personnel but so many more aircrew were needed that the plan continued until March 1945. More than 157,000 aircrew trainees passed through these schools. In addition to ordinary sickness, difficulties arose from the assembly of crews from many parts of the Commonwealth and the varieties of bacterial flora introduced by them.

Problems arose through the use of R.A.F. medical documents. The R.A.A.F. and R.N.Z.A.F. used the same documents. Adaptation of crews to Canadian environment and habits and in particular to the long, cold Canadian winter, had to be made. For instance, a new and more suitable overcoat had to be issued to Australian personnel; the one provided for them at home was too short to give protection against the severe winter weather in Canada. In the United Kingdom, Canadians accustomed to plenty had to adapt themselves to austerity measures due to the war. Learning to fly in a blackout area, when training had been developed in an area with space and light, called for medical advice in relation to morale.

In retrospect it is apparent that varying attitudes and backgrounds added unexpected problems to the application of medical standards and treatment to all those serving in the Air Training Plan. The greatest of these which remained unsolved until the end of the war was the provision of medical care for the families of Commonwealth air force personnel in Canada. No such provision existed in Canada, as the situation had not been foreseen and this resulted in financial embarrassment to overseas airmen. The long period of training aggravated these difficulties. This problem should be anticipated if ever Commonwealth joint programmes are contemplated in the future.

VII. OBSERVATIONS ON THE R.C.A.F. MEDICAL BRANCH

The following observations were made by the historians for the R.C.A.F. medical branch:—

Representation to Higher Authority. The newly developed R.C.A.F. medical branch soon encountered one of the problems common to all medical services in armed forces; it found it difficult to place its advice before sufficiently senior authority to have it implemented. It became evident that representation of medical opinion in important professional matters is necessary at the highest administrative level. The autonomy of a medical service is difficult to define but is of sufficiently great importance to the nation that medical authorities should have the highest representation possible.

Organisation of a Headquarters Directorate. The organisational pattern of the medical branch emerged after much experience, being divided into administrative and professional divisions. Medical and administrative problems came to be so extensive that it was very difficult to combine these functions in one person. The administrative and professional aspects were well handled within the branch by doctors with special qualifications in individual fields. It is frequently assumed that the administrative aspects might be effectively carried out by non-medical personnel and that employment of medically qualified administrative officers is wasteful of man-power. Experience, amply confirmed in civil life, suggests that while the assistance of lay administrators is most valuable, the key medical administrative posts must be filled by medical officers.

Autonomy in Overseas Theatres. In the United Kingdom, where the R.C.A.F. was for a large part of the war almost entirely integrated with the R.A.F., a situation was created which should be forestalled. The R.A.F. was responsible for medical care of Canadians serving with the R.A.F. or in R.C.A.F. units. There were only a few small R.C.A.F. medical units functioning in the United Kingdom or on the Continent, and R.A.F. hospitals provided most of the definitive care. Excellent as this care undoubtedly was, it was given in surroundings, and in a way, sufficiently unfamiliar to Canadians to make many of them dissatisfied. It will be most important in any future conflict where R.C.A.F. personnel serve abroad to see that they are provided with care in their own medical institutions to the greatest extent commensurate with the size of the force and the availability of medical personnel. At the very least, co-ordinate, joint Service hospitals should be established for the treatment of armed forces personnel. Had such a policy been in force throughout the Second World War, many of the differences and frustrations which arose, in spite of every effort to provide liaison between those providing the care and those receiving it, might have been avoided.

Authority of A.F.H.Q. It became evident during the Second World War that overseas formations tended to develop their own autonomy and authority. It was possible at great distances and with inadequate communication and liaison to ignore or to circumvent policies established at National Defence Headquarters. This situation is obviously undesirable. The closest co-operation should exist between formations serving abroad and National Headquarters in order that policies and practices be uniform.

Moreover, despite instances of excellent co-operation, liaison was not adequate during the Second World War either with Canadian formations or with those of our Allies. With rapid advances in medical knowledge such liaison is assuming ever greater importance and the value of exchange officers in Allied Headquarters, from each side, is of great significance.

Medical Man-power. Many problems relating to man-power were encountered in the medical sphere. There was a great shortage of trained specialists which seriously affected the air force medical branch since it only implemented hospitals for definitive treatment late in the war, when other Services had absorbed many of the specialists. It is, therefore, most important to acquire the services of such specialists and to see that adequate provisions are made for their training in future wars. Special attention should be given to the training of officers in the treatment of tropical diseases; such knowledge is of great value in peace-time and would be invaluable in the event of global operations when such diseases might well be encountered. The development of Service hospitals to provide adequate professional opportunities and clinical experience for doctors is an important part of the professional training programme. Such hospitals can also be utilised for the training of radiographers, laboratory technicians, nursing personnel, and medical administrative officers. There should indeed be a training centre for these personnel at or near a Service hospital.

It was observed during the war that some air force medical officers became dissatisfied with their lot in the Service, and some thought should be given to the factors from which this discontent arose. In particular, it may be said to derive from isolation on stations remote from medical centres and other medical officers. Many doctors left their civilian occupations for national service in the expectation of serving overseas. The requirements of the British Commonwealth Air Training Plan made it necessary to retain in Canada, often at isolated stations, a large proportion of the total strength. Consequently, there were very few opportunities for service abroad, and movement was very limited. There was not a great deal of illness on flying stations, and constant attendance upon groups of airmen who were in good health and who had only minor illness served to make even the most enthusiastic of these young medical officers dissatisfied. The alternative for many of them was service on one of the medical boards; some medical men also grew impatient with this form of occupation after a time. With few hospitals until late in the war only a limited number of R.C.A.F. medical officers had much opportunity to have more complicated clinical experience than that offered on medical boards or on a training station. This situation might have been rectified by the inclusion of more hospitals for definitive treatment within the air force medical sphere, or by greater exchange of duty with the sister medical services. Whatever the best remedies may be, they must certainly be implemented, before any future medical service operates on a large scale; the high morale of its medical personnel is indispensable to its efficient functioning.

Some of this discontent might have been avoided had the exigencies of the service been explained as fully as possible to medical officers on appointment. Many had been specifically assured that they would be sent overseas, and air force requirements at home had not been sufficiently stressed. Medical officers realised that many other highly trained Service personnel were not given the opportunity to practise their professions during the war, and the restrictions placed on their own activities might have been accepted more readily had Service requirements been made clearer. Information on Service opportunities should be made as accurate as possible and promises and assurances should not be made when there is the slightest doubt of their being able to be fulfilled.

Immunisation. The control of communicable diseases was a major problem for the Armed Forces, and in the Air Force many experiences with epidemics of scarlet fever, respiratory diseases, and others, showed the importance of quarantining personnel after movement and the value of a sound immunisation programme. Furthermore, adequate housing with proper hygiene, pest control facilities, and education in personal hygiene were shown to be of great importance. The loss of training hours, personal illness and disability cost many times the amount which it would have cost to protect personnel in adequate accommodation and with proper advice. Crowding in barracks was proved to be most unwise and should be avoided at all costs in future campaigns. The medical officers responsible for preventive medicine and hygiene, whether at A.F.H.Q. or at C.H.Q., should have sufficiently high rank to ensure that their advice will not be ignored.

Medical Statistics. A valuable contribution was made in the development of an effective medical record and statistical system and in the production of useful practical medical statistics. These developments were initiated immediately upon the formation of the medical branch in November 1940 and came into full effect during 1941 with the application of modern methods of machine tabulation and the development of standardised forms for securing the basic information. Further extensions and refinements were introduced during the years 1942–44. These included the development of regular reports on key subjects and the production of special releases in particular fields, for example, aircrew medical wastage statistics, rehabilitation data, and industrial disease and injury statistics. The R.C.A.F. undoubtedly provided leadership during the Second World War for Canadian medical services' statistics and gained valuable experience upon which to build future medical records and statistical methods and procedures. Some of the practical results of these efforts are reflected in the air force statistical data in Volume II, Chapter 35, and in those relating to B.C.A.T.P. personnel in Chapter 23 of Volume I of the *Official History of the Canadian Medical Services*, 1939–1945.

Rehabilitation. The development of programmes and institutions for the rehabilitation of the sick and injured was a most satisfactory undertaking from all viewpoints. The impetus of war made possible the advancement of knowledge in the whole field of rehabilitation, and the conservation of man-power was well demonstrated. It was shown that men could be returned to duty earlier and better fitted than was possible without the aids of a properly operated convalescent or rehabilitative centre. The effects of proper diet and nutrition during convalescence were well and repeatedly illustrated, and these lessons need application to armed forces and to civilians alike.

Unification of the Armed Forces Medical Services. Much discussion occurred during and after the war about the need for three separate armed forces medical services. Complete unification initially presents itself as a reasonable and feasible solution but, like many complex problems, closer examination discloses it to be difficult and impracticable. Close integration of the three armed forces medical services is desirable and was achieved to a reasonable degree after the first irritations engendered by separation had passed. Whether continued integration could or should ever lead to amalgamation is a matter which time and experience alone can show. At the close of the war, when Service morale had reached a peak in the Army, Navy and Air Force, it seemed that physical re-union of the three sister medical services was improbable at any point in the future; since that time many former officers have come to believe that such union is desirable, but those with most intimate knowledge of the problems are certain that only close integration is feasible. Certainly a more ready exchange between the three medical services, which would operate more effectively than the war-time arrangement, should be initiated and maintained by whatever devices can be arranged. Joint use of hospital facilities, where economical and feasible, continued use of joint supply systems, frequent exchange of medical personnel, exchange of liaison officers at administrative levels, joint Service committees in all spheres of activity—all of these devices should be developed and encouraged to function for the mutual aid and betterment of the Services, each of which may have men serving on land, at sea and in the air.

In the development of a completely new medical service for the R.C.A.F., tradition had little to contribute and innovations were the order of the day. Despite mistakes and shortcomings which are evident in retrospect the medical branch was established on sound lines and its efforts on behalf of the airmen, whom it was its privilege to serve, can be contemplated with some satisfaction. The important contribution of the wearers of the winged caduceus to all phases of selection, training and operations was made evident to the other branches of the force, and it is now axiomatic that medical considerations be given due weight in the complex business of operating a flying service. In the event of a future conflict, with the inevitable necessity of further rapid expansion, it is to be hoped that the experience of the Second World War will provide a firm foundation on which to build.

VIII. THE CANADIAN DENTAL CORPS

This originated in the First World War and was established as an independent service in 1939. Efficiency and economy were demonstrated by a single unified command. It proved most successful throughout the

Second World War and in 1947 it became the Royal Canadian Dental
Corps.

IX. MAN-POWER AND THE MEDICAL SERVICES

The use of Canada's man-power during war-time required a proper
balance to be kept between the needs of the Armed Forces, industry
and agriculture respectively. In the Second World War this had a
direct bearing upon the functioning of the medical services as regards
recruitment.

EARLY RECRUITING FIGURES

On September 1, 1939 the Canadian Government authorised a Canadian
Active Service Force, which reached about 69,000 volunteers by the
end of the year. Recruiting was then temporarily discontinued. Resumed
for tradesmen in February, the figures rose to nearly 85,000. For the
formation of the 3rd and 4th Divisions in 1940 enlistments rose rapidly,
and 158,000 had been mobilised by the end of July 1940. Some 200,000
had been recruited by the end of the year, of whom 13,000 were
discharged on medical grounds. This gave much work to the R.C.A.M.C.
With the deterioration of the European situation, the Canadian Government in 1940 asked Parliament for special emergency powers and began
the enrolment of National Resources Mobilization Act recruits. With
each successive wave of enlistments revision of the medical standards
became necessary. In September 1939 visual standards had been
lowered. In 1942 they were further lowered, vision being allowed as low
as 20/400ths in either eye, provided both eyes could be corrected to
20/40ths. In 1944 the standard was lowered as to the degree of correction.
Standards for hearing were also down-graded.

It was in 1942 that the first steps were taken towards the development
of the now famous PULHEMS System. This made it possible to
describe relatively quickly the physical standards of an individual and
train medical personnel and others to set them down appropriately in
graphic form. It has been described as 'a graph of the soldier's ability to
work at set levels of performance.' The system is widely used in many
armed forces throughout the world today. With its adoption the standards
of examination both for incoming and outgoing members of the Forces
were considerably improved.

THE CANADIAN MEDICAL PROCUREMENT AND ASSIGNMENT BOARD

This was established to ensure an equitable distribution of medical
personnel during the war. Its composition comprised representatives of
the medical directorates of the Army, Navy and Air Force, the Department of National Health and Welfare, the Department of National War

Services and a lay representative of the Director of National Selective Service. There were five representatives of the Canadian Medical Association, these being also members of the Canadian Medical Advisory Committee. This Board tabulated, analysed and utilised a survey made by the Canadian Medical Association of physicians registered in Canada. They determined the number of doctors available for military service and allocated them in proper proportions to the three branches of the armed forces. At the same time they had to consider civilian needs and the public health services in Canada.

After November 1942, dentists, medical and dental technical personnel were added. The D.G. of Dental Services was a member. Nurses came under the Board in December 1942. From October 1944 the Board arranged post-graduate and refresher training facilities to meet the needs of ex-Service personnel in medicine and public health, and studied placement opportunities in Canada. Representatives of the Association of Canadian Medical Colleges, of the Royal Colleges of Physicians and Surgeons of Canada and of the Canadian Hospital Council were added to the Board.

The Board's work, at times, was hampered by the lack of mandatory or compulsory powers. Local committees usually were able to persuade the person concerned to act as the Board wished in the national interest. Such an organisation will be needed in any future mobilisation of medical personnel.

CIVIL DEFENCE*

In 1938 a committee was set up under the Deputy Minister of the Department of Pensions and National Health to enquire into and report upon the non-military measures which should be adopted against the possibility of air attack, including gas attack. Secrecy was required and the committee recommended that provincial governments and municipal authorities should be taken into the confidence of the Federal Government. It also urged the government to arrange for the manufacture of gas masks, the construction of auxiliary fire equipment and the

---

* In June 1939 there was an arrangement between the Minister of Defence of Canada and the Minister of Health of the United Kingdom for providing Canada with information concerning the medical organisation then being built up in England and Wales in case war broke out. In that month Mr. Elliot, the Minister of Health, sent Sir Arthur MacNalty, Chief Medical Officer of the Ministry, to confer with Government officials in Canada. Discussions covered such subjects as Air-Raid Precautions, anti-gas measures and decontamination, the organisation of the Emergency Medical Services, hospital arrangements for the reception of wounded Service men and air-raid casualties in the civilian population and the provisions for the evacuation of school children and other persons from towns and cities to country districts. Following his mission to Canada, Sir Arthur MacNalty visited the United States of America and had similar discussions with leading Government officials.

Although the medical problems of such vast countries as Canada and the United States differed considerably from those of the United Kingdom, all three countries welcomed this exchange of information and ideas which subsequently was to prove of mutual advantage.

training of instructors. In 1939 representatives explained air-raid precautions to various provincial governments, but they met with a luke-warm response. Subsequently a Federal Air Raid Precautions Officer with general supervisory duties, was appointed. Provincial A.R.P. organisations remained on the whole weak throughout the war, but on the Coasts the committees were charged with blackout responsibilities and were very active. After the fall of France in 1940 air-raid precautions were better organised, especially in the coastal towns. Medical arrangements were well organised and a good warning system with adequate inter-communication was developed.

THE DEPARTMENT OF NATIONAL HEALTH AND WELFARE

Throughout the war various offices of this department carried out specialised duties including health services in war plants, and certain medical investigations, including one concerning fitness for duty as merchant seamen. Adequate hospital facilities at the ports were developed rapidly for convoy survivors. Restriction of narcotics was given close supervision. The Department also dealt with the problems of quarantine and immigration. Of particular value was the Sick Mariners' Service which ministered to the health needs of all Allied merchant seamen using Canadian ports, particularly Halifax.

THE CANADIAN RED CROSS SOCIETY

A total of 16,000,000 food parcels were shipped by the Society to Canadian, British, and Allied prisoners-of-war. These parcels helped many prisoners to survive, especially those taken by the Japanese. The Society also helped to provide blood and plasma and this saved many lives. The Canadian public subscribed $80,000,000 to the Red Cross, and 95 per cent. of its work was done by volunteers.

THE ST. JOHN AMBULANCE ASSOCIATION

The existence of an active St. John Ambulance Association was a very considerable contribution to the efficiency of those recruited by the R.C.A.M.C. and other medical formations during the war. Also the enrolment of women members of the Association as nursing assistants gave valuable aid when there was a critical shortage of man-power. Care was given to injured merchant seamen and survivors arriving at Halifax and other ports. The home nursing service augmented the national resources in a period of crisis. Participation of this organisation in air-raid precautions and Civil Defence should be considered in any future planning. The war brought it increased activity, increased membership and wider functions.

X. ADVANCES IN MEDICINE AND SURGERY

The advances in medicine and surgery between the two world wars were quite as impressive as those in other fields of human activity, and the speed of development was accelerated during both wars. In the second volume of the official history of the Canadian Medical Services from 1939–1945 a detailed study of the experience gained is set forth. This section summarises the chief lessons learned in these two fields.

MEDICINE

ACUTE INFECTIOUS DISEASES

These presented a constant problem for the Armed Forces during the Second World War, causing loss of life, considerable invalidism and much loss of time from duty. Protective measures introduced since the turn of the century helped to reduce the losses and there was no smallpox, little typhoid fever and a reduction in the other acute infectious diseases. Diphtheria decreased when effective immunisation had been undertaken and, after the Royal Canadian Air Force started routine immunisation in 1941 they had, in Canada, only 30 cases of diphtheria, with no deaths, for a period of more than four years. Tetanus was well controlled with toxoid and there was only one fatal case of this disease throughout the war. Few Canadians were exposed to typhus or to yellow fever, but vaccines were available. The development of D.D.T. and the widespread application of sulphonamides and penicillin reduced the hazards from other infectious diseases. But in spite of this there was still a large volume of uncontrolled, rapidly spreading communicable disease in the Canadian Forces. Mass respiratory infections were incurred by the concentration of troops in new circumstances and environment.

Diphtheria. When diphtheria appeared large doses of antitoxin were administered in the potent globulin preparations available from 1944 to 1946. Penicillin in the Mediterranean theatre cleared the carrier rate temporarily but tonsillectomies effected a more permanent cure. Penicillin failed to prevent late complications and despite high hopes proved disappointing in the treatment of this disease. Diphtheria of the skin was adequately treated with antitoxin and penicillin. A severe outbreak of diphtheria in the Royal Canadian Navy in Halifax late in 1940 was controlled by the institution of rigid isolation procedures and the administration of toxoid to certain groups.

Meningococcal Infections. A discovery of note was the prevalence of meningococcal septicaemia without meningitis. During a three-year period 60 cases of meningococcal infection were treated in England. In 30 of these the infection was evident only by the septicaemia and by the eruption on the skin. Sulphonamides and penicillin in 1944 greatly lowered mortality.

Infectious Mononucleosis. Because of its insidious onset and many manifestations this disease was often undiagnosed before the patients were admitted to hospital. Experience showed that a minimum of six weeks from diagnosis was required to prevent complications and prolonged convalescence to ensure adequate recovery.

Infectious Parotitis (Mumps). Occasionally cases occurred with signs of pancreatitis or orchitis only, and presented diagnostic difficulty.

Vincent's Angina (trench mouth). This condition was occasionally confused with diphtheria.

Rheumatic Fever. In Canada during 1941 and 1942 the establishment of new training camps and the arrival in them of thousands of men from all over the world caused a great rise in streptococcal infections. In 1942 in the Forces on the prairies many cases of rheumatic fever occurred with cardiac involvement. These cases were startling because they occurred in large groups in the late spring and early summer. It is evident that they were related to the antecedent respiratory epidemic and while such epidemics are common in Canada every year, rapid movement of troops, with a consequent exchange of bacterial flora, no doubt accelerated this pattern. In respiratory epidemics which preceded these outbreaks of rheumatic fever, type *A 19 haemolytic streptococcus* was the most frequent infector. There appeared to be a close correlation between the incidence of streptococcus epidemics and the arrival of rheumatic fever, one writer putting it at 4 per cent.

'Approximately 4 per cent. of those suffering acute streptococcal upper respiratory infection developed some manifestation of the rheumatic state; these occurred from 20 to 50 days after the onset of the antecedent respiratory infection, large numbers of which occur in the cold months. Ninety per cent. of the cases in the series developed during the first seven months of the calendar year. This is important in view of the large numbers of respiratory tract infections which developed during an epidemic season when troops were housed in large groups together. It may be significant that the highest rates of incidence were encountered in Alberta and Saskatchewan.

'When medical officers met these groups of cases for the first time, they were naturally impressed with their gravity, having in mind the classic descriptions of the disease and the manner in which it occurs in children. In such cases 80 to 95 per cent. are said to have cardiac complications. As a result it was a policy in the Canadian forces, as well as in others, to discharge all such cases on their first attack. This policy was modified in 1942 following a review of over 400 cases; thereafter none was discharged except in the following circumstances:

if after adequate therapy, clinical supervision, and convalescence, there were signs of cardiac involvement; or if signs in any system persisted more than two months. . . .

'While not of great numerical significance, rheumatic fever and its concomitant manifestations or sequelae, were important because they affected younger personnel, wasted much time, and had 25 per cent. cardiac complications. The end result was a high rate of discharge or low PULHEMS activity. The R.C.A.F. experience with rheumatic fever was different and a lower rate of cardiac complications was noted.'

Similar outbreaks of varying degrees of severity were seen in the Air Force and the Navy.

TUBERCULOSIS

The use of radiography of the chest on enlistment assured an armed force relatively free from gross pulmonary tuberculosis. In spite of this 5,000 cases of pulmonary tuberculosis and 1,200 cases of pleurisy were pensioned during the war. The majority of these were discovered during the last year of the war and at the discharge examinations. The average war incidence of pulmonary tuberculosis, including tuberculous pleurisy, was estimated to be 300 per 100,000.

The incidence in overseas troops was much higher than in those serving in Canada. It was largely among recruits from Ontario and the prairie provinces, who had had no previous contact with tuberculosis and were therefore tuberculin negative. The immunisation of recruits in future with B.C.G. must therefore be considered. In the Royal Canadian Navy it was found that 0·47 per cent. of all recruits examined were positive or suspected cases of pulmonary tuberculosis and represented 4·7 per cent. of the recruits rejected for all causes. Since the general incidence of tuberculosis in civil life was about 1 per cent. there was some concern lest half of the existing cases had been missed and as a result a careful survey of all discharge boards was made. Out of a total of 151 men discharged by December 31st, 1943, a percentage of 0·18 suffering from pulmonary tuberculosis was found. As many of them had served some four years this figure was reassuring.

Elimination of tuberculous cases on enlistment and adequate remedial measures for early cases discovered proved of value in keeping a low incidence of tuberculosis in the Canadian Forces during the war. All Services agreed that immunisation of troops from non-tuberculous areas will need to be considered in any future mobilisation programme.

ACUTE RESPIRATORY DISEASES

These were the chief causes of morbidity but the mortality was low. One observer estimated that over a million training days were lost by acute respiratory disease during 1943. Roughly one bed in three was continually used for this disease in the Armed Forces. The rates were variable. They were high when the troops were in transit; on occasion almost all such men would be suffering from some form of acute respiratory infection. On the other hand, seasoned troops living outdoors in battle had fewer respiratory infections, especially during action. The most serious of respiratory infections were the streptococcal epidemics in training camps and scarlet fever was a serious concurrent manifestion of the ravages of acute respiratory infection. In barracks hygienic measures—use of oiled blankets, the oiling of floors, elimination of dust, adequate ventilation and personal hygiene controlled the spread of infection. These measures were employed by all the three Armed Forces.

Influenza. Throughout the war it was feared that a pandemic of influenza might affect the Armed Forces. Repeated surveys were conducted but no major epidemics developed. This was fortunate since no preventive measures were available. However, polyvalent vaccine may be an important factor in the prevention of casualties in the Armed Forces in any future conflict or mobilisation. A puzzling development relating to the virus infections was the condition which came to be known as *primary atypical pneumonia*. Had it not been for the readily available antibiotic in the latter part of the war a pandemic of serious proportions might have developed.

Pneumonia. Pneumonia was a relatively minor cause of death in the Forces. This was attributed to the prompt administration of the sulphonamides and later of penicillin and other antibiotics.

Mucosal Respiratory Syndrome.—'Stevens-Johnson Disease'. This rare respiratory disease made its appearance from time to time in sporadic outbreaks. Its cause was never identified and it had a high mortality rate. It is a condition which needs to be looked for whenever there is a concentration of troops during a mobilisation period; it is possible that some of the modern antibiotic agents may prevent the serious complications due to bacterial infection.

GASTRO-INTESTINAL DISEASES

Peptic Ulcer. A major problem was that related to peptic ulceration. Patients with early manifestations, including dyspepsia and vague gastro-intestinal distress crowded the out-patient services and the wards of hospitals in Canada and overseas. Frequently, when an ulcer had been clearly seen in a young man it would heal so completely that subsequent X-ray examination failed to reveal any sign of scar. This led to some misunderstandings but the policy gradually adopted was to keep men willing to remain in the three Services in a limited capacity, that is, they could not serve where adequate diet might not be available, nor in situations where sudden haemorrhage or perforation might endanger the lives of others.

Surgery was not viewed with favour, but where therapy and dieting failed, operation was found necessary, especially in patients with recurrent haemorrhage.

The Dysenteries. Epidemics occurred in troops stationed in the Middle East. Special precautions were required in the Italian theatre of operations.

Bacillary Dysentery. Epidemic diarrhoea should be regarded as due to bacterial infection and explanations of a more casual nature should not be accepted until proved correct. Sulphaguanidine, with other appropriate measures, was effective. This is a serious disease with certain complications which may require prolonged care.

Amoebiasis. This appeared after the invasion of Sicily in July 1943. Adequate facilities for its diagnosis are important and examination for cysts should be made. Much illness, invalidism and loss of life can be prevented if active investigation is arranged for in the field.

Infective Hepatitis. This disease was a serious problem in all theatres where Canadians served. It caused much wastage in man-power. Patients lost an average of fifty days from duty. Death was rare. Cirrhosis may develop. Measures for control were inadequate, as was the diagnosis of latent cases where jaundice appears at a late date.

NEUROLOGY AND PSYCHIATRY
ARMY

At the close of the Second World War a group of army psychiatrists were invited to contribute their opinions and experience to a joint narrative descriptive of their activities at home and abroad during the Second World War. Psychiatry attracted much attention during this period and the study of mental illness came into prominence more than it ever had previously. At the end of their account those who were concerned with army psychiatry presented the following summary:

Base levels. The conclusions drawn rest on the following basic premises:

1. Modern war demands the total mobilisation of a nation's resources, including its man-power and women-power.

2. Of the personnel mobilised, a relatively small proportion is utilised in the fighting forces that are expected to meet the enemy's forces.

3. Modern war differs from former wars (even from the First World War) in that there is little place in an overseas force for the mentally dull, the inadequate, or the grossly unstable soldier.

4. No test or battery of tests now in use on this Continent or in the United Kingdom will predict with accuracy the soldier's ability to withstand the stress of war.

5. The stresses of war should not be confused with the stresses of combat—the latter are only a small part of the former.

6. The army psychiatrist must, of course, make diagnoses and institute treatment, but above all other things it is his duty to recommend appropriate disposal of the unfit, so that they are not permitted to impede the fighting forces.

7. The psychiatric weeding out of the unfit must be a continuous process from the outbreak of war until demobilisation.

8. The psychiatric service must be united so that uniform policies can be adopted by the forces serving in Canada, at overseas base if there be one, and in any theatre of operation in which Canadians fight.

9. Psychiatric service must be closely co-ordinated with the personnel selection in all areas, so that the maximum use may be made of personnel who are temperamentally unsuited for combat duty, or who have become unsuitable during service.

The first medical screening should, of course, be at the reception centres. This screening should not be too fine, as the best indication of a young soldier's future effectiveness may be determined empirically by his response to discipline, separation from home, and other aspects of Service life, during his first few months in the Service. Suitable intelligence tests should be applied to all personnel prior to enlistment. It has not been proven that cursory psychiatric examination of all recruits serves any useful purpose. The psychiatric examination of new recruits should be limited to the examination of referrals from medical boards and unit medical officers.

A thorough medical examination should be given all soldiers prior to posting for service abroad, regardless of whether the movement of troops is by units and formations, or by reinforcement drafts. At this point, psychiatric referrals should be made wherever indicated, and the recommendations acted upon regardless of pressure from non-medical authorities. This pressure will always be brought to bear in order to avoid last minute depletion of numerical strength.

The following groups should not in any circumstances be permitted to proceed overseas:

1. Chronic alcoholics.

2. Drug addicts.

3. Persons having history of treatment in any mental institution.

4. Persons known to have had repeated convictions for civil offences.

5. Incorrigible soldiers, i.e., those who have repeatedly undergone detention, either with their units or in special detention barracks.

6. Soldiers who are obviously much older or much younger than military age, even though of apparently good type.

The above paragraph might seem superfluous, but throughout the whole of the Second World War, personnel falling into the above groups arrived overseas in large numbers, and spent much of their time in the hospitals, in detention barracks, or in civilian prisons. From 1943 to the end of the war Canadian soldiers in British prisons, added to those undergoing detention in the Canadian Army, more than equalled the numerical strength of a battalion. Most of these had bad pre-war histories, or bad Service histories while in training in Canada, and many of them had both.

Overseas base. At an overseas base, psychiatric casualties may be treated in general hospitals, or in a special neuropsychiatric hospital, or in both. The investigation and treatment in a special base hospital is likely to be better than by a psychiatrist attached to a large general hospital. It is suggested that if an overseas force consists of two corps or more, a special base neuropsychiatric unit is justified.

A psychiatric consulting service must be made available to divisions long before they go into action.

No matter how good the psychiatric screening is in Canada, an overseas force will accumulate large numbers of soldiers who are unfit for combat duty, or for employment in ancillary forces in forward areas. In order to economise in man-power, the better of these should be lowered in category to prevent them reaching forward areas, and should be placed in suitable employment. A few of these can be placed in base units, thereby releasing more fit personnel for forward areas. In order to justify the retention of the remainder overseas, it is advisable to set up special employment units. The numbers and size of these special units should depend on the needs of the overseas service, and should not be dependent on the number of ineffectual soldiers which has accumulated.

In placing at base levels soldiers who are unfit for combat duty, it must be remembered that in future wars important stores and concentrations of personnel at base level will be targets for concentrated bombardment by enemy missiles. Therefore, although a soldier working in a cookhouse at the base in the First World War was free from enemy action, similar employment was not so safe in the Second World War, and in future there may be no line of demarcation between forward and rear areas. Some psychoneurotics of good intelligence did better in active employment on lines of communication and with forward area units, than when they were posted to headquarters units in London during the bombardment from aircraft, V–1, and V–2 bombs.

There should be very close liaison between the Judge Advocate General's Branch and the psychiatric service. Each psychiatrist should receive clear instruction as to his function when called upon to express an opinion in connexion with soldiers undergoing courts-martial or trial by civilian courts. First, the psychiatrist should remain impartial. Whether his services are requested by the prosecution or by the defence, he should never be either the witness for the prosecution, or the witness for the accused, as is so common in civilian cases. In expressing either oral or written opinion to be considered by the court, the psychiatrist should be brief, and his opinion should be as definite as possible.

The services of the psychiatrist should be available when it is necessary to give a pronouncement on the sanity of a prisoner. An important use of the psychiatric service was made in the detention camps, prisons, and reviewing boards where remission of sentences was being considered. A psychiatrist who has special training and aptitude for advising about these problems should be available.

General. In comparison with medicine and surgery, the advances made by psychiatry during the war were not spectacular:

1. Early diagnosis by medical boards and reallocation by the personnel selection branch did prevent many of the psychiatrically unfit from impeding the fighting force.

2. No new disease or clinical entity was discovered. Large numbers of soldiers developed schizoid states as a result of prolonged and severe physical and mental exhaustion. Many of these resembled catatonic schizophrenia, and some of them may have been true schizophrenics. The essential differences between these 'exhaustion schizoids' and true schizophrenics were their excellent response to treatment, and the absence of recurrence; many had served for a period in the North African campaign; smaller numbers appeared in other fields of action; some were returned to

duty with their former units, and carried on to the end of the war, but many did not.

3. Many advances were made in diagnostic and therapeutic procedures.

(a) Wide use was made of electroencephalography, e.g., in differential diagnosis between epilepsy and hysterical epileptiform reactions.

(b) Electro-convulsive therapy was carried out extensively in the United Kingdom, and to a lesser extent in base hospitals on the Continent of Europe.

(c) Abreaction techniques were extensively used in the United Kingdom and in both the Mediterranean and North West European theatres of war. Although the term abreaction was used chiefly for the psychiatric interview following the use of a general or intravenous anaesthetic, similar technique was used without narcosis or hypnosis.

(d) Prolonged sedation (with or without the use of insulin and forced feeding) was employed to good effect in all theatres of war, and in the United Kingdom. The further from the theatre of action, in both time and distance, the less beneficial this type of therapy is.

(e) Leukotomies were not done in Canadian hospitals overseas.

Psychiatric disabilities will account for approximately 30 per cent. of all casualties invalided out of any army during war. Of these, over 80 per cent. show definite evidence of constitutional disposition to psychotic or neurotic breakdown, or have constitutional defects such as mental deficiency or psychopathic personality. In chronic or recurrent cases, where the constitutional factor is prominent, results from treatment are poor. Less than 25 per cent. of cases are rehabilitated to the point where they become useful forward area soldiers.

The above figures are very similar to those given following the First World War. At face value this would appear to be disappointing, and to suggest that the immense expansion of the psychiatric service has served no useful purpose. This is not so. The weeding out of the mentally dull, the unstable, and the ineffectual has been more drastic than ever before. This would seem to be sound policy in the light of the needs of modern warfare. Modern weapons and the thousands of technical instruments now in use demand a higher calibre of soldier than was needed in former wars. The hordes of illiterate soldiers with which Alexander the Great conquered the world would present no opposition to a modern army. In forces where this function of the psychiatric service did not operate, the standard of efficiency fell far short of that in other services of our times.

A comparison of an account of the place of psychiatry in the First World War with the foregoing detailed account and conclusions reveals some outstanding differences. The lessons learned in the First World War, while they were remembered slowly, were eventually applied in the field; diagnostic and treatment services were carried forward into battle areas very effectively. Along with this administrative advance there came several technical advances which improved the care that the psychiatrist was able to give to his patients. The important difference, and the one which led to most controversy, was that the psychiatrist in the Second World War developed a new relationship to administrative authority.

The demand for highly skilled and highly trained soldiers made selection and proper allocation an important function. The close liaison which was established between psychiatry and the personnel selection was important in this undertaking, and in the preservation of scarce fighting man-power. There is little doubt that this liaison was beneficial, and it was generally agreed that it should be perpetuated. The dangers inherent in this liaison are, on the one hand, that army examiners (personnel officers) attempt to assume the rôle of psychiatric diagnosticians; on the other hand psychiatrists sometimes tended to infringe on the territory of the placement officer or the administrative officer. Such infringements are as dangerous as the allocation of an infantry soldier to a tank. By the end of the campaigns in the Mediterranean and European theatres, the functions of the psychiatrist in the divisions, and in the corps, had become more clearly defined. They were useful in conserving man-power, in building morale, in developing treatment units, and for disposal of difficult cases. The conflict between administrative officers, field commanders, and the advisers in psychiatry had resolved itself into satisfactory co-operation.

The psychiatrists in Canada during the last three years of the war were confronted with two major problems: civilian morale and shortage of man-power. In the face of these difficulties, too careful screenings of recruits were sometimes attempted. There was administrative friction, and the solution was found only after some months of difficulty. It has generally been agreed that the best method of psychiatric screening is a test of service, after the obvious cases have been rejected by enlistment medical boards. It was learned by the psychiatrist who confronted these problems, that the fundamental difficulty related to policies of employment of the Canadian during war-time; they also were related to mobilisation, and to lack of appreciation of the rights of citizenship. Early mental hygiene programmes, the inculcation of less selfish attitudes, more independent viewpoints, and a greater sense of responsibility for the community or the country as a whole, have been urged as a result of this experience. The place of the psychiatrist during the Second World War has been outlined. The psychiatrist himself was frequently frustrated at every level of activity, and there was a general failure to appreciate the importance of the work he had to do. The volume of psychiatric casualties alone, 30 per cent., warrants very special consideration of his services. His position, like that of all other medical officers, must be that of an important adviser; to prevent interference by virtue of army rank, it was agreed that he should be placed in responsibility to senior formations, with attachment to the units in which he was to serve. Although the psychiatrist might not agree, in general it would seem that his best work was done as a diagnostician and in the treatment of casualties, rather than on morale and placement. No medical officer in an armed force, and particularly no psychiatrist who deals with sometimes abstruse and philosophical concepts, should step out of the rôle of adviser. It is to be remembered that an administrative officer under pressure of circumstances may accept the responsibility of rejecting medical advice of any kind.

ROYAL CANADIAN NAVY

The Navy did not employ psychiatrists at recruiting centres. When such advice was needed the examining medical officer might choose a Service or civilian consultant. Recruits were entered in an active reserve status and, during training could be eliminated if they did not come up to naval standards. From these trainees the naval bases and ships drew their recruits. Appraisal tests for alertness and aptitude were deferred until the recruit was called for active service. By such methods the loss of trainees was less than one per cent. In the Navy 85 per cent. of all patients passing through psychiatric clinics returned to duty. Men at sea developed a love for their ships and respect for their officers and shipmates. Team spirit was evident and circumstances which took a man out of his ship were an injury to his pride. This, together with good selection of recruits, ensured that mental and nervous disorders were not over-prominent in personnel of the Royal Canadian Navy.

ROYAL CANADIAN AIR FORCE

Psychiatric consultants were available after 1943. In the North West Air Command problems related to isolated life in a remote region. The Eastern Air Command problems chiefly concerned the long patrol duty. In Central Canada a special problem was the treatment and disposal of R.A.F. personnel having flying training. Isolation on the prairies during the long Canadian winters caused psychiatric problems.

Both as regards selection of personnel and morale in aircrews psychiatrists took a lenient view. In particular, refusal to fly on account of 'exhaustion' etc. did not necessarily mean a man's discharge from the Service. At the same time the psychiatric problems of selection of personnel were never fully solved and the subject demands further investigation.

PERSONNEL SELECTION

In September 1941 a personnel selection branch was established to maintain liaison with the R.C.A.M.C. and advise commanding officers in the handling of personality problems. As there was evidence of a man-power shortage it was important to implement this programme at once. At the same time a programme of personnel selection was instituted overseas, but these programmes differed. In Canada the service was concerned with the rapidly moving stream of new recruits and their appropriate selection and placement; in England personnel selection officers were dealing with army units already established and their tasks were largely in re-allocation. Reliance was placed upon the central accumulation of data on a 'Q' card and the use of a punch-card and sorting system was helpful. In 1942 and 1943 Army examiners were stationed at basic training depots, to work closely with medical officers and training officers. They were also placed at special training centres and at officer training units. The success of personnel selection officers in carrying out their duties is indicated by the increasing use made of their services as the war progressed. Their advice was sought and acted upon by commanding officers in the selection of officers for training and the re-allocation of personnel and the disposal of men and women unsuitably placed in the Service. Later, the techniques that had been developed were applied to the Canadian Women's Army Corps. At a later stage in the war this service was used in advising men about to be demobilised. It is to be noted that the service of the D.P. Select developed in the face of opposition and criticism and it would appear that occasionally army examiners failed to remember that they were merely advisers; sometimes they tended to assume the rôle of executive officers. The question of the amalgamation of this branch with the R.C.A.M.C. was not settled at the conclusion of the war.

Personnel Selection in the R.C.A.F. At about the same time as it occurred in the army interest developed in personnel selection in the Royal Canadian Air Force, and in the autumn of 1941 administrative officers were assigned to new duties in this connexion. Valuable work was done on the R.C.A.F. classification test (intelligence) and gradually improvements were effected in the selection methods. The development of a Visual Link Trainer was a valuable adjunct to selection. The emphasis in the air force selection was objective and test-minded.

Correlation of other attempts at selection were never successful. A special flying squad was developed which was helpful in solving special problems at various stages of the war. It is important to note that the institution of a programme of this kind did reduce the number of training failures by providing factual evidence to show a recruit his relative chances of success in various aircrew trades. The programme proved to be effective in persuading crews to accept the trades for which they were best suited. Substituting tests for educational certificates enabled the Air Force to enlist aircrew with less than matriculation standing. This phase of the operation of personnel selection did not have an opportunity to develop fully during the Second World War and it is suggested that particular emphasis should be placed upon it in any future mobilisation period.

VENEREAL DISEASES

The rising incidence of reported venereal disease in the Armed Forces of Canada, combined with the loss of time from duty which resulted, demonstrated the need for greater control. A venereal diseases register was kept overseas from the beginning of the war and proved invaluable. There was a comprehensive reorganisation of control in the Army in February 1943, following a similar step in the Air Force early in 1942. Though no exact data are available, education, legal control measures, prophylaxis, diagnosis, and treatment, helped to check the spread of infection. Nevertheless outbreaks of infection occurred after outbursts of exuberance or during inactive periods.

Syphilis. As regards the treatment of syphilis an adviser in syphilology should be appointed to a senior headquarters post early in any future conflict. There must be immediate establishment of diagnostic standards and treatment routines workable and adaptable to the exigencies of the Service, with adequate personnel available to treat this disease.

Special Treatment of Infections of the Lower Genito-Urinary Tract. The development and clinical application of new chemical and biological agents dramatically affected the treatment of venereal and other infections of this region. A special unit at No. 1 Canadian Special Hospital provided treatment for these patients and a satisfactory régimen for the treatment of urethritis was developed before D-day. In warfare on the Continent of Europe small mobile venereal disease units were organised. These units were provided with their own transport but were attached to casualty clearing stations or field ambulances for hospital beds and for rations and stores. Three such units opened in Europe, one being in Italy. They avoided the evacuation of many cases and provided adequate and early treatment.

DERMATOLOGY

Experience in the Canadian Army with the treatment of dermatological conditions was carefully summarised at the end of the Second World War, and the following criticisms and recommendations were offered.

Defects in the supervision of dermatological problems were obvious during the war, but from the vantage point of history a critical review of the arrangements indicated a situation in which disaster was averted more by individual effort than by administrative planning. At the outbreak of hostilities in 1939, as in 1914, there were no provisions for the proper dermatological assessment of men being recruited for active service. Furthermore, no such arrangements were ever established in the Canadian Army. There was a complete lack of arrangements for dermatological consultations in large troop concentrations in Canada, in the United Kingdom and in the active theatres of war. Sporadic attempts were made to set up such a service but were never brought to completion, except in the United Kingdom where two dermatological specialists were authorised in 1943. The Air Force used civilian specialists for the difficult cases; the Navy had a good dermatological consultant service at its East Coast hospital. No effort was made at any time in Canada to train officers who showed aptitude or interest in dermatology, apart from that in the navy hospital on the East Coast. From 1943, in the United Kingdom, an unofficial arrangement was made whereby a dermatologist visited hospital centres in England to consult on difficult cases, and to arrange transfer for superficial X-ray treatment at the hospital in Leavesden. The establishment of this X-ray therapy unit in England justified itself; the forces in Italy and North West Europe would have been greatly benefited by the provision of similar units of mobile type. There was the excellent example of the British who had well-trained dermatologists at every level, and who had specialists in North-West Europe with trained staffs of dermatologists and graded dermatologists to assist them. The Canadians received valuable assistance from this source, and it helped to raise the standards of diagnosis and treatment appreciably. The Americans were not well organised for dermatology at the outset of the war, but rapidly improved and at the close of hostilities had a splendid organisation with an adequate number of trained dermatologists at every level. The good general standard of treatment which was achieved for the Canadian Forces at home and abroad was the result of the personal interest and enthusiasm of individual medical officers.

In retrospect, the handling of dermatological problems in the Navy, Army, and Air Force left much to be desired. There was no long-term planning for the training of dermatologists in the three Services or for specialists' care of dermatological patients. There were one or two exceptions to this, notably, the excellent dermatological organisation in the Navy on the East Coast and the establishment of two dermatologists in the Canadian Army overseas. No dermatologist was appointed as adviser or consultant in any of the three Services to use the dermatologists available to the best advantage. It is true that civilian dermatologists were used in various centres throughout Canada, but this was a local arrangement and not the result of planning from headquarters.

In spite of these shortcomings in planning, dermatological patients were not neglected in the Canadian Armed Services, but this was the result of enthusiasm and effort by medical officers working without dermatological specialist training. In the future, a planned dermatological service should be arranged for the Canadian medical services, modelled on the excellent system of the British and American Forces. The ideal arrangement would be to have a consultant dermatologist in Ottawa to act as adviser to the three Services and arrange the disposal of dermatologists in the Services to the best advantage. Competent dermatologists should be available at all large enlistment centres for Navy, Army, and Air Force, to give expert advice on all doubtful cases before enlistment. Each command should have the services of a dermatologist as should each large concentration of personnel of all three Services. Every 1,200-bed Service hospital should have a dermatologist on its establishment or one easily available for consultation. Each corps or army should have a senior dermatologist with one or two junior specialists available per division.

History has one important function, that of making the experience of the past available to those who may face identical situations in the future. It is to be hoped that the experience of two world wars will not be overlooked by the Canadian medical services in the future.

Dermatology in the Navy. Certain situations in the Navy during the war created specific skin problems. As a result of experience it was agreed that in war abnormal conditions must be accepted and the diminution of skin diseases was a matter of supervision and education in personal hygiene by the medical officer. The occasional case of a specific allergy to the woollen cloth of a naval uniform was encountered and this led to the release of such a person from the Service.

PREVENTIVE MEDICINE AND HYGIENE

An officer in charge of hygiene was appointed at National Defence Headquarters in 1939. Preventive medicine sections were established in the Navy and the Royal Canadian Air Force at an early date. Throughout the war hygiene officers were supplied to the various active units of the Navy, Army and Air Force.

Immunisation. All troops in Canada were immunised with T.A.B. vaccine from the outset. Late in 1943 T.A.B.T. was made available.

Tetanus toxoid was highly satisfactory and there were only two authenticated cases of tetanus in the Canadian Army. Before the major attack on Europe the First Canadian Army was vaccinated for smallpox and given booster doses of T.A.B.T. and typhus vaccine. There were no deaths from smallpox in spite of constant exposure to this disease in North Africa.

As a result of the immunisation policy in the R.C.A.F. the incidence of diphtheria was strikingly lower than that for the Canadian Army. Both rates improved substantially during the period, the Army from 99 per 100,000 to 22, and the R.C.A.F. from 16 per 100,000 to 1 per 100,000.

Control of Malaria. This was difficult, but some success was achieved in the North African and Sicilian campaigns. See II *Campaigns.*

Control of Scabies. Early in 1943, benzyl benzoate 25 per cent. lotion, controlled this prevalent disease.

Typhus Control. In addition to personal measures, field hygiene sections were equipped with gasoline-driven air compression units, which permitted the dusting of hundreds of persons quickly with 5 per cent. D.D.T. The control of typhus was one of the great advances made in the war.

Environmental Hygiene. Many improvements were made in regard to sanitation, the provision of mobile baths, laundries, kitchens and water purification.

NUTRITION

Surveys of the nutritional standards of troops were made whenever possible. It is desirable that in any future war a comprehensive survey should be made of Canadian Service personnel in operational theatres. A Canadian team equipped with a mobile laboratory was lent to Allied Land Forces, South East Asia. It made nutritional and environmental studies of Indian soldiers in India and Burma and also studied the nutritional standards of a group of captured Japanese soldiers. These studies were, in themselves, of intrinsic value.

One of the great advances of the Second World War was the development of compact rations. Carefully planned and executed ration trials provided the information on which these were established. This kind of study is extremely important and needs to be related to the actual fighting conditions in which the troops will find themselves.

Use of vitamin concentrates. These were used chiefly in the treatment of malnutrition, but sometimes administered after prolonged use of rations deficient in normal vitamin content. An optimum state of nutrition over a long period of time can only be assured by the use of a wide variety of natural food-stuffs, transported, stored, prepared and served by methods which conserve food value.

Feeding of hospital patients. High protein diets for convalescents from injury or surgical operation were instituted and proved of considerable value.

The Standing Committee on Nutrition, Department of National Defence. This committee, representing the three Services, was set up in December 1941. It was composed of civilian and Service experts and advised on the adequate rationing of the armed forces in Canada. It controlled the complicated setting up of ration scales, ration trials and special types of compact rations. There was no widespread or serious malnutrition among the Canadian Forces. This testifies to the Committee's work. This Committee in future should be established early when there is any large concentration of men in armed forces.

PHYSICAL MEDICINE

During the war convalescent units, similar to those developed by British Forces between the wars, proved a useful adjunct to the treatment of casualties. New methods and improved techniques were developed and promulgated. Physiotherapy, occupational therapy and educational facilities added to the value of these units, which were under the command of a medical officer and not of a combatant officer, thus ensuring better co-ordination with other medical formations. The development of casualty retraining centres in Canada was an important and satisfactory advance.

Techniques. High repetition and low resistance exercises were used early in the war. Later, heavy resistance exercise (Watson-Jones' 'rule of thumb' method) was helpful in certain cases. Grouping of similar types of injuries into one platoon for retraining had a good psychological effect. The retraining much reduced the time required to restore the patient to health and there were fewer permanent disabilities. The chief difficulties experienced were to secure doctors trained in physiotherapy and an adequate supply of qualified physical training instructors.

SURGERY

WOUNDS AND INFECTION

At the end of the First World War the position relating to the treatment of wounds was as follows: (1) complete surgical cleansing of the wound, including removal of all devitalised tissues and foreign bodies and provision of adequate drainage; (2) secondary suture; (3) primary suture in the large proportion of feasible cases; (4) importance of rest and immobilisation in the control of the spread of infection; (5) many agents such as Flavine, Dakin's Solution, and B.I.P. were in use.

A large group of cases remained where irrigation for prolonged periods was necessary. Then H. Winnett Orr introduced rigid immobilisation of adequately drained wounds in plaster-of-paris casts. Trueta used this method in the Spanish Civil War, and it was known as 'Trueta's method' at the outbreak of the Second World War. In this war closed immobilisation on an excised wound remained as the basic treatment for all serious wounds and in a high proportion of cases made wounds safe for secondary closure. Its disadvantage was the prolongation of convalescence.

Secondary Suture. There was controversy about the relative value of primary and secondary suture. Towards the end of the war it was standard practice to close all wounds secondarily if their clinical condition seemed to offer an effective result. This applied also to the largest types of wounds. In the last year of the war wounds were treated as early and thoroughly as possible, the injured part immobilised and penicillin therapy begun. As soon as possible the patient was transferred to the base and there secondary suture was done if there was a reasonable hope of success. Penicillin was continued for at least five days after secondary suture.

Primary Suture. With this treatment complete healing is obtained within 10–12 days, pain is minimal, there is no discharge, no necessity for further dressing or operation, and, probably, the result is better. Primary suture, of course, would be a dangerous procedure if sulphonamide or penicillin resistant organisms were present. Even if adequate excision had been done virulent infection might develop.

Wound Infections. Mobile laboratories made careful bacteriological surveys of wounds. This information was of use in the treatment of serious infections.

Gas Gangrene. Thorough surgical treatment of the wound proved the best prophylaxis. Specific anti-sera were valueless. The value of sulphonamides and penicillin in prophylaxis was not fully determined. All patients were given sulphonamide with or without penicillin, blood or plasma and intravenous and intramuscular antitoxin in doses up to 100,000 units of a mixed antitoxin daily. The results seemed satisfactory but were difficult to assess.

WOUNDS OF THE CHEST

Great advances were made in thoracic surgery in the war. An understanding of the complications of intrathoracic trauma, together with the close co-operation of surgeon and physician, are likely to effect the best results in treatment.

The following principles were established. The body and clothing of the wounded man should be kept as clean as possible. The patient should receive at once prophylactic sulphonamide or antibiotic therapy. He should be evacuated at once to a unit competent to deal with shock and to recognise and treat intrathoracic complications. Haemothoraces must be aspirated early and completely and the pleural cavity kept dry by repeated aspirations. It is advisable to inject an antibiotic into the pleural cavity. Pneumothoraces, unstable chest walls, increasing pericardial pressure or cardiac damage should be recognised and appropriately treated.

A patient with a massive wound, or a large foreign body retained in the chest, or one encroaching on some vital structure, that might be benefited by an early thoracotomy, must be distinguished from those that do not require surgical intervention.

Other advances included: the treatment of clotted and infected haemothorax by thoracotomy and decortication; the better use of blood transfusion in resuscitation of patients with chest wounds; the use of sedatives; removal of mucus by bronchoscopic suction; breathing exercises to preserve and restore function and use of antibiotics. Decorticating the lung in cases of clotted and infected haemo-thoraces was the one great technical advance in the surgery of the lung during the Second World War.

ABDOMINAL SURGERY

Perforating wounds of the abdomen must be treated surgically with the minimum of delay. Transfusion of whole blood or serum and replacement of fluid loss by glucose and saline solutions were measures available to every hospital in England and in other theatres of war, and to every medical unit in the field.

The development of the field surgical units, following the experience of the British Army in North Africa, ensured prompt and adequate surgical treatment. They were well staffed by young surgeons trained in urgent military surgery, had a blood transfusion service, were well equipped, self-contained and mobile. As a result mortality rates were lowered. Gastric suction was used and chemotherapy. The latter seemed to have little direct effect in treatment of abdominal injuries uncomplicated by associated wounds of the extremities; penicillin, in the campaign in North West Europe, probably helped; it was given as a routine to all the severely wounded.

The mortality from abdominal wounds in the Italian campaign ranged from 30 to 35 per cent. and reflected the difficult weather and transport conditions in the winter of 1943–44. In North West Europe the mortality rate from these wounds varied from 28 to 30 per cent.

Inguinal Hernia. As man-power shortage developed, hernia was given remedial treatment. In 1943 Physical Standards and Instructions was amended to allow for this. The recurrence rate after operation was only

4 per cent. It was the Canadian experience that 86 per cent. of recurrences occurred during the first year and 56 per cent. during the first six months.

NEUROSURGERY

A special treatment centre was established in 1939 at Basingstoke in England for the treatment of neurological casualties. The plastic surgery unit was housed in the same building. Close co-operation with the departments of plastic surgery and psychiatry contributed to the high calibre of the work done.

Careful investigation of the patient was made. A short-acting anaesthetic agent was valuable; it was important to prevent anoxia. Penicillin reduced the incidence of infection in penetrating head wounds from 6 to 3 per cent.

Work in the unit led to clearer understanding of some types of head injuries; for example, the development of the technique for the treatment of cranio-orbital wounds. Pineal shift, when identified, was the key to the successful treatment of certain types of intracranial damage. The rehabilitation of spinal cord injuries was another important contribution from this centre.

Mobile Neurosurgical Unit. To bring the benefits of early treatment to brain casualties in the field a mobile unit was formed which proved eminently successful. As a result of experience, specific recommendations were made for the equipment and the staffing of such a unit.

The equipment for the production and consumption of electrical power in the unit should all come from one source and an electrical engineer should be responsible for planning the equipment in consultation with the appropriate medical officers. The provision of light waterproof boxes and packing cases is vital for the transportation of equipment. Adequate vehicles for the unit would be two three-ton trucks with a trailer, the trailer to have a generator permanently fixed to it. This unit should also be supplied with a jeep or other personnel vehicle. It was found that Service corps drivers were of no value to the medical activities of the units; if these had been R.C.A.M.C. personnel the unit would have been considerably more efficient. Future planners of such a unit should make every effort to supply truck drivers from within the R.C.A.M.C. Ordnance equipment supplied for the boiling of water broke down quickly and were all too small. The hole through which the fuel came eventually plugged and the unit boiled water with the greatest possible difficulty. The solution of this problem is either to provide sufficient electrical power for the use of electrical sterilisers, or to provide a coal-oil burning stove with a sufficiently big jet to allow the fuel to come through during months of service. Such units were supplied to the British hospitals for autoclaving purposes.

Medical officers of the unit should consist of two surgeons, one anaesthetist, and two internists. While at least half of the operation on the head can be done under local anaesthetic, another anaesthetist would be desirable. At least one of the internists should be well trained, preferably in neurology; a recent graduate was found to be of very little value to this unit.

There should always be nursing sisters in this unit and, in addition, two operating room nurses. It is recommended that the unit should have its own nursing sister for the supervision of ward work.

Other ranks of the unit should consist of one corporal and two operating room orderlies, one clerk and one ward orderly, who should be a corporal, and two R.C.A.M.C. truck drivers.

These recommendations are very specific and come as the result of detailed and prolonged experience in an active theatre of war and the successful treatment of neurosurgical casualties.

ORTHOPAEDIC SURGERY

This was not a separate specialty in the Canadian Forces during the war. Generally the facilities in Canadian army hospitals were good. Each hospital had a physiotherapy staff. Fractures of the femur were successfully dealt with and as far forward as possible. Compound fractures of the femur were given high priority and operated on at an advanced surgical centre. Blood and plasma proved valuable. Persistent bone infection and non-union were rare. A few patients did not make a full recovery of function, the knee-joint being the principal seat of residual disability.

Foot Problems. These were surveyed comprehensively and the following recommendations made:

1. Soldiers' foot problems are part of military medicine and therefore should be carefully taught to medical officers when they first join the Army. Even the most junior medical officer is expected to pass judgment upon foot problems, and his decisions will have a profound effect upon man-power and wastage of personnel.

2. All available information on foot problems should be published in a small brochure for the guidance of the medical officer.

3. *Physical Standards and Instructions* for Canada should be revised to incorporate new knowledge and to give more precise instruction regarding foot problems.

4. A trained chiropodist (other rank personnel) should be on the staff of every medical inspection room and regimental aid post. A school of army chiropody should be maintained to carry out the training of such personnel.

5. Uniformity of practice in the grading of soldiers as far as foot problems are concerned should be ensured.

6. Conditioning centres should be set up to salvage the appreciable number of selected foot cases by physical training.

7. The Army should supply its own orthopaedic appliances and special boots, and not rely on the services of D.V.A.

8. A competent officer should be employed at N.D.H.Q. to supervise foot problems.

9. There is a need for further research.

Injuries of the Knee Joint. Menisectomy proved to be a satisfactory procedure.

REPARATIVE SURGERY

Considerable experience was gained in the field of reparative surgery during the Second World War. The formation of a special plastic unit, in association with the Basingstoke Neurological Hospital for the Army, concentrated this type of casualty in one location, making special experience available. Naval hospitals in Canada developed experience in this field. The Air Force had much opportunity in the plastic surgery wing of the Queen Victoria Hospital at East Grinstead. Many advances were made in reparative surgery as a result of Service experience in three major fields—burns, plastic surgery and facial fractures.

Burns. Tannic acid treatment was given up in favour of covering the burn with a clean dressing, and, if available, a saline compress. From 1943 Colebrook's ointment was applied. Morphine syrettes were useful. Shock was treated with fluids by mouth and intravenous infusions of saline glucose, plasma or blood. Anaesthetics (including intravenous) were given while severe burns were dressed. For the hands and face a dressing of *tulle gras* and saline was used. Saline baths and sulphanilamide were advances in treatment. Skin grafting was employed. When many patients had both hands burned, the problems of nursing became acute. Sometimes duodenal tubes were inserted to give drinking water to the patients. For phosphorus burns the wounds were washed with copper sulphate solution 1 per cent., and the resultant black copper phosphide was then easily seen and removed. The mortality rate from these burns was low, 0·85 per cent. The concentration of patients in a special burns unit lessened deformity and mortality.

Fractures of Facial Bones. The various technical advances (including devising, producing and fitting of prosthetic appliances) in the treatment of these injuries were aided by close co-operation with the Dental

Corps, whose insistence on careful pre-operative prophylaxis maintained a low rate of infection. Only one man died from missile wounds of the face and this was due to uraemia.

General Plastic Problems. These led to the development of new techniques. Cases were concentrated where expert attention was available at an early stage. All soft tissue wounds were closed at once so far as it was possible, resulting in a minimal degree of secondary deformity due to scar contracture.

CARDIOVASCULAR WOUNDS

Wounds of the Heart. Only 4 cases of penetrating wounds of the heart were recorded. All 4 cases lived for 48 hours after operation but died of complications. Diagnosis of such wounds can only be made by suspecting their existence, followed by exploratory operation.

Vascular Surgery. New operative techniques were developed and attention was given to non-operative treatment of vascular insufficiency.

Surgery of the Arteries. Pressure dressings were most satisfactory for control of bleeding. Topical coagulants should be used in first field dressings. The second step in treatment is replacement of blood. After the viability of the limb has been established operative procedures may be considered, such as suture of vessel lacerations, end-to-end suture of divided arteries or insertion of venous grafts. Heparin may be introduced after the insertion of glass cannula into vessels to prevent thrombosis. Prevention of gangrene by stimulation of circulation in collateral vessels was of value. The availability of blood in forward surgery accounted for a good percentage of the successes in vascular surgery. The establishment of vascular centres, which proved so successful in American and British hospitals, would seem to be desirable for the Canadian Forces. In future a vascular surgical team should be available, and surgeons who have special training in this subject should be placed where they would be useful.

UROLOGICAL SURGERY

Urologists were assigned to general hospitals and provided special treatment for renal lesions. All serious wounds of the kidney dealt with through abdominal incision required nephrectomy to avoid the risk of secondary haemorrhage.

Soldiers with spinal injuries resulting in paraplegia and a paralysed bladder were treated at special centres. Cystotomy with closure helped to give some return of bladder control.

SURGERY IN THE ROYAL CANADIAN NAVY

Immersion Foot. Surgical problems were not so numerous in the Navy as a result of shot and shell, but were often related to the problems of those who survived their ships. Immersion foot seemed to be identical with so-called trench foot of the First World War and it resulted from exposure in life boats or rafts, where the extremities were constantly wet and cold. The treatment of such injuries by refrigeration was an advance of the Second World War.

Underwater Blast. The kapok life jacket provided the best protection to the thorax.

SHOCK AND TRANSFUSION

Blood Transfusion. There were no transfusion services available to the Armed Forces at the outbreak of the Second World War. The value of such units was so well known that their development was a major contribution to the medical services. The preservation of whole blood for more than two weeks was difficult and substitutes were sought. The most obvious substitute was blood plasma or serum, and large stocks of the latter were soon built up through the foresight of Dr. Charles H. Best, with the assistance and backing of the Canadian Red Cross Society. Serum or plasma, while devoid of the oxygen carrying power of whole blood, had the osmotic activity necessary to maintain a depleted blood volume when injected in adequate amounts. It also had the great advantage that in the dry or frozen state it could be kept indefinitely without deterioration, a consideration of the utmost importance in war-time conditions. Plasma alone was found to be beneficial when the blood losses were small, but in more serious cases with larger blood loss (30 per cent. or over) blood as well as plasma was equired.

The importance of the Rh. factor was not known at the outbreak of war, and because it was impracticable to cross-match each recipient's blood with donor blood, it was decided to supply only group O blood, which is administered without cross-matching. This proved to be satisfactory and subsequent knowledge demonstrates why some reactions occurred. Since in future group O Rh. negative blood might be the only kind that ought to be supplied, and since only 15 per cent. of the population is in this group, it is doubtful whether the demand could be met. A better solution would appear to be that each man should have his Rh. type on his identity tag, and that a supply of Rh. negative group O blood be available for Rh. negative individuals.

A major problem faced by the medical services was at what point transfusion should be administered because of the difficulty of supply and the necessity of refrigeration. Blood was rarely available further forward than the advanced surgical centres, or six to eight hours after wounding. Reconstituted plasma or serum was given by the field ambulance and continued *en route* to the surgical centre. It is probable that lives were saved by this measure, particularly in wounds of the extremities where pressure dressings can be applied. The aim of transfusion should be the restoration of blood volume with blood or plasma as soon after wounding as possible. Only in this way will irreversible shock (about which so little is known), be prevented. It was learned that early application of a tourniquet above a badly infected wound would help in the resuscitation process.

A common error in many advanced surgical centres was the failure to recognise post-operative shock, and the failure to give the same careful supervision of post-operative care as was given in the resuscitation department.

It was found that after the blood pressure had returned to normal a further 500–700 cc. of blood and plasma was required to have the peripheral veins in the extremities fill normally, for the skin to become warm and for inspiration to cease causing a fall in the blood pressure.

Over-transfusion was rarely seen. The great importance of the blood transfusion service and of the resuscitation teams should be realised in any active theatre of operations.

Shock. Many advances were made in the knowledge of the mechanism of shock, and both civilian and Service teams made their contribution. Development of serum and plasma to replace fluid loss was an early step, and it was demonstrated that the application of heat to the extremities only increased the danger of shock. An outstanding research indicated that the fainting following haemorrhage is due to a decrease in peripheral resistance resulting from an active vasodilatation of blood vessels within muscles, while skin and splanchnic areas constrict. Other investigators showed that the rapid administration of intravenous fluids in the resuscitation of the wounded was likely to produce a more satisfactory result than the slow intravenous drip practised in civilian life.

The importance of the adrenal cortex in the early response to injury and in the subsequent period of convalescence was also recognised at this time.

No. 1 Canadian Research Laboratory. A field medical research unit was established in the fall of 1943. This unit examined problems relating to shock and response to transfusions and other therapeutic measures, and furthermore, certain physiological observations were made on patients without penetrating wounds of the thorax or abdomen, and upon a group with injuries of these areas. Studies were also made on the kidney function and morphology following abdominal and other wounds. It was found that many patients following operation might be excreting a litre or two of urine a day, which on examination, would be shown to have such a low specific gravity that these patients were proceeding slowly into uraemia. It may be necessary to increase fluids to an enormous extent to get an adequate output, so that the urea and potassium and other substances may be cleared by the low specific gravity dilute urine. The amount of sodium iron contained in plasma may well have had a deleterious effect in hindering diuresis.

Field transfusion units and resuscitation officers carried on work in very primitive conditions. They found that the group O blood supplied was generally satisfactory. In the case of chest wounds it was observed that when the external jugular veins were collapsed transfusion was beneficial. Where these were full it was dangerous. It was also learned that in cases of 'thoracic shock' return of blood pressure to normal was much delayed and slower than in other types of cases, and that oligaemia probably did not play so important a rôle as it plays in other types of cases. It was also learned that when abdominal wounds have been resuscitated they should be operated upon at once since they rarely resuscitate well a second time. In one series of cases so dealt with the mortality in 230 cases was only 16·9 per cent.

It was also learned that in burn casualties shock results in haemo-concentration due to the plasma loss. Here, adequate replacement of proteins is essential and haemoglobin determinations by the copper sulphate technique of Van Slyke et al is valuable.

Post-operative circulatory failure and the prevention and treatment of renal failure are the major problems to be conquered in the treatment of battle casualties who have suffered severe or extensive injuries. The obscure state of irreversible shock, so extensively investigated, is not frequently encountered in injured men. As a result of these studies during the Second World War knowledge of the treatment of casualties in such circumstances is now such that it can be precisely taught and expertly practised.

ANAESTHESIA

Personnel. Early in the war the need for additional trained anaesthetists in general hospitals and casualty clearing stations was appreciated and a four-months' course was organised. Late in the war an adviser was appointed to headquarters staff for duties previously undertaken by the consultant in surgery. Had this appointment been made earlier many of the difficulties experienced in providing training, equipment and personnel would have been avoided. The Navy and Air Force appointed consultants in anaesthesia at an earlier date. Field surgical units set up in 1943 required anaesthetists for resuscitation and emergency operations.

Equipment. It is important that hypodermic needles fit the syringes and that gas equipment will operate on the type of gas cylinders available.

Anaesthetics. Inhalation gases were mainly used at first but intravenous pentothal sodium came into use as the war progressed. It was often combined with nitrous oxygen and nitrous oxide and oxygen in critical cases. Intravenous agents were most valuable on ships at sea or in forward units.

Work. Anaesthetists' work in the resuscitation department was almost of equal importance during the war as that in the operating theatre. They were also concerned with the post-operative treatment of pulmonary complications. Deep breathing exercises before and after operation were of value in preventing atelectasis, as also was posturing for drainage of blood and débris from the upper respiratory tract.

Records. The Army record system was inadequately co-ordinated, probably due to defective organisation at headquarters. In 1942 a consultants' committee in anaesthesia was established with representatives from the various Services. It standardised equipment, investigated the cause of explosions and co-ordinated the activities of the Armed Forces in anaesthesia.

Naval Experience. Special problems which had to be considered in the Navy were those created by the cramped quarters and the shortage of trained personnel. Frequently the sea was rough and many were affected with motion sickness, particularly patients after operation. The fear of fire and explosion was always present and prevention was the responsibility of the anaesthetist.

Anaesthesia in the R.C.A.F. The R.C.A.F. programme in anaesthesia was co-ordinated early and well; adequate supplies of equipment and personnel were available to the air force hospitals at all times. Especially valuable lessons were those obtained when a newsletter was sent out periodically from air force headquarters to all anaesthetists. This stimulated the interest of Service anaesthetists in all activities relating to their work and provided an adequate flow of information to headquarters where their activities could be co-ordinated.

RADIOLOGY

The first important advance was the authorisation in September 1939 of enlistment chest films and reference of the findings to the district medical officer before attestation was completed. Eventually all troops proceeding overseas had an enlistment chest film on file. District consultants were appointed to examine films and to make the necessary consultations and recommendations.

The Canadian Radiologists' Overseas Group held regular monthly meetings. The British Institute of Radiology co-operated by lending its centre for this purpose in Welbeck Street, London. This liaison assured uniformity of radiological services overseas. In 1942 a light-weight mobile X-ray plant was devised and adopted for use in the field.

At first, the chairman of the radiologists group advised the surgical consultant overseas. Later, a consultant in radiology was appointed. A standardised technique for the verification of active peptic ulcers was adopted in 1941. Training of radiographers overseas was arranged.

A number of radiologists were trained for service in the R.C.A.F. at the Armed Forces Radiologists' School at Toronto General Hospital. Throughout the war radiologists served at air force hospitals, mainly on the air force stations. Here much work was done on the standardisation of the equipment available. In 1945 a mobile X-ray unit was devised which could be housed on a 30 cwt. lorry; the American Army Field Unit was basic equipment, with temperature controlled tanks for the processing of films and operating from a generator which formed part of the unit.

OPHTHALMOLOGY

For administration of an ophthalmology service and for recruiting specialist personnel it is important to have direct representation of this specialty on a medical directorate. Unfortunately, it was not until late in the war that the Army had such representation on the head-quarters staff. It was regretted that a special eye, ear, nose and throat hospital was not established as in the First World War. This would have concentrated trained personnel, facilitated consultation, trained nurses and orderlies and provided facilities for research.

Visual Standards. Early in the war inadequate vision tests were made; hence, many soldiers had to be re-examined, categorised, and discharged at a later date. As the war progressed, owing to the man-power shortage, visual standards had to be lowered. Allocation of troops to branches where they can do useful work based on visual standards alone is difficult and judgment must be exercised in individual cases.

Night Vision. Experience showed that the elimination of those who have difficulty with dark adaptation could best be made during advanced training when they could be sent for examination and assessment at the dark adaptation centres.

Work of the Consultants. There was a shortage of professional personnel. In any future war early and active measures should establish provision for the supply of trained ophthalmologists. Overseas a travelling consultant was appointed who based himself at the head-quarters of various field ambulances.

In North-West Europe a mobile ophthalmic unit made visits to forward areas from a 200-bed hospital. All its equipment was carried in two trucks and an operating room could be set up in two hours. Eye casualties received prompt attention from this independent unit. In 21st Army Group, this mobile unit treated 25 per cent. of all the casualties in this theatre. In major casualties involving the face and jaw the co-operation of an ophthalmologist was useful. There was a very low incidence of eye infections, due probably to treatment with sulphonamides and later, penicillin and to prompt attention. Excellent first aid was given by field medical officers because of lectures and training given by the forward area ophthalmologists. Lenses were promptly provided—within 12 hours—by the mobile unit. Front line troops could be refracted, spectacles dispensed and men returned to their units with minimal delay.

Eye Diseases. During the early period overseas there was a troublesome epidemic of Kerato-conjunctivitis. Eye injuries were related to training accidents and air raids. An important discovery was that there was a relationship between nutrition and corneal vascularisation; riboflavin deficiency appeared to be a causal factor. Only 204 Canadians became blind as a result of active service; 66 were prisoners-of-war taken by the Japanese in Hong Kong.

Glasses. The wearing of respirators was a problem for those who had to wear glasses. A special type of glasses was generally used, although unsatisfactory. It would have been better if glasses had been supplied both for general use and for respirator use. Contact lenses, except rarely, were unsatisfactory on active service. Among the difficulties of troops serving overseas was the tardy provision in 1943 of a unit for the supply of spectacles. Since British lenses and equipment were used, Canadians continued to be issued with flat lenses, a type considered to be inferior to others.

Royal Canadian Air Force. A consultant advised headquarters on requirements and practised ophthalmology with active hospital facilities. He was assisted by an orthoptist and a refractionist who was either an optometrist or a junior ophthalmologist. This arrangement of personnel at the command medical boards worked efficiently. The ophthalmological unit set up at Air Force Headquarters overseas was of value to the men serving in the European theatres.

The ophthalmologist was concerned with the proper selection of aircrew. Personnel with ocular muscle imbalance were trained and close supervision of the industrial ocular hazards for certain ground trades was maintained. An improved spectacle frame and the adoption of surface-hardened lenses for aircrew improved visual acuity and an improved aviation goggle which could be worn over these spectacles was devised. Study was devoted to the improvement of the lenses provided. Extensive and valuable research was carried out on colour vision, and as a result improved abridged methods were developed for testing colour vision. An adaptation of the Royal Canadian Navy lantern gave an accurate selection. Important research in night vision was carried out. It was found more efficient to put aircrew through a course of visual training at low levels of illumination and to withdraw for further study only those who failed to complete it successfully. In this Service, emphasis was given to the training of junior ophthalmologists in order to provide sufficient trained personnel.

OTOLARYNGOLOGY

Otolaryngologists were employed in the medical services of all three Armed Forces; in the base areas their work was closely related to that of the selection boards. Later most of the officers in this specialty were recruited as specialists and appointed as such to the hospitals. Not until March 1945 was an adviser in otolaryngology appointed to the D.M.S. in London to correlate these services in North-West Europe and in the United Kingdom. In Canada consultants to the Air Force and to the Navy were appointed at an early stage so that there was less difficulty in training and in the distribution of otolaryngologists.

War-time Hazards. Special hazards to the ear, nose and throat during the war were recognised and studied. These require special attention from initial examining boards.

Navy. The advent of sulphonamide and antibiotic therapy made treatment easier. Plastic surgery was important. The firing of heavy naval guns in enclosed towers or emplacements gave rise to special problems of deafness.

R.C.A.F. Auditory acuity demanded careful assessment in aircrew. A study of the effect of flight upon the ears led to the discovery that the common cold presented great dangers to those who were flying at high altitudes and speeds. Otitic barotrauma is a failure of ventilation of the middle ear, when, after being exposed to decreased atmospheric pressure, the ear is rapidly exposed to a sudden increase.

Damage to auditory mechanism from flying was studied and knowledge of specific damage acquired. Permanent damage occurred from inadequate insufflation of the middle ear. Knowledge of the technique of equalising pressure probably saved many airmen from partial deafness.

Research Findings. A mobile sound-proof room was constructed for field surveys by the R.C.A.F. Some thousands of personnel were tested and tinnitus was studied in otological laboratories. As a result a system of pure-tone audiometry was tentatively adopted by the R.C.A.F. as a test for hearing. Data on the percentage of personnel admitted by various hearing-test standards were compiled. The technique of the

U.S. Bureau of Standards for calibration of audiometers was duplicated and used in the Otological Laboratory. Such equipment enabled the three Services to calibrate their audiometers and to pursue research. The field survey showed that noise of aircraft had little or no effect upon the ear in personnel during the war. A significant correlation between pure tone audiometry and articulation test was demonstrated.

DENTAL SURGERY

Jaw Injuries. Plastic and dental surgeons co-operated in the treatment of these casualties. Dental officers attached to field ambulances and field dressing stations gave first aid and treatment. Most of these cases, during active campaigning, came to the Basingstoke Neurological and Plastic Surgery Hospital. Penicillin for the elimination of infection from the oral cavity was valuable during the long fixation required in some of these injuries. Wiring and fixation apparatus, prepared in advance and speedily applied, saved operating time.

Ascorbic Acid and Gingivitis. It was suggested that lesions persisting in gingivitis might be due to a lack of vitamin C and could therefore be controlled by ascorbic acid intake. The administration of 75 milligrams of ascorbic acid daily had a delaying effect on the signs of recurring inflammation.

Dental Pain at High Altitudes. A good deal of such pain is sympathetic and appears due to disturbances of the various sinuses, particularly the maxillary sinus. A properly filled tooth with adequate protection against thermal shock is comfortable alike on the ground and at high altitudes.

MEDICAL RESEARCH

NAVAL MEDICAL RESEARCH

In mid-summer 1940 Dr. Charles Best offered the facilities of the Department of Physiology of the University of Toronto, along with some of those in the Banting and Best Department of Medical Research, to the Navy as a research unit. This offer was accepted and most of the academic pursuits of these two departments put aside for naval medical research. The remainder of its staff, who for various reasons could not wear uniforms, devoted most of their time and effort to the most pressing needs of naval medical service. A vast array of subjects was covered in these studies and some of the most practical and useful contributions were made concerning the problems of nutrition, physical qualities required for special duties (such as acuteness of hearing in ASDIC personnel), visual acuity or colour perception, the development of a remedy for motion sickness, ventilation of ships, engine room noises, colour-blindness, night-blindness and the practical application of such research in mass examination of personnel at large naval bases and training establishments. Studies in conserving and saving life included the perfection of more adequate life-saving jackets, preparation of emergency rations, the development of greased stockings to inhibit immersion foot, and many other projects.

ARMY MEDICAL RESEARCH

A Research Unit was formed in 1943 as A.M.D.8, with responsibility to the Director General of Medical Services for professional matters. It had a close relationship with the Army Medical Research Committee of the National Research Council.

Its studies included night vision, types of field equipment, motion sickness, noise factors in artillery units, foot problems, rations, protective clothing and equipment and industrial hazards, as well as a number of clinical studies.

A Research Unit was set up at Canadian Military Headquarters in London in 1943 to assist in studies in bacteriology, pathology and the use of antibiotics. Work was done on the origin of infective hepatitis, atypical pneumonia, influenza, wound infection and shock and transfusion.

AIR FORCE MEDICAL RESEARCH

Medical research was developed extensively during the war and was closely linked with the National Research Council's Associate Committee on Aviation Medical Research. Sub-committees were appointed to deal with personnel selection, oxygen equipment and protective clothing. Consideration was given to the problems of acceleration and 'black-out' during tight turns in the air. A suit containing fluid was designed by means of which the downward displacement of circulating blood could be prevented. This led to the Anti-G suit, designed and improved by the United States Army Air Force and by workers in the United Kingdom. Other subjects included decompression and motion sickness and vision problems.

THE CONNAUGHT MEDICAL RESEARCH LABORATORIES

Much of the activity of these Laboratories was concerned with the war effort and the prevention and treatment of disease in the Armed Forces. At the same time the Laboratories had to continue their work in the public health field, in the preparation of tetanus toxoid, insulin, liver extract, heparin, diphtheria toxoid, vaccine virus and other products.

As far as the Armed Forces were concerned they provided, among others, typhus vaccine, a combined tetanus toxoid and T.A.B. vaccine and gas-gangrene anti-toxin.

An important function of these Laboratories was the production of dried plasma for the Forces overseas. Their services were further extended to provide complete equipment, including bottles, pyrogen-free distilled water and poly-ethelene tubing. This was an important development because it ensured the standardisation of transfusion equipment in the field.

THE DEVELOPMENT OF PENICILLIN

The National Research Council organised a clinical research programme to be supervised by a committee on chemotherapeutic and other agents. The results of clinical trials stimulated research into the methods of large scale production of penicillin by Governmental and commercial agencies.

In 1943 a Joint Services Penicillin Committee was established to supervise the use of the available supply of penicillin and to train medical officers in penicillin therapy.

CONSULTANT SERVICES

It is difficult to measure the value of the Consultant Services because quality is involved and a comparison between what was and what might have been is impossible. Looking at past experiences in the South African War and the First World War, it is noted that there were many complaints about the medical services in both of these conflicts. There were no real consultants in the South African War and such as there were in the Canadian Forces in the First World War had very little authority and little opportunity to do more than give advice and assistance to individual units.

Consultants began their duties in England in August 1941, and although their duties were, at first, ill defined, they began by making ward rounds at various hospitals and casualty clearing stations, and by giving advice to the D.M.S. on medical policy, placement of officers commanding medical divisions, and recommendations concerning advanced training for officers capable of starting out with specialised duties. The consultants attended regular monthly conferences at the War Office, where they conferred with their British colleagues, including those who were doing active service in the field. As a result of this collaboration they were able to bring consultant treatment closer to the troops by recommending the organisation of new units, such as the field surgical unit. In addition, general policy as to the methods of treatment was laid down, newer drugs were investigated by teams of experts, and close liaison maintained with civilian authorities in England and Canada through the medical research committees, on every phase of treatment relating to war wounds and injuries. The general duties of consultants were:

(1) To advise those on the administrative side on the broad lines of treatment policy.

(2) To keep abreast of new methods and to assess their possible value.

(3) To maintain a constant flow of new information to the officers in the field.

(4) To maintain the level of morale of the field officers, by holding meetings and by arranging short courses of training.

(5) To keep close contact with headquarters in Ottawa, and to arrange a flow of specialists.

(6) To be available for professional consultations and advice in the field and in hospitals.

(7) To undertake the organisation of field research in certain special units.

The effectiveness of the consultant officers in all of the Services may perhaps be illustrated by the fact that there were no Parliamentary enquiries into the medical care provided for the Canadian Forces abroad.

In Canada, consultant services were developed slowly in the Army, but with the formation of the Air Force consultants were appointed very quickly. They were also appointed in the Navy and in each case the duties were similar to those described above.

Brigadier J. A. MacFarlane, who was Consultant Surgeon at C.M.H.Q. throughout the Second World War, puts forward this view of the value of consultant services:

'In whatever form and in whatever circumstances Canada finds herself at war on a future occasion, I am convinced that the purely professional side of the medical services should, in the early stages, be represented by a full and competent board of consulting specialists.'

MEDICAL STATISTICS AND MAN-POWER CONSERVATION

NAVAL MEDICAL STATISTICS

There was a failure to appreciate the value of adequate statistics at the beginning of the war. This was only natural in a situation which developed suddenly and found Canada unprepared. There was no Naval Medical Service at the outbreak of the war and medical examinations were carried out by those who had little knowledge of the physical requirements or of any statistical methods for recording the results.

Some time in 1940, efforts were begun to catalogue and keep statistical records on the number of persons rejected for naval service. It is interesting to note that the rates of rejection, throughout the war, by different examining officers, remained almost constant in the various Divisions. The rejection rates for men and women were found to be similar. For men the rate was 10·17 per cent. and for women 10·15 per cent. Comprehensive statistical tables are available to show the causes for rejection both in men and women. Other tables give the number of hospital admissions by causes, the number of operations, the total number of deaths by cause and those of naval personnel discharged on medical grounds.

ARMY MEDICAL STATISTICS

A considerable amount of information has been obtained by study of the records for the Army, but there are many deficiencies caused by the exigencies of the Service and by individual variations in reporting. Rejection rates were carefully studied. The rates of invalidism and injury have been carefully tabulated, but the user of this information is warned that there may be inaccuracies in the material because of certain gaps in the record system.

Development of the PULHEMS System. During 1942, through the joint efforts of the Army Medical Services and the Director of Personnel Selection, a new method of designating physical and mental fitness was introduced. This new system was designed to register a finer functional assessment of the physical, mental and emotional capacity of the individual in a form that could be easily interpreted by the Directorate of Personnel Selection. It has subsequently been adopted by the Armed Forces of many other countries, including the United Kingdom.

Medical Discharges. These constitute the most important single item in man-power wastage in an armed force. They also constitute a heavy financial burden because of the loss of fully or partly trained soldiers. It was noted that there was a sharp rise in 1944 and 1945, probably resulting from the increased number of injuries received during action.

It is notable that the overall number of casualties, both from battle and other reasons, made a total of 75,775, of which 13,000 or 18·3 per cent. were killed in action, 3,681, or 4·9 per cent., died of wounds, and 0·2 per cent. were classified as fatal battle casualties while prisoners. The total number of wounded, excluding prisoners, was 55,341, of which 6·6 per cent. died. In the First World War the percentage of deaths among wounded for the entire British Force in France and Flanders, excluding gas casualties, was 8·1 per cent. Advances in surgical technique and therapeutic measures might be expected to produce a greater decrease in the percentage of deaths among wounded personnel but these advances were offset by a more serious type of wound. The ratio of those killed in action to those wounded in the First World War was 1 to 5·2, while in the Second World War the ratio was 1 to 4, which indicates a more lethal type of missile. The more rapid collection of casualties in the Second World War would tend to increase the percentage of those classified as 'died of wounds' at the expense of those classified as 'killed in action'. Tables show that only 1·4 per cent. died in general hospitals. The ratio of fatal non-battle casualties to fatal battle casualties, excluding prisoners-of-war, was 1 to 3·6, whereas this ratio in the First World War was 1 to 16. This may be explained by the fact that the British Forces were in contact with the enemy throughout the First World War, but in the Second, the Canadians did not come to grips with the enemy until July 1943, and then only in divisional strength. It was only between June 1944 and May 1945 that the whole force was involved in fighting.

Communicable Diseases. These diseases, while not in themselves serious, were great wasters of men and time. The statistical surveys show remarkable variations in the seasonal incidence of diseases. It can be clearly shown that a greater proportion of susceptibles come from the areas of lower population density, where the possibility of childhood contact with these diseases was less.

Venereal Disease. Statistical information indicates clearly that there was a remarkable rise in the incidence of venereal disease when troops were not in action. In April 1944 the rate in North-West Europe was 54·6 per thousand strength per month, whereas in June, one month after the fighting ceased, the rate rose to 144 per thousand.

A remarkable advance during the Second World War was the institution of treatment with sulphonamides while the men continued on duty; also the introduction of penicillin as a specific treatment for gonorrhoea facilitated the treatment. This policy was successful because the proportion needing hospital care and the number of days spent were both materially reduced. This represented a very real saving in hospital beds.

AIR FORCE MEDICAL STATISTICS

A very comprehensive system of statistics was developed in this Service. The place of medical statistics became generally recognised and firmly established in the branches of the armed forces, but the Medical Statistical Section of the R.C.A.F. was remarkable for its completeness. The basic objectives of statistical methods in aviation medicine were summarised as follows:

(*a*) To provide information on the medical factors which affect the size, character, or composition of the force, including rejection of applicants on medical grounds, discharges on medical grounds, and deaths from any cause.

(b) To provide data on medical factors which influence the effectiveness of the active force and contribute to wastage, including the incidence, prevalence and principal types of sickness and injury; and the incidence, prevalence and distribution of infectious diseases.

(c) To provide indices to assist in the interpretation of recorded statistical data, both for administrative purposes and to further the application of control measures.

In the Air Force not only were statistics under the supervision of this section, but the entire field of medical recording was included. The section was in active operation in December 1940 and the chain of authority ran from the Director of the Service through the head of this section to the principal medical officers in the various commands, and so to the units and unit medical officers. It was discovered that centralisation of statistical activity was advantageous—that a better job could be done where there was unified statistical direction. Most of the information, causes and extent of sickness and injury, medical examination on enlistment, venereal disease, etc., was taken from the unit medical returns sent to the principal medical officers and thence to Air Force Headquarters. The actual tabulation was mainly carried out at Air Force Headquarters. The procurement of personnel adequately trained was a problem. The Air Force did not have its own tabulation equipment, which caused certain delays. The same deficiencies in medical statistics are stressed because of the variation in reporting, and of certain unavoidable gaps which occurred, owing to the exigencies of the Service and to some losses. Extensive data on medical examinations at enlistment, morbidity, discharges on medical grounds, and mortality were selected for presentation in this survey. Carefully prepared analytical material is available with comments on the result of the surveys. As a result of the experience and of these comments, the following observations were made:

'The figures indicate that a large proportion of the male population of flying age was unfit for aircrew training according to medical standards prevailing at the time. It is also clear that under a system of voluntary enlistment, the medical rejection rate increases significantly despite relaxation of physical standards. This reflects a worsening of the physical status of the total man-power in the force.

'A substantial portion of the recorded causes of rejection are not diseases but physiological changes and developmental defects which are not preventable. Among the aircrew candidates, for example, colour blindness and defective visual acuity were responsible for 43·5 per cent.

of all disqualifying defects recorded in aircrew candidates. Neither of these defects is due to disease in the true sense of the word. This fact suggests that "physical fitness" of persons of military age in Canada is not as poor as published data seem to suggest. Perhaps more important, this observation also indicates that medical standards should be subjected to critical re-examination as valid criteria of physical fitness for any task.

'The information available serves also to direct attention to the desirability of knowing something about the total man-power potential in terms of military physical fitness, with the idea of applying a fixed medical selection standards policy. Such a policy would obviate the need for making repeated changes in standards in order to get the required number of personnel to man the required units. Such a plan eliminates certain administrative problems, ensures a uniform quality in physical calibre of candidates enlisted, and resolves many training problems as well.

'The recorded experience in the physical examination of candidates for enlistment suggests that the armed forces should continue to collect data on disqualifying defects in candidates for enlistment in a uniform fashion and that the tabulation and analysis of such data be carried out at a central statistical unit.

'The statistical data presented did not represent the findings of a random cross-section of men and women of the same ages. Information of such character would be advantageous especially if it could be secured by sex, age, education and occupation. This could be accomplished through sampling studies, and the information obtained would be invaluable in the review of medical standards and in medical aspects of planning and personnel assignments.'

Hospital Morbidity. Careful analysis of hospital morbidity led to the following observations:

'A number of striking facts were demonstrated. The seasonal morbidity pattern is common to the two sexes and is strongly marked. Over the whole war period there is a persistent downward trend in both the admission and the wastage (days of care) rates. This trend is quite marked both for men and for women. On the other hand, the average number of days of care per case steadily increases over the period for both sexes—the figures for 1945 being approximately twice those of 1940 for men and of 1942 for women. The net benefit of the sharp decline in admission rate over the unfavourable increases in "days per case" is reflected in the improved wastage rates and perhaps more clearly by the decline in the daily non-effective rate by 25 per cent. for R.C.A.F. personnel and by 20 per cent. for R.C.A.F. (W.D.) personnel.

'Both the morbidity (incidence) and wastage (days lost) rates are substantially higher for women. The admission rate for R.C.A.F. (W.D.) personnel was a regular 60 to 65 per cent. higher than the R.C.A.F. figure. This excess is not due alone to conditions peculiar to women. The average length of stay in hospital was substantially lower for women than for men. The effect of this is reflected in a smaller sex differential in the wastage rates which are but 30 per cent. higher for women than for men.

'The non-effective rates for men and women afford a practical index of wastage due to sickness or injury in convenient form. The figures really interpret the days of care in hospital in terms of the equivalent number of men non-effective daily due to hospitalisation per 1,000 strength. The non-effective rates for R.C.A.F. male personnel in Canada attained their high point early in 1941, during an outbreak of haemolytic streptococcal infections, at 32·6 per 1,000 strength. This peak was never approached subsequently for, despite the increase in the average length of stay in hospital, the admission rate declined so persistently that there was a consistent improvement in the non-effective rate throughout the remainder of the war.

'It is rather remarkable that the peak non-effective rate for R.C.A.F. (W.D.) personnel should also have been 32·5 per 1,000 strength and that it should be attained in the same month (February) although not in the same year, 1943, as the peak for male personnel. The non-effective rate for women presented the same pattern as for males, with a constant improvement over the succeeding years of the war.

'The declining morbidity (admissions) and wastage (days) rates throughout the course of the war is a matter for interesting speculation. This pattern of experience was common to other military forces— with high incidence rates in the early mobilisation period, lower rates following as "seasoned" troops formed a progressively increasing proportion of the total strength.'

Discharges and Retirements on Medical Grounds. A careful analysis of these was made and led to the following general comment:

'*The Implications*. The statistics demonstrate the salient fact that discharges on medical grounds require an annual replacement amounting to 2 per cent. of the total strength of the force each year. Over the years 1941–44 inclusive, something less than 2 *per cent. per year of the total R.C.A.F. strength* were discharged on medical grounds. Only 0·12 per cent. per year of the total strength were discharged due to accidental or war injuries. During the entire period 1939–45, 93·1 per cent. of all discharges on medical grounds among R.C.A.F. personnel were due to disease; only 6·9 per cent. arose from injuries. Among personnel of the R.C.A.F. Women's Division 97·8 per cent. of medical discharges were due to disease.'

Repatriation for Medical Reasons. Repatriation from an active theatre for medical reasons is of considerable significance as a source of man-power wastage. The majority of men repatriated from overseas for medical reasons were subsequently discharged on medical grounds.

Communicable Diseases. A review of these conditions illustrated clearly the value of inoculation against diphtheria. It is worthy of note that there was no case of smallpox among R.C.A.F. personnel, either in Canada or overseas, and there was only one case and one death from tetanus. Investigations conducted during the war supported the con-viction that immunisation by scarlet fever toxin was not effective in controlling the spread of haemolytic streptococcal infection. Clinical studies showed, however, that scarlet fever cases in Dick-positive personnel, who had not received five doses of toxin, had the highest average length of stay in hospital and the highest proportion of severe cases, as well as the highest incidence of complications. There were only seven recorded admissions of typhoid fever or paratyphoid fever among R.C.A.F. personnel—six in Canada and one in the United Kingdom. Only one death was attributed to typhoid fever and this occurred in Canada. In personnel outside the United Kingdom the incidence was substantially higher; twelve cases were reported, with no deaths, in the Middle East and India. It would appear that almost all of these were confirmed cases of typhoid fever.

XI. CONCLUDING COMMENT

From the summary of the work carried out by the Canadian Medical Services two main points emerge. There was general satisfaction outside the Services with the quality of medical care given to the Armed Forces. Mobilisation and build-up of the medical services was accomplished without major difficulties. In spite of the great increase in recruit examinations, in the treatment of the sick and the wounded, good standards were maintained.

The medical services themselves were not always satisfied with the achievements. There were failures of administration and errors of policy, but the results of clinical treatment were on the whole satis-factory.

The arrangement of units in the field sometimes led to strain, but never to breakdown. On the other hand, the commendable innovation in distribution brought the treatment units very close to the areas where the casualties were occurring. This, together with an efficient air evacuation system, saved many lives.

At home the contribution of medicine to the war effort was considerable, particularly in scientific research. The development of new drugs (particularly penicillin) and new protective measures, whole blood and blood substitutes, new techniques and equipment, made a valuable contribution and a great difference to the recovery rates among the wounded. In these activities government departments played a useful rôle. Civilian agencies were of assistance in carrying out some important parts of the programme of evacuating, nursing, and rehabilitating the wounded. The Red Cross played a very significant rôle, especially in the care of prisoners-of-war.

PART III

Australia

The Australian Medical Services

By Brigadier W. P. MacCallum, C.B.E., D.S.O., M.C., E.D., M.B., Ch.M., F.R.A.C.P.

Detailed official accounts of the work of the Australian Medical Services during the Second World War will be found in the following volumes:*

Clinical Problems of War   .   . ⎤
Middle East and Far East   .   . ⎥
The Island Campaigns .   .   . ⎬ Allan S. Walker
Medical Services of the R.A.N. and ⎥
     R.A.A.F.   .   .   .   . ⎦

* Published by Australian War Memorial, Canberra.

CONTENTS

PREFACE

In the preparation of this account the reference material used has consisted entirely of the four Australian Medical War Histories already published. The late Dr. Allan Walker had written *Middle East and Far East, Clinical Problems of War* and *The Island Campaigns* but was prevented by serious illness from completing the last published volume of the series *Medical Services of the R.A.N. and R.A.A.F.*

Dr. Walker himself in the normal course of events would have been the author of this critical analysis and not only added still further to his reputation as a historian of outstanding merit, but maintained the sequence and balance that is so valuable in historical contributions.

The most extensive use has been made of the text and the opinions expressed in his books. In paying tribute to this obvious source of inspiration for the Australian portion of this publication an apology should be made for any faults of omission or commission; inevitably, in dealing even with factual evidence from authentic sources of information, impressions and interpretations will vary. The assessment of what may or may not be regarded as important is, after all, a matter of relativity that to a large extent is influenced by the intellectual and philosophic approach of the individual author.

Much attention has deliberately been paid to the effects of campaigning under tropical conditions. This has not been done with the idea of assuming the credit for any contributions of possible value to medical science in war. The fact that the Australian Forces were, for the most part, engaged in tropical or sub-tropical service throughout the war constitutes perhaps a valid reason for analysing in some detail experiences that were certainly unique in Australian history and probably without exact parallel in the records of other countries.

Many problems were universal in nature and confronted the medical services of other countries, yet the circumstances under which they arose were by no means identical nor was their individual elucidation entirely similar either in process or in result. Australia indeed received most generous assistance from other countries, but the current lessons of the war had often to be learned the hard way. If happily there may be some benefit to posterity from such lessons, the reward of victory will be more complete.

There can be no reasonable forecast of what the future holds, but it seems obvious that in the event of war Australia will have to face the prospect of its armed forces being engaged in tropical service to a greater or lesser degree.

Most grateful thanks are due to various colleagues, professional and Service, for their help in reading appropriate sections of this contribution, their criticism and their suggestions for recasting certain parts.

I. MEDICAL ORGANISATION IN AUSTRALIA

THE INTER-WAR PERIOD

To appreciate the development of the Australian Army Medical Services and to recognise its growing impact on the civilian population, it is necessary to review briefly the period between 1919 and 1939.

It is often hard to recognise the lessons that may be learned from past experiences and sometimes even more difficult to profit by them. Experiences in the War of 1914–18 pointed to the need for internal changes, a need that was all the more important as the probability of total war in the future became increasingly apparent. The first objective, reorganisation of the medical services, was bound up with an important principle—the attainment of a greater degree of independence. Suggestions for reorganisation were not confined to the army services, in which arose a movement in favour of amalgamation of the navy, army and air force medical services under unified control. There were also signs that a wide co-ordination of Service and civilian organisations might be achieved. A third aim in reorganisation was the control of medical supplies and equipment in time of national emergency.

In 1922 a specially constituted conference recommended that there should be a single Australian Medical Corps, with one administrative medical section only, the head of which would be responsible through heads of the Services to the Boards concerned. Ministerial approval of the plan for amalgamation was given, but although there was a suggested unanimity among the Service representatives, the heads of the naval and air force medical services were opposed to the idea and the scheme was not implemented. Further conferences were held, at which naval opinion opposed unification, and strong objections were raised by the air force representatives. In the end, amalgamation of the three medical services was never achieved, although the medical arrangements of air force and civil aviation were brought under the general control of D.G.M.S. Army in 1927 despite a minority protest from the medical representatives of the R.A.A.F. The D.G.M.S. Army thus became responsible to the Air Board for the organisation and administration of the medical services of the Air Force. While the Air Force remained small and the demands of its medical services were few, the arrangements worked with a reasonable degree of satisfaction, although the Air Force Medical Service felt that the position during an important formative period was anomalous and the outcome was not in the best interests of

(95349)

T*

efficiency. The rapid increase of the Air Force and growing demand for independence coupled with strong representations secured the much desired autonomy for the Air Force Medical Service in 1940. Even in retrospect the question of amalgamation is a most difficult one to assess. Tradition, special technical requirements and administrative problems all play important parts in rendering independent control desirable, but on the other hand the economy in man-power, regulation of supplies and general co-ordination of all medical services claimed by the advocates of amalgamation are fundamental in securing the best results from a nation-wide effort. The feeling still remains that it should be possible to produce a formula capable of accomplishing the *desiderata* of a unified medical service.

By 1927 it was clear that a more expanded policy in defence requirements was required. A secret document, the Commonwealth War Book Paper No. 13, was drawn up by the Army authorities which included a plan for the co-ordination of medical services in respect of civil, military, naval and air requirements. Civil medical establishments, medical equipment, drugs and co-ordination of the three medical services in time of war were reviewed and recommendations made. Civil mobilisation of the medical profession was indicated as a possible necessary step in the event of war. The document also dealt with questions of supply, assessment of stocks of drugs, manufacture in Australia of equipment and control of all such stocks. A joint committee representing all medical services met to examine the suggestions made in the War Book and recommended that these, together with additional powers, be vested in the Department of Health, which would then be responsible for:

(1) preparation in peace of schemes for controlling the medical profession and medical supplies,

(2) the implementation of these plans in time of war,

(3) recommendation to the Government of estimated requirements for reserve stocks of medical supplies in peace and special importation of these on the outbreak of war,

(4) arranging for acceleration and increase of local production of medical supplies in Australia.

This method of control proved to be a most contentious matter, and it was not until 1938 that with the formation of the Central Standing Committee, the genesis of what was later to become the Central Medical Co-ordination Committee, was ensured. The question of the means by which doctors would be controlled in time of war was at last settled. It was decided that the Central Standing Committee should co-ordinate arrangements for provision of medical men, material and hospital accommodation, but that on the outbreak of war it should be merged into a Central Executive Medical Committee charged with the executive control of all relevant medical matters. In fact the originally constituted central committee carried on throughout the war. Medical personnel subject to direction included medical practitioners, dentists, pharmacists, trained nurses, voluntary aid members, physiotherapists, instrument makers, X-ray technicians and rank and file for medical military units.

An important component of medical preparedness is the co-ordination of all material necessary for medical and surgical work. It was clearly advisable in an isolated country like Australia to devise methods by which medical supplies should be made available in peace to such an extent as would render the position safe in war. The natural corollary to the formation of the Central Medical Co-ordination Committee was the creation of a sub-committee of this body to deal with medical equipment and all questions related thereto. But before this sub-committee came into being active enquiries in the realm of medical supplies had been instituted. In 1935 a special board formed by the Defence Department had advised that all field medical equipment should be derived from Australian sources, not as hitherto from England. It also began a survey of the minimum essential requirements for war and of the source of supply. Special attention was paid to vitally important drugs.

In pursuance of the co-ordinating policy a questionnaire was sent out to all medical practitioners. This elicited information regarding those available for some public duty in the event of war, for duties of a military nature and for civil duties wherever required.

The army had only three permanent medical officers: the D.G.M.S. and two others. The Australian Army Medical Corps did not possess the advantage of a backing of permanent officers, but depended on the zeal and enthusiasm of its part-time officers, the militia officers who had made part-time soldiering a living interest and had regularly attended camps and exercises. A.A.M.C. training was largely based on R.A.M.C. training manuals. Procedures had been laid down and a complete account compiled of the operative measures of mobilisation. By the time war was actually declared co-ordination of men and material for the purpose of the medical services, including the civilian, had at last been achieved.

MEDICAL EXAMINATION OF RECRUITS

In 1939 and the early part of 1940 great numbers of recruit examinations were carried out by part-time medical officers in such time as could be spared from the demands of general practice. This examination was only preliminary, and a second examination was carried out in the larger centres by a board which had important functions and which was later reinforced by the greater use of consultants in such branches as orthopaedics, skin and other specialties. There is little doubt that initially the primary recruiting examinations were conducted under very unfavourable conditions which resulted in the acceptance of many men who were physically or mentally unsuitable for military service. The need for proper accommodation and adequate equipment was not sufficiently recognised as a prerequisite for the more detailed examination in which the past medical history of the recruit formed an important part. Re-examination also helped to unmask impersonations which undoubtedly took place. Eventually photographs were taken of all members of the forces, but in the early period of the war many of the troops had embarked for overseas before this means of identification could be effected. Finger printing would seem to be practicable and desirable.

The most important innovation in the methods of selection of recruits for the A.I.F. in 1939 was the adoption of radiography of the chest. The method used was that of miniature fluorography. No recruit was rejected on the evidence of a miniature film alone, for where any doubt existed a large film was taken and reviewed. The use of micro-fluorography spread to the navy, the air force and the women's services. Eventually a film was also taken of the chest of every man and woman entering and being demobilised from the Services.

Another important innovation was the introduction of blood grouping tests on every recruit. Each soldier's blood group was recorded in his pay book and stamped on his identity disc.

Preventive inoculation had received much attention before the war. The possibility of using combined vaccines had been investigated but rejected in favour of separate administration of T.A.B. vaccine and the tetanus toxoid, in order to avoid excessive reaction. Initially half the usual full dose of the vaccine was used. It was realised that complete immunity would not necessarily be conferred by these doses. Later on new arrangements were made for the preparation of a strongly antigenic but relatively non-toxic vaccine. Routine 'booster' injections were given every year to all members of the Forces. All personnel going overseas were also vaccinated against smallpox. In the method employed the area, one site only, covered by the lymph was not to exceed 3 millimetres and the skin was repeatedly pressed by the edges of a triangular surgical needle through the drop of the lymph. Scarification was forbidden.

EXPANSION AND ORGANISATION OF THE A.A.M.C.

In the early months of 1940 the Armed Forces expanded rapidly. I Australian Corps was formed and despatched overseas, while in addition there was the mobilisation and maintenance of the militia throughout Australia. All the essential organisation incident to the mobilisation of the A.A.M.C. was carried out by the Medical Directorate. Within the Army Medical Corps itself was a nucleus for expansion. Invaluable work had been carried out in the years just before the war on estimates of the medical material needed annually in Australia. Wastage rates had been ascertained and a year's supply had been obtained in advance. The medical services had the advantage of a complete set of instructions on action to be taken in the event of war. A compact plan for all phases of a military situation was presented in this document, and the mechanism by which the various stages were dealt with was set out clearly. In addition a plan was included for the medical organisation of an expeditionary force. It is impossible to overestimate the value of these preparations undertaken by the small peace-time staff of the Medical Directorate or to disregard their influence on the rapid expansion that was inevitably to take place in the A.A.M.C.—an expansion so great that at the peak of the war against Japan its strength of 32,000 of all ranks represented 8 per cent. of the total strength of the Australian Military Forces.

The organisation necessary to provide a dental service had been considered even before mobilisation began. The problem was colossal; not only were the standards for recruiting vague, but the state of the teeth of Australian people was so poor in 1939 that the principle was adopted that men would be accepted if they could be made dentally fit. Dental units were provided on the medical establishment of a field ambulance, casualty clearing station, general hospital and convalescent depot. A unit was expected to keep about 1,000 men dentally fit, but the task was, in fact much greater, as men were not dentally fit on enlistment. Good dental centres were built in all training camps. Eventually the great expansion of the Services led to the increase of divisional dental units from three to nine, and a hundred units were authorised for home service.

No difficulty was found in providing nurses for military service. The general standard of health was the same for male recruits. Physiotherapists were enlisted as such.

CENTRAL MEDICAL CO-ORDINATION COMMITTEE

Although no official co-ordination of the medical profession was in operation during the War of 1914–1918, indications were not lacking that it was considered desirable by a large proportion of medical men. A further trend in favour of a more effective organisation was stimulated by the ominous threat of a second war, and a co-ordination committee was not only in being but in functional activity when war was declared in 1939. It cannot be sufficiently emphasised that the outstanding success of this measure was due to its establishment during a time of peace. This success would have been even more complete had certain weaknesses been avoided earlier. Although this body was already active in September 1939 it did not function fully until some months afterwards. The first medical units of the second A.I.F. were raised with such speed that the committee was not in a position to control the selection of medical officers. This led to the gain of the medical units at the expense of the teaching hospitals, which lost an unduly high number of their experienced staff. From this it is clear that to be fully efficient in time of war the mechanism for co-ordination should already be established, equipped with full information and endowed with sufficient powers.

Early in 1941 the medical profession as a body showed their practical acceptance of the principles of co-ordination by voluntarily subjecting themselves to the decision of the co-ordination committees and thus anticipated at their own request the later ordinance which legalised medical conscription. In August 1941 an amendment of the National Security Regulations that all members of the medical profession under sixty years of age should be liable for compulsory service was approved. The regulation changed the purely advisory rôle of the committee to an executive one. The Medical Equipment Control Committee, at first a sub-committee of the Central Medical Co-ordination Committee, became an independent body soon after the outbreak of war and assumed control of a very wide field, concerned as it was with both civil and Service requirements.

The Medical Directorate of the Army had already recognised the urgent need for more medical equipment and felt that the official scales for all such supplies required revision. The latter onerous task was undertaken at an early date. In drawing up the revised scales the policy followed was governed by the determination to provide supplies of the numerous kinds of equipment adequate for all types of work demanded of Service medical officers and to ensure that as many items as possible were made in Australia. The soundness of this policy was proved as the war progressed and demands increased beyond expectations. A standard army catalogue including all items on the revised scales was also produced. Further complications were caused by the fact that each of the three Services used a different catalogue. The committee felt that agreement between the three Services on this matter was essential in the interests of efficiency and began to exert pressure towards this end. The drawing up of this standard catalogue for the Army did much to systematise supplies to the Services, and stimulated local production for both Service and civil requirements.

A schedule of essential drugs was compiled, and for all practical purposes a list of 130 was found to be sufficient. Later an A.I.F. Pharmacopoeia containing a list of 174 essential drugs and preparations was drawn up. This with little or no change remained in force throughout the war.

HEALTH AND HOSPITALS

At the outbreak of war there were no army hospitals in Australia. The general principle was laid down that beds should be available in base hospitals for 2 per cent. of the total number of troops in Australia and in camp hospitals for another 2 per cent. The total requirements of 4 per cent. were found to be sufficient except when unusual demands were made.

At the outbreak of war the Australian Army Nursing Service was the only army women's service in existence in Australia. The subsequent formation of the Australian Army Medical Women's Service did much towards releasing men for duty in forward areas and even supplied personnel in the advanced base areas. The formation of these services with large numbers of women in all the military areas in Australia raised special problems of recruitment, accommodation and medical care. Medical examination of women recruits was based on the general lines laid down for men but carried out as far as possible by women doctors, usually working on a part-time basis.

By the early part of 1942 the great expansion of the Army and the more obvious need for conserving resources, so that both civil and military requirements might be more adequately met, had already led to the replacement of many doctors by lay personnel in the Army, thus effecting a considerable saving. Registrars and adjutants in general hospitals, and adjutants in casualty clearing stations had been replaced by experienced laymen; bearer medical officers were no longer appointed to field ambulances, their positions being taken over by men highly trained in first-aid procedures. Medical officers in hygiene sections were replaced by highly trained public health inspectors, and work in some technical specialties such as entomology and bacteriology was being done by scientific technicians instead of medical officers. The shortening of the medical course had been effected at the universities, and women graduates were being used for certain army appointments. At the same time great care was being exercised in calling up doctors for military work, and if a serious emergency occurred final year medical students could be employed in certain capacities under supervision. It was also considered essential that the Central Co-ordination Committee should have full executive powers in the distribution and employment of medical men.

With the changing war situation several new factors had arisen. The increasing numbers of prisoners-of-war, the influx of civilians from evacuated enemy-held countries, the staging of American Armed Forces, with the concomitant risks of disease, and the organisation for civil

defence all led to more administrative work and problems of co-ordination. The inevitable impact on the medical profession pointed to the
necessity for emergency service on a compulsory basis. The necessary
regulations governing the Emergency Medical Services were gazetted in
March 1942. Assignment for duty in this service consisted of the
following categories: continuation with present work; part-time posting
to hospital on first-aid duties; full-time work during an emergency or
as a principal or *locum tenens* carrying out civil practice or as an E.M.S.
practitioner in a country area on a salaried basis. An emergency civil
medical practitioner's service was organised consisting of volunteers and
others whose services were called upon in pursuance of the regulation.
No barrier was raised to any member of the E.M.S. serving in a force
outside Australia. Co-ordination of dentists was effected by a dental
sub-committee of the C.M.C.C., but the proportionately greater number
of dentists available did not require at this stage the introduction of
regulations similar to those needed for the co-ordination of doctors.
The demand for nurses was so great both by the Services and the civil
hospitals that the central committee in 1942 agreed that the nursing
profession should be controlled by regulations similar to those gazetted
for the Emergency Medical Service.

Service requirements of medical equipment imposed more strain on
the mechanism of supply in the years following 1940.

The organisation and stimulation of production were admittedly not
an army function, but the Medical Equipment Control Committee, with
the co-operation of the Department of Supply, brought about admirable
co-operative organisation of the surgical instrument and drug trades,
set up a system of continuous record of quantities of all essential and
important medical equipment, built up greatly increased reserves,
established relations with buying organisations in England and America,
which in association with the relevant Commonwealth Government
Departments facilitated supplies, and enlisted the aid of the medical
profession in the cause of economy. All these angles provided a most
valuable basis for the long-range programme of supplies and the rapid
establishment of adequate reserves that were so essential.

The pharmaceutical panel of the M.E.C.C. had provided an Australian
War Pharmacopoeia which was distributed throughout Australia. While
conforming to all requirements of war-time economy, this offered
therapeutic substances or combinations for all ordinary purposes.
Owing to the shortage of anti-malarial drugs it was found necessary to
conserve quinine, and restrictive use was imposed on the stocks that
were held.

OTHER CIVILIAN MEDICAL SERVICES

The defence of Australia was inevitably bound up with the significance
of the mainland as a large military base. The increasing demand for the

construction of defence works resulted in the formation in 1942 of the Civil Construction Corps. Members of this corps were medically examined, placed in appropriate categories and given treatment when necessary by co-ordinated arrangement between the civil and military authorities.

PHYSICAL STANDARDS FOR SERVICES

In 1941 the original classifications were still official but were later amended. Standards of height, chest measurement, eyesight and hearing were relaxed in 1943. The directions given to examining officers were more detailed, definite guidance was given about specific disabilities, and more use was made of specialists in deciding physical problems in relation to enlistment.

CHANGES IN ADMINISTRATION AND ORGANISATION

The formation of armoured divisions in Australia gave rise to special medical problems. The strategic and political picture altered with the development of the main Australian theatre of war in the Pacific, and in the event there was only a limited employment of armour in isolated instances in the Islands. What the future has in store is, of course, quite conjectural, but it would seem important that army medical authorities in Australia should continue to keep themselves well informed in all technical medical matters concerned with specialised units of such formations.

Experience showed the great difficulties in building a hospital capable of expanding to several times its original size. Rapid expansion of base hospitals was well nigh impossible except by temporary structures for which sites were not always available; moreover, the central necessary services also needed enlargement. Certain of the field general hospitals were established at strategic points to deal with the increased military needs of formations on the mainland as well as of those returning from overseas for rest and further training. The accommodation used in these hospitals varied. In some, huts were already in use for wards and administration; in others, schools were taken over for hospital purposes. In either instance, huts or tents could be used for extending the accommodation. Tents had the obvious advantage of speed of erection and mobility, but their durability was limited, and special proofing was necessary to ensure a reasonable viability in the Tropics. Existing buildings provided immediate shelter, at least in theory, but in actual fact few buildings could be transformed satisfactorily into hospitals without a great amount of adaptation and additional work.

Initially, it was difficult to convince the senior officers of the Ordnance Corps that the equipment of a base hospital in a capital city differed markedly from that of a general hospital in the field.

Convalescent depots and convalescent homes were also needed in greater numbers as hospitals grew. Most valuable assistance was given by the Red Cross Society, which was responsible for the establishment of convalescent homes. Women Service patients were more appropriately treated in such institutions during convalescence.

On account of the great areas involved on the mainland and the varied problems presented it was considered advisable to recommend the appointment of regional consultants. This principle was not immediately accepted but later became imperative in certain sections, and was eventually adopted, with valuable results.

CO-ORDINATION IN 1943-45

The difficulties experienced were mainly concerned with the maintenance of balance between civil and Service medical requirements. In 1944 the Army agreed to discharge soldiers so that they might begin or continue medical courses, if approved by the Director General of Manpower and the Universities Commission. A quota system was applied to the university medical courses under the control of the Commonwealth Government whereby intending applicants were required to intimate their intention before leaving school. Students failing to gain inclusion in the quota automatically came under control of the man-power authorities.

The wastage rate of medical officers in the Services, which was considerable, was hardly equalled by the intake and many establishments for medical units and formations could not be filled. Relief was sometimes given to civilian doctors by assigning a Service medical officer for a short period of private practice, with good results.

In 1943 medical officers over forty years of age were circularised to ascertain who were willing to return to civil practice. Preference was given first to those who had served in a theatre of active operations and then to those with the longest service. Civil needs for nurses and pharmacists also received attention.

The Standing Committee of Service Directors, set up in 1940, advised on the co-ordination of administration and organisation of the medical services of the Armed Forces, and was responsible for the maintenance of a consistent policy.

Although their originally suggested aims and powers were somewhat curtailed, the organisations for medical co-ordination achieved their main objects. They lacked, however, the power of independent executive action. Inter-Service co-ordination was sometimes incomplete. This was particularly the case in hospital resources, and a closer combination of these in base areas and perhaps lines of communications areas would have been advantageous. A common use of consultants and specialists in Service hospitals would be advisable for more effective treatment and for economy. There should be complete co-operation between Services as regards the medical requirements for enlistment, and in securing equal justice for Service medical officers on demobilisation. The important work of these committees might well have been utilised after the war to examine possibilities for the future.

FOOD AND CATERING

The problems of nutrition and the need of technicians and technical advisers led to the formation in 1943 of the Army Catering Corps as an offshoot of the supply services of the Quarter-Master-General's Branch. A medical liaison officer supplied the link between the Medical Directorate and 'Q' Branch, Nutrition. A liaison officer between the A.A.M.W.S. and A.A.C.C. was also appointed to deal with food problems of the Women's Services.

The Australian Military Force ration was compiled to supply 4,500 Calories in a diet of all essential foods.

The feeding of the natives in New Guinea was a difficult and responsible task. Here the problem was two-fold: the feeding of the general native population in Papua and the feeding of the native labour force indentured to the Australian Army. It was found that the ordinary ration scale laid down was too low in fat for native requirements. Marked improvement in their physical condition occurred when the fat ration was increased.

II. MEDICAL SERVICES OF THE AUSTRALIAN MILITARY FORCES

The outbreak of war found Australia in the position of having to develop a relatively large army medical corps from a very small nucleus comprised of the peace-time militia units—field ambulances and hygiene sections—and enlisted personnel, the vast majority of whom had had no previous army medical training. As mentioned, there were only three permanent army medical officers, one of whom was the D.G.M.S.

Initially, the development of the Australian Army Medical Corps followed closely the organisation adopted by the R.A.M.C., and the various Australian units that were formed closely resembled their British prototypes in composition and equipment. As the war progressed it became obvious that certain modifications to cope with new problems or altering conditions were necessary, requiring changes in war establishments and equipment tables and even the creation of new specialised units.

The Australian troops fought under almost every condition of climate and terrain, but were for the major part of their campaigning engaged in tropical service. It was this latter circumstance that was to influence many of the variations that were adopted.

The basic principles enunciated in the training manuals will surely remain unchallenged and will always constitute the important duties of the Army Medical Corps. For these reasons it is essential to maintain a peace-time organisation capable of preserving these first principles, of adapting itself to meet the inevitable problems that future developments may produce, and of forming an efficient nucleus from which expansion can take place in time of war.

ARMY MEDICAL CORPS PERSONNEL

The increased number of technicians required for various purposes necessitated the organisation of special courses of training, a concomitant of any war that is of long duration and involves large numbers of Service personnel.

In the allocation of recruits or enlisted personnel to the medical corps the importance of physical fitness and reasonable intelligence should receive more consideration from the man-power and army authorities. In the field units these qualities are pre-requisites. Far too often men of inferior physical and mental capacity were drafted to the A.A.M.C. owing to the inability or unwillingness of the responsible department to appreciate the duties they would have to perform. Experience in action clearly demonstrated that members of a field ambulance might be, and in fact were, called on for the various duties of nursing, bearing, cooking, building shelters, clerking and driving. The really efficient unit was one in which all personnel had been trained in these manifold activities and were capable of executing them. Even in the units of a more static nature, such as general hospitals, the number of B class personnel that can be reasonably used is limited.

DEVELOPMENT OF NEW UNITS

The exposure of the troops to particular hazards of specific infectious diseases, the development of amphibious operations and the geographical distribution of combat zones in the South West Pacific Area all led to the formation of new units.

ANTI-MALARIA CONTROL UNITS

After the occupation of Syria special units for carrying out anti-malaria work were formed for the first time in the Australian Army. This marked the beginning of a new phase of malaria prevention, and these units did useful work. At the time no one realised how valuable they were to be and the profound influence they were to exert when the Australian troops were engaged in the Island campaigns. On their return from the Middle East they were reorganised into three different types according to requirements, a special tropical scale was provided for jungle operations, and they became known as Malaria Control Units.

They were accepted as an essential part of the order of battle in the various actions that were fought in the South West Pacific Area and followed closely the advancing troops so that malaria control could be promptly instituted.

MOBILE ENTOMOLOGICAL SECTIONS

Mobile Entomological Sections were formed in 1942. They not only helped malaria control units to establish themselves on a scientific basis, but investigated many matters of importance to the Armed Forces, such as studies of repellents, establishment of standards for mosquito and fly sprays and spraying, control of scrub typhus by miticide repellent and the development of aerial spraying by aircraft.

This work was of outstanding value to the Forces undertaking campaigns in areas where malaria, mite-borne typhus and dengue were endemic. It was found to be desirable for mobile entomological sections to accompany malaria control units in the early stages of an advance in order to carry out vector studies.

TECHNICAL APPOINTMENTS

The impact of tropical diseases in general and malaria in particular led to the specific appointment of malariologists to the higher formations in the field. Entomology attained the status of a directorate, but in the final organisation was incorporated in the Directorate of Hygiene and Pathology (including Parasitology). A malariologist and an entomologist advised the Director of Hygiene at headquarters. The fact that subsequent events entirely justified these appointments will surely establish their importance in any similar future campaign.

MEDICAL COMPANY, BEACH GROUP

This was a new type of unit introduced early in 1944 for the needs of amphibious landing operations and had a war establishment of five officers and 74 other ranks. Two surgeon specialists were included in the establishment. The use of beach groups as well as field ambulances was found to give wider scope in the handling of battle casualties, and surgical teams provided ample assistance.

MOBILE OPERATING UNIT

Originally formed in the Middle East, this was not used in the field until the Island campaigns. It comprised four officers and 30 other ranks, with equipment, and could act as a complete unit or as two separate surgical teams for attachment to a field ambulance. Occasionally, supplemented by field ambulance personnel, it functioned as a small hospital.

WATER AMBULANCE CONVOY

The advance along the north-east coast of New Guinea and the distribution of the forces in the Solomon Islands created the need for such additional means, in the latter instance the only means, of evacuating casualties. The medical personnel varied in relation to the size of the craft and the nature of the task, a medical officer being appointed to the large motor cruisers in addition to the prescribed medical establishment.

HYGIENE

The practical application of the important principles of hygiene in the field presented one of the most difficult tasks to accomplish. The unsatisfactory standard in the early years pointed clearly to the intensive instruction and supervision that was necessary at all levels, for it became obvious that the field hygiene section, a divisional unit, was considerably limited in the scope and performance of its duties, which were largely inspectional and advisory in character. This was especially so in a war of movement and when the division covered a wide area. Unit responsibility in matters of hygiene was lacking, and insufficient appreciation of its importance existed in spite of schools of instruction and the efforts of medical authorities. The need for a complete reorganisation was apparent, and it was decided to recommend the abolition of the existing field hygiene section and to adopt a system that would provide an adequate hygiene organisation in each unit, enable inspection and training in the details of hygiene to be carried out within each unit by hygiene personnel, give adequate rank and status to responsible hygiene personnel and provide for the appointment in Army, Corps and Divisional Headquarters of a medical officer with special qualifications and training in hygiene.

The adoption of the new organisation was recommended by the D.G.M.S. An official instruction was promulgated in July 1942, and later in 1942, field hygiene sections were disbanded. Generally the reorganisation worked well, and by mid-1943 improved standards were apparent due to an increase in knowledge and experience of hygiene officers, the influence of schools and training on combatant as well as technical personnel, a general awakening of hygiene consciousness, a stricter enforcement of methods and a greater knowledge of epidemiology. A somewhat similar reorganisation was carried out in the R.A.A.F., also with increasingly effective results. It is axiomatic that the ideal of thorough indoctrination of the individual soldier is the pivot of hygiene training.

There is little doubt that the wider implications of hygiene, which include the maintenance of health and the prevention of disease, will always require the most strenuous efforts from the medical services, not only to provide timely specialised information and advice, but also to secure the intelligent co-operation of all concerned so that the requisite standard of efficiency may be established and preserved. The outstanding importance of hygiene in all aspects of war service cannot be too strongly emphasised, and yet the lessons of past experiences are so often ignored.

TACTICAL USE OF FIELD MEDICAL UNITS

THE FIELD AMBULANCE

Although the composition and war establishment of this unit have been changed since the war, many still regard it in its previous form as the best all purpose field medical unit that could be devised. Its nature and organisation permitted amazing versatility, enabling it to function under all sorts of conditions and, apart from its normal duties, to assume a variety of rôles—casualty clearing station, field hospital, rest station or convalescent depot, according to the particular and local need. The value of having an additional field ambulance at the disposal of corps or higher formations was abundantly proved in various campaigns both in Syria and in the South West Pacific Area.

It was in the first Libyan campaign that the elasticity of the field ambulance showed to great advantage. The extremely rapid advance with the line of evacuation extending over hundreds of miles necessitated a great degree of mobility on the part of the supporting medical units. This was accomplished by combining field ambulances in whole or in part without regard for complete identity, by detaching mobile sections from the individual units, by brigading the ambulance cars of all field ambulances and by making the fullest use of captured transport vehicles.

Mobile sections were budded off from companies and became, as required, quite independent units. They consisted of 1–2 officers and 14–20 other ranks or more according to necessity, with two vehicles plus one or more motor ambulances. These sections proved invaluable for they could and in fact did act as (1) super R.A.Ps. clearing portion of a wide front, (2) advanced A.D.S., (3) A.D.S. or (4) staging post between R.A.P. and A.D.S., A.D.S. and M.D.S., M.D.S. and C.C.S., where distances were great. One mobile section could clear a whole brigade front or a battalion front as circumstances might demand. It was highly mobile and flexible and did not add to congestion of traffic. This type of unit more than justified its creation, especially in mobile warfare as experienced in Libya and Greece, but it was also employed with marked success during the withdrawal in Libya, throughout the siege of Tobruk, in the early stages of the Syrian campaign (although the latter was generally more orthodox in type), and in the South West Pacific Area in a somewhat different guise.

The brigading of the motor ambulances with a shuttle service and forward taxi rank gave greater control, was more economical and ensured speedy evacuation.

The attachment of surgical and resuscitation teams to the field ambulances in the forward areas worked well. The proximity of expert surgical attention to the front line eliminated delay in treatment and resulted in greatly improved conditions of transport for the casualty, matters of prime importance when satisfactory evacuation was prejudiced by long distances or broken terrain. In mobile warfare the necessity for holding certain cases for some days in a dressing station before they could be evacuated sometimes constituted a problem when forward movement was continuing, but this was largely obviated by the scheme of 'leap-frogging', which enabled field ambulances to by-pass one another and maintain contact with the advancing troops.

Experience in the Libyan campaign proved of the utmost value. Techniques of packing and unpacking were consolidated, loading tables were revised. The importance of close liaison was demonstrated and led to the practice of attaching a senior medical officer from the field ambulance to the headquarters of the brigade group to which it was allotted. It was the opinion in some quarters that the number of motor ambulances on the war establishment was insufficient and that despatch riders should be included on the strength of such units. These suggested additions, while of practical importance in mobile warfare and with reasonably good road communications, had no application in jungle fighting, where the only possible form of wheeled transport that could be used was the jeep ambulance and this only on rare occasions.

THE CASUALTY CLEARING STATIONS

Casualty clearing stations were allotted on the basis of one or two per division. They did their best work when stationary and when they could be expected to remain so for some time. Under these circumstances they were capable of emergency expansion to a considerable number of beds and on occasion were called on to provide additional accommodation for very large numbers of sick or battle casualties. The war establishment provided for a light and a heavy section, but in practice the unit was seldom divided in this fashion. The amount of equipment precluded rapid mobility, and adequate unit means of transport could not be provided to make them independent. They possessed no advantage over small field hospitals.

MOTOR AMBULANCE CONVOY

The employment of this unit in the field is limited to conditions where reasonably good road communications exist. Under these circumstances the assistance that can be given in the evacuation of casualties such as occurred in Greece and Malaya is of the greatest value, especially where distances are great. There is less scope for such a unit in jungle fighting, and with the specialised development of evacuation of casualties by air, it may quite possibly be eliminated from the order of battle of an army in the field.

ORGANISATION OF A 'JUNGLE' FIELD AMBULANCE

A factor of outstanding importance in jungle warfare is transport. The whole or part of the line of communication is impassable to wheeled traffic; supplies can come forward only by bearer, e.g., by native porters, or by being dropped from the air either directly (free dropping) or by parachute; casualties can be transported back only by bearer teams. The field ambulance still had to retain its usual functions of mobility, collection and evacuation of casualties. In a region with but few organised roads the time taken to transport a wounded man might be long enough to prejudice his chances of recovery. Multiple posts were, therefore, often necessary, and it was essential to bring a surgical team as far forward as possible. Thus to the customary functions of a field ambulance was added surgical treatment carried out not only in M.D.Ss. and A.D.Ss. but if necessary in each of three sections formed by sub-dividing each bearer company. A unit of 25 beds was found to be the most practical.

In order to maintain efficiency it was found desirable to have equipment of sections interchangeable; certain additional equipment was also necessary. Among the particular items required the most important ones were extra cooking gear, light table tops of the venetian blind pattern, light waterproof tarpaulins or sisalkraft for accommodation, covers and canvas bed-sails for beds. Each section needed about 14 days' supply of medical stores and comforts. The equipment, like the unit, had to be mobile, and this was best ensured by packing it in boxes containing not over 35 to 40 pounds. Bondwood boxes were regarded as invaluable for this purpose. Specially designed boxes were used for dropping by parachute, which was preferred to free dropping.

III. ARMY MEDICAL ADMINISTRATION AND CAMPAIGNS IN THE MIDDLE EAST, GREECE AND SOUTH WEST PACIFIC AREA

As each campaign illustrated aspects of active service that differed owing to the altered tide of battle, the climate and the terrain, changing series of problems were encountered. Brief reference to the main features may, therefore, be of some moment.

LIBYA AND NORTH AFRICA

The initial attack on a fairly wide front was followed by rapid pursuit, a short static phase, withdrawal, beleaguerment in Tobruk, and the final advance in the set-piece of the El Alamein battle. In the first phase the main problems were communications and the long line of evacuation. Field ambulances were used to the full, and the value of the mobile section was clearly demonstrated. Advantage was taken of captured vehicles to supplement the deficiencies of transport. Indeed without them the field ambulances would have been in grave difficulties to maintain the essential mobility. Ambulance cars were employed on a divisional rather than a unit basis. The shuttle service and taxi rank system was found to work well. (*See* p. 582.)

During the siege of Tobruk field ambulances assumed a relatively normal static rôle but still found a use for mobile sections in close support to regimental aid posts. A point that should be remembered was the great value of convalescent depots and rest camps. This was emphasised in all campaigns. Even in Greece steps were taken early to secure convalescence in simply equipped camps for men who did not need hospital treatment.

GREECE

Somewhat similar problems were experienced in relation to communications and the one long line of evacuation. There was the preliminary delaying action followed by the gradual retirement and the final evacuation. Conditions of climate, snow and rough mountainous country complicated the evacuation of casualties. On occasion donkeys and slung stretchers were used. Again ambulance cars were used on the shuttle service and taxi rank system.

CRETE

Owing to lack of equipment the medical service was largely of an improvised and first-aid character.

SYRIA

While the terrain differed little from that experienced in Libya and Greece, much of the fighting took place over very rugged country. The difficulties encountered added more to the responsibilities of the regimental medical officers. In other respects neither communications, distances nor roads presented serious problems, so that evacuation of casualties from the forward area was accomplished with the maximum speed and efficiency. The medical plan there followed a more stereotyped text-book use of units.

SOUTH WEST PACIFIC AREA

The experiences gained in the Middle East were certainly to prove valuable, but more as a basis from which new techniques were developed to overcome the further problems of climate, terrain and endemic infectious diseases. To these were added the previously unfamiliar ones of participation in combined operations, amphibious and airborne. Evacuation of casualties constituted the gravest difficulty that was encountered, and the maintenance of supplies ran it a close second. Although frequently long distances had to be covered, evacuation was gauged by hours rather than miles. In the later stages air transport rendered outstanding service, but even when this was available, transport in the forward areas was often solely dependent on human motive power because of the weather and the nature of the country. The enrolment of native labour to serve as carriers proved to be the answer. Words cannot describe the loyalty and devotion of these men, nor estimate their heroism and strength. Often it required a team of twelve native bearers to carry a stretcher of their own contriving over the most appalling country on a journey that was estimated by the physical difficulties in carrying in preference to actual distances. The adaptation of mobile sections to the needs of the campaign in New Guinea was almost an automatic development. Movement of the fighting troops was at times relatively slow on account of enemy resistance, jungle warfare, the climate and above all the nature of the country. Even so the lines of communication were often lengthy, adding to the difficulties of evacuation and of maintaining supplies. The mobile section gave place to a medical staging post, staffed by a medical officer with limited equipment and a small team, or an ambulance staging post. These posts were established on the line of evacuation at intervals governed by the physical capacity of the stretcher bearer team and provided also for the overnight reception of casualties. Where the situation permitted, jeep ambulances were used in the forward area.

IV. CLINICAL PROBLEMS, MEDICAL

While the safeguards of previously determined physical standards and the medical examination on enlistment should eliminate the unfit or infirm, there were times when, owing to extreme pressure of work under unfavourable conditions, examining doctors accepted as recruits men who for one reason or another were quite unsuitable. There were, in addition to the increased physical and mental strain inseparable from the normal hazards of active service, the dangers from exposure to endemic diseases in tropical countries, to extremes of climate and to conditions of lowered resistance when even minor infectious diseases assumed epidemic proportions. From the outset, hygiene and preventive medicine were recognised as matters of paramount importance that required continually the full weight of medical organisation throughout the war to ensure proper indoctrination. It is a perpetual source of wonder that the average man, divorced from the normal amenities of civilisation, becomes so unhygiene-minded and oblivious of the consequences of failure to carry out commonsense measures necessary for his own protection and for that of his fellows. A severe outbreak of infectious illness, a heavy incidence of casualties from insect-borne disease such as malaria could, in the course of a few days, and on occasion very nearly did, neutralise the fighting capacity of the troops.

There is no doubt that the preventive measures carried out during the Second World War will be applied with increasing success in the future and will cover an even greater range of individual protection.

The routine procedures undertaken during the period of recruit training comprised inoculation against the typhoid and paratyphoid groups of organisms, cholera and tetanus, vaccination against smallpox and a X-ray examination of the chest. As the theatre of war changed, prophylactic anti-malarial drugs were administered to all troops serving in malarious areas. Measures directed to the control of insect-borne disease were given the highest priority and carried into operation wherever there was any concentration of troops.

The far-reaching beneficial effects of these were incalculable, but even so, in the personal equation remained a problem that defied complete solution and, as in the case of malaria, was nearly responsible for a major calamity.

In the ensuing section the description of the important problems affecting the Australian troops will be largely confined to those presented by infections and tropical diseases, skin affections, psychiatric disorders and matters of hygiene.

Other diseases, cardio-vascular, respiratory, alimentary, renal and degenerative, all claimed their victims, but in limited numbers. Under rigorous conditions of service the ordinary ills of the flesh are essentially more lethal. The formation of the Volunteer Defence Corps for home service in 1941 by the recuitment of mostly First World War veterans and elderly men also increased the incidence of the more common diseases usually encountered in civilian medical practice.

When the war began, the majority of Australian medical officers had had little or no practical experience in the tropical diseases they were to encounter during the subsequent years. Very clear and informative Australian Army Medical Services technical instructions were issued as far as possible in anticipation of clinical situations that might arise. The publication of these continued throughout the war, and they were revised to meet the local requirements or to include later developments in diagnosis and treatment. By these means and by attachment to base units for special training the younger medical officers were kept adequately informed and in touch with modern accepted methods.

(1) Infectious Diseases

(a) ALIMENTARY GROUP

BACILLARY DYSENTERIES

When the destination of the Australian troops in 1940 was known to be the Middle East, it was recognised that dysenteric infections would form a major problem as they were endemic there in all forms. Special diagnostic panniers were included in the equipment of all mobile medical units. In spite of every endeavour to prevent the spread of infection, cases of mild bacillary dysentery rapidly appeared and throughout the war remained an active problem which, although usually well controlled, was a constant menace to the health of the individual and the efficiency of the army.

The appalling death-rate from dysenteries among prisoners-of-war in Japanese camps was mainly due to extreme malnutrition, lack of therapeutic agents and the frequency of intercurrent diseases. In contrast, during the years 1939–46 21,015 Australian soldiers on all fronts, excluding prisoners-of-war in Japanese hands, suffered from bacillary dysentery, but only 21 died.

Of the bacilli present the Flexner group predominated; Shiga strains followed with much lower incidence. Schmitz, Sonne and Boyd infections were also found. The relative figures per 1,000 for Shiga and Flexner infections in the Middle East were 1·3/6·5 in 1941 and 2·3/5·65 in 1942. In Australia the proportion was 0·13/1·03 in 1943 and 0·057/0·33 in 1944. In New Guinea the figures were 2·04/6·26 in 1943, 0·716/3·95 in 1944 and 0·221/2·13 in 1945.

Sigmoidoscopy was a routine diagnostic and prognostic method.

The greatest advance in treatment of bacillary dysentery was the introduction of sulphaguanidine. An initial dose of 0·1 gramme per kilo body weight, with four-hourly doses of half this amount until the number of stools fell to five a day. Then the dose was eight hourly until the stools were normal. Treatment did not exceed fourteen days.

AMOEBIASIS

Endemic in the Middle East, in the Far East and in other places where Australian troops were in action, this malady had only appeared occasionally in Australia in small localised outbreaks. There was, therefore, a potential risk to the civil community from carriers, and the medical services had to be familiar with primary diagnosis and treatment.

Only 783 cases were recorded, exclusive of prisoners-of-war in Japanese camps. The rate per 1,000 varied from 0·3 to 1·77, the latter peak being reached in 1941 in the Middle East. Colonic, hepatic and pulmonary types were seen. In Japanese camps, prisoners-of-war suffered from a high mortality rate, which at times reached 20 per cent. Shortage, and often lack of specific drugs caused this grave morbidity and mortality. The fatal cases occurred in men already debilitated who incurred a severe grade of infection and in whom large granulomatous or ulcerated lesions were found. Treatment comprised 8 to 10 daily intra-muscular injections of emetine hydrochloride, 1 grain in 1 c.cm. of water. In chronic or relapsing infections, a course of emetine followed by a course of up to 30 grains of emetine bismuth iodine was given. The usual dose was 1 grain for three successive days, and then 3 grains daily for seven days. During convalescence carbarsone 0·25 gramme twice daily was substituted. This could be given also during the course of the emetine preparations. Yatren retention enemata were found useful. Sigmoidoscopy was a final check.

CHOLERA

Cholera was a possible menace to troops engaged in campaigns in the islands on the northward route to Japan.

In June 1944 all troops exposed to the risk of infection in endemic areas were inoculated with cholera vaccine. Full instructions for hygienic prevention and treatment were circulated. It was emphasised that not only drinking water should be chlorinated, but also water used in preparing food, for cleaning of the teeth and for rinsing mess gear.

Fortunately, epidemic cholera never became a problem in the Australian Forces in the Pacific area, but the preparations made were a necessary precaution. In Malaya, in the working camps, cholera outbreaks caused great loss of life. The attitude of the Japanese authorities to this disease was quite unrealistic. The medical services had to work under conditions of the greatest difficulty, with inadequate supplies of drugs, improvised methods and delays and hardships which materially decreased the chances of survival of the patients. The vaccines supplied gave inadequate protection; in the absence of material and labour the restoration and maintenance of effective hygiene was a herculean task. Inevitably, the mortality was high, ranging from 40 to 50 per cent. and in one camp to 80 per cent.

The camp outbreaks showed the classic picture of cholera—rapid and overwhelming prostration, copious vomiting and purging with characteristic 'rice-water' evacuations. In the early stages sudden faintness was common with tinnitus, deafness and dimness of vision; later, severe muscular cramps were common. Death was in 'coma vigil', or after a phase of fever and delirium. Terminal uraemia was common. The many ingenious improvisations that were devised for intravenous saline saved many lives.

TYPHOID AND PARATYPHOID

Immunisation by T.A.B. vaccine was made compulsory when the Second A.I.F. was first being recruited but the vaccine used was found to give inadequate protection to troops, nurses and other hospital staffs exposed to typhoid infection overseas. In 1940 in the Australian Army in the Middle East the typhoid rate was 0·49 per 1,000 per year. This rose to 1·05 in 1941. In Greece and Syria, cases of a severe type occurred. While a fully potent vaccine was being prepared an inoculation of 0·5 c.cm of the British vaccine was given to all Australian troops in the Middle East. In 1942 the case incidence of enteric fever dropped to 0·50 per 1,000. The rate per 1,000 thereafter did not exceed 0·14 and in 1944 fell to 0·03.

In the latter months of 1942 outbreaks due to the Salmonella group occurred. Although generally mild, *Salmonella enteritidis* caused three deaths. These infections exhibited (1) a continued febrile illness like typhoid; (2) a gastro-enteritis of short duration with rapid recovery; (3) a septicaemic variety with metastatic complications such as cystitis, epididymo-orchitis, periostitis, subcutaneous abscesses, empyema and cholecystitis. An aggluntinating agent facilitated diagnosis in the field. In treatment no specific drug was of value.

INFECTIVE HEPATITIS

Outbreaks developed in the Middle East during the training period in 1940, and also during the campaigns in Libya, Tobruk, Syria and North Africa. The respective yearly rates per 1,000 in 1941 were: in Palestine 11·51, in Egypt, including Tobruk, 22·07, in Syria 43·85 and during the El Alamein operation, in 1942, 36. In the later years the incidence of hepatitis in the Australian Army was low on the mainland, but many cases occurred in the South West Pacific Area, where the monthly rates per 1,000 rose from 0·51 in 1942 to a peak of 9·25 in 1944, dropping in 1945 to 3·53. Most cases occurred in the forward areas. It was difficult at times to distinguish between infective hepatitis and toxic malarial jaundice. Severe forms of the disease caused a number of deaths. In many less severe cases there was considerable time wastage on account of persistent residual symptoms, relapses and prolonged convalescence.

(b) VECTOR-BORNE GROUP

MALARIA

Throughout the war malaria was an important and ever-present problem in the Australian Forces. It was responsible for more sick wastage and hospital admissions than any other cause, indeed possibly than all other causes. As a factor in reducing the efficiency of the troops, it reigned supreme. The efforts of the medical services to secure the fullest support for assuring the required standards of individual and personal protection and general control measures met with difficulties in the early years. Certain changes of major policy in the overall battle against malaria, such as the appointment of specially qualified men as technical advisers, the reorganisation of existing medical units and the formation of others were, however, eventually accepted. The result, combined with a greater individual appreciation that the advice given by the medical service was practical and beneficial, led to a great improvement.

A few cases occurred in Palestine during 1940 and precautions were observed in Greece. At the start of the campaign in Syria in June 1941 the malaria season was just beginning. The Australian troops had not been previously exposed to malaria, nor were they acquainted with the risks likely to be encountered in the country they were about to enter. Great efforts were made to apprise all ranks of this but it cannot be said that a state of 'malaria consciousness' was induced. There was a shortage of equipment such as mosquito nets, and some of the latter were ineffective. Even supplies of quinine were at first deficient.

During the relatively short but arduous Syrian campaign casualties due to sickness, mostly malaria, exceeded battle casualties. Nurses were trained to take blood films from every man with a wound or with a rise in temperature. With the cessation of hostilities the position improved. A mosquito survey of the country was made and troops were stationed in safer areas. The weather was favourable and mosquito breeding was being hampered by the dry summer. Even so, 1,400 cases were reported during the three months following the first entry into Syria. There is little doubt that a war of movement during the period August to October would have caused heavy losses from malaria. At first 5 grains of quinine daily were given as a suppressive dose; later this was increased to 10 grains.

In Egypt before and during the Alamein battle there was comparatively little malaria. In all in the Middle East there were 131 cases in 1940, 2,331 in 1941 and 934 in 1942.

During the first phase of the Malayan campaign the incidence of malaria among Australian troops was low. Control was good in the settled areas, but as jungle training began the incidence increased, and cases had become common when battle stations were taken up. In prisoner-of-war camps protective measures could not be taken and drugs were always difficult and sometimes impossible to obtain. Blackwater fever occurred not infrequently, as did cerebral malaria, and it is estimated that 90 per cent. of all admissions to hospital had had malaria. One lesson that emerges from the experience in Malaya is that thorough training of medical officers in all aspects of the clinical and pathological diagnosis of malaria is essential.

With the change of the main theatre of war for the Australian Forces from the Middle East to the South West Pacific Area early in 1942 three important problems relating to malaria had to be faced. These were: the prevention of the spread of malaria to the mainland; its control in New Guinea and other tropical islands; and the obtaining of anti-malaria supplies from overseas.

In North Queensland and in the Northern Territory scattered endemic foci already existed. The chief danger lay in the introduction of malaria from outside Australia. Troops leaving malarious areas were prevented from entering the Northern Territory and all infected persons were removed from it. This policy was strictly maintained during the remaining years of the war. Troops infected in New Guinea were taken to areas free of anophelines and anti-malaria control measures were maintained.

In March 1942 at Cairns, within the malaria belt and a terminal for troop movement, an outbreak of malaria began affecting about 7 per cent. of the civilian population. With drugs and efficient work by the army malaria control units, in co-operation with the civil authorities, the area was made reasonably safe.

Meanwhile an occupation force had been established in the Moresby area in anticipation of the serious fighting that was expected in New Guinea. It was essential not only to hold Port Moresby, but to make it a safe malaria-free base. The Medical Services had already confirmed that malaria was responsible for most of the morbidity and some of the mortality among the native population. Malignant malaria was the most common variety, benign tertian was also common; quartan, however, was rare. Blackwater fever occurred frequently. In spite of the fact that before the war the Moresby area had been well controlled and relatively safe, a garrison force that had been in occupation since 1940 had consistently suffered from malaria owing to lack of adequate diagnostic and therapeutic facilities and ineffective methods of control. Apart from the native reservoir of infection, there had thus grown up a military reservoir among the troops themselves. The formation of A.N.G.A.U. (Australian New Guinea Administrative Unit) created a powerful ally to the Army in malaria control by regulating the movement of natives and enforcing their segregation from occupied military areas.

By the middle of 1942, however, the Australian forces generally in the South West Pacific Area were in a serious position. The gravity of the situation was intensified by failure on the part of the combatant troops to appreciate the true significance of the risk, with consequent effect on training. Heavy casualties from malaria were to be expected in the impending actions.

Most of the essential equipment in short supply had to be obtained from overseas and, accordingly, in September 1942 a military medical mission was despatched to America and England to obtain adequate supplies of drugs and netting. It advocated the quinine-atebrin-plasmoquine treatment for malaria and the substitution of atebrin for quinine in suppression. Australian experience of atebrin was that 0·1 gramme very rarely caused symptoms; the usual suppressive dose at that time was 0·1 gramme given on four to six days a week. It had also been found that the toxicity of plasmoquine was negligible provided that the dose of 0·01 gramme of the drug was not exceeded. Satisfactory arrangements regarding insect repellent—dimethyl phthalate—and mosquito netting were also made.

The experiences at Milne Bay in South East New Guinea are important in so far that they corroborated the warnings given by the medical services. They were also of value in producing a more energetic and realistic attitude concerning the problem. The land action was only brief. Until the end of August 1942, when the action began, the incidence of malaria was considerable but not crippling. The troops had received scanty training in malaria discipline, but their newness at first saved them. It was after the successful conclusion of the brief sharp action that epidemic malaria attacked the force. The malariologist's report on Milne Bay in July, before hostilities had begun, had stressed the need for at least twice the number of hospital beds usually provided in training areas in the North of Australia and for good laboratory facilities, reserve supplies of all kinds, an active malaria control unit and provision of protection for troops. Even at the end of August difficulties in transport and organisation still left the area with inadequate facilities. In September, when active operations concluded, the rate was fairly steady at 33 per 1,000 per week, but by December a sharp epidemic wave had begun which was responsible for 3,000 cases of malaria during the month. Had this alarming increase in rate continued bounding upwards in geometrical progression, the whole force would have been lost in less than two months. At this stage, in a personal interview with the commander-in-chief, the malariologist to New Guinea Force stressed the necessity for regarding the recent campaign areas as training grounds in dealing with malaria for subsequent operations. He drew attention to a number of important factors that were involved and the corollaries that emerged from them. These were the lack of consciousness of the destroying force in malaria among the troops, that malaria discipline should be an integral part of unit discipline, that no officer was fit to command even the smallest body of men in a hyperendemic malaria area who did not have constantly with him the awareness of his responsibility, that personal protection must be enforced and breaches of discipline visited by punishment, that unfailing supply of all anti-malaria material, particularly suppressive quinine or atebrin, was essential and that such responsibilities were incumbent on all troops whether in forward or training areas. Following this appeal at the highest level, a request for greater priority for all malaria work, particularly increased equipment and stores for malaria control and for additional labour, met with an immediate response. In January 1943 there was already evidence of a dramatic fall in the anopheline index of the area, with consequent reduction in case incidence. Three other important factors should be mentioned: an order that no man should be evacuated from the area for malaria infection except for serious medical reasons, the segregation of native labourers and the resumption of plasmoquine in treatment. Improved conditions were not only gained but maintained. The malaria rate fell to below five per 1,000 per week. Unit discipline was now excellent. Even so malaria was responsible for 8,099 cases in Milne Bay from October 23, 1942 to April 24, 1943. The malaria story of Milne Bay is one of a virtually closed community. The force luckily fought an action while the malaria enemy was gathering strength; it was nearly annihilated by infection, but showed how remarkable a rehabilitation may occur once facilities are available and strong measures taken. A month after the beginning of intensive malaria control in Milne Bay, atebrin was adopted as the suppressive drug for the Australian Armed Forces, but the change was not fully implemented for a time.

In Central Papua, fighting at first took place in the highlands, where there was comparatively little transmission of infection, but culminated in three months of persistent strenuous combat in swampy coastal country where malaria was hyperendemic. Once again there was the cycle of increase of breeding areas, increase of mosquitoes, rising infection rate, the creation of a reservoir of parasites in the blood of the troops and finally an epidemic. The declared overall rate for operational troops in these actions was $22 \cdot 5$ per 1,000 per week, rising to the peak of 48 per 1,000 per week in January 1943. For the same six months period as for Milne Bay the number of patients admitted with malaria to medical units was 11,638; thus there was a total of 20,272 cases of malaria reported in New Guinea for this period, during which the casualties from tropical diseases numbered 29,101, whereas battle casualties were 6,154, a ratio of $4 \cdot 7$ to 1.

When the divisions that had been in action in Milne Bay and Central Papua were withdrawn to the mainland, it was evident that practically the whole force was infected with malaria, and relapses of benign tertian fever were common. Before proceeding on leave the men were instructed to take $0 \cdot 1$ gramme of atebrin thrice weekly during their period of furlough. At this time difficulties were occasionally experienced in various parts of the mainland and New Guinea in establishing prompt and complete control over the primary fever. Where relapses occurred during or soon after completion of a course, a variant of treatment was adopted; intravenous quinine, 10 grains on the first two days of the course, as well as 20 grains by mouth, 30 grains on the third day, $0 \cdot 9$

gramme of atebrin on the fourth day, 0·6 gramme on the fifth day, and then 0·3 gramme for three successive days.

By March 1943 it was necessary to review the whole malaria position. Atebrin in the dose of 0·1 gramme daily for six days a week in hyperendemic areas had already been adopted as a suppressive drug; a smaller dosage of 0·1 gramme for four days a week was used in areas where malaria was endemic. A combined advisory committee on tropical medicine, hygiene and sanitation was formed, comprising representatives of the medical services of both America and Australia. This committee had far-reaching influence, and many important directives were promulgated on its advice. It drafted recommendations covering all phases of an intensive campaign against malaria and drew attention to the dangers of beginning action before anti-malaria supplies were available and before anti-mosquito measures were established. Another point of importance was the necessity to ensure that no troops affected with malaria arriving on the mainland from an endemic area should be sent to a potentially malarious area in Australia. All troops returning to Australia were kept on a suppressive dosage of atebrin for one month and this was discontinued under controlled conditions. All men developing malaria were admitted to hospital, and the full course of standard treatment with quinine, atebrin and plasmoquine was followed up with a further six weeks' administration of atebrin.

A most important step was the establishment of the Medical Research Unit at Cairns. This unit with a staff of entomologists and pathologists was attached to a camp hospital, but had also a research group in a general hospital situated further inland and a convalescent depot nearby. Accurate assessment was made of the progress of men under observation. On volunteers from the Army an investigation was made on the action of drugs on experimentally produced malaria under a variety of environmental conditions.

To obviate the wastage in man-power more hospitals were provided, permitting the local treatment of men with malaria who could be returned to duty after a relatively brief period, thus saving wasteful evacuation to the mainland. The medical services hoped that with the additional measures taken, the improved equipment and supplies, the increased understanding and the better discipline in the forces, operations could be undertaken in hyperendemic areas at a lower cost than hitherto. Since malaria was responsible for about 90 per cent. of the sick wastage due to tropical disease, the problem was largely one of the control of malaria. It was estimated that, out of a military commitment of half a million, a striking force of not more than 95,000 could be maintained in active operation, given reasonably satisfactory conditions of equipment, reinforcements and casualty-rate.

In September 1943 new operations began with landings by sea on the shore of the Huon Gulf and by air to clear the Markham and Ramu Valleys. Junctions were effected and the drive continued north west along the coast. The medical significance of these successful operations is noteworthy. Both the Markham and Ramu Valleys were highly malarious; so too were the coastal strongholds of the Japanese. The advancing troops had to occupy areas defiled by the retreating enemy and infested with heavily infected mosquitoes. It was disappointing to encounter a high malaria rate, which at its peak was comparable with that experienced in the earlier campaigns. The overall rate for opera-tional troops on the Huon Peninsula was 55·3 per 1,000 per week, while that in the Markham and Ramu Valleys was 93 per 1,000 per week. This peak coincided with the period of hardest fighting in which most battle casualties occurred. This great wastage, especially in the latter region, called for strong measures. By this time the work of the research unit in Cairns had shown that experimentally produced malaria would not break through to cause a clinical attack while 0·6 or 0·7 gramme of atebrin a week was faithfully taken. The official dose was already 0·6 gramme a week; it appeared therefore that most of the men were not in fact taking this full amount. To ensure that a full suppressive dose was received, the weekly rate was doubled and the troops in this region were ordered to take 1·2 grammes of atebrin every week. Even allowing for less strenuous conditions of fighting and the assembly in the rear areas of the more heavily infected units the result was striking; a weekly rate in December of 43·7 per 1,000 per week fell in January to one of 14·3 per 1,000 per week. The rate of relapsing attacks remained steady at about 3·5 per 1,000 per week.

In evaluating the significance of the lessons learned from these campaigns it is clear that staging areas for troops undertaking opera-tional tasks in the Tropics should have a low malaria risk and be under efficient medical control, beginning at the earliest possible moment after military objectives have been taken. Anti-malaria supplies during operations must be adequate. Individual and unit discipline is of the highest importance. An officer should report each night to formation headquarters that all malaria precautions have been taken. That discipline can be maintained was conclusively demonstrated in one brigade which throughout many months of arduous fighting had an average rate of 7·6 per 1,000 per week—no higher than that in a forward base after control had been instituted. The routines established in this brigade had a strong influence in determining a general disciplinary standard for the future.

Research had shown that regular daily doses of 0·1 gramme of atebrin suppressed benign tertian malaria, and cured the malignant tertian form. It could therefore abolish the death rate of malaria. From early in

1944 responsibility for measures of malaria control rested with commanders of units and neglect of this duty carried severe penalties.

Dichloro-diphenyl-trichloroethane (D.D.T.) was introduced in 1944 and its production in Australia began. It was effective both in ground work and as an aerial spray. In November 1944 the combined malaria rate, which earlier had been 740 per 1,000 per annum for troops in both base and forward areas in New Guinea, was only 26 per 1,000. Malaria free bases were established from which fresh advances were made.

Preliminary results of experiments at the research unit indicated that the claims made for various sulphonamide preparations were not substantiated. Atebrin, however, was found to be a reliable and effective suppressive drug when taken in doses of $0 \cdot 6$ gramme a week. This dose would suppress benign tertian and would cure as well as suppress malignant tertian malaria. In the next stage of trials field types of experiments were carried out, reproducing as faithfully as possible all the known conditions of extreme physical and mental strain to which troops were or might be exposed. Volunteers were subjected to very heavy infection, a high and effective atebrin level in the blood was maintained throughout, and there was no instance of malaria breaking through. The whole question of the possible toxicity of atebrin had been given the most careful consideration. It was certain that in ordinary suppressive doses, even when taken over a period of months, atebrin was practically non-toxic. The occasional instances of idiosyncracy were few and far too isolated to warrant banning the use of so valuable a drug. The various side effects that were attributed to it in flying operations, greater susceptibility after previous administration, impotence and the like, were categorically disproved.

Experimental work was also carried out with D.D.T. and aerial spraying. Under optimum conditions a dosage of 2 to $2\frac{1}{2}$ quarts per acre of 5 per cent. D.D.T. in oil was found to give better than minimum effective distribution. The ideal method was for the aircraft to fly 100 feet above tree level in straight line runs 100 yards apart, and though cross-winds were preferred, the flight pattern dictated by the topography could be followed with good results. Before the planned combined operations were carried out early in 1945, the routines for air spraying of D.D.T. had been well worked out. In general it was not carried out when planes would risk exposure to hostile anti-aircraft fire, or where the enemy might suspect a gas attack. The indications were the presence of presumably infected anophelines in a newly occupied area, an outbreak of dengue fever, difficulty in applying other control methods to inaccessible areas and an outbreak of dysentery in an area infected with flies. Areas for spraying were selected rather for their proximity to concentrations of native population, or to areas recently occupied by the Japanese, than for the presence of suspected breeding grounds. In the early phases of an operation, reliance was not placed on D.D.T. spraying alone. Pyrethrum spraying was carried out as widely as possible on the day of the landing. Subsequently aerial spraying was undertaken. The beach maintenance area and its surrounding zone were given first priority; thereafter native compounds, main dressing stations, rest camps, casualty clearing stations and transit areas for troops.

During the period 1944–45, from November 1944, when further operations were begun, the incidence of malaria remained within reasonable bounds although the forces were widely spread and much heavy fighting took place under difficult conditions. There was one notable exception to this, the Aitape-Wewak epidemic which will be mentioned later. For the rest, out of about 130,000 troops engaged in forward areas and exposed to malaria infection for periods of from six to twelve months, only 1,256 attacks of malaria were reported over a period of nearly one year. The incidence of the relapse rate of benign tertian malaria was also low. This was important when it is remembered that on January 31, 1945 a review of the records showed that since June 1943 a total of 67,172 men had had malaria.

While the methods evolved for controlling malaria in the field were vindicated in the last years of the war by the excellent results obtained, the epidemics that occurred in the Aitape-Wewak area caused grave concern and provided a chastening experience. Operations began in November 1944 and continued until the middle of 1945. The force had to fight back along a hundred miles of coast and also in the mountainous inland section in an area in which malaria was hyperendemic throughout the whole year. In December an undue malaria rate was noted in certain units, and as a precautionary measure members of the units concerned were given a double dose, 0·2 gramme of atebrin daily. Thorough investigations were made on the spot with the conclusion that conditions of infection were not more severe than elsewhere, that atebrin was not at fault in composition or action and that the outbreak was due to faulty atebrin suppression. All control measures were even more rigidly enforced, and the suppressive dose was raised to 0·2 gramme daily for the whole force until March. Although the initial sharp epidemic subsided after two months, there was a large scale recrudescence in April in spite of what was regarded as the strictest attention to detail. Investigations carried out in the Medical Research Unit at Cairns proved the existence of an atebrin-resistant strain of *P. falciparum* in the Aitape-Wewak area. This was not the prevalent strain and, while no doubt a contributor to the epidemic, was not by any means the responsible factor, for in spite of asseverations to the contrary there must have been breaks in malaria control and discipline. On the other hand, the force was able to carry out the assigned tasks with complete success, and atebrin demonstrated its ability to suppress overt malaria in two-thirds of the troops. The lessons to be learned are the military necessity for continued striving to attain perfection of personal as well as mechanical control of the disease, realisation of the great number of variables involved in solving the scientific problems encountered, the need for constant local technical investigation in every operational area and the desirability of having more than one reliable suppressive drug for use in the field.

Clinical investigations were undertaken in various hospitals to assess the merits of treatment with various drug combinations. However, the standard course of quinine, atebrin and plasmoquine followed by a maintenance dose of atebrin seemed to give results as good as any other method. The standard treatment consisted of quinine 30 grains daily for three days, atebrin 0·3 gramme daily for five days and plasmoquine base 0·03 gramme with 15 grains of quinine daily for three days. Paludrine, which was not available in time for extensive field trials under operational conditions, was also investigated by the Medical Research Unit at Cairns. It was found to be a true causal prophylactic for malignant tertain malaria and was completely successful as a suppressive in benign tertian malaria. In all the experiments at Cairns and in hospitals this drug showed a very low degree of toxicity, and its therapeutic dosage range was wide. It also had the advantage that it did not stain the skin.

The toxicity of atebrin manifested itself in a variety of ways, of which skin lesions were the most common. But even these occurred in relatively moderate numbers of no significance when compared with the necessity of using the drug. Toxic confusion, liver involvement and aplasia of the haemopoietic system were also found, but only in rare instances. The skin lesions resembled lichen planus of a type not seen in civil practice.

The toxicity of plasmoquine was periodically a subject of discusions during the war. Despite overseas reports of abdominal pain and of haemoglobinuria especially associated with previous administration of atebrin, the Australian experience was not unfavourable.

The death rate from malaria was less than 0·5 per 1,000. The only types of parasite of importance were P. falciparum and P. vivax. P. ovale was occasionally seen. Fever which was not promptly controlled, evidence of hyperinfestation and suggestion of a possible metastatic complication of malignant tertian fever were indications for the use of the intravenous injection of 10 grains of quinine. Of all the complications of falciparum infection cerebral malaria and the extremely severe infection just described were most common. Abdominal pains were less common but did occur. Jaundice associated with malaria always suggested the possibility of a relatively severe malignant tertian infection, although it was not infrequently due to a co-existing virus hepatitis. Blackwater fever was seen with increasing rarity as time went on. The treatment favoured was to produce rapid alkalinisation of the urine, using sodium bicarbonate in saturated solution and 4 x molar sodium lactate solution combined in ampoules of 10 cubic centimetres. Two ampoules were injected into a vein initially and at intervals of fifteen to thirty minutes as required. Blood transfusion was also used with great caution and only in cases where blood destruction was severe.

The rare but serious complication of rupture of the spleen was also recorded on a few occasions.

In 1942 the growing number of cases of malaria introduced the infrequent problem of false positive serological reactions for syphilis, sometimes observed in the serum of patients with malaria.

In spite of the widespread infection of the Forces with malaria the aftermath effect on health has been negligible. Among demobilised Servicemen malaria became a diminishing problem which finally disappeared.

From this account it is evident that the organisation of control measures, which became increasingly more adequate and complete, rested on two foundations. One of these was the background of science, the other the principle that guidance was the rôle of the medical services, but that responsibility for carrying out measures for which disciplinary control was necessary rested with the combatant commanders and their deputies.

THE SANDFLY—DENGUE FEVER GROUP

Sand-fly fever

Considerable epidemics occurred in the Middle East during 1940, 1941 and 1942. They followed the usual clinical picture and mostly did not necessitate a long absence from duty.

There was no proof that sandfly fever existed in either Australia or New Guinea.

Dengue Fever

This fever is endemic in certain parts of Northern Australia and has epidemic migratory characteristics. Its importance in man-power wastage affecting a mobile population such as an army was therefore known. In the Northern Territory and in North Queensland epidemics occurred in 1941 and 1942, with an incidence of 10 per 1,000 per week and 25 per 1,000 per week, respectively.

Epidemics also occurred in New Guinea and Borneo. The vectors were not only *Aedes aegypti* and *albopictus* but also *Å. scutellaris*, as transmission experiments proved. Dengue control is largely mosquito control. Protective clothing and repellents are important. Control measures were as those for malaria and success was attained by improved standards.

TYPHUS FEVER

Murine Typhus

During the war murine typhus was not of any importance in Australia, although cases were recognised in widely different areas in 1940–1942.

Mite-borne Typhus

Mite-borne or scrub typhus was a serious problem during the earlier phases of the Pacific Islands campaign, more on account of the severity of the disease itself than because of the numbers involved. The death rate was 9 per cent. in the Services, total deaths being 257 among 2,839 recorded cases. The severity of the disease varied considerably in different localities. Its effects were noticeably more lethal in patients suffering from intercurrent diseases, weakened by severe physical and mental strain and handicapped by age. The prognosis was graver in men over thirty-five years.

The persistence of profound toxaemia, the failure of the patient to respond to specific therapy for malaria or dysentery and the finding of a raised and rising titre of agglutination for *Proteus OXK*, confirmed the diagnosis.

The presence of an eschar varied considerably, reaching 65 per cent. in one series. The site was nearly always on the trunk or proximal parts of the limbs. Enlargement of lymph glands was common. Rapid pulse rate, over 120 per minute, was usually an ominous sign, especially if associated with falling blood pressure. Venous thrombosis was an occasional event, respiratory symptoms were almost always present and nearly all severely ill patients showed bronchitic signs by the end of the first week. Diarrhoea was frequent in the early stages and in a few patients dysphagia occurred. Symptoms referable to the nervous system were always present in all but the mildest infections. Seriously ill patients often were stuperous and inert, the chief problem of nursing being the administration of food, but others were constantly restless and trying to get out of bed. In about a sixth of the cases affection of the 8th cranial nerve was seen, mostly as bilateral nerve deafness from which recovery almost invariably took place. Reflex changes were very common.

T. deliensis and *T. akamushi* were found in nearly all areas in New Guinea and were established as vectors by the United States Typhus Commission. Some species were found only in grass, others in both grass and jungle. In Queensland their habitat was mainly in narrow belts along the edge of scrub or in clearings in the scrub with little or no grass.

Dimethyl and dibutyl-phthalate proved protective repellents. The latter was found to be superior to the dimethyl preparation, particularly in its power to withstand the washing of clothes. Rubbing the drug lightly into the material was sufficient to impregnate it effectively. The standard method of application by which each soldier treated his own clothing by rubbing in repellent by hand at least every fortnight was found to be more satisfactory than any elaborate system. One ounce of fluid allowed about 70 smears, which would impregnate the clothing sufficiently to withstand 7 washings in cold soapy water or 3 boilings. Blankets were also treated by hand or in army laundries.

The results of prophylaxis were very striking and cases showed a progressive decline from the peak incidence of 859 in the week ending December 31st, 1943 to 21 in the week ending 23rd February, 1945.

The incubation period for mite-borne typhus was established at twelve days.

Patients were speedily evacuated to medical units where good nursing conditions prevailed. Drugs were not found to be of special value, but some benefit seemed to follow the giving of para-aminobenzoic acid. The length of convalescence varied considerably.

Tick-borne Typhus

A small series of cases occurred in Tobruk and in Queensland, but tick typhus was not a disease of military importance.

Relapsing Fever

This, though not a serious military problem, caused considerable temporary invalidity in the Middle East. The nervous system was the most frequently affected; recovery was the rule, but residual paralyses were seen in some patients. In 1941–43 382 men were treated, with no deaths. The average stay in hospitals was 42 days. Tick bites were found in at least a third of the patients.

(c) METAZOAN INFESTATION

ANKYLOSTOMIASIS

This was common during and after the first campaign in New Guinea. Ova were found in the faeces in large numbers of soldiers returned to Australia either for wounds, overt illness or rehabilitation. Infection was mainly by *A. duodenale* and *Necator americanus* with occasional instances of *A. braziliense*. Although many of the men had mild symptoms only, there were numbers seen who suffered from a very acute infection. These mostly occurred in the later years and were characterised by severe 'ground itch', marked pulmonary involvement and an acute anaemic state. The best single drug was found to be tetrachlorethylene, but the addition of chenopodium improved its action.

SCHISTOSOMIASIS

This was a medical risk both in the Middle East and in the South West Pacific Area, but there were only two outbreaks, one in 1941 in an engineer unit, where three men passed ova of S. *haematobium*, the other in an Australian Airfield Construction Squadron attached to the American Forces. No deaths occurred among the 226 men infected by S. *japonicum* in Leyte. Treatment with tartar emetic was successful.

(d) OTHER INFECTIONS

CEREBRO-SPINAL MENINGITIS

In Australia in the first two years of the war 269 cases, with a mortality rate of 2·8 per cent., were recorded in the defence forces, as against 1,125 civilians with a death rate of from 20–24 per cent. The disease spread to military camps from a civilian epidemic. The total incidence in troops in the Middle East for the years 1940–42 was 85 cases with 3 deaths, while from 1942–45 in the South West Pacific, there were 34 cases. For the same period 595 cases were recorded for the whole of the Australian Army in Australia. In the early war years treatment was by sulphonamides; in later years penicillin had a marked beneficial effect on both morbidity and mortality. Contacts were put under observation but not isolated.

RESPIRATORY DISEASES

These call for no special comment concerning troops in the field. In camps and training areas they ranked high for sick wastage. No special immunisation treatment was given.

PULMONARY TUBERCULOSIS

Owing to miniature X-ray examination of recruits, which eliminated 1 per cent. with suspected pulmonary tuberculosis, this disease was a negligible quantity. No recruit was discharged from the Services solely on the basis of a X-ray report. In the later years of the war the number of Servicemen needing treatment for this disease increased by accumulation. Although the incidence rate per 1,000 per year for the years 1942 to 1945 was only 1·14, the total numbers over this period were 1,334 in Australia, 74 in the South West Pacific Area and 92 in the Middle East. In 1944 all men and women from the Services with pulmonary tuberculosis were concentrated in one hospital. Treatment was thus coordinated and, by order, patients were kept for twelve months in Service hospitals before coming to a final medical board.

VENEREAL DISEASES

In spite of a more enlightened outlook and increased facilities for diagnosis and treatment, the incidence of venereal disease was high and a constant drain in man-power. In 1942, control of preventive measures was vested in experts in venereal disease, but standards for prophylaxis and treatment were not drawn up until 1943. Incidence in the Middle East ranged from 35·21 per 1,000 in 1940 to 47·22 in 1942. In the Pacific Islands there was no opportunity to acquire infection, but Servicemen risked infection on leave in Australia and the rates varied from 18·93 per 1,000 in 1942 to 17·08 in 1945.

Penicillin altered the therapeutic outlook for both gonorrhoea and syphilis. Treatment was simplified and the duration of stay in hospital much reduced.

(ii) Constitutional and Systematic Affections

NUTRITIONAL CARDIO-VASCULAR CONDITIONS

There were occasional instances of cardiac murmurs and enlargement with oedema in soldiers subjected to hardship and dietetic restrictions. The chief symptoms were loss of weight and exhaustion. Prisoners-of-war in Japanese Camps showed graver disturbances such as oedema, with or without cardiac failure, palpitation, either spontaneous or on exertion, tachycardia, occasionally brachycardia, irregular rhythm due to extra systoles or to auricular fibrillation, dyspnoea, oppression or pain in the chest, dizziness and syncope, definite cardiac failure of the left side of the heart, and ventricular arrest with recurrent Stokes-Adams attacks, sometimes fatal. Sudden death occurred also in men who had not been thought ill. Exact classification in aetiological terms was as a rule difficult; dietetic deficiencies were undoubtedly the underlying cause in most cases. A diagnosis of 'cardiac beriberi' could only be made with associated cardiac failure and radiological evidence.

EFFORT SYNDROMES

Officially, the diagnosis of 'disordered action of the heart', so common in the First World War, was discouraged. Cardio-vascular neuroses were uncommon in the Middle East but increased during the fighting in New Guinea.

PEPTIC ULCER

Digestive diseases were important in all armed forces. The experiences in prisoner-of-war camps illustrated how an occasional or remittent lesion like a peptic ulcer can become a dangerous, permanent and progressive incubus when the vital spark is nearly quenched. It was also seen that peptic ulcer recurred under the stimulus of conditions of service, less flexible than those of ordinary life, particularly in the sensitive or unadaptable types. Most frequent of all the dyspepsias of Service life were those of psychological origin which are probably commonest in civilian life. At the examination of recruits for enlistment, men with a previous history of operation for peptic ulcer or of proven peptic ulcer should be rigorously excluded.

NUTRITIONAL DISTURBANCES

There was no significant lowering of nutritional standards in the Middle East and on the whole Servicemen in Australia maintained a satisfactory grade of nutrition. Fresh food supplements were needed in the Northern Territory. In the Pacific Islands campaigns there were occasions when the diet was unsatisfactory and of low vitamin content. Uncertainty and difficulties of transport as well as the arduous conditions of service contributed to the problem, rather than any intrinsically defective dietary scale.

In general, though malnutrition was seen during the early strenuous periods in New Guinea, clear-cut pictures of specific avitaminoses were very uncommon.

The appointment in 1943 of a medical officer to the staff of the Medical Directorate to act as liaison officer to 'Q' Branch (Nutrition) of the Army proved of undoubted value.

The nutritional disturbances in prison camps, particularly in those under Japanese control, were very considerable. Apart from the general state of sub-nutrition, well defined deficiency states were recognised. These were beriberi, neuritic beriberi, cardiac beriberi, nutritional oedema, encephalopathy, scrotal dermatitis, lesions of the lips, mouth and tongue, painful feet, spastic paraplegia, lesions of the skin, changes in the blood, and eye disturbances. The diets were deficient in protein, calcium, and the vitamins B, A and C. The vitamin B complex and such components as riboflavin and nicotine were probably more important than thiamin.

In any future war despatch of protective foods by the Red Cross Society to prisoners-of-war should rank high in priority.

(iii) Dermatology

It was expected that skin conditions would rank high in disease incidence and man-power wastage, but the number of men affected was much greater than had been anticipated. Throughout the war, wherever it was waged, they caused grave concern. The variable factors of conditions of service, climate and locality each brought their special problems and disclosed aspects that were of particular clinical interest, and in the aggregate emphasised the importance of this section of military medicine.

The lesions most frequently seen in the Middle East were (1) various forms of dermatitis associated with sweating and mechanical or other irritation, (2) pyodermia in forms ranging from indolent ulcers to furuncles and (3) parasitic infections. The so-called 'desert sores' were the centre of considerable controversy. Bacteriological investigation showed that an infective agent, usually a haemolytic streptococcus and often a pyogenic staphylococcus, was present. Although vitamin C was unproven as a significant factor, it cannot be said that this or other nutritional elements may not have been relevant. The rôle of sweat and of sebaceous secretion and of direct sunlight was also uncertain. The lack of any army issue of soap was one contributory factor; others were the need for sterilising blankets by airing and sunlight and the neglect of simple first aid for minor injuries. A frequent and annoying type of septic lesion was due to sandfly bites. Treatment varied with individual preference and local facilities; there was in fact no specific therapy.

Throughout the whole period during which Australian units operated in the Middle East septic sores gave trouble. Exacerbations occurred during campaigns when hygiene and simple care could not always be carried out.

Parasitic infection of the skin included various forms of tinea, scabies and pediculosis. The exact incidence of tinea was impossible to estimate but, though common, was considered to be over-rated. An important complicating factor was over-treatment. Tinea was not, however, of great importance in the Australian Forces. During the later years it was not significant among the many other problems in tropical dermatology, but localised outbreaks in unexpected areas showed that it could not be disregarded. Pediculosis was seen only in moderate numbers, chiefly in the pubic region. Even apart from infected sores and parasitic infection the incidence of other skin diseases was considerable. The acute symptoms settled down well in hospital as a rule, but the lesions tended to become lichenified in many cases and these required long treatment. During the years 1940–1942 the Australian Forces in the Middle East had a constant morbidity rate for diseases of the skin of slightly over 100 per 1,000 per year.

Early in 1942 sensitivity to chrome as a factor of possible importance in dermatitis was investigated. The question of abandoning chrome for vat dyes was discussed, but in fact there was only a negligible incidence of dermatitis due to chrome idiosyncracy and these cases were best dealt with as individuals. Even so it raised the possible advisability of the ultimate abandonment of chrome dyeing for uniforms in the future.

In considering the skin conditions that caused the most trouble during the years 1943–45, both inclusive, particularly in the tropical parts of Australia and in the island combat areas, it is important to realise that although tropical diseases, in particular malaria, were responsible for the most serious depredations in man-power, skin disease became increasingly a cause of sick wastage and indeed for a time provided more casualties than did malaria. The most common conditions seen were sweat rashes, either combined with intertrigo in the flexures or on the hands and feet, *miliaria rubra*, follicular infection, acne vulgaris and tinea. The factors concerned in the high incidence of skin disease in New Guinea and similar areas were the climate, the existence of some skin infections there, the protective clothing made necessary by anti-malaria measures and contact with chemical irritants of various kinds, and eruptions due to drugs. The trying combination of heat and high humidity was present in most areas occupied by troops except in the highlands. This combination was accentuated by the wearing of clothing which covered most of the body and which for durability had to be relatively thick. There was evidence, both clinical and experimental, that *miliaria rubra* can be a prelude to further organic disturbances of the skin and of general bodily function. It thus possesses more than a nuisance value. Special investigations suggested the hypothesis that *miliaria rubra*, tropical anhydrosis and anhidrotic asthenia are three phases of a single disease process of which the essential anatomical feature is blockage of the sweat ducts. The question of soap, the method and frequency of its use and its issue to soldiers gave rise to much controversial discussion. The use of medicated soap was forbidden. In a technical instruction entitled 'Preventable casualties from skin lesions' in 1945 the use of soap was dealt with and advice was given relative to the moderation of its application both on clothes and on the body. Some considerable time previously a recommendation had been made by the D.G.M.S. to the Adjutant General that toilet soap be issued to promote hygiene and prevent skin disease. This was later implemented in part. Although *miliaria rubra* was the commonest lesion of the skin due to environmental causes, it was not responsible for serious disability except in so far as it might be an introduction to severer lesions. Other conditions such as sweat and vesicular eruptions were frequent. Recurrent cheiropompholyx was much more common in New Guinea than in the Middle East and was almost certainly related to disordered sweat function.

Fungus infections were undoubtedly more frequent in New Guinea, being due partly to climatic conditions but more to the existence of large numbers of indigenous parasitic fungi. Heroic and ill-advised over treatment by young regimental medical officers called for timely warnings regarding the evil effects of over-enthusiastic application of strong antiseptics.

Bacterial infections were even more frequent and more important; impetigo, folliculitis, furunculosis, ulcers, supperative infection of the sweat glands and septic processes causing cellulitis were types of pyogenic infections that were seen.

Acne vulgaris was adversely affected by tropical conditions and frequently flared up into acute pustulation with a degree and distribution unusual by civilian standards of practice. These complicating lesions usually rendered a man unfit for subsequent front-line service.

There were several types of so-called 'tropical ulcer' seen in the Islands. Trauma, even slight, was the exciting cause, with infection superadded. The seriousness of such lesions depended greatly on general and local resistance. Among prisoners-of-war in Japanese camps most extensive and dangerous ulcers were produced which destroyed both limbs and lives.

Among the allergic and toxic states that were seen, generalised and exfoliative dermatitis were fortunately not common, but sensitisation rashes of lesser grades appeared quite often. Sulphonamides caused many of these and necessitated a technical instruction warning against their use for local application except when the patient was under observation in a general hospital. Acriflavine was another chemical source of sensitisation.

The most important form of skin lesion due to toxic or allergic action of a chemical substance was undoubtedly the so-called 'tropical lichenoid'. Proof of the association of lichenoid with atebrin is now generally accepted. It did not occur in the South West Pacific Area except in persons taking atebrin and not in any who took less than the suppressive dose. The integrity of malaria control depended on atebrin, and although this side effect had been observed for some two years before any definite opinions were expressed, the small percentage of cases (about 1 in 2,000) justified silence, and the military value of atebrin was never jeopardised by this fortunately uncommon dermatosis. Patients with this condition were considered completely unfit for further service in forward areas or those where atebrin was taken for suppressive purposes.

In the early part of 1945 admissions to hospitals in tropical areas for dermatitis were so high that further efforts were made to attack the problem from the points of view of education and research. In May 1945 skin disease was the largest single cause of casualties in the Australian Military Forces; the rates per 1,000 per year in the South West Pacific Area had risen from 53 in 1943 to 105 in 1945 with somewhat less, but still unduly high, rates on the mainland. Some reduction in this rate was accomplished by adequate instruction of medical officers and orderlies, and by the taking of more preventive measures in units, but there still remained an extensive field in which planned research work should produce good results. Arrangements were in hand to carry out elaborate experimental work, further clinical studies and extensive dermatological surveys of several forward units, but these were never put into effect owing to termination of hostilities in the Pacific.

The official addition of trained dermatologists to hospital staffs was most valuable. More might perhaps have been done in an educational way by using whole-time mobile consultants chiefly for this purpose. As it was, the work done by dermatologists acting semi-officially as regional consultants was most advantageous.

(iv) Psychiatry

While the magnitude of mental problems raised by the war was realised by all interested in modern medicine, there was a feeling that the problem was rather one of disposal and accommodation than of method, that experienced general physicians could handle the psychoneuroses in hospitals and that lessons of the last war could be applied by the junior medical officers in forward areas with some help and instruction. Modern concepts in psychosomatic disorders had not attained general acceptance, and their application in appropriate treatment laboured under this disadvantage. Even with the experience of two lengthy periods in which the stresses and strains of active service could be assessed in relation to their effect on those taking part, there is still a suggestion in some quarters that damage through the violence of war is alone responsible for the mental disorders of Servicemen and Service-women. This attitude is still, to some extent, reflected in the use of the term 'war neurosis' and indirectly saddled the Armed Forces in the early recruiting days with a number of misfits. There were occasions initially when conditions prevented satisfactory questioning and physical examination on enlistment, but, even so, many were accepted whose future value to the Services was already suspect because of constitutional disabilities. The form of *questionnaire* also made it possible for enlisting applicants to give false or misleading information, especially during rush periods.

With this background it is interesting to trace the evolution of the psychiatric services and the developments that took place in later years. In May 1940, following a conference called by the D.G.M.S. to consider 'war neuroses', various recommendations were made. The term 'shell shock' was forbidden and that of 'anxiety state' used in forward areas. The usual terminology was recommended for the ordinary civilian types of neuroses. Acute nervous casualties were to be treated as far forward as possible by regimental medical officers in particular and also by mobile groups of experienced physicians and psychiatric specialists. One interesting recommendation was the need of a psychiatric specialist for each division.

In the Middle East, as the result of a medical conference, the term 'exhaustion' was used for acute neurotic casualties arising in action. For other grades of psychoneurosis such terms as anxiety state, psycho-neurosis or conversion hysteria were employed. These recommendations were used as a basis of current psychiatric practice in the Middle East.

At the end of 1940 the commonest psychiatric disturbances in the Australian Forces in the Middle East were of the psychosomatic type; anxiety states were of the civilian pattern. After active operations had been in progress, fear and exhaustion states were seen in the first desert campaign, and subsequently in the early days of the siege of Tobruk it was found necessary to establish a neurosis clinic. At first patients with nervous disturbances were treated in the hospital, which was within the town area, and later in a non-surgical section on the beach. Both sites were subjected to bombing, and superadded neuroses were seen in patients admitted for wounds or sickness; the latter were more frequently affected, especially those suffering from infections. Subsequently a treatment centre was opened in an underground concrete shelter. This clinic was a divisional centre and no man could be returned to the base for psychiatric illness except through this channel. In the first three months 110 men out of 207 patients treated in this clinic were sent back. A follow-up and more detailed analysis showed that 79 were returned to work within the fortress area, a further 48 treated at base were returned to duty classified as fit for active service with a field formation, a total of over 60 per cent.; a further 48 were classified as fit for base duties. Most of these men recovered quickly from what was only a temporary fear state; in others a morbid fear of shelling and bombing persisted; in others again an anxiety neurosis remained. Anxiety states were by far the most common type of mental illness. Conversion hysteria was infrequent and usually occurred in young men. Few psychotics were seen—four with schizophrenia and one with a depressive psychosis. Of the men examined 58 per cent. were found to have some inadequacy of personality. In 23 per cent. there was a history of previous breakdowns and in 17 per cent. of a severe head injury. As a rule these items in the patient's history had not been disclosed on enlistment. It was found that treatment, to be effective, must be begun promptly near the front line and continued without intermission for an appropriate and sometimes lengthy period.

During the campaign in Greece relatively few acute psychiatric casualties were observed, but the story may have been different had the troops on their return to Palestine been required to carry out responsible or arduous duties in less safe and comfortable surroundings than in training areas.

In the brief Syrian campaign many men suffering from 'exhaustion states' were evacuated to medical units in Palestine, a number with conversion hysteria. Recovery was common and the immediate results of treatment of hysteria were good.

In Australia the psychiatric services of the Army were extended in base hospitals and a three-months' course of intensive training in psychiatry was arranged for medical officers.

In response to a request for more psychiatric help in the Middle East psychiatrists were sent from Australia. Under their guidance a neurosis clinic was established in a convalescent depot and later changed its name to the more desirable one of 'psychiatric centre'. In the first six months of its existence 528 officers and other ranks were examined and 326 discharged. All psychotics were returned to Australia.

In 1942 after the return of most of the Australian Forces to Australia the 9th Division remained to take part in the next phase of the desert campaign. During this fighting fear states were again encountered. The men were treated in units as far as possible. A rest camp was established on the coast, where psychiatric casualties needing treatment were held until the battle casualties had been cleared. The value of early treatment and disposal of men suffering from fear states was well seen in the work of a psychiatric first-aid post established in a field ambulance with a psychiatrist in charge. Most of the cases seen could be treated on the spot, and very few had to be sent back to hospital.

Early in 1942 psychiatric problems arose in the Pacific theatre of war. In New Guinea and other islands the technical experience of the Middle East was repeated. Psychoneuroses were more common in base areas, and the problem of 'B' class men with somatic fixations again arose when they were employed at forward bases. Psychoses were on the whole uncommon, but the relative and absolute increase in numbers of acute psychotic disorders of schizoid or confusional type was noteworthy. Once more exhaustion and fear states were encountered in periods of hard fighting. Infections were again noted as a contributory cause of break-down. The great increase in skin diseases introduced another factor of some importance. In forward bases anxiety and fear states with or without somatic symptoms were commonly seen in the hospitals, but hysteroid and confusional conditions were rare. In the earlier years not many psychotics were seen, but later the proportion of these rose, cases of both acute psychoses and more particularly manic states becoming more common. It was also noteworthy that an increase occurred in hysterical states, some being of gross character. One opinion recorded the fact that the incidence in officers exceeded that of other types of neurosis. The most frequent phenomena encountered were speech disturbances and alteration of consciousness, such as amnesia. Actual fugues were rare.

The acute psychotic states at this time raised a number of problems including the nature and cause of these illnesses, the best method of handling, and the transport of the patients to the mainland. Atebrin was considered a potential cause but could not really be incriminated as the pattern of toxic confusion due to the drug was rather distinctive and confirmed incidence rare. Special wards were built in selected hospitals and staffed adequately. When these facilities were available, convulsive therapy by cardiazol was introduced in order to make the patients more amenable to travel. This proved most beneficial and permitted the subsequent evacuation of patients by air to the mainland in a much more satisfactory condition. Free use of intravenous injections of glucose and saline relieved the dehydration so often present and were considered an essential adjunct in the preparation for air travel. Suppressive atebrin was continued as a routine for all psychotic patients in a malarious area without any adverse effect on their mental recovery.

In the final action in Borneo, where two divisions were engaged over a period of twelve weeks, 360 men were sent to hospital with psychoses and psychoneuroses in the proportion of one to four. At least 60 per cent. of the psychoses were of the schizophrenic type. Battle exhaustion occurred also in the Borneo action, but education of the medical officers and a general understanding of the prophylactic measures, caused a lowered incidence.

At this time analysis of 480 men seen in hospitals over a six-months' period showed that 144 were psychotics, 56 psychopathics, 270 psychoneurotics and 10 mental defectives. Of the neurotic group 206 had anxiety states (including fear states), 25 hysteria and 20 neurasthenia. Another series of 343 psychiatric casualties seen over a period of five months in a hospital revealed that poor or bad home environment existed in 41 per cent.; battle stress was non-existent in half the total number and severe in only 9 per cent.

Among prisoners-of-war those in fixed camps showed a good morale and were greatly helped by the high standard of discipline that was maintained. In the working camps the conditions were usually very much worse, but in general the incidence of mental diseases of all kinds was extraordinarily low.

In Australia in 1943 recruits were prevented from enlistment if they were considered unsuitable from the mental and personality viewpoints and the facilities for treatment of mental illness were extended. These advances culminated in the establishment of a psychological service in the Australian Army at the beginning of 1945. Earlier an Advisory Committee on Psychological Testing gave advice on the selection of staff for highly technical work. This concept was further developed when the rapid expansion of the Armed Services rendered correct allocation of men even more important. Recruits and re-allocated men were subjected to a degree of psychological control.

By the middle of 1943 pre-selection boards for officers were introduced, and the need for vocational guidance of re-allocated men and of discharged men coming under the care of repatriation indicated an increased sphere for the influence of the psychology services. The increasing need for specialised medical advice became evident, and a visiting psychiatrist was appointed to examine men whose response to routine tests suggested mental abnormality. A psychiatrist and a psychologist were also attached to the officers' pre-selection board. Probably the greatest value in these measures lay in a more correct allocation of men and a more satisfactory elimination of the unsuitable or inadequate types on enlistment. In the R.A.A.F. special attention was given to certain aspects of pre-selection, particularly for aircrew, pilots, air gunners and air observers.

Two general hospitals, one in Queensland and one in New South Wales, were used almost entirely for psychiatric patients. All forms of specialised treatment and rehabilitation were carried out and psychiatric patients on discharge from the Services received special care and attention.

The wastage in the Services from mental disorders of all types was great; it is also great in the civilian community at any time. Comparative figures indicate, if anything, a lower incidence of schizophrenics in the Army for similar age groups. Independent analysis of several series of cases showed a number of constant features. In the vast majority there was no history of special combat stress; in fact less than 50 per cent. of cases came from combat zones. Precipitation of a psychosis could be blamed on combat stress in only a very small fraction.

While pre-enlistment conditions in whole or in part were responsible for by far the greater number of breakdowns, age had some selective influence, more in determining acute psychoses than in neurotic disturbances. The drawbacks of an unsatisfactory background are undoubted, and it is regrettably true that a number of mentally unfit were accepted for service during the period of very rapid expansion of the Services. Illness was found to be significant in some series of psychoneuroses, but wounds had little significance. Frustration appears to have been a factor, especially towards the end of the war among seasoned troops who doubted the value of the 'mopping up' campaigns in which they were engaged.

In military psychiatry Australia was at first unprepared, and the number of thoroughly trained experts was small. Prejudice had to be overcome before the value of consultants in this work, especially in forward areas, was properly appreciated. Towards the end of the war the psychiatric services became more adequate. The greatest need was probably the influence of experienced consultants, who could teach by example, circulating through the forward units in the forces, helping to solve problems and seeing at first hand the conditions under which the fighting troops existed.

The special constitution of medical boards for psychiatric cases, the admirable hospital services established and the care given to the mental side of rehabilitation all demonstrate the influence of psychiatric medicine on the medical services of all arms. Medical considerations also reflect upon the causes of mental disorders in the civilian community. Finally, war experience emphasised the growing significance of the mind-body relationship and the need for keen appreciation of the importance of mental health to individuals and to groups.

V. CLINICAL PROBLEMS, SURGICAL

(i) Wound Treatment and Forward Surgery

MIDDLE EAST

Here the conditions under which forward surgery was carried out varied according to whether the military situation was one of movement or not. The chief difference from the practice of the First World War was the attachment of surgical teams to field ambulances. In desert warfare the decision had to be made whether to pass wounded men over a long rough route to a casualty clearing station, or to risk holding up the movements of the main dressing station by keeping them there during the post-operative period.

In the Libyan campaign during rapid movement in advance or retreat, the wounded were removed by road, rail and sea and only exceptionally by air to intermediate units and to hospitals in Alexandria, Kantara and Palestine.

In the campaign in Greece surgery was carried out in field ambulances and one casualty clearing station; in the final retirement, in one hospital. In the Syrian campaign, after the first difficult evacuation of the wounded, they were transferred to hospitals in Palestine. Experience gained in these actions from the end of 1940 to the early part of 1942, led to the following methods of treatment adopted by the A.A.M.C., with only occasional future modifications:

The primary treatment consisted of toilet and excision of the wound. Sutures were only placed in wounds of the skull, thorax, abdomen or large superficial joints like the knee joint, and, after 36–48 hours, in amputation flaps. Sucking thoracic wounds and those of the face and jaw also required sutures. In dressing wounds the space was loosely filled with 'Vaseline' and covered with a few layers of gauze. This was particularly important when a plaster was applied. When this had been done the patient was retained for observation to ensure that the plaster was not constricting the limb and that there was no risk of reactionary bleeding. Instructions were also issued for treatment in the field of fractures of the upper and lower extremities, wounds of large joints, of the face, jaw, mouth, chest and of burns.

The functions of the forward surgeon were limited by considerations of movement and nursing. The establishment of special sections in hospitals—a facio-maxillary unit, an orthopaedic unit and for wounds of the head and chest, emphasised the goal of rapid and complete restoration of structure and function.

Closed plasters gave good results on the whole. Observation in base areas recorded certain drawbacks. In a hot climate the presence of an offensive discharge seeping through the plaster was not uncommon, although this with a coincident rise in temperature and pulse rate did not necessarily mean a serious infection. Prolonged immobilisation in plaster tended to retard healing by secondary intention, where skin loss was considerable. Extensive lacerated wounds sometimes showed a large surface of exposed muscle which closed in and left a small final wound to heal. Others denuded of much skin left unstable scars.

Excision of wounds by surgical teams attached to the main dressing stations of field ambulances was nearly always adequate. When the progress of patients in base hospitals was followed up, an increasing number of young surgeons learned the correct techniques from their seniors.

Sulphonamides were given by mouth to all wounded admitted to a forward operating theatre. The usual dosage was two grammes, followed by one gramme every four hours up to a total of 35 grammes. Close watch was kept of the excretion of urine for any urogenital symptoms. Sulphonamide powder was also applied locally to the wound.

Infections of wounds. In the Syrian campaign only seven cases of gas gangrene occurred among 1,500 battle casualties. Later on more cases occurred in New Guinea. The virulence of anaerobic bacteria appeared low in the Middle East, but haemolytic streptococci were prevalent, especially in 'desert sores'.

Tetanus was practically banished from war surgery by immunisation carried out during recruit training. Regular 'refresher' injections of toxoid were given yearly to all Servicemen and women. One soldier, who had had only one inoculation died from tetanus, and in the concluding stages of the war an occasional instance of localised tetanus was seen following a wound. In 1940 wounded immunised men were given 3,000 units of antitetanus serum. Later 1 c.c. of tetanus toxoid as soon after wounding as possible was given instead.

PACIFIC CAMPAIGN

The Pacific Islands presented great difficulties of terrain and transport, of climate and endemic diseases. While the importance of maintaining the surgical principles already laid down was emphasised, certain aspects acquired additional significance, and the value of adequate early surgical measures was even more apparent. Technical instruction drew attention once more to the important principles of surgery in forward areas—in particular that wounds should be laid widely open and extensively excised with maximal incision and excision of the unhealthy fascia, that the excision of the wounds should be cone-shaped with the base of the cone at the wound of entry and also that of exit if one was present, that all wounds should be left widely open and no sutures should be used. The long interval of time, sometimes up to two days, that on occasion elapsed before wounds received surgical treatment gave additional force to these instructions.

Streptococcal infection had been important in the Middle East, but in the Pacific Islands, staphylococcal infection was more common and troublesome. The type found was *Staphylococcus aureus* coagulose-positive. Salmonella infections occurred; one, *S. enteritidis* was sometimes associated with metastatic suppuration. Anaerobic infections in wounds in the Islands were also found to differ from those found in the Middle East. The chief types were *C. welchii, oedematiens* and *septique* in a ratio of about 3 : 4 : 5. A few rapidly fatal infections were due to *oedematiens*.

The advisable limit of time between the wounding of a soldier and his submission to surgical treatment was previously placed at eighteen hours. This time interval gradually lengthened, and after the first campaigns in New Guinea it was proved that wounds could be excised as late as seventy-two hours after infliction. This delay was not only safely possible, but often essential, owing to the prevailing conditions of terrain and transport.

The administration of sulphanilamide to wounded men was rigidly enforced.

In some of the later Island campaigns wounded could not be moved to settled areas within 72 hours. Extemporised surgical posts had to deal early with the wounded, and forward units had to hold them until their rearward movement was surgically safe. This applied especially to abdominal wounds and compound fractures of the long bones. Extremes of weather conditions, bitter cold and rain on the highlands, intense humid heat in the swampy coastal areas, brought additional hazards.

About 75 per cent. of wounds involved the upper and lower extremities; about half of these were complicated by compound fracture. There were two categories of wounds: those due to gunshot and a larger proportion caused by fragments of grenades, shells and mortars. Bullet wounds inflicted by the small ·273 calibre Japanese bullet seldom did much harm unless they struck bone or damaged a large blood vessel. Sword wounds were usually in the head or shoulder and often of tangential nature. Malaria was not well tolerated by the badly wounded under the unfavourable climatic conditions. Intravenous quinine was given to all seriously wounded men and, in some of the heavily endemic areas, to all with abdominal wounds.

When ascendency in the air and on the sea had been achieved surgical teams and staffs in forward areas worked under favourable conditions and the wounded were evacuated promptly by sea and air.

(ii) Chemotherapy

The history of the war years shows how the older concept of antiseptics continued to influence the local use of sulphonamides for some time, but as the risks and drawbacks became more evident this method was used with greater reserve.

The initial dosage of sulphanilamide, 0·5 gramme given two hours after treatment of a wound and repeated four-hourly for four days, was altered to 5 tablets of 0·5 gramme given twice daily for four days or until the wound was considered to be controlled. Observations carried out on the blood concentration maintained by twelve-hourly dosage of sulpha-pyridine found that this was adequate. It was not so much a matter of dose interval as of the correct selection of patients and the use of sufficient dosage for a sufficient time. The local use of sulphanilamide was found of value when correctly applied. With the greater frequency of skin infection in the Pacific Islands more use was made of local sulphonamide application with the natural consequences of increased local irritation and more frequent sensitisation. This led to the issue of a warning pointing out the danger of producing severe general reaction by the administration of a sulphonamide to a previously sensitised patient and advising that the demonstration of haemolytic streptococci in septic sores was the only correct indication for such therapy.

In 1944, when the manufacture of sulphamerazine began in Australia, it practically replaced the other forms of sulphonamide. The rapid absorption and slow rate of excretion of this drug assured high blood levels with reasonable doses, and its administration was therefore only necessary twice a day. Two dosage rates were suggested, one high, having 8 grammes as an initial dose, the other medium, of 6 grammes. The doses used thereafter were respectively 4 and 3 grammes twice daily for a day, 4 and 2 grammes twice daily for two days, 2 and 1 grammes daily for one day and thereafter a maintenance dose of 2 grammes or 1 gramme if required.

Some of the acridine antiseptics, such as 'Monacrin', proved of undoubted value. A mixture of 'Monacrin' one part to forty parts of sulphanilamide was found very satisfactory by some surgeons as a preparatory application to facio-maxillary wounds before plastic procedures. 'Monacrin' was also found valuable in sepsis of long bones.

Penicillin became available for trial in Australia early in 1944, and its production in Melbourne was successfully undertaken. Early clinical trials were carried out by an investigating team in an Australian base hospital. To begin with, owing to limited supplies, the use of penicillin was restricted to the treatment in general hospitals of certain specified maladies, such as staphylococcal septicaemia or pyaemia, resistant streptococcal septicaemia, septic fracture or joint injuries. Early in 1944, however, trials in the forward area demonstrated the further immense prophylactic value of penicillin in allowing primary suture to be undertaken in wounds after excision and treatment with the powder. Its use was rapidly extended to all cases of infection by organisms sensitive to penicillin, with the assurance that control would be established and that many procedures hitherto extremely hazardous could be safely undertaken. Continuance of parenteral administration where evacuation by air was available made possible the earlier transport of casualties to the base area and thus helped to relieve congestion in the field units or forward areas.

Although sanction was given to early wound closure, this was only undertaken if conditions were suitable, and emphasis was laid on the even more meticulous application of surgical principles and practice.

(iii) Surgery of War Wounds

BURNS

Treatment procedures followed closely those adopted by the Royal Air Force. For burns of the face and fingers the *tulle gras* method; in forward areas tannic jelly, gentian violet or 'Vaseline' gauze was used. The treatment for shock was absolute rest, with raising of the foot of the bed, sufficient warmth, free administration of morphine, hot fluids by mouth or rectum, oxygen and intravenous serum or plasma. Adequate and gentle cleansing of the affected areas under anaesthesia was done in all fixed units receiving patients at a stage sufficiently early for this to be done.

At large base hospitals saline baths and skin grafting were possible. Local applications of sulphonamide powder on a wide area could only be made guardedly, but routine dusting with sulphonamide was done.

WOUNDS OF THE UPPER EXTREMITY

The results in general were satisfactory if the recommended treatment could be carried out completely. The greatest difficulty lay in immobilisation of the limb during transit, especially when the humerus was fractured. Australian experience did not find the 'U' plaster serviceable or comfortable for all fractures of the humerus, although it was satisfactory for fractures of the distal half. The 'hanging cast' gave neither sufficient control nor support. Better fixation was obtained by a long plaster stretching from the iliac crest to the padded axilla and running down the inner part of the arm. Another slab fitted to the posterior and outer aspects of the arm and casings on the lower arm with a window, gave good immobilisation. A bridge of plaster from the shoulder to the forearm, reinforced by Cramer wire, was a valuable device.

Less difficulty was experienced in the forward areas in controlling wounds of the lower part of the arm; excision with immediate application of plaster usually gave good results.

Wounds of the hands were of paramount importance and the incidence was high. It is significant that 10 per cent. of the patients admitted to the Australian Facio-maxillary and Plastic Surgery Unit in the Middle East required plastic treatment for wounds of this nature. In another such unit alone in the last four and a half years of the war 281 men required treatment for injuries of the hands; more than half of these were severe, and nearly a quarter of them were due to burns. In order that the reconstructive surgeon may have the fullest scope to effect the maximum degree of repair, adequate primary treatment is of the utmost importance. This in turn must obviously be based on an essential knowledge of the functional anatomy of the hand. Early technical instructions stressed the importance of avoiding limitation of function and laid down that only devitalised tissue should be removed by débridement or excision, which should be as conservative as possible. The delays that on occasion occurred between the wounded man's first treatment and his eventual arrival at a fully equipped plastic unit had a prejudicial effect on satisfactory rehabilitation, as they did not encourage the patient to maintain either the position of function of the damaged hand, or movement of all the joints of the hand not immobilised for purposes of treatment.

WOUNDS OF THE LOWER EXTREMITY

Compound fractures of the femur, especially the upper part, were serious and were often complicated by wounds of the buttock, pelvis and abdominal contents. Effective immobilisation was best secured by a Thomas splint alone or with plaster. Comfortable transport was obtained by the use of combined methods, such as a split plaster over strapping extension and a posterior slab, with a bent Thomas splint, the whole secured by a final complete plaster from groin to toe. A clove-hitch could be dangerous. A clip or pin on or through the boot was safer, but no such methods of fixation were permitted until the patient reached a main dressing station.

A surgical lesson of the first two years of war was that in the treatment of wounds of the lower extremity the requisites were adequate resuscitation, adequate excision and rigid immobilisation.

During the Island campaigns transport difficulties often necessitated the holding of wounded men in the forward units for lengthy periods. The plaster spica was found to be unsuitable in humid climates owing to atmospheric moisture and sweating, which hindered drying and led to formation of ridges in the case from lifting or moving the patient. Furthermore, when there was so much dependence on carriers, weight became an important consideration. One native porter could carry seven Thomas splints, but only enough plaster for two spicas. Almost complete reliance was therefore placed on the use of the Thomas splint with strapping extension. Unless the site of the fracture was too high for control, these permitted the satisfactory transport of patients not only by air, when this means was available, but also by native bearers on very many occasions.

By 1943 the standardised treatment was excision of the wound, drainage, the use of sulphanilamide with light packing of 'Vaseline' gauze and immobilisation in plaster. This method was, however, restricted to two conditions—where difficulties of transport existed and where a wound of the thigh was recent and sepsis of bone had not occurred.

The introduction of penicillin greatly decreased the morbidity and mortality of serious injuries to the thigh, and chronic bone wounds were largely eliminated.

Towards the end of the war the more favourable conditions that prevailed in transport and the control of infection hastened the use of internal fixation. The introduction of vitallium was an important adjunct to this method. During the Borneo fighting 40 wounds involving long bones were treated by fixation at a forward base, the operation being carried out at the time of delayed treatment, three to seven days after wounding.

ORTHOPAEDIC SURGERY

Disabilities of the feet

The importance of careful examination of the feet on enlistment was not sufficiently realised at first. Men were accepted with foot disabilities, some requiring long periods of hospital treatment or even return to Australia. Foot clinics in Palestine in 1941 helped, by diagnosis and treatment of lesser degree disabilities, to enable men to do ordinary military duties. Proper selection and fitting of the army boots were instituted under a corporal chiropodist in each major unit, who also instructed in foot exercises. Schools of chiropodists were instituted.

Internal derangement of the knee joint

This injury appeared to be more common than in civil life. The main difficulty lay in the after-treatment, and it was found preferable to retain these patients in a hospital area where they could be kept under observation and given graded exercise until they could be discharged to a depot battalion, usually after an average of forty-two days.

Orthopaedic experience

Although orthopaedic hospitals were good, when great distances and difficulties in transport are encountered it is more satisfactory to have as part of the surgical division of a general hospital, an orthopaedic department staffed by orthopaedic specialists, trained physiotherapists and occupational therapists. Both were tried in the Australian Army, and under the conditions of the Pacific War the latter method was probably preferable.

AMPUTATIONS

The total number of Servicemen requiring amputation of a limb was 682 out of 39,803 Australian wounded, as compared with 3,241 amputations in the First World War. Limb fitting by the latest modern techniques was instituted.

Amputations in Japanese prison camp hospitals were mainly for severe 'tropical' ulcers of the legs. The most favourable site was found to be mid-thigh. The ultimate mortality was high on account of severe debility, malnutrition and intercurrent disease.

HEAD INJURIES

Only general conservative measures were carried out at the forward operating centres in the field, the specialised treatment being done by the cerebral surgeon at a base hospital. The advanced surgical team was therefore advised to confine itself to the cleaning of scalp wounds and excision of dirty tissue, removal of obvious depressed bone, excision and cleaning of edges, gentle irrigation of pulped brain and suture of the scalp.

Neurosurgical centres were established in certain general hospitals in the Middle East, and neurosurgical work was carried out by specialist surgeons in all the military base hospitals in Australia. No neurosurgical team was organised during the New Guinea or other Island campaigns. There was no central organisation for neurosurgical work carried out in these campaigns or in the Middle East. It was found that delay for several days was not disadvantageous, but that good results in head injuries depended on the thoroughness of the first surgical procedure, especially on the removal of bony fragments and débris. The presence of focal lesions did not necessarily indicate a bad prognosis. Infection at all depths of the wound was relatively common, and the proportion of abscess formation and discharging sinuses was high. The latter were almost always associated with in-driven bone fragments, which were often sprayed like a jet into the cerebral substance. If these were removed infection usually subsided, and the metallic foreign body which might lie at a considerable distance could be left undisturbed. Sulphonamides, and later penicillin, decreased mortality in infected head wounds.

INJURIES OF PERIPHERAL NERVES

It was an early instruction that divided nerves were not to be sutured. Patients were returned to Australia to ensure continued observation and treatment and to obviate the risk of sepsis.

In the closing phase of the war, with improved control of sepsis by chemotherapy, all important nerves near the wound were explored in the forward hospitals. A divided nerve was sutured two or three weeks after the wound had healed. Sequelae were paralysis of muscles or loss of sensation. Residual pain (causalgia) was noted in battle casualties, sometimes disappearing after five weeks, sometimes lasting two years.

WOUNDS OF THE CHEST

These wounds were treated conservatively unless (1) air was being sucked into the pleural cavity; (2) a tension pneumothorax existed; or (3) there was a pleural effusion. Suture was considered the best and only reliable method of closing a sucking wound, especially when a long and difficult journey had to be faced. Where simple silkworm gut sutures would not close the opening, a flap was made under local anaesthesia. The pleural cavity was kept dry.

Few chests became infected in the Middle East. Sulphonamides were given by mouth.

The removal of foreign bodies from the chest should only be done in a well equipped base hospital.

There was more risk of staphylococcal infection in New Guinea than in the Middle East. Such infection almost invariably led to clotting of the blood in traumatic pneumothorax; this was treated by early aspiration with or without air replacement. Penicillin in the pleural cavity lessened the risk of pleural infection and was a standard practice.

The transport of patients from the forward areas presented difficulties in maintaining the half-sitting posture. A wooden framework backrest covered with a blanket and attached to a Stokes litter proved very satisfactory.

In the field hospital patients were instructed in the Brompton Hospital type of breathing exercises by physiotherapists.

WOUNDS OF THE ABDOMEN

Recovery from these wounds in the Middle East and New Guinea was 50 per cent. as a rule; in one small series it rose above 70 per cent. in the Middle East. Facility of transport, terrain of the combat area, tactical situation and climate affected the results. Examination of one series showed that men who recovered and were ultimately sent on to the base averaged nine hours from their first-aid treatment in an aid post, whereas those whose transit had averaged thirteen hours died.

Ten hours appeared to be the critical period; after this the results deteriorated. The general condition of the patients was an important and determining influence in all abdominal work. Severe shock meant delay and resuscitation to a point where operation was practicable; this in turn depended on the severity of the wound.

Resuscitation and blood transfusion were important.

In New Guinea the adverse factors were the delays before patients reached an operating unit due to the nature of the country, the lowering of the patients' resistance by malaria, the limited supplies of blood and the short supply of sulphadiazine.

The recovery rate can be improved if patients are promptly received, operating facilities are good, bed accommodation is given for an adequate period after treatment and there is smooth transport to a base hospital. The need for keeping patients for at least a week after operation caused deep concern in some areas. Where an operating unit was semi-stationary arrangements for holding patients during the anxious first post-operation days could be made without embarrassment, but one critically injured man could hold up a unit. In the desert campaign the loose union of two field ambulances solved this problem temporarily, as parts of the unit could adopt a 'leap-frog' manoeuvre. The position was different in jungle warfare; there transport by land was equally difficult for different reasons, but high mobility of units was not required, nor indeed was it usually possible.

PLASTIC AND FACIO-MAXILLARY SURGERY

Great assistance and valuable advice was received from authorities in England, where also selected Australian surgeons received the requisite training. A special facio-maxillary and plastic unit was formed in the Middle East and incorporated with the surgical division of an Australian general hospital. Later, more units were formed in Australia. There was personal contact of general and dental surgeons with these units.

Psychologically the beneficial effects of skilled plastic surgery were inestimable in men whose future mental and physical approach to life depended on the degree of successful repair. Men with extensive scarred areas from previous lesions should not be enlisted for service. This proviso particularly applies to vulnerable areas of the legs, axillae, hands and neck.

ANAESTHETICS

Of necessity there were considerable variations in the administration of anaesthetics under Service conditions. In the forward areas dental officers and medical orderlies in times of stress had to give anaesthetics and did so both skilfully and efficiently.

Often equipment was either lacking or in short supply, and improvisations had to be made. Later apparatus and agents were available in fixed units, and more mobile units were well equipped for anaesthesia. Special analgesics were used. 'Pentothal Sodium' was mainly reserved for use in forward areas. It was invaluable for battle casualties.

Manual of Army Anaesthesia. This was issued in 1942 to all medical units, and described the various forms of apparatus and their maintenance.

Inhalation anaesthesia continued to be the standby where ether of good quality was available. Chloroform was of value particularly at night with naked lights in a theatre and in Japanese prisoner-of-war camps. Nitrous oxide and oxygen anaesthesia were unsuitable under field conditions and were little used, even in base units.

(iv) Blood Transfusion

In Australia the greatest advance during the period that elapsed between the two world wars was the establishment of blood transfusion services throughout the country, particularly by the Australian Red Cross Society. Pioneer work on blood storage was undertaken and blood banks were established. Conditions affecting the best methods of prolonging the life of the blood corpuscles and the most suitable maintenance temperature were subjects of special investigation.

At the beginning of the war a blood transfusion section was formed for the Australian Army. Apparatus designed by A.A.M.C. officers was adopted as standard use and with slight modifications was used thoughout the war. This equipment fulfilled the following purposes:

1. Collection and immediate transfusion of a volume of citrated blood.

2. Enabled blood collected aseptically to be stored at a suitable temperature for ten days or more and minimised risk from infection and haemolysis.

3. Provided storage of physiological solutions, particularly glucose-saline, which could be produced in bulk by commercial firms, or, if needed, under Service conditions, and could withstand prolonged keeping, rough handling and tropical conditions.

4. Permitted storage of serum collected aseptically.

5. Provided means of administration of intravenous injections of such drugs as antibiotics, analeptics, anti-infective agents or anaesthetics.

6. Provided special surgical technique of suction or irrigation, e.g., for thorax, alimentary tract or the bladder.

The 'Soluvac' in the Australian set was a mass-produced infusion set, a modification of the original gravity-feed infusion sets. It had a large one litre container.

BLOOD GROUPING

The mass grouping of the blood types of all troops in the Australian Forces was undertaken as a routine on enlistment. Each soldier's blood grouping was recorded in his pay book (later 'record of service' book) and stamped on his identity disc. The accuracy of the grouping was of a very high order, and although cross-checking for compatibility was advised, no accidents due to incompatibility occurred. The notation adopted was a combination of the Moss and International— that is, AB1, A2, B3, O4.

PREPARATION OF SERUM

Preparation of serum both 'dry' and 'wet' was undertaken by the various transfusion services. Pooled serum was later to become the mainstay for infusion fluids replacing blood. A valuable asset of liquid serum was its ability to be kept successfully at ordinary temperatures. In the earlier campaigns the preference for 'wet' serum was fairly general.

BLOOD TRANSFUSIONS IN THE FIELD

Although blood banks were established in field hospitals, the policy in the Australian Forces was to favour a decentralised method relying on a high standard of efficiency in all field medical units. Small blood stores were used, but blood was also obtained from walking wounded. This decentralisation had the dual advantage of disseminating knowledge of techniques throughout the medical services and lessening the difficulties of transport.

Seven per cent. of the casualties in the Libyan Campaign of 1941 needed transfusions. A transfusion team was formed and worked in the field ambulance main dressing station. Blood was collected either from walking wounded or from members of the ambulance staff. Groupings were accepted from pay books or identity discs without cross-typing.

In Syria two serious problems arose, namely (1) the risk of infection and (2) the transmission of malaria. In (1) haemolysis took place in a batch of stored blood kept from four to eight days, due to infection by coliform organisms and streptococci. Three fatal cases occurred. A committee of experts made recommendations for the complete preparation of stored blood with rigid technique to ensure asepsis. These were promulgated in detailed instructions by all Services.

As regards (2) the problem of transmission of malaria, the use of stored blood was first thought to be the answer. This was not always possible, and for a time at least, owing to the unfortunate happenings already mentioned, it was not regarded with whole-hearted enthusiasm. When blood was taken from donors, if time permitted the donor exposed to the risk of malaria was given 10 grains of quinine or 0·2 gramme of atebrin six to twelve hours before blood was collected. The recipient was given 0·2 gramme of atebrin at once or 10 grains of quinine by mouth or intravenous drip. If the donor was found to have malaria a standard course was given to the recipient. In all instances a follow-up course of 10 grains of quinine or 0·3 gramme of atebrin in divided doses twice a week was given for two weeks.

In 1942, during the battle of El Alamein, blood requirements were largely met by the British Blood Transfusion Service. Blood was also stored in refrigerators in the main dressing stations of the Australian field ambulances, where a stock was built up by the resuscitation team during the twenty-four hours preceding an attack. Blood, serum and plasma were all available during this action. A noticeable feature of the transfusions at this time was the frequency of reactions. These were largely controlled by intensive care in cleaning the apparatus and continual testing. Not all patients could stand a rapid rate of transfusion well, and reactions were more commonly found after transfusions given in the middle of the day. Jaundice occurred in some patients, especially if a large volume of blood was given and more particularly if the blood was some days old.

In the Japanese prison camps blood transfusion was often only possible by ingeniously devised extemporary measures to ensure asepsis. The technique of using defibrinated blood was used at times; on other occasions when citrate was available numbers of transfusions of citrated blood were given.

In the Pacific Islands campaigns blood was sent by air from Sydney to Port Moresby in New Guinea in specially designed cork-lined ice boxes. Blood from universal donors was collected into the standard 'Soluvac' flask using saline citrate anti-coagulant. In the latter months of the war in Borneo, the supply of blood and serum for the forward area was ensured and maintained by a blood transfusion unit attached to a general hospital on Morotai. Transport of blood in the Islands was by air. After arriving at the airfields its distribution to its final destination was often by jeep over rough roads or by native carriers. Blood would last up to a week under proper conditions of transport and refrigeration. Serum was of more practical value than blood for immediate use for battle casualties. The use of transfusion in amphibious landings was illustrated in New Guinea and again in Borneo, when initially two standard transfusion panniers were included in the equipment of surgical teams and packed in loads weighing 40 lbs—a suitable weight for native carriers. Each package contained all essentials. Serum infusions were used, and as no stored blood was available, donors were obtained from troops near the main dressing station. In later phases of the campaign surgical teams worked under much more settled conditions with refrigeration and a small resuscitation ward. Stored blood was available but was never kept for more than twenty-four hours.

MALARIA AND BLOOD TRANSFUSIONS

The problems of fighting in a malarious country experienced in Syria became intensified in New Guinea, where the weekly malaria rate reached almost astronomical figures at times and even in 1945 was 22 per thousand per week. There were obvious advantages in using blood collected in non-malarious areas from donors who had never incurred the risks of infection; advantages too in the use of serum with its almost unlimited 'life' under even poor storage conditions, but local conditions could not be expected to permit the invariable use of either. At the Medical Research Unit in Cairns careful experiments had clearly demonstrated that, even when known malarious blood was used, no symptoms occurred provided that a standard course of anti-malaria treatment was administered to the recipient. Indeed the situation often arose when the blood of the patient was more potentially malarious than that of the donor. Accordingly the routine was established of giving the following anti-malaria course to each patient after transfusion: 1st, 2nd and 3rd days 40 grains of quinine daily, 4th and 5th days 0·6 gramme of atebrin daily, 6th to 9th days 0·4 gramme of atebrin daily, and 10th to 12th days 0·2 gramme of atebrin and 0·02 gramme of plasmoquine daily.

SERUM AND PLASMA

In Australia serum alone was used for transfusion, largely because its preparation was easier, the therapeutic results were good, serum was more stable in the liquid form, and it had lighter weight and less bulk than blood. Not one instance of contamination was reported throughout the war. 'Merthiolate' was added in a concentration of 1 in 10,000 to increase the serum's resistance to infection, without any toxic effect.

VI. MEDICAL SERVICES OF THE ROYAL AUSTRALIAN NAVY

PRE-WAR PERIOD

In the Australian Navy the medical services were modelled originally on those in the Royal Navy, from which doctors and sick-berth attendants were drawn until the permanent medical services were established in 1917. From 1928 onwards certain modifications suitable to Australian conditions were instituted. Opportunities for specialising and attending post-graduate courses were given to naval doctors. Technical instructions were issued. The dental services were expanded. A naval doctor was appointed to each destroyer and medical officers were changed when and where possible. This was found to develop efficiency and increase the attractiveness of service.

In 1935 sick-berth staff were trained and provided a valuable nucleus for expansion in war-time. The importance of capable and competent sick-berth staff, especially on small ships which do not carry a doctor, cannot be over-emphasised. To obtain these the provision of incentives in the form of specialised training with additional privileges and opportunities for promotion was of considerable value. In 1945 the highest rank held in the sick-berth branch was that of wardmaster lieutenant, and with greater responsibilities the various war establishments were further increased, carrying also a larger proportion of senior grades.

Initially there were few female nurses, partly owing to the fact that the Navy made use of civilian and military hospitals and partly because the sick-berth staff on board ship must be male. In contradistinction to the army or air force medical orderly, the naval sick-berth rating was in every sense of the word, a nurse. The medical needs of the Navy in time of peace could be met almost entirely by a male staff, but with the general war-time expansion and the development of shore-based hospitals administered by the Navy, the need for female nurses became paramount, and the Women's Royal Australian Naval Nursing Service was formed in 1942 when a number of trained nurses was recruited. Also some members of the W.R.A.N.S. received sick-berth training, thus allowing additional male personnel to be released for sea-going duties.

RECRUIT EXAMINATION

All men entering the Navy were volunteers, selected for particular branches. Common causes of rejection were sub-standard development, deformities and visual, dental and speech defects. The naval physical standards for men and women were higher than those of the Army as recruits who broke down were more serious liabilities and difficult of disposal.

MEDICAL SUPPLIES

Medical stores and equipment will always constitute a problem in sea-going units. During the course of the war medical supplies were frequently revised in view of the demand for new products and to meet the rapidly expanding requirements, especially those of warfare in the Tropics. The R.A.N. supplied Allied Navies in the Pacific area and the Australian Station, so the needs of the Royal Navy, the United States Navy, the Royal Netherlands Navy and the Free French Forces had also to be met. The Medical Equipment Control Committee, on which each Service had its representatives, obtained and distributed medical supplies.

For the action first-aid bag the addition of cotton wool and lint cut into 4 in. squares and packed in a bundle, and of more triangular bandages and splints, were found desirable. Acriflavine was useful and replaced picric lint and boric lotion for burns. The introduction of the simple 'Soluvac' outfit provided an ample supply of blood serum, which was carried by all ships and establishments. Dried plasma was supplied in the later years of the war from both American and Australian sources. Generally wet serum was the standby. The tubunic ampoule or syrette of morphia was in short supply and not extensively used. It had its faults, but, if these can be corrected, this form of administering morphia may well be the future choice, and stocks should be maintained. In the later years of the war supply ships accompanied the fleet. They had refrigeration space. Drugs, dressings, etc., were packed in units calcu-lated to supply so many men for periods of fixed days.

CONDITIONS OF SERVICE

With the increase in the number of ships and in ships' complements, additional technical staff and new equipment, maintenance of satis-factory hygiene and ventilation became difficult and refrigeration, washing and sleeping facilities inadequate. The Navy was also subjected to frequent and violent changes in climate with little opportunity of becoming conditioned to them. Although sometimes cold weather in winter in the Mediterranean was intense, greater discomfort due to heat and fatigue was suffered in the Tropics, leading to physical deteriora-tion, with salt deficiency and heat exhaustion. For ships' crews serving in the Tropics additional salt had to be provided in the diet. Here also the incidence of communicable diseases and skin affections increased. The general health improved with a diet sufficient in vitamin B and vitamin C, adequate refrigeration, facilities for washing and laundry purposes and unlimited supplies of water.

EXPERIENCE IN ACTION

The space for sick bays was inadequate as compared with that in the United States Navy. Air-conditioning ventilation is essential, as well as proper isolation for infectious cases.

Medical arrangements for action were governed by two main principles:

(1) Distribution of personnel and stores should be on as wide a base as possible with each action station self-contained.

(2) During an action only first-aid and life-saving procedures should be carried out.

Each dressing station should have: (a) an independent lighting system, (b) its own supply of fresh water, (c) its own means of sterilisation, and (d) its own transfusion apparatus, splints, instruments and dressings. The Hedley stretcher and the Stokes litter were found satisfactory. Stretchers should be of exchangeable pattern. Sick-bay accommodation was generally inadequate. It was important for as many naval ratings as possible to be instructed in first aid in order to give emergency treatment and preferable to decentralise medical personnel and supplies. Sub-divided equipment should include adequate supplies of morphine, stretchers, splints, secondary lighting and a portable torch with head adjustment. Individual canvas bags for the sick-berth personnel should contain morphine solution, hypodermic syringe, gauze pads, bandages, cotton wool, triple dye, acriflavine, tourniquets and a pair of scissors. Adequate quantities of plasma and wet serum should be available.

SALT DEFICIENCY AND HEAT EXHAUSTION

These conditions became serious problems in ships operating in tropical waters.

The clinical states of salt deficiency were as follows: heat exhaustion proper, or heat shock; heat exhaustion with abdominal pain; heat cramps, either acute and severe or chronic and mild; with gastric symptoms; dyspeptic, vomiting or emetic type; alimentary symptoms; apyrexial diarrhoeic type; vomiting—diarrhoea—pyrexial type; low-grade pyrexia. Heat exhaustion was due to extremely high heat and humidity resulting in inadequate heat loss by evaporation. The symptoms were shock with diminished sodium chloride excretion in the urine. The safeguard of prophylactic salt administration against the occurrence of heat exhaustion was often not given sufficient prominence. Stokers were often affected. The patient might faint or collapse on duty because of salt deficiency. With a routine daily ration of additional salt, prognosis was good and recovery the rule. In the treatment of severe cases the environment had to be cool, and the sodium chloride deficiency corrected by intravenous infusion of an isotonic (0·9 gramme per cent.) solution of sodium chloride. In heat exhaustion with abdominal pain the patients were put to bed in Fowler's position, given continuous intravenous drip of normal saline (1–2 litres), and later given salted fluids by mouth when the diagnosis was confirmed. In incipient heat-stroke the onset may be sudden. A quick reduction of temperature and saline fluid by mouth are necessary. Heat-stroke proper did not occur in the Royal Australian Navy. It was with the purpose of avoiding this dangerous condition that almost exaggerated care was taken in the diagnosis, treatment and prevention of salt deficiency cases.

The remaining types responded well to general measures with or without intravenous infusion of normal saline and prophylactic salt, two grammes daily.

TREATMENT OF CASUALTIES

Intravenous anaesthesia when practicable was useful. The greatest proportion of casualties consisted of burns and shock; the number of wounds was comparatively small. For this reason blood products and substitutes, particularly plasma and serum, were more in demand than whole blood. While both wet serum and dried plasma were used for blood transfusions, the preference was rather for the former on account of less weight and space that was required. Many sick-berth attendants became extremely proficient in administering transfusions.

One very real problem in the Pacific theatre was to ensure that sufficient stocks of plasma were carried to meet repeated emergencies. This was all the more essential when action took place a long distance from a base or supply depot.

BURNS

By March 1945 standard treatment comprised immediate injection of ½ grain of morphine, repeated as required and replacement of fluid loss by intravenous plasma. Dead tissue was then cleared away, the area dusted with sulphanilamide powder and sterile vaseline applied with a fairly firm bandage. All serious surgical wounds had penicillin. An air-cooling unit in the sick bay was beneficial. First-aid treatment of phosphorus burns required prolonged immersion in an alkaline solution until all traces of phosphorus had disappeared. Protective gear and anti-flash clothing were valuable, but lost protective power if washed. The gear should consist of an overall with a hood or cowl which could be quickly drawn over the head. It should have strong fastenings, for preference zips, with a broad waist belt capable of carrying small items of equipment.

VII. MEDICAL SERVICES OF THE ROYAL AUSTRALIAN AIR FORCE

EXPANSION AND ORGANISATION

At the beginning of this narrative it has been shown how in pre-war years the Medical Services of both the Royal Australian Navy and the Royal Australian Air Force, on account of complex and technical considerations, were strongly opposed to the view that one medical corps should provide the medical services for all three Fighting Services. It was also noted that early in 1940 the Australian War Cabinet agreed that the D.G.M.S. of the Army should relinquish control over the R.A.A.F. Medical Service and that all medical matters of co-ordination should be considered by a standing committee of the three Directors of the Medical Services.

The inauguration of the Empire Air Training Scheme made it imperative to reorganise the Medical Directorate to cope with the rapid expansion that was to take place. The value of previous liaison with the Royal Air Force was apparent and influenced the reorganisation, which followed closely the policy and machinery adopted by the R.A.F. When in due course the Empire Air Training Scheme reached fruition and a continuous stream of Australian personnel was flowing to the United Kingdom or Canada, the advantage of similar systems in administrative matters resulted in much saving of labour and in greater efficiency.

Initially the recruiting of medical officers was hampered by the uncertainty as to the part that the R.A.A.F. would play in overseas campaigns; and the more definite prospects offered by service in the Army, which was also calling up large numbers of doctors, including specialists from the Army Medical Corps Reserve, made it increasingly difficult for the Air Force to obtain an adequate supply. When the rôle of the R.A.A.F. was determined at the Ottawa Conference on the Empire Air Training Scheme, it was realised that the R.A.A.F. would require large hospital units in Australia and, with the formation of R.A.A.F. squadrons overseas as well as locally, that medical officers would be necessary in increasing numbers for service abroad. This stimulated the recruitment of medical officers. At first they were attached to a recruiting centre for training. Then a section was formed for intensive training of medical officers and nursing orderlies. In 1943 a separate unit for medical training was established and specialist courses in a number of subjects were arranged.

At the outbreak of war all nursing in the R.A.A.F. was carried out by males who were given general and special training before being posted to units for duty in medical sections and sick quarters. The number of suitable men available was inadequate to meet the expanding requirements and, even with the formation of the R.A.A.F. Nursing Service, whose members took over the responsibility of the nursing in all the larger medical units, some additional means of supply had to be provided. In February 1942 it was therefore decided to enlist sick-quarter attendants and nursing orderlies in the W.A.A.F. This made it possible to employ male medical orderlies in posts more compatible with their previous experience and training and to use them in the field medical units and the small isolated units. Owing to the shortage of laboratory and X-ray technicians courses of training were arranged for specially selected personnel.

Medical equipment and supplies were reorganised at the end of 1940, to meet the increasing demands consequent on the growth of the Empire Air Training Scheme and the formation of many new units.

The reorganisation included the development of stores depots and preparation of specific tables of equipment for every type of unit. These establishment tables formed the basis for unit provisioning and supply throughout the war. The Medical Equipment Control Committee co-ordinated the demands of the Services, as already described.

R.A.A.F. MEDICAL UNITS

Initially, the medical services were restricted to small sick quarters at each of the main R.A.A.F. permanent stations. With the development of the Empire Air Training Scheme many more training stations were set up in Australia and full use was made of civilian hospitals. Temporary base hospitals were formed near each capital city. When Army base hospitals were constructed in Sidney and Melbourne the R.A.A.F. transferred the base hospitals to them. There they functioned as independent units separately administered. Also 200-bed R.A.A.F. hospitals with adequate technical facilities were developed at three of the large centres. Later, separate wards or parts of wards were set aside in army hospitals in the capital cities for the Navy and Air Force. There was, however, insufficient accommodation for air force patients in army hospitals so that the existing hospitals had to be maintained throughout the war. Additional hospitals had to be constructed in country centres, and some increased accommodation for air force patients was provided in the army base hospitals.

When Japan entered the war the R.A.A.F. was reorganised on a mobile basis for service on the mainland of Australia or overseas. For the medical care of units so employed medical receiving stations were formed. These were a type of field general hospital and served with the R.A.A.F. in that capacity both in the operational areas of Australia and in the Island campaigns. When the Wing became a basic tactical unit, it became necessary to provide an integrated medical service for it. This led to the formation of the medical clearing station, a unit that had a capacity of 40 beds but was capable of expanding to 100 beds if necessary, and combined many of the functions of the field ambulance and casualty clearing station. It was completely transportable by air and accompanied the Wing wherever it went. These arrangements in the field worked well and with the availability of transport provided an adequate medical service.

The great expansion of the R.A.A.F. brought with it a host of admini-strative problems, many of them medical in character, so that it became more and more essential to have medical representation on the head-quarters of areas, command training groups and operational groups. These formations administered their own units directly and continued to do so until late in 1944, after which a wing headquarters administered three squadrons, a repair and salvage unit and a medical clearing station, with a section of a malaria control unit when operating in malarious areas. The medical clearing station was self-contained. It included a prefabricated hut for use as an operating theatre, X-ray plant, incubator, refrigeration, medical supplies for three months and an allocation of motor transport. All the equipment was compact and designed for transport by air, requiring sixteen C-47 transport aircraft for this purpose.

Each Group was allotted a medical receiving station and a malaria control unit when operating in malarious areas. The medical receiving station was modelled on similar lines to the analogous R.A.F. field hospital unit. It had a capacity of from 100–200 beds. A physician, a surgeon and 8 nursing sisters were included on its staff. These stations admitted and treated all patients evacuated to them through the medical clearing stations. Normally they retained all who were expected to be fit for return to duty in the operational area within three months and evacuated to base hospitals the long-term cases or those which for various reasons warranted the transfer.

It was originally intended to establish rehabilitation units for each of the major formations. However, wide dispersal and geographical considerations made this plan uneconomical. Only three such units were formed and serviced the three biggest formations.

MEDICAL STANDARDS

With the inauguration of the Empire Air Training Scheme in 1940, when uniformity of medical standards for aircrews throughout the British Commonwealth became necessary, R.A.F. standards, with a few exceptions, were adopted by the R.A.A.F. This uniformity was maintained throughout the war. In the R.A.A.F. no modification of standards in visual acuity or heterophoria was approved, nor was the medical category of 'Colour Vision Defective Unsafe—Daylight Flying, Non-Operational' ever accepted. In 1943 the R.A.A.F. adopted the recommendation of the Medical Directorate that visual acuity of fighter pilots should be a minimum of 6/6 without glasses. Aircrew selection boards, including a medical officer, solved difficult problems in special cases.

In 1943 for 'Universal Service Personnel' called up compulsorily and allocated between the air force and army, a more basic minimum standard was accepted by the R.A.A.F., including a Visual III class, and certain more general standards were adopted for the two Services. The air force, however, continued to maintain higher physical standards, especially visual and auditory, in special technical musterings.

The employment at the outbreak of war of full-time medical staffs familiar with aircrew and ground staff examinations at recruit centres maintained a uniform medical standard for enlistment and promoted efficient selection.

Psychological consideration was given to the selection of those training as pilots, air observers and air gunners by the Flying Personnel Research Units.

A fuller appreciation of many medical problems affecting instructors and pupils during the period of flying training was gained when permission was given for a number of medical officers to take a course in flying. Cases of visual defects, air sickness and psychological defects diagnosed among trainees in Australia were appropriately treated. Air sickness and psychoneuroses were important causes for repatriation among personnel sent to Canada for further training, the figures being 15 and 28 per cent. of medical repatriation cases respectively.

DISTRIBUTION OF R.A.A.F.

The Empire Air Training Scheme led to the distribution of air force personnel in many countries. A number of Australian squadrons operated overseas under R.A.F. administration and command. R.A.A.F. medical liaison officers were attached to appropriate headquarters in England, Canada and India.

On the operational side the R.A.A.F. was represented in practically every theatre of war. With the later exception of the units serving in the S.W.P.A. the medical care of casualties was largely undertaken by the R.A.F. and army medical units.

In 1943 No. 10 Operational Group R.A.A.F. was formed. Here for the first time the R.A.A.F. had a complete medical organisation of its own in the field with a medical clearing station, medical stores component and malaria control unit with each wing. A medical receiving station was allotted to the group or to smaller formations acting independently or in isolated parts. Later the name of the Group was changed to First Tactical Air Force and as such took part in combined operations with the Australian military forces for the first time in the Borneo campaign.

Experience of the R.A.A.F. in the South West Pacific Area concerned *inter alia* certain special problems. For long overseas flights a collapsible rubber dinghy was installed in the pilot's seat. Prolonged sitting on this caused a macular eruption on the buttocks. A cushion devised by one of the medical officers obviated this trouble. The emergency rations supplied from Australia contained an excessive amount of dehydrated food which could not be eaten without a liberal supply of water. The American ration did not contain dehydrated food, and it was issued to Australian aircrews. The use of anti-glare spectacles was discouraged as it led to diminished visual acuity. The demand oxygen system was more satisfactory than the American one including the B.L.B. mask. Combined operations in the Borneo landings showed the need for a more complete autonomy of the medical services. Experience confirmed the view that an air force medical unit which included a surgical team capable of speedy establishment should accompany the early landing forces and be ashore within forty-eight hours to deal with air force casualties; medical units should land as entire units with independent tentage and water supply.

MEDICAL ASPECTS OF SURVIVAL

When an airman baled out or made a forced descent, especially in enemy territory, his chance of making a safe return depended to a great extent on his health and strength and pre-flight preparation. Long-sleeved shirts with sleeves rolled down and long trousers were compulsory. They afforded protection against malaria and burns. The standard R.A.A.F. flying helmet was not popular because of faulty design and heat. The tropical flying helmet which came into service towards the end of the war was much more satisfactory. Goggles gave considerable protection from burns and injury. The flying gauntlet glove was regarded as clumsy and too hot. Most aircrews preferred motor transport driver's gloves with part of the flare removed, or anti-mosquito gloves.

Earlier emergency kits were not satisfactory; the dehydrated and compressed rations were unappetising. It was felt that a more logical approach was by instructing aircrews on how they could live in the jungle. Later kits contained items that experience found were essential. The contents of the R8/70 aircrew survival kit devised in 1943-44 are shown in Appendix A. The most important rule for a jungle kit was that it should be worn securely attached to the body. Boots and gaiters were advisable. The American army boot was excellent for jungle wear. The R.A.A.F. issue boot with 'Kromhyd' sole was satisfactory but failed to stand up long to rough usage. Fleece-lined flying boots were unsatisfactory for jungle wear; they had also been unsatisfactory in the desert. Malaria, dysentery, dengue and scrub typhus were likely risks. Prophylactic drugs were included in the escape kit and instructions given as to their use, and in first aid to the aircrews. Most squadron medical officers regarded the aircraft first-aid satchel as unsatisfactory and requiring complete revision.

In the South West Pacific Area protection against cold was not a serious matter even when aircraft were ditched in the sea. Thirst was the important problem. The usual way of storing water on aircraft was by carrying sealed cans in the rubber dinghy. In addition filled water bottles were carried, and instructions were to salvage water from the aircraft in preference to food.

Sunburn increased dehydration. Aircrews were advised against undue exposure by removing clothing in the dinghy and to use any means available to cover their faces and hands.

EVACUATION OF CASUALTIES BY AIR

When war was declared in 1939 the air transport of casualties was an accepted principle; and although air ambulance units were formed and indeed functioned with considerable success, there were initially many difficulties to be overcome, and it was not until the later years that evacuation of casualties by air reached the peak of its employment and efficiency.

Among the disadvantages of specific air ambulance planes was their limited use. They were not economical between engagements, and their maintenance constituted a special problem. However, in spite of restrictions these air ambulance units rendered excellent service.

The fact that so many transport planes were returning to their bases from the forward areas completely empty after delivering their loads prompted the next stage in the development. Stretcher fittings were introduced as normal equipment, and with the use of oxygen and the carrying of trained medical personnel, air evacuation of casualties entered on a new phase.

In New Guinea in 1942 there were few ambulance aircraft available to fly back the numerous casualties during the Kokoda Trail campaign and the subsequent fighting on the north east coast. Then the use of returning transport for casualty air evacuation became an immediate necessity. In the course of 70 days some thirteen thousand patients were carried by these means. On the other hand the sudden necessity to transport large numbers of sick and wounded men by air found the Australian and American medical services unprepared. There was no organisation or medical personnel available to care for patients or planes. Patients were often improperly prepared for flight. There were insufficient supplies of blankets, medical equipment and oxygen; indeed the latter were often entirely lacking. Members of the plane crew mostly had to undertake any medical attention that was necessary.

Soon after this, in 1943, the first medical air evacuation transport squadron, an American unit, arrived in New Guinea. Instructions were given that air evacuation should henceforth be carried out by the Air Force and be under the control of these squadrons when they were available.

In March 1944, after training with the American squadron, the R.A.A.F. formed its first own medical air evacuation unit and later 2 full strength units. These carried out all Australian evacuations, from forward and operational areas to the Australian mainland, without a single loss. A third unit operated solely in Australia.

The practice was for transport aircraft which had carried troops, supplies or munitions to the forward areas to be back-loaded with patients. A team consisting of one nursing sister and one medical orderly was carried on the forward flight to provide for the care of the patients on the return journey.

The medical air evacuation units classified the cases for evacuation, superintended the loading of the planes, cared for the cases during the flight and supervised their unloading. The Service requiring evacuation was responsible for collecting its cases and for providing shelter and medical treatment at the points of emplaning and deplaning. The unit also acted as the co-ordinating agent between the Services concerned for the supply of the requisite number of planes. The final decision as to the suitability of patients for air evacuation rested with the commanding officer of the air evacuation unit.

In the Pacific theatre flights were of many hours' duration, sometimes lasting a day or more. Sisters and trained medical orderlies therefore accompanied the patients. Ninety per cent. of the evacuations were carried in the two-engined transport C.47. Earlier types fitted with metal brackets took 18 stretcher cases. Later types had webbing fittings carrying 24 cases in American litters or 19 in Australian stretchers. Stretcher cases were always loaded head foremost at the front of the plane. Before departure the following points were carefully checked:

1. All wounds and fractures were adequately supported and all wounds recently dressed.

2. Tuberculous chest patients were wearing gauze masks; psychotic patients had been properly sedated and restrained.

3. All patients had recently defaecated; catheter cases had received attention.

4. Patients had had a light meal with adequate fluids.

Medical equipment was carried by each flight team, including a plasma set and portable oxygen apparatus.

Fifteen per cent. of all cases evacuated by air from New Guinea were psychiatric in nature. It was found that patients who had had a course of treatment with cardiazol or similar drug travelled the best. Many psychiatric cases had marked dehydration and did not travel well.

Sodium amytal was found to be the drug of choice for sedation. Intravenous sodium amytal administered just before the patient was loaded on to the ambulance was the best method, as it achieved a quick result and could be better controlled. If further sedation *en route* was necessary, oral 'Sodium Amytal' or 'Nembutal' was used. Morphine was unsatisfactory. Paraldehyde *per rectum* was useful; the intramuscular route was not favoured, although good results were obtained by using this method in combination with oral 'Sodium Amytal'. Restraint of maniacal cases was secured by straps of soft material, such as triangular bandages or towels. Straight jackets were not advised nor was the use of tight clothing and blankets because of the aggravation of dehydration.

Chest cases travelled well provided oxygen was available. Slow ascent and descent were necessary for cases of pneumothorax. Air evacuation of patients with upper respiratory infections and pneumonia was found to be inadvisable. In cases with cardio-vascular disease the type of lesion was not as important as the cardiac reserve, nor the increased demand on the heart as the effect of anoxia on the heart muscle. All cases of anaemia and scrub typhus travelled well.

Patients with head injuries only travelled well with oxygen. Anoxia occurred even at low altitudes. Patients with recent abdominal wounds involving the gut with subsequent repair experienced no ill effects provided the aircraft could fly at moderate height.

Patients were not nearly so prone to air sickness as might have been expected. Several factors probably contributed to this, the prone position, the loosening of all tight clothing and the administering of oxygen, mild sedation and glucose. Generally speaking air evacuation proved to be the ideal method of transporting casualties and was economical of time, personnel, transport and material. Because flights were more frequent than visits by hospital ship, fewer holding hospital beds were required and combat areas could be more speedily cleared. Air evacuation was also valuable where the terrain, distance and endemic disease areas made travel by land undesirable or impossible. Rapid air transport was much appreciated by the troops in the forward areas and added greatly to their morale. With few exceptions even seriously ill patients could be moved safely provided adequate attention was available by trained flight personnel. With the cessation of hostilities large numbers of prisoners-of-war in Japanese camps were repatriated by air.

AVIATION MEDICINE

In 1940 a Flying Personnel Research Committee was set up in Australia to study matters, both medical and of kindred interest, relating to aircrews—e.g., selection, flying performance, operational efficiency, comfort, safety, survival, escape and evasion. Sub-committees worked on problems of flying training, clothing, orthoptics, acoustics, motion sickness, high altitude, anti-G, tropical service and fatigue. An aviation medicine section was formed in each Initial Training School. One most important feature was the application of aptitude, co-ordination, high altitude, night vision and ocular muscle balance, tests. Those showing some muscle imbalance were given orthoptic instruction, with excellent results. This orthoptic training was also extended to operational pilots who for various reasons developed ocular imbalance. Much original work was done on visual acuity, colour and night vision. Decompression chambers were built for training in conditions encountered at high altitudes and in the use of oxygen. The Cotton aerodynamic anti-G suit with graded air pressures was adopted by the R.A.A.F. in 1942, and in 1944 three squadrons were fitted with it. Research was also carried out into anoxia detection, motion sickness and acoustics. A panel worked on the problems of survival of aircrew after bale-out in tropical areas, in addition to designing suitable flying clothing and protective kits for tropical service.

It was found that no adverse effects were caused by anti-malarial drugs on dark adaptation, susceptibility to motion, G tolerance or high-altitude tolerance, and that no breakdown in anti-malaria measures would be caused by the anoxia and cold likely to be experienced by troops who were transported by air. The physical and psychological aspects of tropical fatigue were investigated as well as the industrial hazards of benzol and toluol poisoning among workshop personnel.

APPENDIX A

The R8/70 aircrew survival kit developed by 'Mission X' and packed in Brisbane in the 1943–44 period contained:

R8/71   Medical Pack in plastic bottle
Sulphaguanadine tablets
Atebrin tablets
Salt tablets
Benzedrine sulphate
Sulphadiazine powder
Adhesive compresses
Iodine swab
Tweezers
Ophthalmic ointment (boric acid)
Toothbrush

R8/72   Survival Pack in plastic bottle
Chocolate rations
Chewing gum
Bouillon powder
Razor blades
Leader kit

Fish hook kit	Saw blade
Fishing line kit	Prophylactics
Sewing kit	Sharpening stone
Compass	Matches

G6E/271 Signalling mirror
R4/189 Canvas satchel

The plastic containers were intended to serve as water bottles after removal of the contents. It was said that the space in the containers was so confined that it was necessary to employ Asiatics to pack the kits, as Europeans did not possess the necessary manual dexterity.

VIII. MEDICAL EXPERIENCES RELATING TO AUSTRALIAN PRISONERS-OF-WAR

In any war of long duration the fluctuation of the campaign will inevitably result in the capture of personnel and material even from the side that eventually emerges victorious. Australia was particularly affected in this respect on two occasions; during the evacuation from Greece and the capitulation in Singapore.

The lot of any prisoner-of-war is not a happy one, influenced as he is by the psychological and physical circumstances of his capture, subjected to the rigours of a humiliating existence and distraught by the uncertainty of the future. He needs all the toughness of mind and body that he can produce together with a spiritual faith that stimulates him and exalts him in the face of his sufferings.

The personnel of the Army Medical Corps, however, have a great advantage. At least they can, with great effort, continue to apply their specific skills in spite of the worst conditions and altered surroundings.

In the detailed Australian History it is rare to meet instances of humane treatment that was genuine or of reasonable duration in any prisoner-of-war camp. Mostly it is a record of continuous striving for better conditions, an unending, often ineffectual, attempt to obtain not only amenities but the vital necessities to maintain life and health. In this struggle both in Europe and the South West Pacific Area the medical profession played a notable part. Although in German and Italian prisoner-of-war camps conditions were far from satisfactory, it is fair to say that at their worst they did not approach those under Japanese control, which will go down in history as an everlasting memorial of the shameful conduct of a modern nation.

HYGIENE

One of the earliest tasks ranking equally in importance with the care of the sick and wounded was the necessity of demanding the highest possible standard of hygiene. This was a matter requiring not only constant representation to the authorities concerned, but also training and indoctrination of the prisoners themselves. The beneficial effect of this on health and even on morale was very noticeable. The proximity of prisoner-of-war camps to native compounds and villages in Malaya, Burma and Borneo which contained a potential and actual reservoir of serious epidemic diseases constituted an additional hazard that was always grave and often decimating in its effect; it was uncontrollable by the medical personnel, handicapped as they were by the lack of drugs for either treatment or prophylaxis. To this was added the callous indifference of the captors, who apparently regarded their prisoners as expendable and made little or no attempt to ameliorate their condition or even to maintain some semblance of physical well-being that would yield a better standard of work.

RATIONS AND DIET

In all main theatres of war there were clear indications at an early stage that both the nature of the ration and the quantities supplied to prisoners would fall far short of what was required for bare subsistence. In the European prisoner-of-war camps the daily ration varied, in some camps being low, in others reaching a more adequate level. In the Far East the standard ration scale approved by the Japanese yielded 2,296 Calories but was unsatisfactorily balanced and notably lacking in many essential requirements. In practice, however, this ration scale was seldom implemented. The diets were supplemented by Red Cross food parcels, but these were an uncertain source of supply and were often looted. Even the right of the men to receive and use them to the best advantage was not recognised without a struggle.

MALNUTRITION AND DEFICIENCY DISEASES

Inevitably, physical states attributable to malnutrition were very rife, and beriberi in all forms was common. In the Far East the menacing scourge of deficiency diseases assumed even greater proportions, aggravated as it was by exposure to tropical climate, oppressive hardship and infectious disease. Moreover, the Japanese compelled their prisoner working parties to undertake the most arduous labour under appalling conditions. The combined effect of all these noxious influences can be readily understood and the almost superhuman task that in consequence confronted the medical personnel.

It was a challenge that was immediately accepted. Apart from maintaining the care of the sick and wounded the urgent problems that demanded attention were those dealing with diet, nutrition, hygiene and infection. In the brief description that follows emphasis is mainly upon what happened in the Far East, for it was there that the greatest numbers were involved and the worst overall conditions prevailed.

Food was the dominant consideration in the maintenance of health and strength of body. Fortunately a number of experts on nutrition were with the Australian Forces in captivity. From the very first the great risk of serious malnutrition was clearly realised, and close study was made by the physicians of the initial signs of dietary disorders as well as of the developed clinical syndromes. The forecast was made that unless substantial appropriate additions were made to the ration scale, serious manifestations of deficiency diseases would quickly appear, beginning with beriberi. The importance was realised of avoiding an excess of carbohydrate in relation to thiamin in a dietary. The early onset of the thiamin and riboflavin groups of deficiency was expected; only too soon was this prophecy fulfilled.

A nutritional advisory committee was appointed and rendered valuable service in checking constituents of the diet and advising in the selection and provision of supplements. This account of the work done to combat malnutrition of course merely concerns the A.I.F. The measures adopted by the A.I.F. and its medical services were technically similar to those adopted by the British Forces, for while the Australian administration shouldered its own medical problems there was free interchange of information and opinion.

Various measures were undertaken to supplement diets. A yeast centre was established after obtaining the original cultures from the Japanese. Potatoes, sweet potatoes and rice were used with the addition of gula malacca in place of ordinary sugar. Rice polishings were used when obtainable. One of the methods of making soya bean palatable and effective as a food was by preparing *tempe*, which was a product containing soya bean, preferably unhusked and partially predigested by fungus action. The soya was crushed and mixed with cooking oil and then cooked. Riboflavin was obtained as a constituent of an extract from 'telang' grass or the Malayan wild passion vine. The residue from the production of surgical alcohol by fermentation of sweet potato and gula malacca made a substitute for 'Marmite'. The Japanese encouraged unit and group gardens, which furnished all ranks and units with a highly valuable means of providing additional food.

As the incidence of deficiency states increased the burden cast on the medical administration grew, for it was necessary to meet the needs of many of the men admitted to hospital and even those being treated as out-patients. A definite policy for treatment had to be adopted. For example—'Marmite' was used only for the treatment of beriberi, keratitis and retrobulbar neuritis, spastic paraplegia and dysentery and, in general, for patients requiring dietary supplements who could not take rice polishings. A specific dosage was also determined.

Special food for hospital patients was distinctly limited in supply and had to be controlled with care. By local purchase limited supplies of eggs, greens, sugar and oil could be obtained from time to time. The economy and wisdom with which the dietetic affairs of hospitals were managed on Singapore Island are worth noting, for special diets were devised for certain conditions such as beriberi, peptic ulcers and pulmonary tuberculosis.

INFECTIOUS DISEASES

Matters of hygiene required close attention from the outset and throughout the whole period of captivity. By degrees an increasingly efficient scheme of sanitation was introduced, and general measures became more effective as the troops realised their importance.

The most important measures were those directed to the control of dysentery and similar diseases and of malaria. The early period was full of difficulties. On Singapore Island the whole area allotted to the prisoners was partially destroyed, dirty and covered with débris. Flies were breeding profusely. Education of the troops themselves as usual was not easily accomplished, but lectures, visual instruction with posters and the influence of hygiene picquets helped to maintain hygienic discipline. By the time these tired men could be rallied to the fight against disease, dysentery had already gained a foothold in the camps, and a long struggle lay ahead before any mastery could be gained.

When in the course of time the various parties were despatched to work in other places, in particular on the Burma–Thailand Railway, the conditions under which they were forced to exist exposed them to such privation and disease hazards that, despite the most heroic efforts of the medical service, very many perished or were rendered permanently invalid. Meagre supplies of essential drugs could not cope with out- breaks of dysentery, cholera, malaria and diphtheria. The combination of malnutrition, deficiency disease and debility with even minor injury, resulted in the occurrence of tropical ulcers that not infrequently necessitated amputation of the leg in order to save life. Skin disease was common and severe in character. There were many cases of hookworm infestation. By contrast the incidence of pulmonary tuberculosis was extremely small owing to the care in selecting recruits and to the use of X-ray examination at enlistment.

HOSPITALS

In all the prisoner-of-war working party camps hospitals were estab- lished. A noteworthy feature was the introduction of a system of ward mastering whereby the services of combatant officers were obtained to manage wards. The ward master was in a position of authority by virtue of which he organised the various services of the wards, supervised the details and, by keeping the domestic affairs and nursing procedures running smoothly, did much to raise and maintain the morale and physi- cal condition of the patients. The insufficient number of trained medical orderlies to deal with the care of sick men was thus more effectively employed.

In the Singapore area the hospitals gave a remarkably complete general medical service. Special departments were competently staffed and afforded essential treatment, often undertaking valuable research. Much ingenuity was displayed in devising instruments and apparatus. Media and vaccines were prepared. Specially improvised methods were devised in the ophthalmic, ear, nose and throat, dental and X-ray departments. Almost every type of surgical operation was undertaken with a remarkable record of success. Tropical ulcers were throughout a serious malady, often demanding some radical operation such as excision of teddons or muscle, removal of sequestra or even amputation. Good results were obtained in less severe forms by removal of sloughs and the application of iodoform. A solution of copper sulphate, carbolic acid and water was also found useful after cleaning or excising the ulcer.

Necessity is certainly the mother of invention. All sorts of hospital articles were made, including special instruments ranging from bamboo needles to retractors, suction pumps, proctoscopes, surgical alcohol and catgut and even to an ophthalmoscope. An artifical limb factory was set up and was of immense value with the ingenious and painstaking prostheses that were produced. Even artificial eyes were made.

Cases of psychological disturbances occurred but did not reach a substantial number.

At the time of liberation special arrangements were made regarding adequate preliminary treatment for beriberi, malaria and dysentery before evacuation. Further arrangements were made concerning fitness to travel and dietary requirements. The needs of each individual were assessed, and the men were drafted accordingly. On return to Australia all ex-prisoners-of-war were fully investigated in hospital, given appropriate treatment and rehabilitated. Many of the prisoners-of-war repatriated in 1944 from Europe undertook further service in the South West Pacific Area.

If there is any lesson to be learned from this portion of medical history, it is surely that proper action should be taken by the United Nations to ensure reasonable civilised treatment of prisoners-of-war in the future. A veneer of civilisation is insufficient guarantee against the perpetration of atrocities, and the varying standards of national behaviour require elevation to an agreed human level. (*See* also United Kingdom p. 156.)

PART IV

New Zealand

The New Zealand Medical Services

By Sir Duncan Stout, C.B.E., D.S.O., M.B., M.S.(Lond.), F.R.C.S.(Eng.), F.R.A.C.S.

Detailed official accounts of the work of the New Zealand Medical Services during the Second World War will be found in the following volumes*:

War Surgery and Medicine
New Zealand Medical Services in
    Middle East and Italy.   } Sir Duncan Stout
Medical Services in New Zealand
    and the Pacific.

The New Zealand Dental Services   T. V. Anson

---

* Published by the War History Branch, Department of Internal Affairs, Wellington, New Zealand.

CONTENTS

PREFACE

This contribution covers the whole range of the activities of the New Zealand Medical Services, both in New Zealand and overseas.

It deals with all the Services, Navy, Army and Air, and the experience of our prisoners-of-war. Emphasis is laid on general planning and organisation and an overall picture of our experiences is given rather than a chronological account of the different campaigns in which New Zealand Forces took part.

Experiences in the treatment of war wounds and in war surgery are recorded. Infectious and other diseases of importance to our Forces during the war are described, as are the important aspects of hygiene and sanitation.

The medical administration in New Zealand, both civil and military, is given particular attention.

The integration of our Forces with those of the Commonwealth, and in the Pacific with those of the United States of America, is described.

The New Zealand Medical Corps was proud to be associated with other members of the Commonwealth and Allied Forces and acknowledges with gratitude the great help given, especially by the Royal Army Medical Corps, under whose helpful control our Corps worked in the Middle East and Italy.

It is hoped that the New Zealand contribution to this volume will be of value to the other Medical Services of the Commonwealth.

I—ARMY MEDICAL ORGANISATION IN NEW ZEALAND

HISTORICAL BACKGROUND

BEFORE the War of 1914–18 compulsory training for army service had been in force in New Zealand for some years and was reintroduced after the war in 1921.

The war-time Army medical organisation continued until November 1923 though Army hospitals and convalescent homes had ceased to function in 1922. The administration then reverted to a Territorial basis, with three training depots, two in the North Island and one in the South.

The depression that followed some years after the war led to the abolition of compulsory military training in 1931. The Medical Corps was reduced to a small number of loyal enthusiastic volunteers who attended the annual camp. Fortunately there was an improvement in the two years prior to the war, especially as regards the number and quality of the medical officers, and the D.M.S. did his best to develop the Corps. Nevertheless in May 1938 the strength of the medical units amounted only to 43 officers and 254 other ranks. There were only three regular force personnel attached, including only one qualified instructor.

The training during the period was limited to that of the three army field ambulances and the ambulance unit at the Otago University and such experience as medical officers obtained as R.M.Os. at army camps. There was no training in, or study of, the problems of war medicine and surgery or of military hospitals, nor were there any hygiene units.

Fortunately some experience of war conditions in the War of 1914–18 remained, especially among the senior officers, and there were many First World War personnel still in the reserve when war began.

ARMY MEDICAL ADMINISTRATION IN NEW ZEALAND

CENTRAL ADMINISTRATION

Prior to the war the New Zealand Medical Corps was entirely a Territorial Service with a skeleton administration under a D.M.S. and three military district A.D.M.Ss. and a Matron-in-Chief, each receiving a small honorarium.

On the outbreak of war a D.M.S., an A.D.M.S. and a small office staff were appointed full-time officers at Army Headquarters; the district A.D.M.Ss. were appointed half-time and later full-time; the Matron-in-Chief became full-time in April 1941.

Medical officers were appointed at the mobilisation camps as required. Later a Deputy Director of Hygiene and a full-time A.D.M.S. (Air) were appointed.

THE NURSING SERVICE

The Nursing Service had reverted in 1922 to a peace-time basis and had an establishment of a Matron-in-Chief, a principal matron, four matrons and 62 sisters, though no special army training was carried out. The majority of the sisters had had army service and all the seniors at the outbreak of the war had Service experience in the First World War.

OPTICIAN SERVICE

This service was set up in the latter half of 1942 and optician units were attached to the main camps. Well equipped and staffed units were also sent overseas to Fiji, to the R.N.Z.A.F. Islands Group, to the Pacific Division and later one was despatched to Italy. Opticians also assisted at recruit medical boards.

DENTAL SERVICE

The Army Dental Service was placed nominally under the D.M.S. for administrative purposes, but in general acted under the Adjutant General as the dental service wished strongly to be independent. Dental treatment was carried out in the camps, well equipped dental hospitals were set up in the three main mobilisation camps and dental sections were attached to various other units.

There was a Dental Sub-Committee of the National Medical Committee.

HYGIENE IN NEW ZEALAND

A hygiene officer of the Health Department was appointed as Director of Hygiene, and local Health Officers acted as local advisers to the Army in the different districts as regards hygiene and camp sanitation.

Camp regulations were drawn up to ensure healthy living conditions, to prevent overcrowding, for the drying and airing of clothing, for adequate sanitary facilities and for a full and varied diet.

A School of Hygiene was established at Trentham camp to train sanitation personnel and hygiene sections were set up in the camps.

RECRUITMENT OF MEDICAL PERSONNEL IN NEW ZEALAND

During the War of 1939–45 the recruitment of personnel, including that of the Medical Corps, was on a voluntary basis until conscription was introduced in June 1940. The medical officers were recruited entirely from the civilian medical profession, the majority being without any previous military experience. The other ranks of the Medical Corps were civilians from every walk of life.

TRAINING IN NEW ZEALAND

Recruits were trained in camps sited near Auckland, Wellington and Christchurch before being sent overseas. Later a special camp for the training of armoured units was set up at Waiouru in the centre of the North Island, where a large area of undeveloped land was available for manoeuvres. The Medical Corps units were assembled and some preliminary training undertaken at Wellington and Christchurch, the hospital units and convalescent depot at the former and the field units at the latter. The training of the Field Medical Units carried out in New Zealand was according to the R.A.M.C. routine and manuals. A nucleus of trained Territorials, both officers and O.Rs., was available for the field units in particular, and any prolonged training was unnecessary. The hospital units already had well trained officers and sisters with hospital experience, and several officers with First World War experience. As long as some administrative experience and knowledge was available little in the way of training in New Zealand was necessary before sending medical units overseas.

The 2 N.Z.E.F. was mobilised from September 1939 onwards in three Echelons, each consisting of a composite brigade with an attached field ambulance, regimental medical officers and a proportion of ancillary units. A Field Hygiene Section accompanied the First Echelon which left New Zealand on January 5, 1940 for Egypt.

The first hospital and the convalescent depot proceeded overseas on May 2, 1940 with the Second Echelon which, following the fall of France and the threat of war with Italy, was diverted from Egypt to England, thus depriving the First Echelon of New Zealand hospital services for several months longer than was intended.

The second hospital went to Egypt with the Third Echelon on August 27, 1940, as did the third hospital with the Fourth Reinforcements on February 1, 1941. All the units of the Second New Zealand Expeditionary Force had proceeded overseas by this date.

The medical units sent overseas provided the full complement for the Force as determined at that time, and the C.C.S. was the only major unit added later on in the Middle East.

Before the first troops had embarked decisions were made in New Zealand concerning the development of medical and hygiene services in the Middle East, as well as the diet of the troops. The G.O.C. took especial interest in these matters for both he and the D.M.S. had personal experience of the Middle East area and its problems in the First World War.

A *training depot* for medical personnel was set up at the end of 1940, controlled at first by combatant staff and later by the medical corps, and all reinforcements, both officers and men, were trained there for overseas service. Men were also trained for the Pacific Force and for home service.

Camp hospitals were established to care for patients requiring less than 48 hours treatment. Contagious diseases hospitals were set up in the camps for men suffering from venereal disease.

The general control of sick personnel in New Zealand and the sick and wounded returning from overseas was in the hands of the Adjutant General, who set up a Sick and Wounded Branch to keep a check on these personnel and arrange for their many requirements.

The incidence of sickness in the camps in New Zealand generally was low. There was an epidemic of influenza in September and October 1939, 20–25 per cent. of different units being affected but no deaths were reported. Other mild epidemics occurred from time to time, usually among newly mobilised personnel. There were 4,700 cases in 1940 and 9,000 cases in 1942, but less than 2,000 in any subsequent year. Measles and mumps were the only other epidemic diseases of any consequence.

Mild outbreaks of gastro-enteritis and dysentery occurred. There were 89 cases of cerebro-spinal meningitis in camps out of a total of 1,036 cases in the Dominion as a whole. Venereal disease figures varied from 15 per thousand to 30 per thousand per year. Preventive measures were adopted and treatment centres established in all camps.

The total number of deaths among troops in New Zealand was 441, of which 148 were from accidents.

PREVENTIVE INOCULATION

Inoculation of the troops against the typhoid group, vaccination against smallpox and inoculation against tetanus were carried out in New Zealand from the beginning. The typhoid inoculation consisted of two injections of T.A.B. vaccine manufactured in New Zealand.

There appears to have been some difficulty concerning the vaccine owing to the low incidence of typhoid in New Zealand. It is said that an old bone abscess was used at one time. The British vaccine supplied in Egypt proved to be satisfactory. Vaccination against smallpox was carried out and repeated if no positive reaction occurred. Some interference with training arose and at first, in some cases, the vaccination was carried out on the troopships. This proved unsatisfactory under tropical conditions and later all vaccinations were done in New Zealand.

Tetanus toxoid was given in two doses to all troops. This was considered to give immunity against tetanus, but did not preclude the giving of A.T. serum following wounding.

These preventive measures were repeated overseas at intervals, determined both by the length of period between injections and by the local incidence of the diseases concerned.

Injections against typhus and cholera were also given to the troops in the Middle East, again repeated at appropriate intervals.

Anti-diphtheritic inoculations were given to hospital, particularly nursing, personnel later in the war following the occurrence of diphtheritic infection of wounds.

EQUIPMENT IN NEW ZEALAND

The Army medical equipment and stores retained after the First World War consisted of field ambulance and regimental equipment only, with appropriate medical supplies.

This was kept in store but was utilised to a great extent for training during the inter-war period. After dispensing, during the depression, with the services of the quartermaster the stores became sadly depleted and out of date. In spite of strong efforts of the D.M.S. to correct the position the equipment and stores were still in short supply when the war began and all the medical units had to be sent to the Middle East unequipped. Fortunately the British Army was able to supply the units in time and very efficiently.

Home defence called for a marked increase in the Territorial Force and several field ambulances as well as field hygiene sections were formed. Medical practitioners also helped in a part-time capacity. Three divisions with thirteen field ambulances, four field hygiene sections and four motor ambulance convoy sections were mobilised in New Zealand. The civilian hospitals were organised to take over the treatment of the sick and wounded. There was an acute shortage of medical officers and the staffs of medical units were below strength. Civilian practitioners and non-qualified officers were used as far as possible. When the Japanese threat lessened, the forces were reorganised and considerably reduced.

A Home Guard was formed in August 1940 and continued to serve until December 1943.

The *hospital ship service* was under New Zealand command during the war.

II. CIVILIAN MEDICAL ORGANISATION IN NEW ZEALAND
NATIONAL MEDICAL COMMITTEE

In 1936 an Organisation for National Security was set up by the Government of New Zealand and a National Medical Committee was constituted as part of the organisation. This committee's work covered the medical examination of recruits, care of the sick and wounded in New Zealand, and medical care of the civilian population in any emergency. The members were the Director General of Health (Chairman), a member of the Department of Health, the D.M.S. of Army and Air and a nominee of the British Medical Association. The Committee was an advisory body under the Minister of Health, not the Minister of Defence, and predominantly a civilian organisation. It regulated the supply of professional personnel to meet the needs of the civilian population and the Armed Services. Its personnel remained unchanged throughout the war.

The Committee determined, with the concurrence of the Minister and Cabinet, that medical boarding of recruits and hospital treatment in New Zealand should come under the civilian authorities.

Army camp hospitals were only responsible for patients requiring not more than 48 hours in hospital. The Army, however, assumed the responsibility for treating patients with venereal disease and also for carrying out dental treatment in the camps throughout the war.

MEDICAL BOARDING IN NEW ZEALAND

Medical classification of recruits was undertaken by the Department of Health. The country was divided into eleven districts under part-time regional deputies. Medical boards were constituted, each with two medical officers, a dentist, and, later, an optician.

The regional deputies having approved the boards' findings, submitted them to the Army authorities.

The medical standards and system of classification were drawn up before the war; they were based on the Hill Report, as revised in 1933 and were further revised in 1940 as the result of experience and criticism from overseas concerning the unsatisfactory nature of some of the reinforcements.

The results were much superior to those of the First World War, owing to more detailed and careful examination of the recruit. X-ray examination of the chest, blood pressure and cardiac efficiency tests, and dental and optician examinations were valuable.

STANDARDS OF RECRUITS

The recruits had to be fit for service in any part of the world. For O.Rs. the age limit was 21 to 40. The lower age limit was enforced but the upper limit was relaxed in the case of volunteers, especially for officers, but the standard of fitness was maintained.

Recruits were graded as follows:

Grade I.   fit for active service in any part of the world;

Grade II.   fit for service in New Zealand;

Grade III.   unfit for service except clerical or other sedentary work in New Zealand;

Grade IV.   permanently unfit for any service.

X-ray examination of the chest was carried out for the Third Echelon and afterwards, only a few of the Second Echelon being covered. Chest specialists and radiologists examined all doubtful cases. Officers of the Mental Hospitals Department checked the lists of recruits to remove any known mental defective. Psychiatric examination of recruits was not undertaken as it was held to be wasteful and unnecessary and liable to make the men 'psychology-conscious'; but psychiatrists were consulted when necessary.

Remedial treatment was carried out for a relatively small number of recruits with minor disabilities, and was limited to conditions which could be relieved in one month. At first treatment was compulsory but this was discontinued. It appears that the experiment was not successful, partly because too much stress was laid on the time element and too little on the efficiency of the surgical treatment; there was also too much accentuation on such treatment as tonsillectomy.

Medical boarding of returning Servicemen was carried out in New Zealand by the same civilian boards that examined recruits, to determine whether medical treatment was necessary, or whether there was any disability warranting a pension. The Serviceman was retained in the Army on full pay if only a short period of treatment was necessary, but in longer cases he was discharged and put on pension.

Dental examination and treatment were given to render the returning Servicemen dentally fit. An X-ray examination of the chest was carried out to exclude tuberculosis, which condition was pensionable if arising within two years of discharge.

As many as 141,000 Boards were held in the Auckland area alone. On the whole the work was done satisfactorily and the Code of Instructions proved sound. The psychological element caused the main difficulty as this was difficult or impossible to assess in a brief examination. Undoubtedly too much attention was paid to minor physical disabilities and the standards too rigidly adhered to. Of nearly 58,000 volunteers just over 24 per cent. were unfit for service overseas. Of 110,000 later recruits nearly 35 per cent. were unfit, and as older men were called up this percentage increased.

MAORI RECRUITS

X-ray chest examinations of Maori recruits were carried out from the beginning as it was known that the incidence of tuberculosis in the Maori race was high. The value of this X-ray examination was proved. It was impossible to detect early signs of tubercle in any other way, especially in crowded and noisy board-rooms. The absence of any marked greater incidence of tuberculosis in Maoris serving in the Middle East showed that few cases had escaped diagnosis in New Zealand.

Maori recruits were also prone to disabilities of the feet. There was a tendency to flat feet with dropping of the arch. The main trouble, however, was that the ordinary Army boot was unsuitable for the broader Maori foot and caused cramped toes and the development of corns. Broader boots, though often recommended, were never supplied.

RECRUITMENT OF MEDICAL OFFICERS

The recruitment of medical officers was put under the control of the National Medical Committee at the beginning of the war to ensure that the claims of both Army and the civil population were met. Ministerial approval had to be obtained before any medical practitioner could leave New Zealand during the war. Medical students who had completed two years study were compelled to finish their course and serve as house surgeons for a year before they could be accepted for service in the Armed Forces. Later the period was shortened to nine, and then to six months.

Although doctors and dentists came under the compulsory service regulations and were liable to be called up in the ballot there could have been few who were not volunteers, and many volunteering were not permitted to join the Forces.

There were in the original units a number of senior medical officers whose ages ranged from the late forties to the middle fifties, especially in the hospital units. Almost all of these officers had served in the First World War, many in the Middle East, and their knowledge of Service conditions and treatment of wounds and of diseases endemic in that area was of great value to the Force.

The Medical Corps was for this reason particularly well equipped to carry out its responsibilities in the Middle East and had many officers capable of higher command. The many officers and men who had had long periods of Territorial training were also of much value, particularly in the field units, and from their ranks the senior administrative posts were filled. This led to some difficulty for many of these medical officers were specialists and their employment in administrative work weakened the hospital staffs.

Throughout the war there was a shortage of civilian medical practitioners and the Army frequently appealed for reinforcements. The requirements in each area were reviewed to determine how to make the best use of the personnel available. The provision for the Pacific Force, the mobilisation of three divisions and the formation of the Home Guard increased the shortage of doctors, but when the threat of invasion receded and the Pacific Forces were recalled, all serious difficulties ended.

In October 1943 there were 285 medical officers in the Army, 44 being in New Zealand, and 53 in the R.N.Z.A.F., 41 being in New Zealand.

Nursing and Ancillary Staff. After the first six months, enlistment into the Army of masseurs and chemists, laboratory and X-ray technicians, was controlled so as to retain sufficient for civilian work.

Enrolment of nursing sisters was also controlled and arrangements made to call up nurses equally from each district or hospital. There was never any lack of volunteers. A certain proportion of senior nurses was retained in every area of New Zealand.

During the war 300 New Zealand registered nurses were in England. This depleted our resources, so permission for others to leave the country was withheld. The age limits for service overseas were 25–45 years. The first group (18) of nurses left with the First Echelon in January 1940, each transport carrying three nurses. This practice was continued throughout the war. Meanwhile extra nurses were trained in New Zealand hospitals.

As many as 375 sisters were serving at one time in the Middle East and Italy, in the Pacific and on hospital ships. During the whole period of the war 602 served overseas while 65 of the N.Z.A.N.S. served in New Zealand. A civil nursing reserve of registered nurses and voluntary aids was established in New Zealand in March 1943 to help in the hospitals.

The training of voluntary aids was instituted in 1940 with the help of the Red Cross Society and the Order of St. John, and by May 1940 1,000 girls had had their first period of 60 hours' hospital training. The employment of V.A.Ds. in the Army began in 1941, both at home and overseas, the first contingent leaving in December for the Middle East.

By February 1944 there were 268 V.A.Ds. overseas, 50 in military camp hospitals in New Zealand and 119 on air force station hospitals in New Zealand.

N.C.Os. AND O.Rs.

Volunteers of excellent quality provided a nucleus of N.C.Os. and O.Rs. for the medical units. They proved themselves adaptable, capable and able to improvise and live and work under difficult conditions. Among them were chemists, physiotherapists and technicians, as well as men of administrative experience. Some were later granted commissions as Registrars and company officers, with some saving of medical officer personnel. Others such as chemists and physiotherapists, were also granted commissions.

COMBATANT TROOPS

For combatant troops the age limits 21 to 40 proved generally satisfactory. In the forward area men over 40 usually did not stand up to the conditions of service as well as the younger men. There were many officers over 40 both Regular and Territorial, but very few in the over 50 group. Although many of these proved suitable for administrative work at the Base, generally, and especially in the forward areas, few were as suitable as the younger officers. War is undoubtedly an occupation for younger men.

HOSPITAL TREATMENT IN NEW ZEALAND

On the recommendation of the Advisory Medical Committee, the Cabinet decided, in November 1939, that the Health Department should have full responsibility for hospital treatment in New Zealand of all patients of the Armed Forces needing hospital care for more than 48 hours. The Health Department and the Hospital Boards became responsible for them until they became fit for full duty, including convalescent treatment when necessary and for the organisation and control of convalescent hospitals.

This decision was determined by the need to save medical and nursing personnel by concentrating the work in the civilian hospitals, and also by economy in building. Any enlargement of accommodation required would be available to the hospitals after the war. There was also some political antagonism to military control. Liaison was established between the Army and the hospitals by the appointment by the Army of a Hospital Officer and clerical staff in each main centre, and later by the Sick and Wounded Branch of the Army. The provision for convalescence was never adequately met and the majority of patients convalesced in their own homes. This caused delay in returning to camp. There were two hospitals under the Department of Health available for convalescent orthopaedic and other special long-term cases. Three convalescent depots were completed at the end of 1941 to come under Army command. Two functioned, the third being taken over by the Americans.

THE RECEPTION OF CASUALTIES IN NEW ZEALAND

This was arranged by the Department of Health. A clearing hospital of 288 beds was established near the wharves at Wellington where all the patients, except the serious cot cases admitted directly to the Wellington Hospital, were medically boarded and sent to their respective districts, either to their local hospitals or to their homes.

Their care was undertaken by the local hospital, and the Pensions Department assumed responsibility as soon as the patients were discharged from the Army. Generally full army pay was granted as long as hospital treatment was being given.

Certain types of patients were sent to the specially staffed and equipped hospitals in the main centres. Facio-maxillary cases were sent to Christchurch, head cases to Dunedin and Auckland, while major orthopaedic and psychiatric cases went to the four main centres.

Patients suffering from anxiety states were sent to Hanmer Hospital and Rotorua was used for convalescents requiring massage and physiotherapy.

As the patients usually became civilians while in hospital and were not segregated, records of their progress in New Zealand have been difficult to obtain. The dispersal of the patients to their homes also made it difficult to keep a check on them, and this seems to have led to some delay in treatment of such conditions as nerve injuries. The dispersal of patients to the district hospitals conserved medical man-power and ensured that the fresh accommodation provided would act as an enlargement of the civil hospital accommodation. On the other hand the military hospitals and annexes set up during the War of 1914–18 had the advantages of continuity of treatment and better supervision of the patients requiring further treatment.

Although in general the treatment of Service and pension patients in New Zealand was carried out satisfactorily, there were certain deficiencies due to some lack of elasticity and co-ordination.

Many more of the lighter cases could readily have been treated in camp hospitals, and the arrangements for convalescence led to much wastage. Full use was not made of ex-Service officers in treating Service personnel in hospital. In any prolonged war one hospital controlled by the Services could well act as a valuable training centre for Service medical personnel.

The *psychiatric patients* on return to New Zealand were examined by a psychiatrist and admitted to the public hospitals in the four main centres or referred for out-patient treatment to local hospitals. If necessary, patients were certified and admitted to the mental hospitals.

The *neuroses patients* were quickly returned to regular employment, and, except for being kept on pension for varying periods, caused no serious trouble.

The number of neurosis cases dealt with by the War Pensions Board up to 1946 was 7,080 of which 363 were psychotics and 105 epileptics.

The *amputee cases* were all fitted with their artificial limbs in Wellington on their return to New Zealand. Private firms had made and serviced nearly all limbs until 1943 when the Rehabilitation Board took over a large firm with its plant, and entrusted its operation to the Disabled Servicemen's Re-establishment League. An orthopaedic surgeon was appointed to go overseas for experience and then supervise the work in New Zealand. Facilities for the fitting and repair of limbs were also made available in the other three main centres. In all 491 amputees of the War of 1939–45 were fitted with artificial limbs.

A *Plastic Surgery Unit*, an Army unit, was trained in England and established in one of the main civilian hospitals for the treatment of men invalided from overseas. It functioned under civilian hospital control, but the dual control proved unsatisfactory and it became a wholly civil unit early in 1945, and treated both Army and civilian patients.

The *Disabled Servicemen's League* undertook the training of many disabled men in different trades and occupations in six main centres and also on a farm.

Blind Servicemen were cared for by the Rehabilitation Board and a St. Dunstan's Home was set up in Auckland, where training in suitable occupations was instituted.

DISABILITY PENSIONS

A pension was granted for all disabilities arising during service overseas and for all disabilities attributable to or aggrevated by service in New Zealand.

War disablement pensions were granted generously and by March 1957 a total of 43,089 had received at least a temporary pension out of 145,000 returned personnel, and of the 66,000 home Servicemen, 10,500 had received a pension.

Of the conditions giving rise to late disability the most interesting was amoebic dysentery.

Pensions were administered by a War Pensions Board of three members, one being a medical practitioner, and an Appeal Board of a judge or magistrate and two medical practitioners. The Social Security Department handled the administration of the benefits.

CIVIL EMERGENCY

Medical arrangements for any civil emergency were planned throughout New Zealand. Two handbooks, one for urban and the other for rural localities, were issued. The local authorities undertook the local planning and control, and compulsory enrolment was ordered in 1942. The Army co-operated in the scheme. A medical section was organised which was to work independently of the public hospitals. A large emergency reserve of 20,000 beds was established by the Hospital Boards.

Local controllers were appointed in the different local areas and four group officers appointed to cover the whole of the country. The nursing services were under the Director of Nursing Services in the Health Department.

The Department of Health set up a Public Health Emergency Precautions Service to control matters of public health, acting through the Medical Officers of Health. The medical section of the E.P.S. was organised by the local members of the medical profession, and an excellent booklet of instructions was issued in 1941.

Medical supplies in New Zealand were put under the control of the Director General of Health at the outbreak of war, the Medical Officers of Health acting as local controllers. An advisory committee of representatives of the four principal importers of medical and surgical supplies was set up in Wellington. Supplies in New Zealand were short and it was difficult to arrange for adequate supplies from overseas, though eventually stocks were received from the U.S.A. The use of drugs was controlled, a special formulary was drawn up and doctors and chemists urged to conserve all supplies. Efforts were also made, with some success, to manufacture drugs in New Zealand.

A Joint Council of the Order of St. John and the New Zealand Red Cross Society was set up in 1938 to be the sole expending agent of the

National Patriotic Fund Board for the sick, wounded, distressed and prisoners-of-war. In addition to money from the Patriotic Fund the Council also received grants from the Goverment to defray the cost of food parcels for prisoners-of-war.

Sub-committees were appointed, all of voluntary workers. Sewing and knitting parties were set up all over New Zealand to provide stocks of comforts and medical dressings and supplies, which were distributed overseas to medical units and to the troops.

Red Cross Commissioners were appointed in the Middle East and in London. Convalescent homes in New Zealand were administered. Over a million parcels were sent overseas to prisoners-of-war. Supplies were also provided for the American Forces established in New Zealand.

Rehabilitation of Medical Officers. Provision for the rehabilitation of medical officers after serving overseas was made at the end of the war. Post-graduate bursaries, with an allowance of £250 a year plus fares, fees and books, were awarded to suitable young medical officers with long service overseas who wished to study for higher degrees, or follow special courses of study. Short refresher courses in New Zealand were also provided, and medical officers acting as house surgeons at the public hospitals were assisted by the Department of Health. The British Medical Association acted as adviser to the Rehabilitation Board on these matters. Altogether 151 doctors availed themselves of the post-graduate bursaries. Courses included those for F.R.C.S. 66, M.R.C.P. 53, M.R.A.C.P. 9, M.R.C.O.G. 9, and F.R.A.C.S. 6. In addition, 72 grants were made for special courses of study and 47 grants to subsidise the salaries of house surgeons.

Members of the New Zealand Army Nursing Service received 10 post-graduate bursaries for overseas study and 89 for study in New Zealand.

Thirty-six New Zealand Medical Corps other ranks were among the 169 ex-Servicemen and women granted bursaries to study medicine at the University of Otago.

III. MEDICAL ORGANISATION OF 2 NEW ZEALAND EXPEDITIONARY FORCE IN MIDDLE EAST FORCE AND CENTRAL MEDITERRANEAN FORCE

The medical organisation of the 2 N.Z.E.F. in M.E.F. was based on the policy of New Zealand personnel being treated, as far as possible, by their own medical corps, both in the field and at the base; and, as necessary, on the lines of communication, so that the New Zealand Medical Corps should provide a complete chain of medical attention and nursing. This policy could not always be carried out, but it was firmly pursued. Apart from the difficulties associated with segregation during a period of active operations, especially when evacuation was difficult and the numbers of casualties excessive, it had many advantages. The patient was usually happier and more contented with his own medical units; he understood the working of the units and was given his normal diet. He had the fellowship of his own people, both patients and staff, and he had no difficulty with his mail and his local news.

In general, he fitted in readily with the environment that was, except for being a patient, a normal one. This does not imply that he was not very well looked after in other hospitals or was not happy there. In fact in many cases New Zealanders were extremely happy in British and other hospitals. They were often treated almost as pets, and had to be almost forcibly extracted from their pleasant surroundings!

Some patients were sent to British hospitals for treatment in specialist units not otherwise available, such as neuro-surgical, facio-maxillary and chest units. We also relied upon many other units of the British Army Medical Services such as M.A.Cs., ambulance trains, hospital ships, ambulance and other planes, and the blood transfusion service. We were also serviced generally by the Army organisation and equipped and supplied by it with all kinds of stores and rations.

Again, we had attached to our units at various times, and often for long periods, British and other special units and personnel, particularly field surgical and field transfusion units and neuro-surgical and ophthalmic units, all of which rendered us invaluable service.

Fortunately, we were able at times to reciprocate in caring for British and other patients in our medical units. In fact, our 3 N.Z.G.H., while stationed at Beirut, had comparatively few of our own personnel as patients. Our C.C.S. while working in the Western Desert dealt with large numbers of casualties other than our own troops, as also did our field ambulances.

PROVISION OF MEDICAL UNITS

At the beginning of the war these consisted of three field ambulances, a field hygiene section, two general hospitals, one of 600 and one of 1,200 beds, and a convalescent depot. The hospital provision was altered, on the recommendation of the D.D.M.S. 2 N.Z.E.F., strongly supported by the D.M.S. M.E.F., to three hospitals of 600 beds, two to be expanded to 900 beds. This alteration was advised because of the likelihood of changes in the siting of the hospitals, and this forecast was proved to be correct and the provision of the three hospitals amply justified.

All the units were based on the R.A.M.C. establishment of personnel and equipment in every particular, and regimental medical officers were likewise provided.

Later in the war the medical chain was completed by the formation of a C.C.S. which was first set up in Syria and was in full operation at the battle of Alamein. The C.C.S. was preceded by a Mobile Surgical Unit based on the units attached to the British Army in France before Dunkirk, and equipped to deal with all types of wounds, including those of the head and chest. It gave good service during the second Libyan campaign, from which fortunately it emerged practically intact, and was then incorporated into the C.C.S. as the light section. Later the C.C.S. was one of the first in the British Army to be equipped as a mobile unit.

In the Middle East several smaller medical units were established as the need arose. Rest homes were provided in Cairo, one for nursing sisters and W.A.A.Cs. and another for officers, and a rest home for O.Rs. was established on the sea coast at Alexandria.

A Base Hygiene Company was formed early in Egypt to deal with the base camps and later in the war in Italy the Field Hygiene Section was enlarged by incorporation of anti-malaria and anti-typhus companies, into a Field Hygiene Company to cover all aspects of hygiene and preventive medicine in the Divisional area.

Camp hospitals were also set up in the base camps both in Egypt and in Italy, and they did a great deal to relieve the hospitals by providing accommodation and treatment for large numbers of patients suffering from less serious conditions. A training centre and depot for medical reinforcements was attached to the camp hospital in Egypt.

Difficulties in equipping field units and efficiently providing the numerous medical units with supplies led to the establishment of a Depot of Medical Stores attached to Headquarters 2 N.Z.E.F. at the Base camp. This was especially valuable as our Depot dealt with equipment supplied from private gifts and also that purchased through the Joint Council of St. John Ambulance and the Red Cross as well as the normal army supplies. The staff of the Depot had full knowledge of the needs, and especially the priorities, of the different medical units at different periods.

Apart from the major medical units smaller specialist units were formed.

A Venereal Disease Treatment Centre was established at the base camp hospital early in the war and Ablution Centres were associated with it. Later two centres with a R.A.M.C. establishment were formed and attached to two of the general hospitals. One of these was changed to a Mobile Unit with a special establishment and equipment for service with the divisional units, the first unit to be so constituted in the British Army.

A Field Surgical Team was formed during the pre-Alamein period.

A Field Transfusion Unit was formed also during the same period and continued to function until the end of the war. The first F.T. officer was the Pathologist of one of the general hospitals and subsequent officers were specially trained to carry on the work.

A Plastic Surgery Unit of both medical and dental officers was trained in England under Sir Harold Gillies and Sir Archibald McIndoe. Part of the unit was attached to the 2 N.Z.E.F. centred in one of the hospitals, also with trained medical officers in each of the other two hospitals. The main section was attached to a civil hospital in New Zealand where it dealt with the casualties evacuated to New Zealand and also with civilian patients.

STAFFING OF MEDICAL UNITS

Orthopaedic surgeons were appointed originally to the staffs of each of the three hospitals but it was not found possible to maintain this arrangement. At one period all three hospitals were without the services of an orthopaedic surgeon and for the greater part of the period in Italy only one orthopaedic surgeon was available, though fortunately general surgeons were able to cope with the situation.

No neuro-surgical unit was available. A neuro-surgeon and a neurologist were attached to the British neuro-surgical unit in Cairo for a period of 9 months, and they were available in one of the New Zealand hospitals in Cairo for some time before and after their attachment to the British unit.

There was no chest unit, patients being dealt with in our own hospitals. Some patients were admitted to British chest units both in Egypt and Italy.

There were no special ophthalmic units. Ophthalmic surgeons were attached to the staffs of our hospitals but, as in the case of the orthopaedic surgeon, in the latter part of the war individual hospitals were often without their services.

Ear, nose and throat surgeons were similarly attached and again the supply was insufficient to ensure regular staffing.

No special psychiatric unit was formed though psychiatrists in the medical corps were consulted and reported on individual cases and on psychiatric problems.

There were few specialist anaesthetists in New Zealand before the war and this again rendered it difficult to fill the positions overseas. Some younger officers were trained overseas and rendered satisfactory service.

Radiologists and technicians were attached to the hospitals but shortages again arose during the war and new staff had to be trained.

Experienced physicians and surgeons were available in excellent quality and number at the beginning of the war and the hospitals, when formed, were very well staffed. As the war progressed these staffs were depleted by the natural wastage through illness and by promotion to other branches of the corps so that there arose at frequent intervals urgent appeals for reinforcements from New Zealand, sometimes for physicians and more often for surgeons. The original staffs of the medical units had taken a considerable number of the senior men in the profession, and the necessity to provide medical personnel for the Pacific theatre of war and for the defence of New Zealand itself made it difficult to provide satisfactory reinforcements. There was also an impression in New Zealand, even in the National Medical Committee, that the Medical Corps in the 2 N.Z.E.F. was more than adequately equipped in hospitals and personnel to do its work, and that one hospital overseas was superfluous. The shortage of medical officers became very marked during the campaign in Italy and two physicians and one ophthalmologist were seconded from the R.A.M.C. The training of young surgeons was of great help but practically all specialist staffs were in short supply in Italy. The institution of the Social Security scheme in New Zealand at the beginning of the war added to the difficulties of adequate medical staffing in the civilian sphere, and this reacted on the availability of medical personnel for 2 N.Z.E.F. In the medical profession itself, specialisation had not reached an advanced stage in New Zealand before the war, and this again made it difficult to fill specialist posts in the hospitals overseas. On the other hand the broad experience of the New Zealand medical officer rendered him well able to deal with the work and problems he encountered. The war accelerated the development of specialisation in the profession in New Zealand, as to a lesser degree did the War of 1914–18. It is hoped that this will not mean a deterioration of the capacity of the average medical practitioner.

At first the Field Ambulances were staffed largely from men in the active Territorials, the majority being young active men in general practice, but including many specialists, as well as capable physicians and surgeons. Later, some of these were appointed to the staffs of the hospitals but there was always present in the ambulance staffs men capable of dealing with medical and surgical problems. The N.Z. Medical Corps' policy was always to ensure that in every field ambulance there should be one officer capable of handling major surgery, quite apart from the attachment of surgical teams in Field Surgical Units. The Mobile Surgical Unit and later the C.C.S. were both staffed adequately with well qualified and specialist personnel.

In general, the N.Z. Medical Corps had among its members medical officers and nursing sisters experienced in, or capable of rapid training in, practically all the problems of surgical or medical treatment met with during the war.

The Convalescent Depot was staffed with the general practitioner class of medical officer and stress was laid on having mature men able to sum up the convalescents and sustain their morale. The use made of the Convalescent Depot in 2 N.Z.E.F. differed considerably from that in the British Forces. In the 2 N.Z.E.F. the Depot was primarily used for the convalescent treatment of hospital patients, both medical and surgical, and recreational facilities were provided freely. Patients were sent from the hospitals with limbs still in plaster splints and in a condition quite unsuited to any marked physical activity. Military training was quite a secondary consideration, though physical training was undertaken when possible. This was in marked contrast to the British Convalescent Depot where rehabilitation in a military atmosphere was considered to be of prime importance, and where physical training under fully trained instructors was well carried out. The introduction of instructors of this type into the N.Z. Convalescent Depots would have been of considerable advantage.

The Rest Home established in Egypt and the Rest Camps in Italy were of great benefit. The Divisional Rest Camp, such as was set up during the Alamein period, proved its value by holding the physical exhaustion cases in the forward areas. The Field Ambulances themselves carried out the same function in Italy, where rest camps were also provided.

The New Zealand Forces Clubs were also used for the convalescence of officers in Italy.

IV. MEDICAL ADMINISTRATION AND CAMPAIGNS IN THE MIDDLE EAST

ARRIVAL OF FIRST NEW ZEALAND TROOPS IN EGYPT

The First Echelon, consisting of an infantry brigade with ancillary troops, including artillery and a Field Ambulance and Field Hygiene Section, landed in Egypt in February 1940. A small staff advance party, including a medical officer, had arrived a short time before. With the Echelon were the nursing sisters who had been allocated to the different transports.

CAMP ARRANGEMENTS IN EGYPT

The formation of the main camp in Egypt at Maadi near Cairo was well in hand when the First Echelon arrived. The troops were housed in huts with overflow in tents, and hutments were available for kitchen and mess rooms and for headquarters office accommodation, as well as for stores. Large areas of desert were available for drill and manoeuvres, and a railway to Cairo was about two miles distant.

The main difficulty was that of sanitation. The use of native labour called for special measures of cleanliness and medical examinations for detecting disease.

The Force developed the base area. Some of the troops were trained for desert warfare and were stationed in the Western Desert at Baggush before and during the First Libyan Campaign, but were not involved actively in the campaign. The Field Ambulance personnel gained experience of desert conditions and dealt with a number of casualties. A camp hospital was set up in Maadi and a Convalescent Depot at Ismalia.

On the whole the health of the troops was satisfactory. A series of Health Regulations was drawn up in Egypt in 1940 which gave adequate guidance in solving the problems encountered.

SECOND ECHELON IN ENGLAND

The Second Echelon formed part of the garrison of England during the Battle of Britain, and medically, had few problems. 1 N.Z. General Hospital was well sited in a newly built E.M.S. hospital in the country. It dealt with camp sick and many civilian bomb casualties from London. It also had to treat severe bombing casualties from a nearby aeroplane factory.

The field units had experience in manning positions in Southern England and in attending to casualties from bombing. A few New Zealand medical officers and sisters resident in the United Kingdom were recruited there but, apart from two other medical officers, no further New Zealanders were recruited in the United Kingdom for the N.Z.M.C. during the war. This policy was followed at the request of the D.G.M.S. R.A.M.C. who pointed out the great difficulties the United Kingdom had in supplying M.Os. for the Services, as well as for the numerous E.M.S. and civilian hospitals dealing with the large numbers of casualties from bombing. Almost all the New Zealand medical men resident in the United Kingdom were young men studying for senior degrees or gaining further hospital experience—just the type and age most suitable for the Army or E.M.S. hospitals, as indeed they would have been for service in our own 2 N.Z.E.F. During the later years of the war, the New Zealand Medical Corps in the C.M.F. was at times very short of well trained physicians and surgeons and would have eagerly welcomed New Zealand men of that type who were in the United Kingdom. But it is gratifying that young New Zealanders did provide much well appreciated help to the army and civil medical staffs in the United Kingdom throughout the war, and so relieved their kinsmen in a time of great stress.

ADMINISTRATION AND BASE UNITS IN EGYPT

Administration in Egypt was reorganised at the end of 1940. A 2 N.Z.E.F. Headquarters was set up in Maadi apart from the Headquarters of the 2 N.Z. Division. This necessitated the appointment of an A.D.M.S. N.Z. Division in addition to the D.M.S. 2 N.Z.E.F., who exercised control over the whole 2 N.Z.E.F. Later in the middle of 1941, the Consulting Physician and the Consultant Surgeon were given independent appointments and detached from the staff of a hospital. The decision not to send a hospital unit with the First Echelon led to difficulties in Egypt, which were accentuated by the sending of the Second Echelon with its attached hospital unit to the United Kingdom. It was soon realised that some hospital provision was necessary, in spite of the fact that an efficient British hospital was receiving our patients and employing a New Zealand staff to look after them. The only personnel available were those of the 4th Field Ambulance, and by using them the Field Ambulance was necessarily thrown out of action both as regards training and possible active operations. On the other hand the staff attached to the British Hospital gained very valuable experience, especially in hospital administration, and this was passed on later to other members of the N.Z.M.C. A hospital staff was assembled and a building, which remained as a New Zealand hospital throughout the war, was procured at Helwan. Two extra surgeons were flown from New Zealand to strengthen the unit, and later Australian medical officers and Australian and British sisters were attached at different periods until 2 N.Z. G.H. arrived and took over the hospital, the temporary unit being disbanded. Thus a valuable lesson was learnt in that adequate provision of medical services, including hospitals, must be provided for any combatant force. Unless circumstances are exceptionally favourable it is not advisable to rely on any other force to provide such services.

CAMPAIGN IN GREECE

This problem also arose during the Greek campaign, the first operations to which New Zealand troops were committed. The A.D.M.S. (Divisional) did not proceed to Greece with the first flight of troops, though on arrival he had to accept responsibility for arranging medical services for the forward areas. D.M.S. 2 N.Z.E.F., who had control of 1 N.Z. G.H. sent to Greece, did not arrive in Greece until much later. In the meantime difficulties arose as to the siting of the hospital and the sending of further base medical units. There is no doubt that if he had been permitted to proceed to Greece earlier he could have helped considerably in solving the local problems. In any case he would have appreciated the local position. In Greece the D.M.S. B.T.G. was faced with several problems especially associated with the lines of communication. The only medical units he had were Field Ambulances, two C.C.Ss. and 600-bed General Hospitals. The hospitals were very well equipped and staffed base hospitals, eminently suitable for base hospital work in such a base as Athens, but quite unsuited to lines of communication work in the centre of Greece. Their elaborate staffs and bulky and heavy equipment made them difficult to handle and to move. They were over-equipped in every way for L. of C. work. The D.M.S. needed smaller hospitals with less equipment and smaller staffs, as were later constituted by the R.A.M.C. 1 N.Z.G.H. at Pharsala, where

Caesar and Pompey fought, was able to do very little serious medical work as all serious cases, quite rightly, were sent on by train to Athens. During the retreat the hospital lost practically all its valuable equipment, and only good fortune saved the staff.

The field units learned their first lessons of active warfare, and also the wisdom of displaying the Red Cross to secure protection for their patients and personnel. The Field Ambulances dealt with many battle casualties, especially in the Servia area, where the evacuation of the wounded proved difficult. Excellent work was also done during the hurried evacuation to the Thermopylae line and later to the beaches, from which, fortunately, the ambulance units were evacuated largely intact, though without their heavy equipment. The ambulances transferred their patients to the Australian and British C.C.Ss. where forward surgery was carried out, utilising the efficient Australian M.A.C. There were few good roads and the greater part of the Force had to retreat along the main road south from Larisa, with inevitable congestion and vulnerability to attack by German planes, which had practically complete control of the air after the small British air force had been eliminated.

Misunderstanding arose with regard to the destruction of equipment, owing to a corps order not having taken the medical aspect into consideration and to lack of knowledge of the terms of the Geneva Convention. Fortunately little damage was done.

The Navy was successful in evacuating the greater part of the Force from beaches scattered over the eastern coast of Greece from the east of Athens to the southernmost tip of the country, a brilliant achievement.

The breakdown of railway evacuation added to the difficulties, as did the absence of wireless in medical units. The general health of the troops was excellent, the rations were good and no malaria was encountered as the season for it had not started.

CAMPAIGN IN CRETE

The N.Z. Division was evacuated to Crete, where two of the three brigades and detachments of other arms remained to take part in the defence of the island. The Division lost nearly all its equipment in Greece and all its artillery, and the Field Ambulances were in like plight. The Field Hygiene Section had also lost its equipment. In general the field medical units had to function with what equipment had been carried out of Greece by the personnel, and with what few supplies were available from 7 British General Hospital in Crete. One 15 cwt. truck was available to each field ambulance and eight ambulance cars were available for the whole force, another three cars arriving later. There were few telephones and none in the medical units.

Roads were few, the main ones running along the northern coast. That across the island to Sphakia was narrow and hilly and faded out a few miles from the southern coast. The lack of transport and the condition of the roads made it impossible to evacuate any serious cases from Sphakia, though many sick and wounded struggled courageously across the island. Absence of transport also made it difficult to evacuate cases from the forward areas to the hospital at Canea. Thus, as in Greece, all the severely wounded men not evacuated early by hospital ship were captured. Treatment of the seriously wounded was difficult in the disturbed conditions and no blood transfusion was available. Medical supplies were limited, partly because of loss at sea and partly because of the bombing of 7 British General Hospital.

The siting of the Medical Units proved difficult, especially on account of the unusual type of paratroop attack. It was difficult to site the units away from the main roads which were bombed and machine gunned. Road junctions were also dangerous. One unit sought protection under a culvert, which was also a target for the planes. Separation from combatant troops was desirable yet protection from the paratroops was necessary. 7 British General Hospital was bombed before the main attack and then became a target for bombing and machine gunning. Both the hospital and our own 6 Field Ambulance adjoining were captured by paratroops and the staff and patients rounded up and escorted away towards a German assembly area, only to come in contact with our own troops and suffer several casualties. These incidents caused doubt as to whether the Germans adhered to the Geneva Convention, especially as one of our medical officers was shot dead by a paratrooper during the attack, and the hospital ship *Aba* was bombed at sea during the same period. On the other hand ambulance cars and trucks with prominent Red Cross markings were not molested. The battle casualties were very heavy and the mortality high. Many wounded and other troops, including medical personnel, became prisoners-of-war.

The health of the troops in Crete was good in spite of some reduction in rations. The malaria season, as in Greece, had not begun. Some dysentery was present during the last days of the campaign and water supplies from the wells became contaminated. In spite of the severity of the fighting and the heavy casualties little anxiety neurosis was noted in Egypt after the withdrawal.

As a sequel to the difficulties during the evacuation the employment of down-graded men in the Division was considered inadvisable by the combatant officers. Similar conditions, however, were not experienced again during the war.

REORGANISATION IN EGYPT

The Division was re-equipped satisfactorily in Egypt. Reinforcements arrived quickly from New Zealand and training was resumed in the base camps and then in the Canal Zone. The medical units were reorganised, with many staff changes. The Mobile Surgical Unit, a gift of Sir Arthur Sims, was provided with an official establishment and staff, and the re-equipment was completed.

PROBLEMS OF STAFFING

During this resting phase several problems arose. In 2 N.Z.E.F. the establishments of medical units were based strictly on the R.A.M.C. manual.

There was provision for a fixed number of senior officers in the hospital units and rank was granted accordingly. In the R.A.M.C., however, medical officers with senior qualifications were granted major's rank automatically if they could be classified as specialists, and young men who had recently gained higher qualifications were in general granted the rank. In our hospitals there were many medical officers who had held higher degrees for many years, and who were leading men in the profession, yet had only the rank of captain. This anomaly was never corrected, but in time the senior rank was obtained by most of the affected officers by their promotion to senior appointments. The promotion of higher grade specialists to Lt.-Colonel rank was, in the latter part of the war, granted to two of our officers, who were employed to a great extent as consultants in ophthalmology and psychiatry. These are problems that necessarily arise in what one may call a citizen army. The promotion of N.C.Os. also provided problems at this period as so many men holding this rank came over in the reinforcements, and so were competing with men with long experience in the corps in the Middle East. This problem was in general solved by the reduction to the ranks of the reinforcement N.C.Os.

Owing to the loss of M.Os. in Greece and Crete a shortage of specialists arose, and two New Zealand surgeons were obtained from the United Kingdom.

There also arose an excess of graded men owing partly to the employment of Egyptian labour at the Base Camp.

At that time the Convalescent Depot sited at Moascar was rendered ineffective by heavy bombing of the Canal and was moved back to the Base Camp.

SECOND LIBYAN CAMPAIGN

The N.Z. Division was involved in the Second Libyan Campaign at the end of 1941 and became one of the original divisions of Eighth Army, which was formed at this time. Arrangements were made for the Medical Corps to service the Division as far as its medical units would allow, the only deficiency in the New Zealand medical chain being a C.C.S., which had not yet been formed.

Three field ambulances and the Mobile Surgical Unit were attached to the Division, the Mobile Surgical Unit acting as a light section of a C.C.S. attached to the field ambulances. An A.D.S. was attached to each brigade. Evacuation from the field ambulances was carried out by a British Motor Ambulance Convoy to a medical centre behind the Libyan frontier at the railhead, from which evacuation to the Base was arranged by train, air, or coastal road, with a relay of hospitals on the line of communication, including 2 N.Z. G.H. at Garawla. A 200-bed detachment of 3 N.Z. G.H. was set up at Alexandria and the other two N.Z. hospitals, 1 and 3 N.Z. G.H. were sited in the Cairo area.

In the forward area arrangements had been made to have medical relay posts set up every 25 miles, but the fluid nature of the battle soon rendered this quite impossible. The separate field medical units could not be protected, and eventually all three M.D.Ss. and the Mobile Surgical Unit were congregated in one wadi where they were held captive by the enemy for some ten days, the majority of the personnel being taken away to Italy as P.O.Ws. before relief came. All medical units, except one A.D.S., were captured at one time or another during the campaign.

Lack of wireless was again a great disability and prevented the captured medical centre from making known its plight and its shortage of food and water. Evacuation of casualties over the Desert was rendered very difficult by the marauding mobile units of both forces, and also by the changes in the position of medical units necessitated by these conditions. The rough desert terrain made the journey very irksome for the patients, especially at night. Casualties were heavy and, although the Mobile Surgical Unit proved very efficient and the units were well staffed for carrying out surgery, the conditions under which they worked prevented satisfactory results.

Shortage of water proved serious and abdominal cases in particular died of dehydration. Blood transfusion was not available in the forward areas nor were other intravenous transfusions. Food also was short and had to be strictly rationed. In general the medical units had no difficulty with the Germans, but found the Italians less co-operative and guilty of pilfering.

Altogether 44 per cent. of the medical personnel were taken away as P.O.Ws. and there was a heavy loss of equipment and transport. The lessons of the campaign were that more medical supplies were needed, and that less equipment would have rendered the field units more mobile. More transport (lorries and ambulances) were necessary and they should have had larger Red Cross markings. Wireless was again considered vitally essential for field units in the Desert. The attachment of surgical teams had proved of great value and it was considered that their use should be extended even to brigade groups. At the hospital on the L. of C., where seriously wounded cases were dealt with, it was considered that more blood transfusion should be given in the forward areas and more provision made for holding serious cases in the L. of C. At the Base few men with abdominal injuries were seen, but the others generally arrived in good condition. The condition of the wounded was evaluated at a surgical conference held in Cairo after the campaign. Special consideration was given to the value of blood transfusions, the success of the Tobruk splint for fractured femur, the treatment of secondary haemorrhage, the necessity to conserve as much of the limb as possible in amputations and the desirability of treating head injuries at the Base.

REORGANISATION IN EGYPT

On return to Egypt reorganisation and re-equipping had again to be undertaken, and fresh reinforcements from New Zealand had to be integrated into the Division. Fortunately these came quickly, but after that no further reinforcements arrived for over twelve months because of the extra commitments in the Pacific following Japan's entry into the war.

Serious casualties were returned to New Zealand expeditiously by the N.Z. Hospital Ship *Maunganui* and the Netherlands Hospital Ship *Oranje*.

The first W.A.A.Cs. arrived from New Zealand at this time, supplementing the staffs of the hospitals. Convalescent Homes were instituted in Cairo and Alexandria for sisters, officers and other ranks. A Depot of Medical Stores was set up in Maadi and a separate Red Cross administration was established. Special V.D. treatment centres were established at two of the hospitals.

A Motor Ambulance Convoy, an A.S.C. unit, was formed from ambulances handed over by the Australians and from others donated by the U.S.A., New Zealand and Scotland.

A Plastic Surgery Unit, for use in New Zealand and in the Middle East, and whose personnel had been trained in England, was formed and a section set up in one of the hospitals, where a saline bath unit was installed.

Some medical personnel captured in Libya were returned to Egypt at this time and were all sent back to New Zealand, as there was at first some uncertainty as to whether they could, under the Geneva Convention, be re-employed in the same theatre of war. Many, including senior medical officers, were later posted to the Pacific Forces. 1 N.Z. C.C.S. was finally established, absorbing the Mobile Surgical Unit as its light section and, after being fully equipped, was first used when the Division was sent to Syria.

CLASSIFICATION OF INVALIDS ON HOSPITAL SHIPS

At this period misunderstandings arose as to the classification of invalids for return to New Zealand by hospital ship, and the Germans intimated that the *Oranje* would not be entitled to protection under the Geneva Convention because she had carried personnel not in the proper categories. The nomenclature used purely for hospital ship purposes, clashed with the ordinary R.A.M.C. classification of invalids. A new classification cleared up the difficulty, though no alteration was made in the type of patients sent by the hospital ships.

DIVISION IN SYRIA

After training in combined operations in the Canal Zone the Division was sent to Syria to man the defensive positions between the Lebanon and Anti-Lebanon mountains, chiefly in the Baalbek area where the field medical units were at first sited. Later, one of the units manned a small hospital in Aleppo when some of the troops were stationed on the Turko-Syrian border.

The C.C.S. was established at Zahle, 2 N.Z. G.H. at Nazareth, 3 N.Z. G.H. at Beirut and the Convalescent Depot, along with the Advanced Base, at Kfar Vtikin in Palestine. Special training was carried out by the field medical units and an underground dressing station was constructed. The main medical problems encountered were malaria, sandfly fever and venereal disease. A complete anti-malaria organisation was set up within the Division, and officers were trained at the British Malaria Field Laboratory. The heavily infected areas were mapped out and preventive measures adopted, including special clothing and nets and cream. Swamps were drained and sprayed. Controlled brothels were set up and inspections carried out, and warning against venereal disease given to the troops.

DIVISION RETURNS TO WESTERN DESERT— PRE-ALAMEIN

There was now a rapid return of the Division to the Desert, following the success of Rommel's attack in Libya in May 1942 and the fall of Tobruk. The Division, with two field ambulances attached, was rushed to Mersa Matruh. Twenty A.F.S. (American Field Service) ambulance cars were attached, to begin a long association with the Division. Then followed the battle of Mersa Matruh when the Division was encircled at Minqar Qaim by the Germans and forced its way out of the trap during the night back to the Alamein line, the line previously prepared for the defence of Egypt. During the withdrawal casualties were evacuated satisfactorily in spite of the difficulties encountered. Individual R.M.Os. also took out groups of casualties independently.

The two field ambulances were then stationed behind the Alamein line, with evacuation by British M.A.Cs. to a medical centre, formed by a British C.C.S., at Gharbanyat. Then followed several battles to defend the line, the New Zealand Division suffering very heavy casualties. The M.D.Ss. were assisted by surgical teams from a British C.C.S. and later by an attached British F.T.U. Some evacuation to Cairo was carried out successfully by both ambulance and ordinary transport planes. Two of these planes were brought down. Blood transfusion was now used extensively, the excellent transfusion service based in Cairo proving very efficient. The early surgical treatment of the casualties at the M.D.S., the short lines of communication both to the medical centre and to the Base Hospitals, the excellent splinting of fractures and the use of blood and sulphonamides, all contributed to excellent results of surgical treatment. It was found that evacuation by plane was detrimental to patients suffering from abdominal injuries, and to those with chest injuries involving disturbance of respiration. As a result of this observation these patients were held at the operating centre for 10 days, and beds and better nursing facilities were provided. This gave improved results. The patients with abdominal injuries were dealt with by exteriorisation of the damaged colon, by gastric suction and continuous intravenous glucose and saline infusion, as well as by blood transfusions. This treatment had become stabilised. Sterilised dressings, including vaseline gauze and *tulle gras*, had been made available from the base in Cairo, and sulphonamide medication, both by mouth and locally, was used systematically. Tannic acid treatment of burns had been discarded in favour of local and general sulphonamides, and saline baths. Pentothal was used freely as an anaesthetic, with good results.

The health of the troops, in spite of the rigorous conditions, was generally good, but there was a rather high sick rate from dysentery, and later a severe epidemic of infective hepatitis.

The Hygiene Section did not function at first because of lack of transport, but later had to contend with a serious plague of flies as the terrain became fouled, both from native camps and then from the troops, especially in the enemy lines.

Hepatitis had been present in the enemy troops for some time, and New Zealand troops occupied ground which had been occupied by the Italians. Investigations pointed to the disease being spread by intestinal infection, and this was confirmed later. The disease, though not fatal, caused severe debility and required a long convalescence of 4 to 6 weeks. However, from evidence obtained later, it seems that the health of the New Zealand troops at that time was infinitely better than that of the enemy forces. This probably contributed to the exhaustion of their forces and the eventual victory at Alamein. Brigadier Ardagh stressed the reasons for the success achieved in the treatment of casualties at that period:—

(a) Early collection and evacuation from place of injury to the nearest station providing surgery.

(b) Provision of resuscitation at A.D.S. and/or M.D.S.

(c) Provision of efficient surgery as nearly as possible within the optimum period of six to twelve hours.

A summary of the lessons learnt was:

(1) The importance of a considerable increase in the number of ambulance cars in the forward area.

(2) The value of early blood transfusion, with the attachment of a F.T.U. to the operating M.D.S.

(3) The need for the attachment of at least two surgical teams and a nursing section from a C.C.S. to the M.D.S. to ensure skilled surgery and post-operation nursing.

(4) Early air evacuation is dangerous for patients with abdominal injuries and for those with chest injuries and having distress in respiration. It is eminently suitable for all other cases.

(5) Wireless inter-communication between medical units is desirable in mobile warfare.

(6) The value of sterilised dressings forwarded from the base.

At this time the question of psychoneurosis and its association with army classification was considered. Men from the forward areas suffering from anxiety states were being described as Battle Casualties. This was illogical, and it was decided that only casualties actually associated with battle injury should be described as Battle Casualties. A new designation of physical exhaustion was adopted to describe the condition of men suffering from battle strain.

BATTLE OF EL ALAMEIN

The Division was withdrawn for special training before the battle of El Alamein as it had been decided to attach it to an armoured corps during the battle.

During the training a medical plan of evacuating casualties through the minefields was worked out. This was successfully used during the battle and it subsequently became the standard plan in Eighth Army.

For the battle A.D.Ss. were attached to the brigades. The M.D.Ss. were largely concentrated around the Alamein railway station where two underground dressing stations were constructed. The N.Z. operating

M.D.S. with two surgical teams attached, was alongside the road further east. Behind the M.D.Ss. was the medical centre at Gharbanyat, alongside the old inland road, where three C.C.Ss. were grouped, including 1 N.Z. C.C.S.

A British Field Ambulance was sited just in front of this group and sorted out the cases, dealing itself with the light cases and evacuating them back beyond the C.C.Ss. Ample ambulance cars were available and evacuation from the medical centre was by train, air or road, the road cases going to Alexandria and the others to Cairo or the Canal Area. F.S. Units and F.T. Units were more freely available and the New Zealand Forces had their own F.T.U. for the first time.

A rest station was set up by one of the N.Z. M.D.Ss. on the coast end of the medical centre and light cases, especially the physical exhaustion cases, were dealt with there, the first time they had been treated in a M.D.S.

ADVANCE TO TRIPOLI

In the advance to Tripoli, following the battle of Alamein, the three Field Ambulances continued to function as at the Alamein period. Surgical teams and the transfusion unit were attached to the active M.D.Ss., which often leap-frogged each other, leaving one of their number behind to nurse, and then evacuate, the serious casualties following operation. The Division rested for a period in the Bardia area and prepared for the advance on the Agedabia area, where it was given the task of carrying out a left hook over difficult sandy country. For this manoeuvre elaborate preparations were made to enable major surgical operations of all types to be performed, and casualties carried forward or held and nursed deep in the desert, extra ambulance cars being provided. The C.C.S. was sited at Agedabia at that time, and then moved on to Tamet where it dealt with many casualties from the British Divisions in the coastal zone. In the final advance to Tripoli—another left hook—full use was made of evacuation by transport planes, and medical units were set up at all the landing strips to hold and nurse patients and make arrangements with the Air Force for their evacuation. The M.D.Ss. of the Field Ambulances had surgical teams and F.T. Units attached and carried out all the necessary major surgery, including abdominal surgery. Serious mine casualties occured at that time, but other casualties were relatively light. Good use was made of air evacuation, and medical officers proved excellent liaison officers with the Air Force.

At Tripoli Field Ambulances were at first used for hospital work until the C.C.Ss. and general hospitals were able to take over. The Field Hygiene Section helped in the management and control of sanitary arrangements in the city, where fortunately the water and sewage systems were intact. British hospitals were soon functioning in satisfactory buildings, and later on 3 N.Z. G.H. was brought from Beirut to set up a tented hospital around one of the old forts not far from the large civil aerodrome.

The Division moved on to Medenine urgently when Rommel threatened attack following his temporary success against First Army.

MEDENINE

The Field Ambulances set up their dressing stations around Medenine and the light section of the C.C.S. combined with sections of British Field Ambulances to form an operating centre at Medenine, where the forward surgery was undertaken. The main body of the C.C.S. was moved back to Ben Gardane where British C.C.Ss. were sited to form a medical centre from which casualties were evacuated back by road to Tripoli.

Fortunately the German attack was a disastrous failure and there were few British or New Zealand casualties.

BATTLE OF MARETH

Then followed the Mareth battle when the Division, with other troops under command to form a corps, again carried out a left hook to the Tebaga Gap through very difficult sandy terrain. The main evacuation route to Medenine was in the hands of the enemy, and the route over the desert was so rough that serious casualties could not be sent that way.

Provision was, therefore, again made to do all the necessary surgery at the M.D.S., with attached surgical teams and F.T.Us., and extra nursing staff supplied from the C.C.S. Ample blood supplies were carried. A landing strip was prepared by the Field Ambulance personnel near the M.D.S. and the serious casualties flown out, largely by transport planes, to Medenine where the N.Z. C.C.S. and two British C.C.Ss. were functioning as a forward medical centre. The Field Ambulances dealt efficiently with the heavy casualties from N.Z., British and enemy forces, finally sending back a large convoy by the main Hallouf road to Medenine after the Indian troops had cleared the enemy from the area. The transport planes carried back the serious casualties and brought supplies, including blood, to the Forces.

After the defeat of the enemy by the left hook at Tebaga the Division, with its field medical units, went ahead to Gabes, and the C.C.S. came up from Medenine with the two British C.C.Ss. to set up another medical centre behind Akarit where the next battle was fought. The N.Z. Division was not primarily involved, but pushed through after the main attack and passed quickly up into Tunisia to the Enfidaville area, where the enemy again made a stand. The field ambulances went with the Division and dealt with the few casualties, mainly mine injuries, sustained. The C.C.S. dealt with the heavy casualties from the British divisions. This was one of the two C.C.Ss. undertaking surgery. During the advance to Tripoli British units had been attached to the C.C.S., partly to replace the surgical team and F.T.U., which had been sent forward to the Division. The British teams consisted of a F.S.U., a neuro-surgical unit, an ophthalmic unit and a F.T.U., all of excellent quality. The neuro-surgical unit consisted of a section of the first neuro-surgical unit formed for work in forward areas, the other section being attached to a British hospital at Tripoli. The unit, under Major Eden, did outstanding work and proved beyond question the advantages of operating on men with head injuries in forward areas, especially to prevent infection, the main cause of secondary morbidity and mortality in head wounds.

The ophthalmic unit dealt with wounds of the eye and extracted foreign bodies with an electric magnet. Difficulties were encountered in dealing with the many non-magnetic fragments.

The association of the three C.C.Ss. in one group was one of the outstanding medical successes of the war, and the sorting out and distribution of the patients to the different C.C.Ss. was well carried out.

ADVANCE TO ENFIDAVILLE

In the advance to Enfidaville the C.C.S. moved up to El Djem, some distance behind the active M.D.S. at Sidi Bou Ali, and the M.D.S., with its attached F.S.U. and F.T.U., acted as the forward operating centre for the Division as well as for other troops in the area. Later the C.C.S. moved up to the same area, took over the major surgery and remained there until the end of the campaign. The field ambulances were busily engaged during the attack on Takrouna, where the R.A.Ps. and A.D.Ss. worked well under difficult conditions. The M.D.S. at that time also carried out the major surgical work and dealt with large numbers of casualties.

RETURN TO EGYPT

After the campaign the Division moved back to Cairo by stages, and the field ambulances went with it. The C.C.S. halted at Tripoli for a while, assisting in the treatment of British battle casualties and malaria cases from Sicily, and then moved to Cairo. 3 N.Z. G.H. and a section of the Convalescent Depot remained at Tripoli, assisting in the treatment of British troops and proceeded to Italy shortly after the Division had landed there.

On the return of the Division to Maadi the medical units were given instruction in the prevention and treatment of malaria, a disease which had caused so many casualties in Sicily. Young medical officers from the Division were attached to the hospitals to acquire experience.

The release of men of the three Echelons for furlough leave to New Zealand came into operation for all except medical officers. Married men were given preference and balloting by the single men took place for the remaining places in the first draft. The granting of leave after a period of three years overseas would appear to have been a reasonable reward, but the return of the men to the environment of New Zealand and their families proved to be psychologically disturbing, both to the men themselves and to the population in general.

In effect few of the furlough men returned to the Middle East. It was generally felt that their places should have been filled by fresh recruits. This experience shows how unwise it would be to send troops back to New Zealand in any future war, except for home service or discharge.

The Divisional troops were prepared for the Italian campaign and were marched from Maadi to a concentration area at Burg el Arab, ready for embarkation from Alexandria. The marching was part of a hardening up process in preparation for the campaign, and many of the men suffered from foot fatigue after the march.

V. MEDICAL ADMINISTRATION AND CAMPAIGNS IN ITALY

The Division crossed to Taranto without mishap, and was stationed on flat land alongside the inner harbour. Malaria precautions were taken at once. A M.D.S. was established in a school at Taranto and functioned satisfactorily. A British hospital and an Indian C.C.S. were also available there. 3 N.Z. G.H. and the Convalescent Depot, were sited in the medical clinic area at Bari, a very large and elaborate hospital centre just being built to serve a large area of Southern Italy. Arrangements were quickly made to staff and equip the hospital, and a Convalescent Depot was established in an old school building in Casamassina, a small town inland from Bari. The winter climate necessitated the use of buildings.

BATTLE OF THE SANGRO

After a short period at Taranto the Division moved up to take part in the Battle of the Sangro, and the Field Ambulances moved up with the troops. Buildings were used wherever possible. Transport was rendered difficult because of the condition of the roads.

The medical chain for this battle consisted of an operating M.D.S. based at Attessa, to deal with the casualties, a medical M.D.S. quartered at Gissi, another small village in the hills, and an A.D.S. in the Sangro river valley to collect cases as they were evacuated over the river. R.M.Os. and stretcher bearers went across the river when the advance started and established R.A.Ps., and later an A.D.S. and ambulance cars went across. At first evacuation was very difficult as one of the two bridges had been destroyed and the river was flooded. Dressing stations sent over the river were set up in small buildings. Fully established A.D.Ss. were not employed.

Later, the operating M.D.S. was formed by another Field Ambulance well across the river at Castelfrentano, where the casualties from the Orsogna battle were received. The treatment and evacuation of these casualties proved difficult in the open exposed country. Most of the surgery, including abdominal surgery, was performed at this M.D.S. Extra surgical teams were supplied, including one from the Paratroop Brigade attached to the Division. From the M.D.S. the casualties were evacuated to the N.Z. C.C.S., set up in a schoolhouse at Vasto not very far away, but their transport at times was difficult. A British Field Surgical Unit and a Transfusion Team were attached to the C.C.S. Head injuries were referred to 5 British C.C.S., also stationed in Vasto, as it had a neuro-surgical unit attached.

Casualties were evacuated by road from Vasto to Termoli which was the railhead at that time, and where two British C.C.Ss. were eventually sited to act as holding centres controlling the train evacuation. Damage to the bridges over the Trigno interfered with train evacuation at one time. The winter weather, including a period of snow, held up the advance. The Division was learning that the Italian winter, though not prolonged, could be relatively severe. Nursing sisters were attached to the N.Z. M.D.S. for the first time during the war and proved their worth, particularly in nursing men with abdominal injuries. From Termoli casualties were evacuated to the Hospital Centre at Bari where 3 N.Z. G.H. was well established with a British General Hospital, which later had a chest centre attached, alongside.

CASSINO

After the stalemate at Orsogna the Division moved across the peninsula to the Cassino front and medical units were established, though not without difficulty as the best sites had already been occupied by the American Army. The wet weather and the mud hampered the setting up of the units and road metal had to be used in large quantities. Again an operating M.D.S. was established while another M.D.S. held minor sick. Two A.D.Ss. were set up on the plain towards Cassino. The Division was used as the nucleus of a Corps and the medical units had to deal with heavy casualties. Malaria precautions were taken, as the area was malarious, and their effectiveness was shown by the low incidence in the Division. Mepacrine tablets were taken regularly. The weather at Cassino again held up operations and the fighting was stubborn. The Division was moved to the mountain sector inland from Cassino after the failure of the first assaults.

The C.C.S. was at Presenzano, within easy distance of the active M.D.S., and this made it possible for the severely wounded men, including those with abdominal injuries, to be operated on at the C.C.S., where British Field Surgical and Transfusion Units were still attached. Men with head injuries were referred to an American Field Hospital nearby, where a neuro-surgeon was available.

From the C.C.S. evacuation was by road to 2 N.Z. G.H., now established at Caserta, the neuro-surgical cases going to the British unit attached to a British Hospital at Naples. All the other wounded men were dealt with by the N.Z. hospital at Caserta except those with fractured femurs, who were sent on to the N.Z. hospital at Bari as soon as possible for penicillin treatment. Evacuation to Bari was by hospital train. At 3 N.Z. G.H. Bari, which acted as the Base Hospital during the whole period in Italy, patients were held and treated until they were ready for discharge to the base depot in Italy, situated between Bari and Taranto, or to the Convalescent Depot at Santo Spirito, close to Bari.

Patients medically boarded for evacuation to New Zealand were first sent to 1 N.Z. G.H. Cairo for transfer to hospital ship. Later N.Z. hospital ships were sent to Taranto to embark the invalids.

After the Cassino battle the Division rested for a while at Arce, the C.C.S. moving forward to Frosinone.

BATTLE FOR FLORENCE

The next active period was the battle for Florence in which the Division was involved in some heavy fighting in the main thrust from Siena.

Lines of communication now became somewhat elongated, the base hospitals still being sited mainly in the Naples area, while some were in Rome. The difficulties of evacuation were mostly overcome by the use of air transport from an airfield on the western shore of Lake Trasimene, from which patients were flown to Rome and Naples.

The Field Medical Units worked in rotation and an increasing number of seriously wounded men, including those with abdominal injuries, were operated on in the M.D.Ss., with surgical teams and transfusion units attached.

The C.C.S., sited at Siena, dealt with large numbers of casualties and evacuated them by road to British units near Lake Trasimene, for eventual air evacuation to the hospital at Caserta.

RETURN TO THE ADRIATIC

After Florence was captured the New Zealand Division returned to the Adriatic front to take part in the battles around Rimini and later in the Po valley.

1 N.Z. G.H., which had been sent across to Italy as a 600-bed unit, leaving a small 400-bed hospital behind at Helwan, had been sited at

Molfetta on the Adriatic coast, where it partially relieved 3 N.Z. G.H. at Bari. It was then sent forward to Senigallia, north of Ancona, to serve the Division at Rimini, and was well established by the time the Division was in action. The hospital was set up in buildings of an old health camp. Huts and tents were used for extra accommodation for patients and staff.

The field units were actively involved behind Rimini and after the advance, treated many of the seriously wounded men. The N.Z. F.S.U. and F.T.U. were both attached to the field units. The C.C.S. was not used at first, but it supplied a surgical team to the Canadian C.C.S. nearby which was undertaking the major forward surgery.

The value of the newly established smaller British hospital units was demonstrated at that period, when neuro-surgical, ophthalmic and chest units were operating in one of these hospitals close alongside the C.C.Ss. This was undoubtedly a great advance in the treatment of specialist types of wounds, and the attachment of a general surgical team made provision for cases of multiple injuries.

Later, when the Army entered the Po valley, the C.C.S. was located in a large school at Forli, and the forward evacuation was such that nearly all the major surgery was carried out there, where normally the F.S.U. and F.T.U. were attached. The field units dealt with some casualties, especially during the battle for Faenza. Conditions in the Po valley during the winter brought fighting to a standstill, and the greater part of the Division was brought back to the Fabriano area for a few weeks' rest, before a further attack was made.

Communications with the Po valley rapidly improved so that during the second period in the valley the railhead had reached Forli, and it was possible to send casualties by rail or road through to the hospital at Senigallia. They were rested on the way, when necessary, in a British hospital unit.

Air evacuation now became available, and patients were flown not only to Senigallia but also to Bari for admission to 3 N.Z. G.H. This proved so satisfactory that many of the wounded had their primary wound treatment at Senigallia and Bari, and delayed primary suture of all suitable cases was routinely carried out with great success.

With the rapid advance across the Po valley towards Trieste the lines of communication became extended. The field units had to leap-frog behind the Division, split up into sections, and deal with the casualties or hold them pending evacuation. Fortunately casualties were few. The C.C.S. later moved to Mestre outside Venice but again the field units went forward and lost contact until eventually the C.C.S. moved to Udine.

At Udine air evacuation was used when available. During this period 2 N.Z. G.H. at Caserta was off the line of evacuation of New Zealand casualties and was largely used to deal with British cases, thereby easing the work of the British hospitals in the Naples area. It had been planned that the whole hospital would be moved to the Po valley when circumstances warranted it, but the campaign moved so swiftly that all that could be done was to send forward a section of the staff to reinforce the C.C.S., first at Forli, and then at Mestre and Udine.

END OF FIGHTING IN ITALY

When the campaign was over and the enemy had surrendered the forward medical units dealt with accidental injuries and sickness, and set up rest camps for the Divisional troops. A marked increase in the incidence of venereal disease occurred at that time and continued while the troops were in the Trieste and Florence areas.

The Division moved from Trieste first to Trasimene and then to Florence, the field medical units accompanying it. The C.C.S. moved across to Assisi. Medical units were then reorganised for duty in Japan but when Japan surrendered only occupation duties remained. The C.C.S. became incorporated in a small hospital at Florence and a Rest Home was set up nearby.

VI. DEMOBILISATION OF 2 N.Z.E.F. STATISTICAL DATA AND EVACUATION OF CASUALTIES

DEMOBILISATION OF MEDICAL UNITS

After the end of the Italian campaign there was a gradual disbandment of the medical units. The Field Ambulances were disbanded at Trasimene, 1 N.Z. G.H. at Senigallia. 2 N.Z. G.H. was moved back to Egypt to take over the Helwan hospital from the Section of 1 N.Z. G.H. which had been left behind there. The section of the Convalescent Depot which had been sited at Senigallia was disbanded, and the Santo Spirito section continued to deal with patients referred from 3 N.Z. G.H., which remained in action at Bari until nearly all N.Z. troops had left Italy. It was then disbanded.

The depot of medical stores which had been sited at Bari, with a section at Senigallia, dealt with all the medical equipment handed in by the disbanding units. It also arranged with the British depot for stores to equip the New Zealand Force being sent to Japan and to collect and send to New Zealand the complete equipment of 3 Field Ambulances, a C.C.S. and two 600-bed general hospitals. The winding up in Italy was expeditiously carried out and 98 British Hospital at Bari dealt with the last patients after 3 N.Z. G.H. had closed. The H.S. *Maunganui* took on patients for evacuation to New Zealand at Taranto on February 11, 1946. This marked the end of the New Zealand medical services in Italy.

DEMOBILISATION IN EGYPT

In Egypt 2 N.Z. G.H. at Helwan was closed and a 100-bed expansion at 15 British General Hospital for New Zealand patients was staffed by N.Z. Medical Corps. Similar arrangement were made later at 63 British General Hospital. The *Maunganui* cleared all the patients on February 15, and the N.Z. Medical Corps terminated its six years' work in the Middle East.

STATISTICAL DATA

During these six years over 4,000 officers, other ranks, sisters and voluntary aids served in the N.Z. Medical Corps, assisted by regimental stretcher bearers, A.S.C. drivers, dental officers and orderlies, and chaplains.

The average sickness rate per 1,000 varied from a maximum of 3·5 per cent. in October 1942, when infective hepatitis was rife, to 1·12 in October 1943. The percentage of the Force under the care of medical units varied from 13·41 in November 1942 to 3·29 in November 1943.

The battle casualties totalled 21,684, of which 5,414 were killed or died of wounds. The heaviest casualties occurred during the pre-Alamein period, when there were 3,597 wounded with 936 deaths. The Second Libyan Campaign accounted for 2,784 battle casualties with 884 deaths. At Cassino there were 2,286 wounded with 456 deaths while in Crete there were 2,209 casualties with 674 deaths, much the largest percentage of fatal wounds.

The rates of killed and died of wounds to wounded steadily decreased during the war from 1 to 2·5 in Greece and Crete, and 1 to 2 in Libya, to 1 to 5 in the final period from the Senio to Trieste. This reflects both improved conditions and improvement in medical treatment.

Deaths from disease in the troops in the Middle East and Italy throughout the whole six year period numbered only 188, the main causes being meningitis 29, heart disease 17, pneumonia 14, appendicitis and peritonitis 13, and septicaemia 12. These figures show a remarkable decrease from those of 1 N.Z.E.F., which for just over four years were 1,579 deaths.

In the Medical Corps the casualties were 9 officers, 2 sisters, 6 W.A.A.Cs. and 44 O.Rs. killed or died from accidental injury or disease, 11 officers and 61 O.Rs. wounded, while 32 officers and 492 O.Rs. were made prisoners-of-war. The Force was fortunate in that few casualties occurred at sea, in spite of the hazards of the Mediterranean, and the presence of raiders elsewhere on the long lines of communication to New Zealand.

The *Chakdina*,which was not a hospital ship, was sunk with the loss of many wounded outside Tobruk, the only loss of this kind. Relatively few of the troops were otherwise lost at sea, though two medical officers were lost on relief ships during the evacuation of Greece.

EVACUATION OF CASUALTIES

Evacuation to Base Hospitals varied according to the means available and the length of time required. New Zealand patients were often treated in other hospitals, either on the line of communication or at the Base, and were not admitted to New Zealand hospitals until the major part of the surgical treatment had been undertaken.

The condition of the patients was adversely affected by ambulance car evacuation over the rough Western Desert during the Second Libyan Campaign. Evacuation by train was satisfactory, as was evacuation by hospital ship. Air evacuation was very satisfactory for all patients except those suffering from abdominal injuries, or chest injuries accompanied by respiratory distress. Its benefits were negatived to some extent by the inability of the planes to take ordinary stretchers.

In the forward areas stretcher-carrying jeeps and bren carriers were used with success and four-wheel drive ambulance cars proved of great advantage, especially in the Desert and during the winter in Italy. The New Zealand Forces were very well served by American Field Service cars during the period pre-Alamein to Tunis, and, again in Italy by the British Ambulance Convoys at different periods, especially in the Second Libyan Campaign, and by the Australian ambulances in Greece. After the Alamein period New Zealand had its own Ambulance Convoy under the command of the N.Z.A.S.C.

EVACUATION OF CASUALTIES TO NEW ZEALAND

Casualties were evacuated from the M.E.F. and C.M.F. to New Zealand by means of hospital ships and transports. Those needing medical attention or so incapacitated as to be unable to fend for themselves in transports were returned by hospital ship. The others, including lightly wounded and sick, were sent back on returning transports. There was close co-operation between Australia and New Zealand in the use of hospital ships.

New Zealand provided one hospital ship, S.S. *Maunganui*, which had been well equipped in New Zealand. She arrived in the Middle East at the end of the campaign in Crete and was thus able to evacuate the Greek and Crete casualties. She continued to evacuate cases from the M.E. and C.M.F. until the end of the war, except for a short period when she was refitting in the United Kingdom on account of a broken shaft.

The Australian hospital ship *Wanganella* evacuated many New Zealand casualties at different periods.

The Netherlands ship *Oranje*, a large modern liner, was fitted out as a hospital ship at Sydney, and its services were offered to the United Kingdom, Australia and New Zealand with the ships' complement and some medical personnel, the remainder of the medical staff being supplied by Australia and New Zealand. Later, United Kingdom personnel took the place of the Australians when the Australian troops left the Middle East, and the New Zealand complement was increased at the same time. During the latter part of the war the *Oranje* was used to carry patients between Italy and South Africa, and then between Italy and the United Kingdom. British hospital ships also assisted in evacuating a number of casualties to New Zealand.

There was no serious hold-up in the evacuation of casualties from the Middle East during the war and no consequent overloading of the bed capacity of the general hospitals.

From the Pacific theatre many seriously wounded men were flown back to New Zealand from New Caledonia, and in the area of operations American hospital ships were used. Returning transports carried the less serious cases as well as the graded personnel back to New Zealand.

VII. GENERAL HYGIENE IN THE MIDDLE EAST AND ITALY

CLIMATIC CONDITIONS AND CLOTHING

The climatic conditions in the Middle East differed greatly from those to which the New Zealand soldier was accustomed, especially during the summer months, but generally the troops acclimatised well.

The excessive heat at midday was countered, when possible, by a period of rest. Sunstroke and heat exhaustion were of little or no importance, for, since it had been found that excessive sweating leading to salt deficiency was in fact the cause of heat exhaustion, saline drinks were provided in the excessively hot weather, with excellent preventive results.

The clothing provided proved eminently satisfactory. Cotton drill shirts and short trousers, with long trousers for use after sunset to protect against mosquito bites, and stockings and boots were worn during the summer. Battledress was worn during the short winter. The ordinary slouch hat was worn in Egypt, while the field service cap was worn in the winter. The beret was adopted later.

Before the Greek campaign sun helmets were issued to the troops, but they were soon returned to store as unnecessary. It was common for the troops to dispense with head covering in Egypt even in the heat of summer. Shirts were often discarded and sunburn was not encountered. Acclimatisation and the dry climate prevented any ill effects.

Battledress was worn in the Greek and Crete campaigns.

The climate in the Western Desert was trying on account of the hot dry winds—the khamsins—and the moving sand and plagues of flies. It was made worse by the frequent lack of adequate supplies of water.

However, whenever the troops were stationed near the sea bathing and cool breezes improved conditions considerably.

In Italy winter was the difficult time. Contrary to expectations it was sharp, wet and severe, though short in duration. The Po Valley was very wet and cold, the normal winter temperature being about zero Centigrade. In summer the climate was pleasant and the heat not excessive. Drill was still worn in the summer and battledress in the winter.

In the winter provision was made for the supply of clean dry woollen socks with the rations when wet conditions were encountered. This satisfactorily prevented the occurrence of trench foot, which at one time had a rather high incidence in the American troops. The absence of puttees and the prevention of damp cold changed the picture completely as compared with that in Flanders in the First World War.

Adequate warm underclothing, pullovers and balaclavas were available, as well as blankets and ground sheets.

At the Base camp in Egypt huts were available, with tents as required. In the Desert tents and bivouacs were used. In Italy tents were again used, but buildings were secured, whenever possible, especially in the winter.

Mosquito-proof bivouacs were provided in Greece and again in Italy. Mosquito nets were also made available, but the supply was not always adequate.

DIET IN 2 N.Z.E.F.

The diet of the troops in the training camps in New Zealand was excellent in quantity, quality and variety and special attention was paid to this subject by the D.G.M.S. On the question of rations for the Expeditionary Force it was decided that the Australian ration should be adopted for the transports and that the British ration, with certain modifications, should be adopted for Egypt. This was specifically decided so that the New Zealand soldier should not have any preferential treatment over his British comrade. Slight adjustments were those prompted by the different habits and tastes of the New Zealander, especially his preference for jam and butter instead of cheese and margarine. Less tea was also included. The rations in Egypt, though based on the British scale, varied continually according to the resources of the country, and were adjusted to save the importation of food from overseas. Buffalo beef from the Sudan, for instance, was supplied when available.

At the Base camp in Egypt a sum of sixpence a head per day was available for the purchase of extras for the different messes, but when the troops were in the Desert this allowance ceased, though every effort was made to provide adequate rations, and extra vitamin tablets were given to make up for the scarcity of green vegetables.

The troops were warned against the consumption of food and drinks which might lead to intestinal infections, especially dysentery, and itinerant vendors were not permitted in the camps.

An ice cream plant was installed at Maadi Base Camp in order to ensure a supply of uninfected ice cream to the hospitals and, as far as possible, to the troops. Fruit unprotected by thick skins was prohibited and even melons were not allowed except when bought from reputable firms. The nature of the campaigns in the Desert was such that it was seldom necessary for the troops to continue on iron rations for more than a few days, though certain supplies, particularly vegetables, were difficult to obtain and to keep fresh. With the iron rations ascorbic acid tablets were supplied.

In Greece the hard rations, particularly biscuits, caused considerable damage to artificial dentures—a sad commentary on the dental deficiencies of the New Zealand soldier.

In Crete a full ration could not be supplied, but there was no real deficiency.

In Italy satisfactory rations were always available, with fresh foods and vegetables in good supply.

COOKS

Arrangements were made, on the arrival of the first troops in Egypt, for men to be trained in the British Army Cookery School in Cairo; also for the institution of a N.Z. School of Cookery, some members of the staff being provided from British Army personnel from Aldershot. This latter school continued to function throughout the war and was instrumental in the training of an adequate number of cooks able to undertake field cooking and improvise under difficult conditions.

In the hospitals male cooks were on the establishment and dietitians, when available, were later added to the staff.

HYGIENE AND SANITATION

Hygiene and sanitation were considered to be of the highest importance to the New Zealand Forces, both by the Medical Corps and the Higher Command.

It was realised that men normally accustomed to a high standard of hygiene in civil life would be more likely to suffer from crowded and insanitary surroundings, especially under abnormal climatic conditions, with associated endemic diseases.

In New Zealand camps overcrowding in sleeping quarters was guarded against and good sanitary services provided, though there were deficiencies in the early stages of rapid provision of camp accommodation, due to lack of consultation with the medical services.

Provision was made in New Zealand to educate men in the essentials of hygiene and to make them aware of the dangers of disease in the Middle East. A Hygiene Section, under a former Medical Officer of

Health, was attached to the First Echelon and organised sanitary services in the Base camps on arrival of the troops in Egypt. Drainage difficulties occurred at Maadi camp as the ground consisted of impermeable rock strata with only a shallow covering of sand. The leading of sullage water into large evaporating pans proved the solution to this problem. Deep latrines could not be dug at this camp and bucket latrines were used, the excreta being incinerated and buried.

Mess rooms and cookhouses were screened against flies with varying success, and efforts were made to provide ample hot water for the cleansing of mess utensils. Large water tanks in the camp were covered to protect them from contamination. Before use the water was chlorinated.

Showers were freely provided, as were camp swimming baths. Frequent chlorination was found essential. Later other Advanced Base Hygiene Sections were set up as required.

At the end of 1942 an Italian shower unit was captured and proved to be a great boon to the troops. There can be no doubt that shower units should be part of the normal equipment of any army under whatever climatic and other conditions it operates. The Hygiene Section attached to the Division greatly enlarged its scope as the war progressed. Malaria and typhus sections were set up in the Division in Syria and Italy. Early in 1944 a Field Hygiene Company was formed, incorporating both the malaria and typhus sections, and the O.C. was appointed D.A.D.H. on the staff of Divisional Headquarters.

Training in hygiene was available at the British M.E. School of Hygiene in Palestine, and full use was made of it. The Hygiene Section itself provided regular courses of instruction to unit officers and N.C.Os. Divisional orders promulgated hygiene instructions and advice.

In the forward areas deep trench latrines were used when conditions and the type of ground made it possible to construct them. Otherwise incineration was carried out with the use of petrol tins and petrol and oil. Urinals were mainly soakage in type, with funnel superstructure. Refuse was disposed of by burning and burial, special care being taken in the disposal of food tins, owing to the menace of flies. Fly control was of prime importance, especially in Egypt and the desert campaigns. Proper control of sanitary services usually sufficed to keep the pest under control and fly-proofing of cookhouses, mess rooms and latrines was normally carried out as facilities allowed. The worst experience of the Division was at the Alamein line when the flies bred in no-man's-land and in areas previously occupied by the enemy troops. Vigorous measures had to be taken with fly traps and insecticides to control this plague. Later in 1944 the advent of D.D.T. made control much easier.

Dead animals caused trouble in Italy, tar and oil being used for spray and the animals buried.

A mobile laundry and bath unit was first formed in the Division in Syria in 1942. In the Base Camp at Maadi a laundry was established almost from the beginning.

Water supplies were always considered as of the first importance and chlorination was regularly used, with de-tasting when possible.

A pipe line was built from Alexandria far into the Desert and the old Roman aqueducts were tapped and used freely, though the water was apt to become very salty. Local wells were tested and used in every country. Water carts were part of normal unit equipment and water cans were of much value, especially in the Desert campaigns, where the German jerrican proved very serviceable. Similar cans were later provided by the British Army. Lice control was carried out and disinfectors were available in the Field Hygiene Section. Disinfestation of refugees was undertaken in Aleppo and in the Desert of prisoners-of-war. Typhus inoculations were given before the Italian campaign and D.D.T. was freely used in Italy in buildings and also to impregnate underwear. Mosquito control was carried out throughout the war, especially in Syria and Italy, where the incidence of malaria was high.

In the New Zealand Force hygiene measures were of particular importance as New Zealanders had little or no immunity against diseases due to food contamination, such as dysentery, typhoid or hepatitis. Despite rigorous precautions the incidence of dysentery and hepatitis was relatively high. The incidence of malaria, on the other hand, was very low, showing that the preventive measures taken were effective.

VIII. INCIDENCE OF DISEASE IN NEW ZEALAND FORCES OVERSEAS

HEALTH OF MAORIS IN 2 N.Z.E.F.

The war showed clearly that in certain respects the Maori personnel differed from their European fellow countrymen in their susceptibility to disease.

It is well known in New Zealand that tuberculosis is much commoner in the Maori race. Fortunately, provision was made to carry out X-ray examination of the chest for all the Maori recruits. This disclosed, as expected, a high incidence of the disease. During their service overseas, however, the incidence was not unduly high, i.e., 13·5 per 1,000 as against 7·4 per 1,000 in the whole Force.

After their return to New Zealand the incidence in the Maori personnel was 1.73 per 1,000 for the four years 1945–49 as against a European incidence of 0·95 per 1,000, whereas the annual incidence of new civilian cases in 1948 was 3·6 for the Maoris and 0·77 for the Europeans. These records seem to support the view that in the same environment there would be little difference in the incidence of tuberculosis in the two racial elements.

Venereal disease was also prominent in the Maoris both in civilian and army life, due largely to their social background. On the other hand the Maoris showed a definite relative immunity to certain diseases, especially to infective hepatitis, which was so prevalent in the New Zealand Force.

Again, there was a relatively very low incidence of anxiety neurosis and the allied disease of dyspepsia. The morale of the Maori Battalion remained very high throughout the war in spite of heavy casualties. Since the war also there has never been any neurosis problem among the Maoris.

GENERAL INCIDENCE OF DISEASE IN 2 N.Z.E.F.

In general the incidence of disease in the New Zealand Armed Forces throughout the war was relatively low.

In the camps in New Zealand there was no severe epidemic and very few deaths. The commonest causes of admission to camp and general hospitals in New Zealand were, in order of frequency, influenza and the common cold; diseases of the bones, joints and muscles; diseases of teeth and gums; tonsillitis; skin diseases; P.U.O.; venereal disease; scabies; ear and nose diseases and diseases of the nervous system. Most of these conditions—the ordinary ailments of civil life—were among the twenty most common causes of sickness in 2 N.Z.E.F. Diseases overseas included infective hepatitis, dysentery, malaria and sandfly fever—diseases endemic in the Middle East to which New Zealanders possessed little or no immunity. Devastating diseases of previous wars such as typhoid and typhus fevers caused relatively few cases of sickness, due in part to artifically induced immunity, while pneumonia, which caused many deaths in the War of 1914–18, was relatively harmless, partly because of improved treatment.

Expressed as man-days, skin diseases, infective hepatitis and dysentery and diarrhoea caused the greatest wastage, with malaria, pneumonia and venereal disease next in order. This is in accord with the experience in the British Army in the Middle East.

Some minor disabilities proved of more importance overseas than they did in civil life. For instance, asthmatics did not acclimatise well in the Middle East and, except for a few who were able to work at the Base, they had to be returned to New Zealand as unfit. Old infections of the middle ear commonly flared up, as did chronic infection of the nasal sinuses. Men subject to seborrhoeic skin diseases were unsuited to the climate of the Middle East. The dyspeptic, in general, proved an unsatisfactory soldier.

New cases admitted to medical units each day averaged 2 per 1,000 and the percentage of the Force in medical units varied from 3 to 13, the sickness cases averaging 4 to 5 per cent.

Invalids evacuated to New Zealand showed no special variation from civilian experience, nor did the mortality from disease overseas which accounted for 188 deaths, as against a total of 1,579 in the War of 1914–18.

There was considerable wastage from down-grading for minor disabilities of various kinds, especially functional nervous disorders.

In the Pacific Force the experience was similar to that in the Middle East and tropical diseases caused little concern.

Accidental injuries were responsible for much disability in the Forces throughout the war and accounted for almost as many hospital admissions as did battle casualties.

INFECTIOUS DISEASES

Infectious diseases endemic in the Middle East caused considerable morbidity in 2 N.Z.E.F., as was to be expected in a force with little or no immunity. On the other hand the Force never suffered from any of the epidemics of diseases usually experienced in New Zealand, such as influenza or measles, though in New Zealand and on transports these diseases did occur.

Dysentery was prevalent in 1 N.Z.E.F. while it was stationed in the Middle East and 2 N.Z.E.F. had the same experience. There could have been few troops who did not suffer at one time or another from an attack of diarrhoea, usually soon after arrival in Egypt, despite good sanitation and hygiene. The hospital admission rate was about 4 per cent. of the Force annually. The majority of the cases were of the Flexner type and few were severe. In Italy the incidence was less but New Zealand troops had a higher incidence than those of the British Army. The introduction of sulphaguanidine for the treatment of the disease brought about a dramatic improvement in its relief and cure. In the Pacific dysentery was less severe and the incidence lower than in the Middle East. Here again the majority of the cases were Flexner in type.

Amoebiasis was infrequent in the Force in Egypt but more cases occurred in Syria, while in Italy the relative incidence was much higher. Special investigations in one of the New Zealand hospitals in Italy showed that the infection was present in 250 out of 4,600 hospital patients. Very few cases were diagnosed in the Pacific. In a pensions survey in New Zealand it was reported that 148 cases of amoebiasis were found in returned Servicemen in New Zealand up to the end of 1949. By 1952 few new cases were reported.

Z*

Typhoid fever, which was a serious problem in Gallipoli in the War of 1914–18, caused little trouble in the War of 1939–45, though it was found that the inoculations of vaccine given in New Zealand did not give fully satisfactory results in the Middle East. One epidemic occurred in the Base camps late in 1943 and a small one among W.A.A.C. personnel in Syria in 1942. It would appear that to be successful a vaccine must give immunity against the specific strains of the disease endemic in the area concerned.

Infective hepatitis was the major scourge of 2 N.Z.E.F. as far as infection was concerned and the New Zealand soldier appeared to be particularly susceptible. In the War of 1914–18 there was also a marked incidence of jaundice in Gallipoli and in Egypt. Between August 1942 and January 1943, 2,500 cases occurred among 30,000 New Zealand troops, the great majority being in the forward areas. Although the disease was relatively mild in type and only six deaths occurred, convalescence was prolonged by the resultant debility, and recurrences were frequent.

Investigations into the disease were carried out by Kirk, a New Zealand medical officer, who formed the opinion that the disease was spread by flies from excreta and that the infection was introduced by the gastro-intestinal tract. This theory was finally confirmed by experimental work carried out later in the United States.

New Zealand troops suffered another epidemic of hepatitis in Italy and again showed their susceptibility to this infection. There was no epidemic at the time among the civilian population either in Egypt or Italy which showed the immunity acquired in an endemic area. There were many sub-clinical cases during the epidemics. There was a markedly lower incidence of the disease among the Maoris. Experience showed that a convalescence of some six weeks was necessary to ensure satisfactory recovery.

Many of the cases did not exhibit jaundice and persistent dyspepsia was often the main sign of the disease. Enlargement of the liver was usual, as was food intolerance.

The relationship of serum jaundice to infective hepatitis was investigated and the two were thought to be different.

Malaria. The New Zealand Forces served in many highly malarious areas during their campaigns, yet the incidence of this disease was very low, being approximately 2 per 1,000 during the malaria seasons. This was due to two main causes. First, the Division escaped the malaria seasons in Greece, Crete and Tunis, and to a great extent also in Syria, though precautions were taken against infection. Secondly, by the time the Division went to Italy, the Army generally had been alerted by the serious malaria infection in Sicily, preventive measures were being more efficiently carried out and mepacrine administration had been introduced. The use of D.D.T. and other insecticides had also been widely adopted and malaria control was very active.

In Egypt a small number of cases occurred, usually during the Nile floods, but in Syria more cases arose. In Italy the Division was never in a highly malarious area for long and the incidence was never high. It was much lower than that of any other section of the British Army.

Again, in the Pacific campaign our troops were fortunate, as the base camps were in New Caledonia which was free of malaria, and the active campaign period in the Solomons was not prolonged. Lessons had by then been learnt from the experience of the Americans and from the research work carried out by the Australians. Carefully prepared plans were carried out to free the areas from the mosquito, and atebrin was regularly administered to the troops. This resulted in a very low incidence of the disease. Less than 700 cases of malaria occurred in the New Zealand Pacific Force of over 12,000 men, and of these only 120 were recorded in the Solomons, the remainder developing in New Caledonia and in New Zealand. No deaths occurred and no cases were evacuated from the area because of malaria.

Malaria was made a notifiable disease in New Zealand early in 1944, in which year 397 cases were notified; but by 1948 the number had dropped to 12. Since then the problem has ceased to be of any importance, though precautions are taken to spray overseas aircraft on arrival in New Zealand. There are no pensioners from malaria as all ex-Servicemen ceased to have any recurrent attacks within three years of returning to New Zealand, the great majority within one year.

Dengue fever was experienced by the Pacific Force. It was learnt that the main danger lay in infection in urban areas, and that the disease was unlikely to cause serious concern to a force engaged in jungle warfare or camped in rural areas.

Sandfly fever was responsible for about 2,000 cases in 2 N.Z.E.F. in the Middle East, and proved a debilitating disease. A severe epidemic occurred in 1941 in a hospital sited on barren sand near Cairo.

Typhus fever, though always a menace in the Middle East, was responsible for only six deaths in a total of 11 cases in 2 N.Z.E.F. In June 1943 part of the Force was inoculated against the disease and most of the troops were inoculated before being sent to Italy. Booster doses were given every six months.

An anti-typhus squad was formed in the Division during the winter period in Italy and disinfestation was carried out regularly.

Ankylostomiasis was encountered by the Pacific Force during the campaign in the Solomons but no serious trouble arose, the infection quickly dying out. It was considered that there was little danger of the disease being introduced into New Zealand by the troops.

Cerebro-spinal fever did not occur in epidemic form in the New Zealand Forces during the war. Meningitis of all forms, however, including tuberculous, accounted for 18 deaths in 2 N.Z.E.F. in the Middle East, the highest single cause of death from disease, whereas in 1 N.Z.E.F. there were 115 deaths, 109 from cerebro-spinal fever.

Poliomyelitis was experienced in 2 N.Z.E.F., 40 cases occurring in an epidemic from November 1940 to July 1941, with 4 deaths and 19 cases of paralysis. In all, 66 cases with 8 deaths were reported in 2 N.Z.E.F. during the war.

Diphtheria was of low incidence in 2 N.Z.E.F. except for two small epidemics in 1 N.Z. G.H., one at Helwan in December 1942, the other at Senigallia in the winter of 1944–45. In the latter 150 cases were diagnosed and routine swabbing revealed four carriers among the hospital staff.

Infection of gunshot wounds was a serious complication and this was seen particularly at Senigallia. Twenty-four cases of post-diphtheritic polyneuritis occurred.

Arrangements were made to Schick-test and, if necessary immunise, all nursing sisters and voluntary aids in the Middle East. It was recommended that this should be carried out in the future in New Zealand before these personnel proceeded overseas. Altogether four deaths, including that of a nurse, occurred from diphtheria.

During the war many infections were not diagnosed specifically and were classified as 'P.U.O.' (pyrexia of unknown origin). Many of these cases were of short duration and were dealt with in the forward areas.

Patients whose pyrexia was of longer duration were referred to the Base and efforts made there to determine the exact diagnosis. At times sandfly fever was suspected as being responsible for many of the cases. A group of cases diagnosed later at the Base included such conditions as otitis media, sinusitis, prostatitis, pyelitis, rheumatic fever, catarrhal enteritis, bacillary dysentery and infective hepatitis. In 2 N.Z.E.F. nearly 3,000 cases were classified as P.U.O. in four years.

RESPIRATORY DISEASES

Respiratory diseases were not common though there were between 300 and 600 cases of pneumonia admitted to hospital yearly.

Influenza, except for a small epidemic in March 1940, did not affect the overseas troops though several large outbreaks occurred in the training camps in New Zealand. A serious outbreak occurred among reinforcements on their way to Egypt. This outbreak was completely checked on their arrival in Egypt by isolating them from the other troops.

Pneumonia. The incidence increased in the wet weather and was highest between January and June 1944 in Italy. The introduction of the sulphonamides in the treatment of pneumonia reduced complications and lessened the severity and the mortality of the disease. Epidemics of atypical pneumonia occurred in Italy both in 1944 and 1945 and these cases were finally diagnosed as Q fever. In all there were 2,012 cases of pneumonia in 2 N.Z.E.F. in the Middle East, with 10 deaths, whereas in 1 N.Z.E.F. there were 578 deaths from pneumonia as well as 20 from pleurisy and 152 from influenza (often with complicating pneumonia).

Asthma caused few admissions to hospital but the climate of Egypt proved unsuitable to these cases and the majority were evacuated to New Zealand.

Pulmonary tuberculosis did not occur in large numbers in 2 N.Z.E.F. In all 729 cases were recorded up to 1949. Unfortunately none of the First Echelon and few of the Second Echelon troops had had X-ray examination before proceeding overseas. This was of considerable importance in the light of the development of the disease later, as between 2 and 3 recruits per 1,000 were rejected on account of an active tuberculous lesion shown in X-rays of men reported fit on physical examination. Of the 729 cases recorded no less than 495 enlisted in 1939 and 1940, 140 in 1941 and only 94 in 1942–45. Only 115 cases were invalided back from the Middle East, the remainder being discovered in routine X-rays on discharge in New Zealand, or developed signs later in New Zealand.

In the Navy, however, the incidence was much higher and the disease was of more importance owing to the crowded conditions in warships.

Among the New Zealand prisoners-of-war the incidence was also considerably higher and 155 cases were reported, with 4 deaths. Experience during the war proved that with X-ray examination of recruits the disease was relatively unimportant and that the incidence was less than that in the civilian population.

VENEREAL DISEASE

The incidence of this disease in troops serving in the Middle East and Italy was a matter of some concern and every effort was made from the beginning to minimise its effects by education and preventive measures. Fortunately the incidence was not as high as that of the War of 1914–18. The disease was less virulent, and, of more importance, the treatment available was incomparably superior.

The introduction of the sulphonamides and, later, penicillin enabled gonorrhoea and soft sores to be satisfactorily coped with, though there was a period in Italy when sulphonamide resistant strains caused trouble until penicillin became freely available.

Syphilis was at first dealt with by the arsenical compounds but finally penicillin again was used with success, especially in clearing up primary lesions rapidly.

The highest incidence of the disease occurred after hostilities ceased in Italy, mostly in Trieste and Florence. The irresponsibility of the troops and the dislocation of the life of the civil population resulted in a lowering of moral standards. A register of cases was kept to ensure adequate treatment.

Views differed on the question of controlled brothels. In Cairo they were finally put out of bounds. It was thought that this action reduced the incidence of disease. In Syria brothels were instituted and given careful medical inspections. The incidence of disease was very low.

In Italy brothels were not controlled, though medical examinations were carried out in Florence.

The establishment of venereal disease treatment centres undoubtedly proved successful, especially when one was attached to the Division. The New Zealand Forces were the first to set up a mobile unit.

The total number of cases of venereal disease in 2 N.Z.E.F. was 6,842. The rate per 1,000 per annum varied from 11·8 in 1943 to 115·8 in 1945.*

Apart from infectious disease the New Zealand Forces' main medical problems related to the neuroses, skin diseases and dyspepsia.

NEUROSIS AND PSYCHOSIS

The problem of neurosis became prominent overseas very early, long before any active military operations were undertaken. The change from civilian life and occupation to the life and surroundings in a desert camp, under trying climatic conditions, was sufficient to bring about a condition of neurosis in men constitutionally and psychologically unstable, and thereby unable to adjust themselves to army life. The great majority of the cases of neurosis were of this type, and relatively few resulted from battle stress in normally adjusted men. Strong emphasis was placed on the importance of training and discipline in reducing the number of cases of breakdown, and welfare measures such as good food, sports, entertainment and leave were given full consideration. The neurosis often expressed itself in complaints of minor organic disabilities such

---

* In Japan the incidence of the disease was at first much lower than it had been in Italy, but by 1948 the rate was higher than that ever recorded in 2 N.Z.E.F. The other Occupation Forces in Japan had similar experiences. Brothels were placed out of bounds, but this had little effect.

as backache, painful feet, headache, gastric complaints and other psychosomatic symptoms. In periods of stress at the front the incidence of neurosis increased, especially when the stress was prolonged and the living conditions unpleasant, but there was a marked decrease when the victorious advance started after the battle of Alamein. This change was noted throughout the war, there being few cases when the campaigns were progressing satisfactorily. Unit morale was found to depend a great deal on the C.O. and the medical officer, and also on the higher command. This was illustrated by the improvement in morale brought about by the explanation of the campaign given to the troops by General Montgomery before the battle of Alamein. Few cases of hysteria were encountered.

The Maoris showed little liability to nervous disorders except under prolonged battle strain.

Treatment was generally unsatisfactory, except in cases of physical and nervous exhaustion in the forward areas. A period of rest and sedation in rest centres in the forward areas often restored men quickly and allowed them to rejoin their units. At the Base men evacuated from the forward areas seldom returned to their units and were boarded to base duties or for evacuation to New Zealand. It proved difficult to provide congenial employment at the Base for the large numbers of these men, and from time to time some had to be re-boarded and evacuated to New Zealand, where it was considered they were more likely to recover and to be usefully employed. The return to their families and ordinary home surroundings and to the type of civilian work they had done before enlisting was generally sufficient to restore them to their ordinary pre-war state of health. From every point of view the retention of large numbers of these men overseas was uneconomic in man-power and generally harmful to the individual.

There were comparatively few psychiatric cases.

On return to New Zealand the psychotic cases were admitted to the main hospitals and, if necessary, to the mental hospitals. The neurosis cases required little in the way of hospital treatment though the number receiving pensions was considerable. In all, one in every six or seven down-graded men suffered from neurosis, and the number boarded in New Zealand after their return from overseas was double that of those actually invalided to New Zealand during the war.

By 1950 few men were not working—probably less than 2 per cent., and the number receiving pensions was rapidly diminishing. Pensions for neurosis had been granted to 1·75 per cent. of the men enlisted.

At the end of 1953 only 28 per cent. of these remained on pension, and only 53 or 2·55 per cent. were not satisfactorily rehabilitated.

DYSPEPSIA

Dyspepsia proved an important cause of disability and invaliding. Most of the cases were functional in origin—one of the manifestations of neurosis. The percentage of duodenal and gastric ulcer cases was not high. Unfortunately, detailed investigation to exclude ulceration tended to accentuate and fix the neurosis. Seldom did a patient recover sufficiently to be fit for further service after the investigations had been undertaken. The only hope of preserving a dyspeptic soldier for full service was to diagnose the condition quickly and to treat him either in the forward medical units or for a very brief period in hospital.

These men were as a rule unsatisfactory for service at the Base and the great majority had to be evacuated to New Zealand, where they generally recovered satisfactorily, though occasionally ulceration was diagnosed later.

SKIN DISEASES

Skin diseases were common in the New Zealand Forces overseas and accounted for 13 per cent. of all men invalided back to New Zealand, the largest number being affected by eczema and dermatitis. Seborrhoea was common in the Middle East. Desert sores were troublesome and resistant to treatment. Tinea was uncommon though precautions were taken to prevent its spread in shower rooms. In the Pacific Force skin diseases, mostly eczema and dermatitis, were common. Insect bites caused much disturbance and skin infection. Tropical ulcers were also relatively common.

DOWN-GRADED MEN IN 2 N.Z.E.F.

The problem of down-grading personnel overseas was of considerable importance and large numbers were involved.

The categories at first used were similar to those employed in the original medical examination of recruits, but a fresh classification was later adopted in the Middle East to enable men with minor disabilities to be employed in special tasks in the forward areas. It was found necessary to down-grade and even return to New Zealand many men on their arrival overseas. The element of neurosis was common, often associated with relatively minor disabilities. Satisfactory employment at the base for these men proved difficult and their condition tended to deteriorate.

Medical boarding was carried out in the general hospitals and by specially constituted boards at the Base Camp, the findings of the boards being confirmed by the consultant physician or surgeon.

Only a limited number of down-graded men could be employed at the Base, especially in Egypt, where native labour was used for many camp services, particularly sanitary services.

In September 1941 (a quiescent period) in a group of 600 down-graded men, other than those on the New Zealand roll, the disabilities were: foot disabilities 126, functional nervous disorders 70, accidental injuries 66, arthritis 41, cardio-vascular 36, eye 33, otitis media 25, deafness 24, fibrositis 20, mental dullness 19, dermatitis 15, asthma 14, battle casualties 12, respiratory 11, organic nervous disorders 11, gastro-intestinal 10, other conditions 67. Whereas, in a group of 465 men boarded for evacuation to New Zealand, there were: functional nervous disorders 76, organic nervous disorders 29, accidental injuries 33, battle casualties 31, arthritis 37, gastro-intestinal 25, peptic ulcer 17, otitis media 24, asthma 21, skin 21, respiratory 23, rheumatic fever 11.

IX. WOUND TREATMENT

At the beginning of the war the technique of primary wound treatment laid down during the War of 1914–18, and continued in the treatment of civilian injuries afterwards, was carried out by the army surgeons. After the surgical cleansing of the wound the closed plaster treatment, as developed during the Spanish civil war, was employed. Very soon the sulphonamides were used as bacteriostatics, both locally to the wound and parenterally by the mouth and, later, intravenously and intra-abdominally.

Penicillin, when introduced in the latter half of 1943, gradually displaced the sulphonamides, and with its help the regular delayed primary suture of wounds was introduced. However, the primary efficient surgical treatment of the wound remained the essential element in wound treatment.

The severity of the wound depends on the missile and mines were responsible for particularly severe wounds, including the loss of many limbs. Gross injuries, especially to muscle, were often associated with severe infection, often anaerobic in nature, and injuries to large blood vessels were commonly associated with gangrene.

Abdominal and head injuries caused a heavy mortality. The removal of skin was at first overdone, and the extent of muscle removal increased in Italy, where wound infection proved to be more severe.

The closed plaster treatment, though beneficial primarily, proved to have disadvantages later, causing delay in healing, and wasting and loss of function in the limb. The sulphonamides applied locally proved to have a preventive but not a curative action in wound infection. Parenteral administration was, however, held to be of definite value, but only for a limited period and mainly again as a preventive measure. Penicillin proved a much more satisfactory agent for combating infection, especially when given early, and also when introduced into the pleura. Blood transfusion not only acted favourably in saving life from loss of blood, but in raising the resistance of the patient and his tissues to infection.

Infection was present in many forms. Recognition of its danger in the frequent dressings of wounds and in cross infection in hospitals led to infrequent dressings and strict precautions during dressings. Primary suture was used in abdominal and head injuries, and in face wounds, under suitable conditions.

Delayed primary suture was carried out routinely during the last year of the war, when penicillin was more freely available, and proved very successful. Plastic repair was also undertaken. Sterilised dressings, often of vaselined gauze, were used freely and prepared at the Base for the forward areas. Preservation of all viable tissues, including bone, was carried out.

New Zealand experience confirmed that the removal of soiled and devitalised tissue from the wound, the relief of tension, the provision of rest for the tissues and the individual, the replacement of lost fluid and blood, the protection of the wound from contamination, and finally its complete closure to prevent that contamination and allow of early restoration of function, were neither new nor strange but had to be relearnt by a new generation of surgeons. This may possibly have to be relearnt again.

FORWARD SURGERY

In France during the War of 1914–18 forward surgery was carried out at C.C.S. level.

In North Africa rapid movement and poor communications, combined with the relative immobility of the C.C.S., forced the field ambulances to take on the burden of forward surgery and they had to be re-equipped accordingly.

Surgical potential was ensured by the provision of at least one surgeon on the staff of a field ambulance, and by the attachment of surgical teams. These teams were staffed and equipped as independent units as far as the surgical work was concerned, but were dependent on the parent field ambulance for all services.

These F.S.Us. proved of the greatest value to the British Army and in time became recognised units, with an establishment of staff and equipment.

In the N.Z. Forces a surgical team was used in Greece and Crete. During the Second Libyan Campaign a N.Z. Mobile Surgical Unit, similar to the Head and Chest Units sent with the first British troops to France in 1939, was attached to the Division, working in association with the field ambulances. This unit was afterwards incorporated into 1 N.Z. C.C.S. as its Light Section. A surgical team with equipment was detached from one of the New Zealand hospitals and attached to a field ambulance just before the battle of El Alamein, and the light section of the C.C.S. was similarly attached at that time. Thereafter in periods of activity the same arrangements were made and eventually the surgical team was officially constituted as a F.S.U.

The C.C.Ss., some of which, including the N.Z. C.C.S., had been provided with transport and so converted into mobile units, then began to fulfil their original rôle as far as the British Army was concerned. The New Zealand Field Ambulances, however, continued to carry out much major surgery throughout the war.

Field Transfusion Units were organised in the Middle East by the excellent British Transfusion Service. At first British Transfusion Units were attached to New Zealand field ambulances until a N.Z. unit was formed. Whole blood, plasma, serum, glucose and saline fluids were supplied by the Transfusion Service to the forward areas.

At the battle of El Alamein the organisation of forward surgery was very efficient. Units were well staffed, and casualties were smoothly evacuated to the surgical centres at the field ambulances and then to the grouped C.C.Ss. Air evacuation was used to some extent but there were few ambulance planes, and unprotected transport planes were subject to enemy attack.

Nursing sisters had been attached to the C.C.Ss., and beds had been made available to the field ambulances and F.S.Us. to enable men with abdominal injuries to be held and nursed after operation, as their early evacuation by air had proved calamitous.

In the long advance to Tunis air evacuation was used freely.

In Italy buildings were used if possible. Evacuation was difficult owing to the destruction of the railways and the deterioration of roads.

At Cassino men with abdominal injuries did better with a longer period of resuscitation, whereas early operation proved best for traumatic amputation and large missile wounds. Lesser wounds were dealt with more freely in order to make delayed primary suture possible at the Base. Specialist units—neurological, ophthalmological, faciomaxillary, as well as chest units, had forward sections close to the C.C.Ss.

In the final period in Italy evacuation by air was a special feature and many men had their primary surgical treatment at the Base hospital.

PRIORITY OF OPERATION

The priority of operation at the beginning of the war was:

(1) Bleeders
(2) Sucking chest wounds
(3) Abdominal injuries
(4) Serious wounds and traumatic amputations
(5) Head injuries
(6) Light wounds.

Later, abdominal injuries were placed below the serious wounds. The degree of urgency in the surgical treatment of wounds was a matter on which opinions differed. Some considered time was all important, and this led to the performance of the greater part of surgery at the field ambulance level where there was a lack of staff, particularly as regards post-operative nursing. Others considered that the better staffing and equipment, the more peaceful conditions and especially the nursing at the C.C.S. level outweighed the time advantage in a great proportion of the cases. The local conditions, however, usually decided the question. Operation at the field ambulance level was sometimes essential owing to poor facilities for evacuation. The employment of the surgical potential of all forward units in times of great activity was naturally the ideal to be aimed at, but the greater the proportion of casualties dealt with in the C.C.Ss., the better. The presence of a senior experienced surgeon in all forward units was of great advantage, and the New Zealand Consultant Surgeon was usually employed at the C.C.S.

The type of operating theatre used during the North African Campaign usually consisted of two E.P.I.P. tents joined together sideways, one to act as the operating room and the other as the shelter for patients awaiting operation, and for supplies. Each operating team had its own theatre. Electric lighting was generally provided either by the parent unit or by the operating team itself.

The control of haemorrhage in the Aid Posts was effected by pressure and bandaging, with very occasional application of forceps. Tourniquets were not often used as it was considered that they did more harm than good. Splinting was carried out mainly by the use of plaster. The Thomas splint was employed for the lower limb and Kramer splints were used for temporary first-aid splinting.

Resuscitation consisted of rest, fluids and the transfusion of blood, plasma, serum, or glucose-saline. Anti-tetanus serum was administered in doses of 3,000 units to all wounded men.

A pre-operation ward, where resuscitation was carried out and patients sorted for operative treatment, was usual in both the field ambulance and the C.C.S. Post-operative care consisted largely in the continuance of resuscitation, and the administration of gastric suction and intravenous fluids to men with abdominal injuries. Evacuation was carried out as soon as possible, except for those unfit to travel and for those with abdominal injuries. The problems of shock were studied assiduously during the war. The British Blood Transfusion Service carried out excellent work both in the preparation of blood and other intravenous fluids, and in the supply and administration in the forward areas and at the Base. Blood grouping of the individual soldier was carried out in New Zealand at enlistment.

As regards anaesthesia, intravenous pentothal was commonly used as was cyclopropane in special centres.

Gas gangrene, though not so common as in the War of 1914–18, caused anxiety. Fortunately, penicillin proved to be of value in its treatment.

X. SURGERY OF WAR WOUNDS

Head injuries were dealt with successfully by neuro-surgical units. After-effects have not proved to be as serious as had been expected.

Nerve injuries were common. Operative treatment for their repair was carried out after return to New Zealand. The results generally have been disappointing.

Chest injuries caused a heavy mortality on the battlefield. The sucking chest injuries demanded urgent attention and were first priority cases in the forward areas. At first a firm pad kept in place with strapping was used to close the sucking chest. Later, stitches were used to secure a pad of vaseline gauze more securely, while some cases were stitched. It was noted that sepsis was apt to develop in these wounds, especially in Italy. At the end of the Italian campaign the treatment of chest cases had become stabilised as regards early treatment. The chest wounds, particularly the sucking wounds, were adequately excised and injured rib and foreign bodies removed from the wall and pleura. Suture of the muscles closed the chest, and a pad was anchored by a few loose skin sutures. Penicillin was then instilled, no drain being used, but the chest kept dry by repeated aspiration. Blood transfusion was limited in amount to replace actual blood loss and shock largely treated by rest, warm drinks and the removal of fluid from the chest, the patient being nursed flat until the condition of the circulation warranted the sitting posture. The serious cases were held in the forward areas until the stormy crisis was over. The importance of respiratory exercises as a preventative and curative treatment of atelectasis and the patchy pneumonic changes that occurred in chest wounds was stressed, and the exercises became a routine in these cases. The removal of foreign bodies at the base hospital was carried out commonly from the seventh to the fourteenth day in about half the cases reaching the special chest centres. Decortication for clotted haemothorax was done between the third and fourth weeks, though cases requiring this were not common. Convalescence was accelerated by high protein and vitamin diet, and by blood transfusion in anaemic cases.

The treatment of haemothorax was at first conservative, with delayed tapping; then tapping was carried out early and repeated frequently. When penicillin became available it was injected into the pleural cavity at every aspiration. Rib resection and drainage were required for any marked infection.

Abdominal wounds were the cause of serious mortality, a number of these casualties dying on the battlefield. Of a group of casualties, including those brought in dead to field units and those dying in the field units but not operated on, there was a mortality of 50 per cent. in New Zealand troops. Of those operated on there was a mortality of 36 per cent. The main features of the treatment during the war were adequate resuscitation with blood, early operation, careful exploration of the abdomen, exteriorisation of colon injuries, continuous post-operative gastric suction and glucose and saline infusion—no evacuation until the condition was stabilised. Most of the liver and kidney injuries were treated conservatively, as were the late abdominal injuries. Early nursing of the patients post-operatively was carried out in the horizontal position in the latter period of the war. Drainage was employed in all doubtful cases and definitely for wounds of the colon, pancreas, duodenum, biliary passages, bladder and retro-peritoneal injuries. Thoraco-abdominal cases were mostly operated on through the chest wall.

Fractures. The treatment of fractures gave generally good results. Sepsis was at times troublesome but treatment by careful excision, penicillin and delayed primary suture gave excellent results in the latter part of the war. The early development of the Tobruk splint—the Thomas splint incorporated in plaster—led to excellent splintage of fractures of the lower limb. Plaster splints were used for upper limb fractures; Kramer splintage was also available.

Bone fragments were preserved more and more until, in the latter part of the war, it was routine to preserve them all. Excision of the patella in compound fractures was commonly carried out. Fractures of the feet were common and created difficulties in treatment. They were finally treated conservatively, with early active movement. Carpal fractures frequently led to permanent disability.

Amputations were common, especially of the lower limbs, following mine wounds. At first early amputation was performed through the sites of election but this quickly proved disastrous and as much as possible of the limb was preserved initially, and secondary amputation, if necessary, carried out later. Primary suture also proved dangerous, but delayed primary suture, especially when penicillin became available, was very satisfactory. Careful and free wound excision was found to be essential in traumatic amputations.

Secondary amputations were indicated in cases of gangrene following destruction of the main vascular supply, in massive gas gangrene, in severe and life-endangering infection and in severely damaged and infected feet for which there was no hope of eventual satisfactory function. Re-amputations were only carried out when any danger of infection had passed.

Vascular injuries were common and damage to the main vessels of the lower limb led to many amputations. The popliteal artery injuries were especially serious and few limbs were saved in these cases. The ligation of the main vein, as recommended by Makins, was given up. Fasciotomy of the calf proved of some use in the serious vascular injuries of the lower limb. Arterial repair by suture was carried out in some cases.

OTHER SURGICAL AND SPECIALIST CONDITIONS

Burns. The treatment of burns changed markedly during the war. At first the tannin treatment was used but this proved unsatisfactory and dangerous. This was followed by local suphonamide and *tulle gras* dressings, then sulphonamides were given orally so that dosage could be controlled. Finally penicillin displaced the sulphonamides. Local treatment of the burns themselves became more and more gentle and dressings infrequent. Saline baths were used, especially for the deeper burns. The marked swelling seen in burns of the hands was dealt with by the use of pressure dressings. The shock so frequently seen was treated by the giving of blood plasma in large quantities for the first 48 hours. Whole blood was often needed in the later stages associated with high protein diet, iron tonics and vitamins, to counter the anaemia and debility so often present.

Skin grafting for the deeper burns was carried out as early as possible, both as a temporary dressing and as final treatment.

Plastic surgery was carried out freely, both for men suffering from burns and for those whose injury involved loss of tissue, especially of the face and jaw. The dental surgeon assisted greatly in these cases.

Accidental injuries of all kinds were very common in the New Zealand Forces. At times they were more frequent than war wounds. Motor transport had much to do with this as did the use of petrol for lighting fires. Games such as rugby football contributed a large quota.

Knee joint injuries were common, especially cartilage injuries, for which operation proved satisfactory provided muscular exercises were carried out before and after operation. Wounds of the knee joint in general did not give rise to much anxiety and, except for the excision of the fractured patella when associated with compound injuries to the joint, were treated conservatively.

Wounds of the hip joint, if infected, gave rise to serious trouble and prolonged illness.

Foot disabilities were prevalent. Minor disabilities were found to be of little significance provided physical training was graded wisely, especially on enlistment. The boots supplied were at times unsuitable, especially for the Maoris, most of whom possess a wide flat foot. Major surgical procedures for foot deformities were banned—wisely.

Hernia was relatively common but caused little disability. Operation proved to be warranted for the simple hernia in young men, but not for recurrent hernia in older men.

Varicose veins also proved of little moment, but repeated injections often led to serious disability. It was learnt that the only worthwhile treatment was to carry out efficiently the Trendelenberg operation in men with deficient venous valves.

Eye diseases were not serious though much work was necessary in attending to minor complaints and supplying spectacles. Eye wounds were serious and often resulted from non-magnetic missiles. Fortunately sympathetic ophthalmia was not encountered in the New Zealand Forces. A neurasthenic element was present in the Middle East associated with minor eye complaints. In the Pacific Area eye conditions of any severity were uncommon. An optician unit proved of value in the Middle East and also in the Pacific.

Ear, nose and throat conditions were in general not serious in nature, though of common occurrence. Otitis media of old standing was prone to recur in the Middle East. Otitis externa was very common and refractory to treatment both in the Middle East and in the Pacific Area. Nasal conditions tended to be aggravated in the Middle East, and often arose after swimming. Nasal sinusitis and polypi tended to be refractory.

It was considered that dust, dirt, sweat and the drying air were the chief causes of the incidence of ear, nose and throat diseases in the Middle East. Operative treatment overseas was restricted to cases of urgency, and to those which would normally lead to the increased efficiency and lengthened service of the soldier without too much hospitalisation.

Battle casualties mainly consisted of blast injuries to the middle ear, and these were common. It was soon learnt that local treatment of the ear by instillation or syringing was dangerous and almost always led to infection. When local treatment was discontinued, sulphonamides were given and men referred to specialists at the Base; the majority healed satisfactorily. Deafness leading to pension often resulted from otosclerosis undetected at the original medical examination.

XI. THE NEW ZEALAND ARMY IN THE PACIFIC

A garrison force of a brigade was sent to Fiji early in the war. Two light field ambulances and two hospitals were established as well as a small convalescent home and two hygiene sections. No major medical problems arose and the health of the troops was satisfactory. This Force was relieved by United States troops and on return to New Zealand formed the nucleus of a force of a division of two brigades which proceeded to New Caledonia to relieve and assist United States troops.

Later the Force took part in three landings in the Solomon Islands at Vella Lavella, Treasury Islands and Green Islands from an advanced base on Guadalcanal. Few casualties resulted from the operations. The medical units of the Force comprised three field ambulances and a C.C.S. stationed in the Solomons, and a general hospital and a convalescent depot in New Caledonia. Smaller attached units were two field surgical units, a malaria control unit, an optician unit and a motor ambulance convoy.

Conditions in New Caledonia were very suitable for New Zealand troops and, apart from dengue fever, their health was excellent. The United States rations proved to some extent unpalatable to the troops.

In the Solomons the wet and tropical climate was irksome. Malaria, skin infections and hookworm were encountered in minor degree.

Problems of equipment and transport, and operations and evacuation of casualties in the jungle had to be dealt with, and valuable lessons were learnt. The protection of dressings from moisture and the necessity to pack equipment so that it could be man-handled were of special importance.

Evacuation of casualties from the Solomons was by landing craft and later by air from the forward areas, and then by hospital ship or air to the base in New Caledonia.

Prefabricated hospitals were sent over from New Zealand and erected in New Caledonia and Guadalcanal.

Malaria was the main medical problem. Other problems were in general similar to those encountered in the Middle East.

Small garrisons were also sent to Tonga, Norfolk Island and Fanning Island.

In the Pacific theatre the battle casualties were: killed 85, died of wounds 12, wounded 187. Deaths from sickness and from accident respectively were: Pacific Force 16 and 34, Fiji 4 and 6, Tonga 5 and 1, Norfolk 1 and 2. Total sickness 26, accident 43.

Medical Services of Royal New Zealand Navy

The New Zealand Naval Medical Services comprised a small number of medical officers drawn largely from the volunteer reserve, and sick-bay personnel on the ships of the N.Z. Navy and at the naval bases in New Zealand. The majority of New Zealand personnel, however, were seconded to the Royal Navy.

Nursing sisters were seconded from the Army Nursing Service to the small naval hospital and training school established at Auckland, and a sick-berth branch of the W.R.N.S. was also formed.

A small number of casualties were dealt with at the battle of the River Plate, in the Solomons and in the South West Pacific.

The medical boarding of recruits, who totalled 14,000, and the invaliding boards, were carried out by naval medical officers.

The principal causes of invaliding, in a total of 762 cases, were:— neuro-psychiatric and mental disorders 182, pulmonary tuberculosis 114, wounds and injuries 75, and gastric and duodenal ulcer 48.

The relatively high incidence of tuberculosis was the only striking feature. The congested living conditions on the ships was partly responsible for this. Experience concerning neurosis was similar to that in the Army.

Total deaths, including New Zealand personnel attached to the Royal Navy, was 672, of which 494 were from enemy action, 125 from accidents and 53 from sickness. Of the latter 9 died while Ps.O.W. in Japanese hands.

The rate of deaths from sickness was only 1·23 per thousand.

Royal New Zealand Air Force Medical Services

The medical service of the Air Force was administered as part of the Army Medical Service until it became a separate service in May 1943. The service was responsible for the selection of aircrew recruits, the training of aircrew in the physiology of flight and the care of flying personnel during training and active operations in the Pacific theatre. Most of the trained pilots were seconded for duty with the R.A.F. in the main theatres of war, especially in Britain. The medical officers and orderlies of the Air Force were comparatively small in number, and active operations were limited to the Pacific theatre where as many as 8,000 Air Force personnel, including aircrew, were on service at the beginning of 1945.

Nursing sisters were seconded from the Army and V.A.Ds. of the W.A.A.F. were also attached. An important evaluation of the selection of aircrew was made during the war. This showed that young recruits straight from school and young farmers made the best pilots. The Air Force had their own Sick and Wounded Branch, under medical control.

In the Pacific theatre air stations in Fiji, Tonga and Norfolk Islands had medical personnel attached and the main Pacific Force had an advanced medical base at Santos in the New Hebrides. Two small hospitals with nursing sisters attached were established, one at Santos and another at Guadalcanal. Medical officers and orderlies were attached to the different flying units and kept in close contact with the flying personnel so as to counter the strain of flying operations.

Malaria control was the main activity. Deaths in the Pacific theatre were:—by enemy action 256, by flying and non-flying accidents 82, by sickness 7. There was relatively very little sickness.

New Zealand Prisoners-of-War

During the war 8,000 New Zealanders were taken prisoner in Greece, Crete and the Western Desert. Medical personnel were in proportion and were able in general to carry out their medical duties in captivity, especially in Germany.

In Greece temporary hospitals were set up at Corinth and Kalamata. A main prisoner-of-war hospital was established at Kokkinia near Athens where medical officers and orderlies helped their Australian and British colleagues to care for the serious casualties evacuated from Crete. In Crete New Zealand medical personnel struggled hard to establish satisfactory conditions in the prison camps. The dreadful conditions at the Salonika transit camp also called for strenuous efforts by our men to help care for the large number of sick prisoners.

Those captured during the Second Libyan and pre-Alamein campaigns were taken to Italy, where at first conditions were very unsatisfactory, but later N.Z. medical personnel were able to take a great share of the work in the hospitals. Some protected personnel were exchanged from Italy.

In Germany medical officers and orderlies were allowed to carry out their professional duties in hospitals, camps, and with working parties, with very satisfactory results.

Red Cross food parcels proved of inestimable value to all the prisoners, especially the sick and wounded.

The incidence of sickness and death was not excessive except as regards tuberculosis, for which a special hospital was established.

Red Cross medical supplies, including instruments, were of great assistance.

Deaths from sickness totalled 105, a rate twice as high as in 2 N.Z.E.F. in the Middle East. There were no serious epidemics.

Two hundred and ninety-two deaths were recorded, half of them due to drowning following the sinking of two ships transporting prisoners across the Mediterranean. Twenty-five were shot in attempts to escape.

PART V

India

The Indian Armed Forces Medical Services

By Lieutenant-Colonel B. L. Raina, A.M.C.

Detailed official accounts of the work of the Indian Armed Forces Medical Services during the Second World War will be found in the following volumes:*

Administration
Medicine, Surgery and Pathology
Campaigns in the Western Theatre
Preventive Medicine } B. L. Raina
Statistics
Medical Stores and Equipment
Campaigns in the Eastern Theatre

---

* Published by the Combined Inter-Services Historical Section, India and Pakistan, Delhi.

CONTENTS

MEDICAL SERVICES OF THE INDIAN ARMED FORCES IN THE SECOND WORLD WAR

MILITARY medicine is a part of the historical development of medical science and the concepts of warfare of the time. The Indian Army Medical Corps is, inevitably, the result of such a development. It was formed by amalgamating the Indian Medical Service (I.M.S.), the Indian Medical Department (I.M.D.) and the Indian Hospital Corps (I.H.C.).

To appreciate fully the development of the Army Medical Corps, it is necessary to recall briefly the organisation and development of the medical services in India from the middle of the 18th century.

INDIAN HOSPITAL CORPS

Little is known concerning the medical organisation that served the Indian troops during the latter part of the 19th century. In the days of the East India Company, each unit had its own small dispensary, with a few drugs and dressings. Gradually, these dispensaries developed into small regimental hospitals, known as 'Line Hospitals'. These hospitals were non-dieted and ill-equipped.

In 1881 Station Hospitals for British troops were started in the Bengal Army. The original staff was mainly recruited from the personnel of disbanded Regimental Hospitals. These personnel were enrolled into the Army Hospital Native Corps (A.H.N.C.) as compounders, dressers, ward servants, cooks and *bhistees*. They were classified as hospital attendants and their pay varied from Rs. 4 to Rs. 9 per month, depending on their calling and their grade. Rations were free only when employed on field service.

In 1895 the Presidency Armies were abolished and one system of administration was enforced for the whole of India. In 1898, the A.H.N.C. was reorganised as the Army Hospital Corps (A.H.C.) with 10 companies, each under a Divisional Principal Medical Officer. The Commissariat (Supply and Transport Corps) recruited *Dooly* bearers to carry casualties. The Frontier Force Regiments were authorised *Kahars*, who were locally engaged through the Regimental '*bania*'. In 1901, the Army Bearer Corps (A.B.C.) with 32 companies, was formed, and the *Dooly* bearers and *Kahars* were enlisted in it. Each company had *sirdars*, mates and bearers under the command of an Assistant Surgeon. In 1903 the A.B.C. was reorganised to form 10 Divisional Companies. The duties of these Divisional Companies in war were to carry stretchers and *doolies*. In peace stations they were employed on general duties in

721

hospitals and in Divisional Headquarters. At the outbreak of the First World War, the ranks of Havildar, Lance Havildar, Naik, Lance Naik and Bearer were introduced. Their pay was also increased and varied from Rs. 9 to Rs. 18 per month. They were entitled to good conduct pay, follower's scale of clothing and, after 1917, free rations at the follower's scale.

In October 1918 Station Hospitals for Indian troops were authorised. The war orderlies and followers were then locally employed by the medical authorities. There was no provision for clerks or storekeepers for the Indian Hospitals. The organisation for providing personnel for Indian and British Hospitals was completed. Bearers for both were provided by the Army Bearer Corps (A.B.C.). Followers for the British Hospital were provided by the Army Hospital Corps (A.H.C.), and hospital storekeepers and their assistants by the Supply and Transport Corps. Hospital writers, clerks and storekeepers were civilians. The multiplicity of agencies for recruitment was not conducive to efficiency. On June 1, 1920, the A.H.C., A.B.C. and the subordinate personnel of Indian Station Hospitals were, therefore, combined and the Indian Hospital Corps (I.H.C.) was formed with 10 Divisional Companies, one for each of the Military Divisions into which India and Burma were then divided. In May 1929 the I.H.C. was reorganised into five companies on a Command basis. The I.H.C. included Clerical, Store, Nursing, Ambulance and General Duty sections. To centralise records, the I.H.C. Depot was formed at Kirkee in 1935.

INDIAN MEDICAL DEPARTMENT

Early in the 19th century a scheme for the training of boys from the Upper and Lower Orphan Schools as compounders and dressers, and ultimately as sub-assistant surgeons, was started in Bengal. Similar schemes were organised in Madras and Bombay. Until 1827 there were two departments, Apothecaries and Dressers. In 1827 the dressers were re-designated as Assistant Surgeons. This branch consisted of Europeans and Anglo-Indians.

Indian Hospital Assistants were first employed in 1868. They were educated at Government expense and were taken from all classes of Indians between the ages of 16–20 years. (Training at Government expense was discontinued from 1932.) In 1900 Senior Hospital Assistants were granted the Viceroy's Commissioned ranks of *Subedars* and *Jemadars*. In 1910 these Hospital Assistants were re-designated as Sub-Assistant Surgeons.

INDIAN MEDICAL SERVICE

Prior to 1896 each Presidency had its own Medical Service. The Bengal Medical Service was formed on January 1, 1764, and the Bombay and Madras Services in 1767 and 1779 respectively.

In April 1896 the then three Presidency Medical Services were combined to form the Indian Medical Service (I.M.S.). The I.M.S. was primarily a military service and its officers were responsible for the medical care of the Indian Army. However, the members of the service appear to have been eligible for all posts for which any scientific knowledge was required. These medical officers were regularly posted to senior appointments in the Assay Department and Botanical Gardens, and were frequently posted to appointments which were quite different from their profession. Among these 'extra-professional employments' were as a cotton agent, a postmaster, a superintendent of a school of art, a naturalist, a political agent, a commissioner and a conservator of forests.

The I.M.S. officers were seconded to the Civil Service and staffed all higher civil medical appointments. The service provided medical aid throughout the country and was responsible for the direction of public health and the administration of jails. The service virtually laid the foundations for the scientific study of modern medicine, the public health services and medical research in India. Many of its contributions to medical research were outstanding and of enormous benefit to India and the rest of the world. No medical service can have done more for its country than did the I.M.S.

Secondment to the Civil Service took place after the officers had learnt their military duties and only if there was an excess over the requirements of the Army. Seconded officers were liable to recall to military service. Military medicine involves no new basic medical concepts, but the rapid development of organisation and the speed with which preventive and curative measures have to be applied demands flexibility of plans, improvisation, a vigilant outlook and an urgency not always met with in civil life. Thus, to the Civil Service these officers brought experience of organisation and administration acquired through rigid discipline, and skill to deal with problems expeditiously. On their return to the Army, they brought varied professional experience gained in different parts of the country. Both the military and civil medical services, therefore, benefited by this arrangement.

INDIAN ARMY MEDICAL CORPS

The Second World War created a different situation for the Army Medical authorities in India. They were ill-prepared to meet the requirements of the Defence Services whose size and rate of expansion had not been clearly foreseen. Despite unfavourable circumstances, an efficient organisation was built up. It was, however, realised that the shortage of doctors and nurses, and the training of I.H.C. personnel would present a difficult problem. Hence, in 1943 the Medical Personnel (Army in India) Mission recommended that a homogeneous Indian

Army Medical Corps should be formed and so Government orders to form the Indian Army Medical Corps (I.A.M.C.) with effect from April 3, 1943 were issued. The corps was formed by combining the I.M.S., I.M.D. and I.H.C. into a single corps, with its own officers and men, and it grew rapidly into a well-knit and well trained corps.

The first woman medical officer was commissioned in the I.M.S. (E.C.) in April 1942 and women have been in the service ever since.

ORGANISATION OF THE MEDICAL SERVICES

Medical Officers of the Navy and Air Force are seconded to these services from the A.M.C. Each service has its own Director of Medical Services (D.M.S.), who is the adviser to his Chief of Staff and who is responsible for the efficiency of the medical services under him. In addition, there is now a Director General, Armed Forces Medical Services (D.G. A.F.M.S.) in the Ministry of Defence. Briefly, the D.G. A.F.M.S. is responsible for recruitment of officers of the A.M.C., the Dental Services and the Military Nursing Services, provisioning and supply of medical stores, issue of technical instructions, medical research and consideration of medical matters common to the three Services.

TRAINING

Before the Second World War, I.M.S. officers recruited in India were attached to Military Hospitals where headquarters of I.H.C. Companies were located. They received professional training at the hospital and military training at the I.H.C. Company. Officers recruited in the United Kingdom, after initial military training, attended a Junior Officer's Course at the Royal Army Medical College (R.A.M. College) Millbank, London. Officers with five to seven years' service were deputed to the R.A.M. College to attend a Senior Officers' Course, which included clinical training in civil medical institutions. After the completion of the course, selected officers were permitted to study special subjects, such as Pathology, Hygiene, Medicine and Surgery at the R.A.M. College. Officers, if they wished, were permitted to take study leave to obtain post-graduate qualifications. In India, officers were sent to selected civil and military hospitals and institutions for specialist training.

During the period September 1939 to April 1942, medical officers given Emergency Commissions in the I.M.S. received initial military training for two weeks at the I.H.C. Companies and were then deputed, by selection, for further training in Field Medical Units or for specialist training and appointments. Under this scheme, the minimum requirements of training were adopted in order to meet the urgent man-power demands. The need for expansion of training facilities was felt, and a Medical Wing was started at the Officers' Training School (O.T.S.),

Mhow in April 1941. The Wing was organised to train 100 officers at a time. The training was mainly confined to military subjects such as organisation of the Army and tactical handling of medical units. In 1940 a Training Field Hygiene Section was established at Rawalpindi. Later, the Army School of Hygiene was established at Babina for the training of Medical Officers and other ranks as well as a Field Ambulance Training Centre at Secunderabad. A V.C.Os.' and N.C.Os.' school was sanctioned in December 1941, and located at Poona, for the training of a large number of I.H.C. personnel for duty with field medical units. In 1942 it was realised that the Medical Wing of the O.T.S., Mhow, did not fulfil the training needs of the military medical services. It was therefore decided to establish an Army Medical Training Centre (A.M.T.C.) for the co-ordination of post-graduate medical education of officers and technical training of I.H.C. personnel. The A.M.T.C. came into being in December 1942. It was formed in Poona by the amalgamation of the Medical Wing of the O.T.S., Mhow, the Field Ambulance Training Centre, the V.C.Os.' and N.C.Os.' school and, later, the Army School of Hygiene, Babina. The course for officers was of three months' duration and included military training and clinical medicine and surgery, with special emphasis on medical problems in the field, and hygiene. Technical training of Laboratory Assistants and Technicians, Dispensers, X-ray Assistants and Radiographers, Blood Transfusion Assistants, Sanitary Assistants, Dental Technicians and Dental Hygienists was also conducted at the A.M.T.C.

Reference may be made to the nursing services. The number was totally insufficient for both civilian and military needs. The Auxiliary Nursing Service was formed and other measures (including training schemes) were taken to meet urgent demands. Even after vigorous efforts the needs could not be fully met. The necessity to accelerate the output of nurses in peace-time is obviously imperative. The achievements of the nursing services were remarkable. They gained sixty-two decorations and mentions in despatches. Their employment in field units was a major development in the care of the sick and wounded.

ARTIFICIAL LIMB CENTRE

After the First World War it was realised that war amputees must be provided with artificial limbs and that these would require to be kept in constant repair. There were very few firms in the country making artificial limbs, and the Government placed contracts with them.

After the outbreak of the Second World War, it soon became evident that the State would have to take over the responsibility for the manufacture and repair of artificial limbs to ensure that they were of good quality. A factory was, therefore, started in Poona in the middle of 1944.

It was decided that eventually all the component parts of artificial limbs should be manufactured in India. To begin with, parts such as joints had to be imported, as manufacturing these on a large scale would have taken considerable time. The factory not only supplied artificial limbs, but other orthopaedic appliances, such as surgical boots, boots for foot drop, knee caps, walking calipers and hernia trusses.

In 1945, Medical and Electrical and Mechanical Engineer (E.M.E.) Officers and E.M.E. tradesmen were sent to the United Kingdom for training in the preparation and fitting of artificial limbs. In the same year experts from Roehampton visited India and assisted in organising the Centre on modern lines. In January 1947 the Centre was moved to Lahore as most of the raw materials required for artificial limbs were available in the Punjab or neighbouring States. After Partition, the Centre was moved back to Poona.

The Artificial Limbs Centre is now one of the largest in the world. When it was first started it catered for the needs of disabled servicemen only, but since 1951 the Centre has also provided civilians with artificial limbs and surgical appliances on payment of charges fixed by the Government. Even people from neighbouring countries have been fitted with artificial limbs at the centre. The Centre has a well-equipped walking, training and rehabilitation wing, where thorough training in the use of artificial limbs is given.

MEDICAL STORES ORGANISATION

This Organisation has passed through various stages since its inception. Its history goes back to 1888 when a few Medical Stores Depots were established for supplying medical stores to military units. These Depots were civil and quasi-commercial institutions. In 1894 they were brought under the control of the Government of India, Defence Department, their administration being vested in the Surgeon General to the Government (later D.G.I.M.S.). There were five such Depots existing at that time. The D.G.I.M.S. was responsible for the necessary civil and military commitments of India and also of overseas forces. To this end, he consolidated all demands for medical equipment and stores, and undertook their procurement and distribution to the various Depots. The Armed Forces Medical Stores Organisation was created during the Second World War and had very little time to consolidate its experiences as it was drastically reduced shortly after the cessation of hostilities. The problems of the Stores Organisation in the post-Second World War period were confined to the disposal of surpluses, reorganisation of the peace system of accounting and establishment of various procedures for the proper functioning of the Depots and Units, such as accounting, stock-verification, packing, store preservation, indenting, disposal of surplus and unauthorised holdings of units, revision of scales compatible with their needs and revision of the war-time medical vocabulary of Medical Stores.

MEDICAL DIRECTORATE

The beginning of a properly established army medical service in India may be traced to the year 1895, when the Indian Army was organised into four Commands each with a principal medical officer of the rank of Surgeon Major-General attached. A Principal Medical Officer for His Majesty's Forces in India was appointed about 1907, and five years later this appointment was re-designated as the Director of Medical Services in India. At the outbreak of war in 1914, the Headquarters staff was augmented. In 1920 the medical branch of the Army Head-quarters emerged as the Medical Directorate under the Adjutant General. The staff of the Medical Directorate included the director of medical services, a deputy director of medical services who was also the director of hospital organisation, and a director of hygiene and pathology. In addition, there were a chief woman superintendent, a director of medical organisation for war, two assistant directors of medical services and four deputy assistant directors of medical services. This organisation was changed in 1937 and consisted of the director medical services, a deputy director of medical organisation for war, a deputy director of hygiene and pathology, a deputy director of dental services, an assistant director of hygiene and pathology, a chief principal matron, two D.A.Ds.M.S. and an officer supervisor.

With the outbreak of the Second World War, the work of the Medical Directorate increased considerably. Plans had to be made to provide medical services not only for the Army in India but also for the overseas forces based on this country. A large number of recruits for the rapidly expanding Indian Army had to be medically examined, many field medical units raised and equipped and medical personnel recruited and trained. The increasing problems of hygiene, malaria and nutrition had to be effectively tackled. The machinery of medical administration had not been geared to undertake the tasks which faced it, as all the preoccu-pations of India Command before the war centred mainly on the defence of the North West Frontier. The task of the Medical Directorate was rendered more difficult as it had depended so far largely on other agencies for the provision of personnel, transport, ordnance and medical stores. This feature made organisation and planning no easier. Personal liaison with the various agencies became the only way for meeting the requirements of this fast expanding service. It seems that the Director of Medical Services, initially not a principal staff officer, was not always kept in the picture in respect of planning for the expansion of the armed forces or their disposition. This occasioned many awkward situations as the medical services were generally the last to obtain such information. Experience showed that it was imperative that the medical services should be kept informed of the situation right from the initial planning stage.

The work done by the Medical Directorate during the Second World War was impressive. Its scope of work and responsibilities increased enormously as the war progressed. In May 1941, the Director of Medical Services assumed the function of provisioning of medical stores which until then had remained the responsibility of the Director General Indian Medical Service. Officers of the Indian Medical Service in civil employment were recalled, and recruitment to the emergency branches of the Indian Medical Service and Indian Medical Department was instituted. An I.M.S. Dental Branch was formed. Training centres for field ambulances, field hygiene sections, light field ambulances, etc., were established in various stations. New establishments for field units, embodying modifications considered necessary in the light of experience gained in the various theatres, were introduced. An Army School of Hygiene was started at Babina in Uttar Pradesh. Specialist units, e.g., ear, nose and throat, ophthalmological, mobile surgical, dental, etc., were raised and mobilised. When the Allied offensive in Burma gathered momentum and casualties started pouring in, the General Headquarters Casualty Evacuation Organisation was established to deal with the problems involved. Medical arrangements for the famine-stricken in Bengal were organised by the Medical Directorate. A hospital town was established at Jalahalli to provide hospital cover for the extensive operations contemplated in South East Asia. Finally, the Medical Directorate was made responsible for the release of personnel and disbandment of units on the conclusion of hostilities.

At the outbreak of hostilities the Medical Directorate in India consisted of six sections with a total strength of 86 (including 10 officers). Many new sections were created and by August 1945 the strength of the Medical Directorate had risen to 100 officers and 555 subordinate personnel. There was a proportionate expansion of the staff at the headquarters of various commands in India to meet the increased volume of work connected with the raising of units and their mobilisation, as well as recruitment and other tasks.

RECRUITMENT

MEDICAL OFFICERS

The strength of medical officers at the beginning of hostilities was 631, the number actually employed in the military services being 366. The remainder were employed by civil medical services. In addition there was an authorised strength of 300 Army-in-India Reserve of Officers (Medical). At the outbreak of war it was clear that the total strength of medical officers available would be quite inadequate.

The emergency commissioned officers cadre was to provide the bulk of medical officers for war-time duties. The conditions of recruitment had to be considerably changed in order to ensure the free flow of recruits for the emergency cadre. The strength of medical officers in garrison hospitals was scaled down. By the end of September 1942, in spite of all these measures, there was a shortage of about 793 officers in relation to the then existing target. The rate of wastage was appreciable and a considerable number of medical officers were lost in the campaigns in Burma, Malaya and the Far East.

NURSING SERVICES

The nursing services had also presented similar problems. There was an acute shortage of trained nurses for the army. In this case the shortage was never made up and various auxiliary services had to be instituted to ensure that at least a minimum number was available. The A.N.S. (I.) was inaugurated on September 24, 1941, and in all 2,787 nurses joined the service for the army and civil defence duties. On August 1, 1945, the actual strength of the A.N.S. (I.) serving was 1,709, which included 1,500 for general service in India and abroad. They were not fully trained nurses. They were given training in selected hospitals, both military and civil, so that they could carry out their duties efficiently.

INDIAN HOSPITAL CORPS

The rank and file of the medical services was formed by the Indian Hospital Corps (I.H.C.) which was established on June 1, 1920. In September 1939, the corps had a strength of 8,645 and an authorised reserve of 3,522. The war naturally demanded a rapid expansion in the corps, and it was anticipated that even in 1941 the additional requirements would be in the region of 21,000. Demands from overseas units for reinforcements were higher than anticipated. Recruitment to the corps was carried out by the army recruiting organisation. In the beginning, owing to the low standards required and unsatisfactory terms of service offered to recruits, they came mainly from illiterate classes. Some were also selected from those considered unfit for other arms of services. It is surprising how long it took to appreciate that the work of the I.H.C. personnel was of a highly technical nature and required certain essential basic qualifications as well as aptitude. The basic standards, terms and conditions of recruitment, especially in pay and prospects, were considerably improved, and recruitment thereafter became fairly satisfactory. On the formation of the I.A.M.C. in April 1943, the corps had a strength of 86,268. By October 1945 it had reached a strength of 147,100.

COMMITMENTS

At the beginning of the war in September 1939, the Indian Army had a strength of approximately 352,000, including British troops numbering about 67,000. In addition an air force of about seven squadrons was based on India and there was a small navy. The then existing plan of operations had allotted the tasks of frontier defence, internal security and coastal defence to the army. In addition, the army maintained a general reserve which was primarily meant for external defence. This formation had a strength of approximately one division with most of the supporting and ancillary personnel, and was organised into three independent brigades under the command of Headquarters Deccan District. This force was actually despatched to the Middle East before the beginning of the war, and subsequently became the 4th Indian Division.

These commitments of India were to expand beyond all estimates as the war progressed and enveloped almost the whole world. Increasing commitments were met by expanding the army to about eight times the pre-war strength. General mobilisation was not ordered either at the beginning or during the course of the war. Recruitment continued satisfactorily under a scheme of progressive mobilisation, and the intake covered requirement. By May 1940, it was apparent that the pace of expansion had to be speeded up to meet the growing commitments at home and abroad. With the fall of France and the spread of war to the Middle East, India's commitments in the western theatre had increased, especially when operations in Iraq and Iran were undertaken. In the autumn of 1941, two Indian divisions were in Malaya. For the operations in Iraq and Iran, India had despatched about three and a half divisions. All requirements of administrative and auxiliary units for these formations were also met by India. By the end of 1941, India had overseas the equivalent in numbers of 15 divisions, a force larger than that sent by any other Commonwealth Country.

Japan entered the war in December 1941 and after a short-lived campaign, Malaya and Burma passed under Japanese control. In addition to the loss of experienced fighting formations, 33 medical units, including nine hospitals, were lost in this theatre. Increased commitments coupled with these losses imposed a considerable strain on the medical man-power situation, which remained critical, with no visible signs of improvement. By the end of 1942 the Japanese advance appeared to have been held, but the potential threat of invasion still remained. Plans were now made to convert India into a base for operations against the Japanese in South East Asia and for providing supplies to China. India was to receive, maintain and train far larger forces than ever before for the fight against the Japanese. Although planning work began early in 1943, it was not until the formation of South East Asia

Command in November 1943, that the size of the force that had to be based on India was known. It became clear that the administrative arrangements set up for the forces operating in the west would be totally inadequate to meet the commitments in the east, which grew to enormous proportions by the time hostilities ceased in 1945. No part of this fresh task was in any way connected with frontier defence or internal security, for these had been completed much earlier and required no further expansion. By the end of September 1945, the army had expanded to 2,644,323. Over 500,000 were under training, and 600,000 were in depots and on L. of C. duties. The majority of these were directly or indirectly connected with the South East Asia Command operations.

Ratio of medical services to troops of the Army-in-India and Indian Army Overseas—1939-1945.

Date	Total Army-in-India and Indian Army Overseas	Total medical services Army-in-India and Indian Army Overseas	Ratio of medical services to troops
31 December, 1939 . . .	361,325	13,566	1 : 27
31 December, 1940 . . .	558,046	28,889	1 : 19
31 December, 1941 . . .	1,020,392	62,527	1 : 16
31 December, 1942 . . .	1,827,417	81,306	1 : 22
31 December, 1943 . . .	2,362,156	120,139	1 : 20
31 December, 1944 . . .	2,560,574	157,589	1 : 16
31 December, 1945 . . .	2,644,323	174,740	1 : 15

The medical services in India were responsible for (i) the raising, equipping and training of such medical units as were necessary for the field force; (ii) the maintenance of the supply of trained personnel as reinforcement for these forces; (iii) the provision of a full medical service for the Army-in-India as well as for the Navy and Air Force; (iv) the creation of a provisioning establishment which would be capable of supplying the needs of the Army-in-India and the needs of the civil population in countries from which the Japanese were ejected until such time as the civil administration was established; (v) the reception and treatment in India of casualties from the forces based on India operating in overland or overseas theatres, a task which necessitated the provision of adequate transportation facilities and base hospitals; and (vi) subsequent disposal of casualties unfit for further service to their depots in India or to the United Kingdom, the latter being a task which necessitated an adequate provision of hospital ships.

The magnitude of India's war effort can only be realised when viewed against the background of the serious shortcomings that had to be faced. The vast extent of the country with its limited transportation system constituted a big problem. Although India is twenty times as large as the United Kingdom, it had only the same mileage of rail track and about one-fourth the rolling stock. For a country about as large as Europe there were only seven harbours. The railway, telegraph, telephone, and road systems, which were fairly adequate for peace-time conditions, were quite inadequate for the huge expansion entailed by war. There was hardly any marginal reserve for food, housing or storage. The financial policy of the then Government of India precluded development in many spheres of national life. These were some of the serious problems for a country which found itself a base for war in the east as well as the west.

FIELD MEDICAL UNITS

The medical organisation in India for a field force at the beginning of the Second World War did not differ materially in principle from the one that had existed for the operations on the North West Frontier of India. But it did not take long to realise that the organisation evolved for positional warfare in a mountainous terrain like the North West Frontier was hardly suitable for situations likely to be encountered in a warfare involving highly mobile and mechanised forces in different terrains. A thorough remodelling of the medical arrangements for the field, therefore, became inevitable. Existing units had to be reorganised and their establishments changed, while new units had to be evolved and perfected. These improvements and modifications, however, took time and were completed, in some cases, only at the very late stages.

Each battalion on mobilisation had one medical officer on its strength. For duty with the regimental medical officer (R.M.O.), the unit provided an orderly trained in first-aid and sanitation work. The smaller units had no medical officer on their establishment, only trained orderlies. Sick personnel attended the nearest medical inspection room. The R.M.O. was responsible to the officer commanding (O.C.) for the maintenance of the health of the troops. Technically he came under a senior administrative medical officer, usually the Assistant Director of Medical Services.

The field medical units included the field ambulance, the casualty clearing station (C.C.S.), the staging section, the general hospital, the field hygiene section and the motor ambulance section (M.A.S.). Ancillary units such as the mobile X-ray unit, the field laboratory, the convalescent depot and the advanced depot medical stores were also available. Specialised units like the E.N.T., mobile surgical, and anti-malaria units, etc., were formed as the war progressed.

FIELD AMBULANCES

The field ambulance was the most important forward medical unit and concerned itself mainly with the early treatment of casualties and their evacuation to rear areas. The Indian field ambulance was organised at the beginning of the war on the basis of experience gained during the First World War as well as on the operations on the North West Frontier, and comprised a headquarters and two companies. The headquarters was designed to form a main dressing station (M.D.S.), while the two companies formed the advanced dressing stations (A.D.Ss.). An A.D.S. was equipped to deal with casualties received from the regimental aid post (R.A.P.), but only undertook the most urgent treatment, such as the treatment of shock, arrest of haemorrhage and the immobilisation of fractures. Usually stretcher bearers evacuated casualties from the R.A.P. to the A.D.S. Casualties from the A.D.S. to the M.D.S. were evacuated in motor vehicles wherever the terrain permitted; otherwise by animal transport (A.T.) or river craft. The field ambulance was essentially a mobile unit and as such could only provide the simplest accommodation and treatment. Patients requiring more elaborate care were evacuated to the rear units, which were equipped to deal with complicated cases. In addition to the A.D.S. and the M.D.S. the field ambulance staff also established casualty clearing posts and rest stations, wherever necessary.

Considerable alterations had to be made in the organisation, allocation and deployment of the field ambulance. Its tactical use also underwent considerable modification in the light of experience. The realisation of the importance of forward surgery—a lesson learnt fortunately early enough in this war—necessitated the use of the mobile surgical unit along with the M.D.S. as a forward surgical centre. It was possible to use the field ambulance in various rôles on the line of evacuation with minimum improvisation.

Changes in the organisation of the fighting forces during the course of the war necessitated modification of field ambulances to suit the changed establishments of formations. The light field ambulance for use with armoured divisions came into existence, with headquarters and four sections, each capable of division into two independent self-contained half-sections so that they could be widely deployed. Their increased mobility enabled them to keep close to the fighting forces. The parachute field ambulance grew out of the parachute medical detachment. The headquarters and four sections were fully mobile. The mobile surgical units (parachute) were attached to this field ambulance for operational requirements.

CASUALTY CLEARING STATIONS (C.C.S.)

The casualty clearing station was usually organised in a light section of 50 beds, a heavy section of 150 beds and an administrative headquarters which could be attached to either. The heavy section was capable of further division into two half-sections of 75 beds each. An operating team and later a mobile X-ray unit were attached to the unit. Casualties from this unit were usually evacuated to a general hospital or to a convalescent depot. The tactical use of the unit in an advance was to move the light section forward to take over casualties from the field ambulance. The heavy section in the rear disposed of its casualties to general hospitals or convalescent depots and then moved forward to join the light section. It was customary to use the C.C.S. in echelon during an advance so that while one section was functioning, the other was packed up to move forward.

STAGING SECTIONS (S.S.)

The staging sections were sited on the line of communication (L. of C.) to provide rest and refreshment for casualties on the move, as well as urgent medical aid. In the early period of the war separate Indian and British sections were set up. Towards the end of 1940, combined sections catered for both Indian and British troops. These sections were peculiar to the Indian Army and usually released the field ambulance from the task of providing personnel and equipment for rest stations. In all, 124 staging sections were established and some of these were changed from one type to the other.

HOSPITALS

Three main types of hospitals were organised during the war, *viz.*, the Indian General Hospital (I.G.H.), the British General Hospital (B.G.H.) and the Combined General Hospital (C.G.H.). The I.G.H. consisted of a headquarters and a varying number of sections (each of 100 beds). The B.G.H. was exclusively for British personnel and had an establishment similar to that of the I.G.H., but the number of sections usually did not exceed six. The C.G.H. was a new type introduced in the early months of the war and consisted of a headquarters and six sections, five Indian and one British. In all cases provision was made for further expansion and specialists were authorised on suitable scales. Later it was found necessary to increase the headquarters staff when the number of sections was increased. In all, 117 general hospitals were set up in India, and these included 37 Indian, 9 British and 71 combined general hospitals. In India, base general hospitals for Indian and British troops were provided on separate establishments, but generally followed the main pattern of British and Indian general hospitals. The number of sections in these hospitals varied from 8 to 15. The necessary complement of specialists was authorised. There was an acute shortage of nursing officers during the whole period of the war, and allotment of nurses to the various hospitals had sometimes to be reduced to half. By January 1942, members of the Auxiliary Nursing Service (India) were available for service overseas, and these nurses were posted to overseas hospitals in place of nursing officers. The hospitals were mobilised in sufficient number to provide bed accommodation. Provision was also made for the expansion of the hospitals in an emergency. The hospitals were usually located at the bases or on the L. of C.

CONVALESCENT DEPOTS

The need for convalescent depots was felt as early as 1940, but until June 1942, there were only two field convalescent depots. Others were to be mobilised and opened as required. Each unit had two medical officers. These units were found very useful and, in times of emergency, could accommodate ambulant cases from hospitals. The establishment was considerably modified to suit the needs, and units for service in India and overseas were speedily set up. In all, 33 convalescent depots for Indian troops and 19 for British troops were established during the war.

MOBILE SURGICAL UNITS (M.S.U.)

Experience in the Middle East revealed that a single surgeon attached to a C.C.S. or a hospital was unable to cope with the work during a heavy influx of casualties. Often two additional surgeons were required. The most economical way of meeting this situation was not by increasing the number of surgeons on the establishment of the general hospital or the C.C.S., but by setting up specialised units. A self-contained mobile surgical unit was thus formed. With the establishment of forward surgery as an essential life-saving measure, it was found that these mobile surgical units were extremely useful as they could be pushed as far forward as the M.D.S., or even further if needed. The staff of these units consisted of one surgeon, one anaesthetist, one nursing sister and a few other ranks. The intention was to bring surgical aid as far forward to the casualty as possible in order to avoid the risk of long evacuation. Thus, very little time was lost between the infliction of a wound and skilled surgical treatment. The provision of these units not only speeded recovery but also lessened the period of inevitable discomfort to the wounded, and increased the morale of the troops. The mobile surgical unit was usually a corps unit and was allotted on the basis of two per division. In all 24 mobile surgical units were set up.

FIELD TRANSFUSION UNITS (F.T.U.)

Transfusion units ensured the supply of blood and blood products at the most forward medical units. Specialised field transfusion units were also employed with mobile refrigerators and a staff trained in transfusion work.

MAXILLO-FACIAL SURGICAL UNITS (M.F.S.U.)

Maxillo-facial surgical units had existed in the British Army as early as November 1941, and came into existence in India by March 1943. These units were attached to general hospitals.

X-RAY UNITS

The X-ray unit or mobile X-ray unit was attached to a general hospital or a C.C.S. and was under the administrative control of the O.C. of the hospital or C.C.S. to which it was attached. The mobile X-ray unit had motor transport for an X-ray plant and a generating set. Ninety-seven X-ray units were set up.

MOBILE OPHTHALMIC UNITS (M.O.US.)

The ophthalmic units included a specialist in ophthalmology and a limited nursing staff. Twenty-nine ophthalmic units were provided. The normal allotment was one unit per division.

FIELD HYGIENE SECTIONS

At the outbreak of war it was decided to provide field hygiene sections on the basis of two per division. Of these, one was to be a divisional unit and the other a L. of C. unit. Subsequently this scale was found inadequate, especially where the L. of C. was lengthy or difficult, and the scale of three per division was sanctioned. The field hygiene section normally consisted of a headquarters and three sub-sections, each of the latter being capable of working independently. The personnel included bricklayers, carpenters, tinsmiths, sweepers, and trained supervisory staff of non-commissioned officers (N.C.O.) and an officer trained in hygiene. The equipment of the sub-sections was so designed that each could carry out its technical work independently. The duties of a field hygiene section were partly supervisory and inspectorial and partly executive. The former included the inspection and supervision of the purification of water, disposal of human and animal waste products, general sanitation of the camp and supervisory control over all other problems of hygiene. The executive functions mainly were: control of epidemic diseases, disinfection, disinfestation and the provision of sanitary appliances until such time as the unit sanitary organisation was able to function. In addition, these sections trained regimental sanitary personnel and carried out sanitary schemes which were beyond the limited scope of the unit.

ANTI-MALARIA UNITS (A.M.U.)

The need for malaria control and research when troops were deployed for operational duties in malarious areas had been accepted since the First World War when malaria decimated operational troops in Macedonia and in East Africa. These units, however, were not organised in the pre-war years nor were they used in the North West Frontier operations. Wherever it was necessary to undertake anti-malaria measures, the duty was usually assigned to the field hygiene sections. The R.M.O. was responsible for personal prophylaxis as well as for such other limited anti-malaria measures as were possible in the camps.

The situation did not materially alter at the beginning of the Second World War, and it was only in March 1941 that the anti-malaria unit was formed. The unit consisted of a medical officer trained in malariology, an assistant surgeon and a small staff of ward servants and laboratory assistants. These units were to work in conjunction with the field hygiene sections whose resources were not adequate to include the work of malaria control. This problem was one which necessitated efficient and continuous anti-larval measures and an adequate supervisory organisation. Civilian labour was employed to undertake major works in connexion with anti-malaria measures. The field hygiene sections were involved in frequent and rapid moves, and these units could hardly discharge such functions. When divisional areas were taken over by L. of C. during an advance, there was a definite time-lag before the latter could get effective control over the area. During the active malaria season this time-lag was really a critical period. Many major malaria outbreaks occurred owing to infection contracted during such periods. It was decided to provide a permanent and trained supervisory anti-malaria staff to carry out uniformly efficient malaria control. Accordingly a fully fledged unit with a headquarters and four sections for work in different areas was organised. Adequate transport to facilitate the task of the unit, which usually covered a wide area, was also provided. In addition to the permanent staff of the unit, provision was also made for civilian labourers to be attached temporarily to the unit, and powers were given to the O.C. to recruit local labour to undertake major works. The number of anti-malaria units required in a certain area was decided, not on the strength of the formations deployed in the area, but on a regional basis. A preliminary survey was made of the areas to which formations were likely to move. Information as regards malaria in enemy occupied areas into which the troops were likely to move was obtained beforehand and the number of anti-malaria units was calculated on the basis of this data. However, the normal allotment to a corps was usually six, of which three remained as corps units and one was allotted to each division. Lightly equipped 200–400 bed hospitals (Malaria Forward Treatment Units) were also formed.

FIELD LABORATORIES

Another unit which came into existence during the war was the field laboratory. Though used in a skeleton form in the North West Frontier Province, its emergence as a fully fledged unit occurred during the war.

It was decided to set up one field laboratory to serve two general hospitals on the assumption that general hospitals would always be grouped together. This allotment had subsequently to be changed when it was found that one field laboratory could hardly cope with the laboratory work of two hospitals, especially in the eastern theatre, where over 60 per cent. of cases required laboratory investigations. Steps were taken to provide more field laboratory units and their allotment was increased to one per five sections. A specialist in pathology was usually in charge of the unit. Sixty field laboratories were set up during the war.

OTHER UNITS

Other units included ambulance trains, ambulance coaches, hospital river steamers, hospital ships, hospital carriers and trooping parties. This group of units was involved in evacuating casualties from abroad to India and conveying them from one part of the country to another. The hospital ships were unarmed and were protected under the terms of the International Conventions. Air-conditioned wards were usually provided in hospital ships operating in tropical waters.

AIR EVACUATION

The outstanding development relating to the evacuation of casualties during the war was evacuation by air. The varied terrain—desert, mountains, jungles, rivers, chaungs, beaches—led to the use of every type of transport from hand carriage to water and aircraft. Notable advances were made in reception, evacuation and distribution of casualties, especially in air evacuation. During the retreat from Burma 1,900 sick and wounded were evacuated in ten days by air. In the beginning air evacuation was on a limited scale, and mostly to meet emergencies. By the end of the war a large scale, continuous, well developed air evacuation organisation had been developed. The recorded evacuation of casualties by air during the fighting in South East Asia in 1944 and 1945 was 178,367. This method reduced the period of evacuation from weeks to a few hours, with a consequent saving of life and suffering. By 1945 patients with gunshot wounds of the head reached the neuro-surgical unit at Comilla in India within a few hours of being wounded in North Burma. This volume of air evacuation was possible owing to air supremacy. Experience suggests that for the evacuation of casualties the use of aircraft marked with the Geneva Red Cross emblem and special airstrips similarly marked, is desirable.

DISEASES DURING THE WAR

In the early years of the war most of the trained personnel and reserve medical supplies were allocated to the Middle East, Iraq and Persia.

Japanese victories in South East Asia and the ultimate withdrawal of the Indian and British troops, along with about 500,000 civilians from Burma in 1942, created a grave situation. The annual sickness rate on the Indo-Burma front in 1943 rose to 1,196 per 1,000. Hospitals were taxed to the utmost capacity as the accommodation available was about one-sixth of the need. The medical services were strained almost to breaking point.

Subsequent fighting on the Indo–Burma front was carried out in areas notorious for a high incidence of ill health and infectious diseases. These areas included some of the most highly malarious regions of the world, with an annual rainfall as high as 200 inches. Facilities for treatment as far forward as possible in the field were provided to reduce evacuation of casualties to the base. Research teams were established to study urgent problems. The resources of the whole country, including many departments and civilian institutions, were harnessed. By 1945, 1,163 medical units, including 374 specialist units, had been raised; hospital beds were increased from 13,321 in 1939 to 197,539 and 9,393 medical officers, 4,104 nurses and 152,469 other ranks were serving in the medical services.

Malaria, dysentery, diarrhoea, venereal diseases, minor septic conditions, common colds and skin diseases stand out prominently as the principal causes of morbidity. They accounted for 70 per cent. of all admissions in 1942, 66 per cent. in 1943, 59 per cent. in 1944 and about 48 per cent. in 1945. The most important single cause of morbidity was malaria (418 per 1,000 in 1942 and 479 in 1943). During 1943 and 1944, injuries due to enemy action also increased.

MALARIA

It may be recalled that malaria had played an important part in deciding the fate of military campaigns from very early times. The Walcherian expedition of 1809, the First Burma Campaign (1824–26), and the incidence of the disease in Macedonia, Egypt, East Africa and Mesopotamia in the First World War are well known examples. During the Second World War, history once again repeated itself in Burma, the South West Pacific, the Middle East, North Africa, Sicily, Italy and in East and West Africa.

On the Indo–Burma front during 1943 and 1944 morbidity figures revealed that, statistically, every soldier was hospitalised more than once. For every 10 persons sick from all causes about 3 to 5 suffered from malaria alone. It is estimated that the daily average of malaria cases in 1943 and 1944 was 5,560 and 3,606 respectively. In three months, October to December, 1942, 18,000 cases were evacuated from the Eastern Army. These figures, however, do not reflect the very high regional morbidity in certain formations.

The anti-malaria organisation which was evolved during the war must be considered against this background. It had to cope with a huge and complex problem, and was accordingly comprehensive in its scope. Anti-malaria units, malaria forward treatment units and research units were set up and large malaria control projects started. In Manipur base alone, 600 miles of drainage were constructed and maintained during 1944, while 454,292,148 lbs. of D.D.T. were sprayed and 801 million tablets of mepacrine distributed during 1944 and 1945. All the troops east of the line Gauhati (inclusive) Shillong (exclusive) and Chittagong (inclusive) were given suppressive mepacrine. New insecticides, repellents and other personnel protective measures and suppressive mepacrine considerably reduced the wastage of man-power due to malaria. Thus, in 1945 malaria incidence was reduced to one tenth of what it had been in 1943 and the daily malaria sick rate in A.L.F.S.E.A. dropped from 0·95 per 1,000 men per day in March 1943 to 0·20 in March 1945. According to the report, *The Utilisation of Hospitals and Man-power*, by the Operational Research Group India, an average of 8·5 days was required for the treatment of a case of malaria in 1945, compared with 40·6 during the Dardanelles Campaign in 1915. In the Middle East Force in 1943 this figure was 24·4 (including stay in convalescent depots) and in 1944 it was 20·6.

A large amount of work on mosquito ecology was done during the war. Some new observations were also made. For example, in Assam, an additional carrier, *A. leucosphyrus* was found in heavily wooded valleys. It was observed that in the pre-monsoon periods *A. minimus* was the carrier; during monsoons *A. leucosphyrus* carried on the transmission and after the rains *A. minimus* returned again. Two additional carriers were also observed in Arakan, *A. jeyporiensis var cadiensia* and *A. phillipinesis*. Although *A. jeyporiensis* appeared for a short period (March and April) it began transmission early, raising the gametocyte rate in the local population, and enabling *A. minimus*, the latecomer, to start intensive transmission. This overlapping of two species *A. minimus* and *leucosphyrus* also occurred in other places such as the Kabaw Valley and led to an unusually high incidence of the disease.

The high relapse rate of benign tertian malaria and the varied and severe manifestations of malignant tertian malaria gave rise to serious problems which remained unsolved. About 50 per cent. of benign tertian cases relapsed either within the first three months or between the sixth and the ninth months of the primary attack. It was difficult to decide whether a particular relapse was a true relapse or a fresh infection. The relapses were usually related to multiple infection, incomplete treatment of the primary attack and/or deficient immunity.

The formation of malaria forward treatment units made it possible to treat malaria patients as near the forward areas as possible. This obviated the necessity of evacuating cases and enabled the malaria casualties to return to their units in reasonable time. Later, anti-larval measures were almost completely replaced by suppressive mepacrine and residual D.D.T. spraying. Great stress was also laid on personal protective measures. Their effectiveness was variable, and depended on the living conditions of troops and the infectivity and biting habits of mosquitoes. In stationary units and camps in Assam, these measures were generally successful, especially the use of mosquito nets. In operational areas, where a large number of persons were on night duty and exposed to a high infectivity rate of *A. minimus*, protective clothing alone proved to be ineffective. The incidence of malaria in the 23rd Indian Division in the Kabaw Valley in 1943 is an apt example. In the latter part of the campaign the reduction in malaria, sometimes attributed to the personal protective measures, was probably the result of D.D.T. spraying and suppressive mepacrine.

For effective control it was obvious that mere advice and orders were not enough. Success depended on medical leadership, on how far the medical services could persuade the commanders to accept and enforce their advice, and to what extent the soldiers could be convinced of the utility of preventive measures. It was established beyond doubt that the incidence of malaria was directly related to the interest taken by the commander and the discipline enforced in a unit.

That malaria influenced the conduct of the war is indisputable, yet it is true also that malaria was not deliberately employed as a weapon of war, though it was certainly reckoned with in tactical planning. The controversial subject of the use of malaria as a weapon of war is hypothetical. Nevertheless, malaria was a decisive factor in some battles, such as the one around Imphal where the Japanese died in hundreds, in Tamu and the Kabaw Valley and where their forces could not maintain their supply lines because of sickness.

The development of a separate anti-malaria organisation gave rise to some comment. It is often forgotten that the scope of hygiene and anti-malaria measures had widened considerably during the war. The urgent, manifold and difficult anti-larval operations, before the advent of D.D.T., made the task all the more exacting. It was obvious that the hygiene officers alone could not undertake the responsibility for both hygiene and anti-malaria operations without affecting the efficiency of the one or the other. The anti-malaria organisation, was, therefore, developed in response to the pressure of circumstances. The need to eliminate malaria as the most dangerous foe in the campaign was urgent. 'Theoretical considerations had to give way to this primary necessity. Organisationally the dominant need was to ensure the speediest possible development of an efficient plan for the conquest of malaria, and that could be ensured by having two parallel organisations of hygiene and anti-malaria rather than by expanding the former to cover the functions of both'. The anti-malaria and hygiene policies were, however, integrated at G.H.Q. It must be stated that the successful tactical moves and the subsequent re-occupation of Burma, through highly malarious areas, were made possible by the anti-malaria organisation which was evolved.

During the early part of the war the treatment of malaria was on the lines recommended by the League of Nations. In 1942, the system of giving quinine for two days, mepacrine for five days, rest for two days and pamaquin for five days was introduced. The work of Shannon, as well as the experience in other theatres of war, suggested that treatment with mepacrine alone was satisfactory if a sufficient dosage was given at the initial stage to ensure a high mepacrine blood level rapidly, and small maintenance dosage thereafter. Controlled and successful trials of this procedure resulted in the introduction of the all-mepacrine treatment. In areas where suppressive mepacrine discipline was not enforced all the patients recovering from malaria were given a maintenance dose (0·1g. daily for 42 days) after discharge from the hospital. Experience had shown that the tendency to primary relapse in B.T. malaria was noticeable in the first six weeks after recovery and the second relapse about six months after the initial attack. The six weeks daily maintenance course was designed to cover this early relapse and also to cure all cases of M.T. infection. At the time, the stock position of mepacrine did not permit a longer maintenance period. The aim up to 1945, however, was that when sufficient mepacrine was available, all cases which had relapsed twice should be placed on continuous suppressive therapy, no matter in what part of the country they were located. A trial of combined treatment with quinine and pamaquin, ten grains each, thrice daily for ten days, given concurrently, was instituted for B.T. relapse patients. It was noticed that 34 per cent. of the 384 cases so treated relapsed within three months. These results and the danger of pamaquin haemoglobinuria indicated that it was not justifiable to continue this treatment. The all-mepacrine treatment was found relatively the best available. The problem of B.T. malaria relapses still remained unsolved, although much was learnt about the treatment of M.T. malaria. The necessity for immediate diagnosis and treatment of cases of cerebral malaria had to be frequently emphasised. Ransome, Gupta and Paterson introduced the routine management of cerebral cases in Fowler's position combined with drip-hydration and nutrition by the Ryle's tube. The incidence of black-water fever on the Indo–Burma front was low, being 0·01 per 1,000 from January to September 1945. This was attributed to the use of mepacrine. The aetiology of black-water fever was not clear. It was suggested that the main cause may be renal ischaemia and anoxia. The experience gained during the war led to malaria control schemes and later to malaria eradication programmes in India.

DYSENTERY

Next to malaria, diarrhoea and the dysenteries were the most common ailments. The highest incidence of dysentery in Indian troops per 1,000, was as follows: Burma and S.E.A.C., (excluding Ceylon) 49·42 (in 1942); Ceylon 24·64 (1944); Sudan and Eritrea 24·86 (1942); Persia and Iraq 29·50 (1941); Egypt, Western Desert and North Africa 28·77 (1942).

Sulphaguanidine was not available for general treatment of bacillary dysentery until 1943 but supplies progressively increased. The policy was to allow full supplies for forward areas and to retain the balance for use in the base and garrison hospitals. All cases in forward areas were thus ensured treatment with sulphaguanidine. Some cases were also treated with other sulpha drugs, especially sulphathiazole. Succinyl sulphathiazole was available in small quantities only and its use was reserved for surgical cases involving intestinal operations. With the introduction of sulpha drugs bacillary dysentery ceased to cause anxiety. The treatment of amoebic dysentery, however, continued to be difficult. Until 1945, anti-amoebic drugs were in short supply. It was, therefore, a case of using whatever was available; with the result that cases of amoebic dysentery were treated with 12 injections of emetine hydrochloride followed by arsenical preparations, if available; otherwise, an additional six emetine injections were given. This treatment was repeated in relapse cases and it happened that some of the relapsed cases received upwards of 100 injections of emetine. The relapse rate unfortunately was high and a large number of cases of chronic amoebiasis among British troops had to be evacuated to hospitals in the United Kingdom. It was alleged that these cases had not been treated satisfactorily. While admitting the justification for the criticism, it was urged, in extenuation, that India at the time could give no other treatment, as drugs such as chiniofonum, emetine bismuth iodide (E.B.I.) and diodoquin were not available. As the supply situation improved a standard treatment was introduced in 1944. The need for a fresh outlook was, however, obvious and special emphasis was given to the importance of the initial attack being taken seriously, early diagnosis established and treatment instituted without delay. A complete clearance examination, repeated three weeks after the discharge of the patient from hospital was considered essential at the termination of the treatment. The value of sigmoidoscopy was stressed, and to ensure its routine practice in all hospitals, sanction was given for the provision of a sigmoidoscope in each hospital of 300 beds and over and of two in hospitals of over 1,200 beds. The results of the standard treatment were gratifying and this was attributed to the establishment of a well-regulated system of therapy and follow-up. The course of treatment outlined was a compromise between the patients' requirement and the drugs available and consisted of six injections of emetine and chiniofonum retention enema.

The research for effective amoebicides, however, continued unabated. Two research teams, at Ranchi and Poona, were set up to test the drugs and to report on their efficacy. By the middle of 1945, liberal supplies of E.B.I. became available and encouraging reports on the value of diodoquin were received. It was also noticed that amoebic ulcers were complicated by an advanced degree of secondary infection which indicated the necessity for previous treatment of chronic amoebic dysentery cases with sulphasuxidine and later with penicillin. The standard treatment was modified accordingly. The new treatment recognised E.B.I. as the drug of prominent value. Emetine injections twice or thrice were permissible only for relieving initial acute symptoms. The E.B.I. therapy was supplemented by the administration of oral diodoquin or enemata of chiniofonum and the treatment was completed with the administration of an arsenical preparation for a short period. Emphasis was maintained on the importance of early examination and treatment, and sigmoidoscopy on its termination.

TYPHUS

The concentration of troops in Assam and the campaign in the Kabaw Valley and other mite-infested regions brought into prominence the menace of scrub typhus. Between July 1943 and October 1944, nearly 3,000 cases were evacuated from the Burma front, with a mortality of about 10 per cent. In the ensuing campaigns troops in larger numbers were to be employed and they were understandably apprehensive of the risks involved. In view of these considerations, research organisations were set up to study the problem. The G.H.Q. Field Typhus Research Team, Medical Research Council (M.R.C.) Typhus Team, the U.S.A. Typhus Commission and others investigated the problem. *Trombicula Deliensis* was established as the vector in these regions. Several strains of *Rickettsia Tsutsugamushi* were also isolated. The extreme prostration in most cases, the rash, the frequency of respiratory complications, the association of malaria, the temporary nature of cardiac affections were some of the important features observed. It was also noticed that it was dangerous to move the patients after the fifth day of the disease. In the absence of any specific treatment (before the introduction of chloromycetin) the patients were treated on general lines such as skilled nursing, fluid and salt balance and adequate nutrition. If cyanosis set in, it was found necessary to give oxygen.

INFECTIVE HEPATITIS

The incidence of infective hepatitis in India and Burma did not assume the same proportions as in the Middle East. The features of the disease, however, were identical.

Incidence was low among the Indian troops. This might be due to the fact that they had acquired an immunity in early life. Mortality among Indian troops was higher than among the British owing to their lower protein intake and poor nutritional reserve. Post-arsenical jaundice, common both among the Indian and British troops, was found to be due to the transmission of the causative agent through the syringes used for injections. It appeared to be of greater severity than true infective hepatitis, showed longer duration, greater liability to haemorrhages and was associated with higher mortality.

NUTRITION AND DEFICIENCY DISEASES

The war-time food supply position created serious problems. They were accentuated by recruitment of men of low nutritional status. The latter problem was more marked. Soon after the declaration of the war, it was impossible to depend on the old sources of supply of men with characteristically fine physique. Men of inferior physical and nutritional status had to be recruited. To make them fit for battle and raise their stamina and resistance to disease called for a thorough nutritional reconditioning, which considerably taxed the ingenuity of the medical services. The general food situation made the problem more complicated.

The total energy value and vitamin content of military rations was worked out to a reasonable degree of accuracy, and it was thus possible to determine whether or not a particular scale of rations was conducive to the promotion and maintenance of health. The requirement of troops such as the Long Range Penetration Groups, and patrols in tropical and sub-tropical regions necessitated the preparation of ration scales specially suited to them.

Scurvy did not affect the fighting men. Correct planning of military rations and the liberal use of vitamin preparations were to a great extent responsible for this phenomenon. The Japanese success in South East Asia cut off food supplies from Indo-China, Thailand and Burma. Shortage of shipping aggravated the problem of supply to the forces fighting in Burma, which lay at the end of a long and difficult line of communication. Problems also arose with the new developments in strategy. Jungle warfare, long range patrolling commandos, and para-troops made new demands, for the troops had to be away for considerable lengths of time from their bases and had to be maintained on rations which, besides being palatable, would provide adequate nutrition. The consideration of bulk and weight was important in such rations, and in the absence of a well developed food-processing industry in India much reliance had to be placed on imported commodities. In the Assam–Burma regions, where the troops were necessarily exposed to diseases such as malaria, dysentery and ankylostomiasis, malnutrition appeared among the Indian troops and necessitated the evacuation of considerable numbers from the forward areas. A large proportion of the sick suffered from multiple vitamin deficiencies, especially of the B vitamins. Attempts to cure them with simple purified vitamins were generally unsuccessful. These cases responded to improvement in rations, mainly fresh protective foods and those of high protein value. The British troops under similar conditions reacted differently; they recovered more quickly and completely than their Indian compeers, and this led to the belief that the unfavourable response of the Indian troops to the conditions met with in the Burma campaign was in some way connected with the difference in the rations. The poor haemopoetic reserve and poor animal protein intake appear to have been mainly responsible for the breakdown of health of Indian troops. Over 1,000 British troops were invalided for sprue and about three times as many suffered from the disease during 1943-45. It was suggested that this condition was caused by defective biosynthesis due to changes in the intestinal flora and the breakdown of the enzymic system related to phosphorylation, which was in turn due to deficient co-enzymes embodying known or unknown members of vitamin B complex.

The notable characteristic of the Indian ration was its deficiency in animal protein and vitamin content, which led to emphasis on the need to supply meat to Indian troops. Owing to their dietary habits special consideration was given to the provision of fresh meat, but there were many difficulties in providing it. Although dehydrated meat was prepared in India for the use of Indian troops, it fell far short of solving the problem. The need for building up the nutritional reserves of the troops and for replenishing them during the campaigns was quickly recognised, and special attention was given to appropriate ration scales for this purpose.

The morale and efficiency of troops depend to a considerable extent, not only on a scientifically planned dietary but, on the manner of its preparation and presentation. Recognition of this led to improvements in catering in the Army and ultimately to the establishment of the Indian Catering Corps.

Strenuous efforts were made by the Directorate General of Industry and Supply and the Department of Food, to meet the demands of the Armed Forces. Not only were dehydrated vegetables, fruits, meat and meat products manufactured but products such as cheese, fruits and vegetables were tinned; jams and marmalade, refined salt, white pepper, bacon, oatmeal, raisin and nut blocks, amla sweets, lemonade powder, pearl barley, yeast and yeast concentrates, egg powder, golden syrup, vitaminised margarine, hard boiled sweets, sugar cubes and other such products were also produced.

In Assam and Burma, a malnutrition anaemia syndrome appeared in some cases and these responded to the improvements in rations, mainly fresh protective food and proteins of high biological value. Diarrhoea, anaemia and loss of weight, were the outstanding features in some cases. Loss of weight was so great in a large number of such cases that they were reduced to a bag of bones. These cases were labelled as marasmus syndrome. Recovery was slow and most of the patients required more than four months of treatment in hospital. Vitamins, iron, liver extracts, yeast, high protein diet and transfusion (whole blood and red cell concentrates), were all advocated as cures. Anaemia treatment centres were opened to treat and study such cases in the Central Command and the Southern Army in 1943. A marasmus investigating team was set up in 1945 to work in No. 145 I.B.G.H. (I.T.). The marasmus syndrome was limited to the Indian troops only. The British troops, on the other hand, suffered from sprue, or sprue-like syndromes.

HEAT EFFECTS

The loss of water and salt caused by a hot humid climate led to a number of cases of heat effects and dehydration.

SKIN DISEASES

Minor septic conditions ranked fourth among the sick casualties on this front. Prickly heat, septic abrasions, insect bites and fungus infections of groin and foot accounted for most of the skin diseases.

Such a wide prevalence of skin diseases was greater than had been anticipated. A pre-war establishment of seven dermatologists treated not only skin but also venereal diseases; they were equipped for combating the latter but not the former. As the army expanded, more and more troops were affected by skin diseases, (including scabies, classified as a non-dermatological disorder) and venereal diseases; but the establishment continued to be unaltered until early in 1943, when an adviser was appointed to help in what had by then become an administrative problem. Later in 1943, dermatology and venereology were separated, each specialty having an adviser, and the problem was then to find or train specialists and nursing staff in dermatology. Technical instructions were issued to acquaint regimental medical officers (R.M.Os.) and others with the rudiments of dermatology, including treatment for the commonest affections, in the hope that early recognition and adequate simple therapeutic measures would diminish the pressure on hospitals, for in most theatres of war ten per cent. of the beds had to be allocated for skin diseases, including scabies.

The great increase in dermatological work was not attributable to campaigning in unhealthy terrain; a similar increase occurred in Europe in the First World War. Most cases of inflammation of areolar tissue admitted to surgical wards began with some lesion of the skin that had not been skilfully treated in the early stage. Infection of the skin was the usual sequel to some defect in skin hygiene, the prevalence of scabies being outstanding. Prickly heat caused serious complaints mainly because the lesions usually turned septic after scratching. Adverse climatic conditions were responsible for the occurrence of jungle sores, prickly heat and widespread fungus infections.

VENEREAL DISEASES

The venereal diseases were acquired mostly in the base areas or during leave. The introduction of sulphonamides and later of penicillin considerably reduced the number of 'man-days' lost due to gonococcal infection.

NEUROLOGICAL DISEASES

Among the neurological diseases, meningitis, acute poliomyelitis, epilepsy, peripheral neuritis, neurological complications of malaria, heat-stroke, late effects of head injuries and neuropathies observed in prisoners-of-war (P.O.W.), were of special interest.

PSYCHIATRIC DISORDERS

Psychiatric disorders presented a major medical problem and it is estimated that from 10 to 15 per cent. of all casualties showed psychiatric symptoms. Arrangements for special treatment had to be made for these casualties. Practically the whole of this work grew up during the war as few facilities existed in the Indian Army in peace-time. In pre-war days patients whose psychiatric disabilities did not clear up with the simplest treatment were discharged from the army. Such a method of disposal was, of course, out of the question in war. Advance in psychiatric work took two forms; the training of psychiatrists and mental nursing orderlies (M.N.Os.) and the provision of special accommodation. An expansion of the establishment of psychiatric specialists from 4 to 86 naturally involved a variety of training schemes. Thus, in time, treatment of every type was available. In the forward areas, under the divisional psychiatrists, patients received early treatment; about 25 per cent. of these were returned to duty. On the lines of communication and in the base areas the number of beds reserved for the care and treatment of psychiatric patients varied between 3,000 and 4,000. Where possible out-patient clinics were set up. Accommodation was a serious problem. Specially designed 25-bed wards (capable of expansion) were built as part of many general hospitals in all areas. In addition, there were several bigger centres in Comilla, Calcutta, Ranchi, Moradabad, Poona, Secunderabad and finally, a 1,000-bed hospital at Jalahali 'hospital town'.

The types of illness showed certain points of interest. Psychiatric symptoms were common as an accompaniment of malaria and, now and then, of typhus. Among Indian troops conversion symptoms were more frequent than among British soldiers, in whom anxiety states were generally more prominent. Schizoid episodes were often found, and with adequate treatment responded well. The medical regulations laid down that patients with psychotic symptoms must be boarded out of the army. Experience with this short-lived type of schizophrenia, however, was such that the old policy had to be changed.

The training of the Indian M.N.Os.—a new departure—served a valuable purpose during the war. It was anticipated that these M.N.Os. would be welcomed in the civil mental hospitals after the war and this, in fact, did occur.

The sickness rate per 1,000 of psychiatric patients on the Indo–Burma front was 1·41 in 1942, 3·10 in 1943, 4·28 in 1944, and 5·33 in 1945. The rise in incidence was due to the altered conditions in which fighting took place. Exhaustion, malaria, dysentery, etc., were generally found in association with psychiatric disabilities. It was rare to find a patient with a clear cut clinical picture. The absolute morbidity rates for psychosis, psychoneurosis and not yet diagnosed (N.Y.D.) mental diseases during 1945 were 0·86, 1·20 and 3·26 respectively on this front. It often happened—more often than not—that the diagnosis was revised when the patient reached the hospital. Not all the patients were seen in the first instance by a psychiatrist—this was not possible—and so strange terms were often affixed. One 'label' found—happily a rarity—was 'N.Y.D. Lunatic'!

OTHER DISEASES

In addition to the diseases and disorders mentioned above reference may be made to arsenical encephalopathy, brucellosis, hill diarrhoea, ankylostomiasis, leishmaniasis, leprosy, *Salmonella Enteritidis* as the cause of enteric fever, tuberculosis, pulmonary eosinophilosis and cholera, as being of special interest. Plague, relapsing fever, yellow fever, filariasis, dengue and sandfly fever did not present any military problems. It may, however, be added that a great deal of work was done on plague in India during the war. It was found that the mortality due to plague could be lowered with the use of sulphathiazole, sulphadiazine (and later streptomycin), especially when given in combination with anti-serum. It was also observed that a vaccine of living non-virulent organisms gave better protection than a killed vaccine in experimental animals.

MORBIDITY PATTERN

The pattern of morbidity rates in Ceylon was almost the same as in Burma, except for the extent of sickness in some cases.

The major diseases remained the same in Burma as in Ceylon, with the only difference that their individual rates were very much lower. In Egypt, however, enemy action casualties occupied a very important position during the period of hostilities from 1941 to 1943. The total annual morbidity rates were of the order of 603·12 per 1,000 in 1941, 582·34 in 1942, 438·33 in 1943, 409·18 in 1944 and 330·34 in 1945. The major diseases constituted about 30 to 35 per cent. of all casualties each year, except in 1944, when the relevant figure was 28 per cent. Non-enemy action casualties accounted for 92 per cent. of all admissions to hospital in 1941, 96 per cent. in 1942, 94 per cent. in 1943, 98 per cent. in 1944 and about 100 per cent. in 1945. It may be noted that malaria was the most important single cause only in 1943, when the rate was 38·21 per 1,000. In other years this position was occupied by either minor septic conditions or venereal diseases.

During 1940 and 1941, the years of maximum concentration of troops in Sudan and Eritrea, the major causes of morbidity among Indian troops were mainly battle casualties, venereal diseases, dysentery, diarrhoea, minor septic conditions and malaria. Enemy action was responsible for about one-fourth of all casualties in 1941. Venereal diseases, dysentery, diarrhoea and minor septic conditions each caused higher admissions than malaria in that year. During these two years, the overall rate of morbidity was comparatively very low. It was only 59·29 per 1,000 in 1940 (September to December) and 390·76 per 1,000 in 1941.

It seems remarkable that in Persia and Iraq the major diseases should follow an almost similar morbidity pattern, viz. malaria, venereal diseases, minor septic conditions, common cold, dysentery and diarrhoea. This morbidity pattern was disturbed in 1945, when venereal diseases were the cause of maximum admission. Dysentery and diarrhoea, though contiguous, varied somewhat from year to year. Thus malaria remained the most important single cause of hospital admissions almost throughout. Overall morbidity rates continually fell over the period from 742·82 per 1,000 in 1941, to 357·47 per 1,000 in 1945. During the same period the malaria rate was reduced from 117·45 to 26·56 per 1,000. Battle casualties, which were 4·19 per 1,000 in 1941, the year of maximum engagements in this area, were reduced to about 1 per 1,000 for each of the later years. It will be apparent that sick casualties were responsible for the greater part of the overall rate each year. The above-mentioned major diseases fluctuated between ratios of 38 per cent. (in 1945) and 46 per cent. (in 1941) of all admissions. The overall morbidity rates of the B.O.Rs. were consistently higher than those of the V.C.Os. and

I.O.Rs. The incidence rates for B.O.Rs. in respect of venereal diseases, minor septic conditions, dysentery and diarrhoea were also higher than in I.O.Rs. They were, however, lower for malaria and the common cold.

INVALIDMENT

Of the various individual causes of invalidment, tuberculosis occupied a high position. Its rate was never less than 10 per 10,000 and shot up to as high as 17·38 per 10,000 in 1943. It was observed in 1945 that the relaxation of the standards of medical examination of recruits allowed enrolment of many individuals suffering from diseases and defects which often, after a comparatively short period of service, proved to be a cause of invalidment. Large numbers of recruits were invalided with less than four months service from such diseases as advanced pulmonary tuberculosis, partial blindness, deafness and deformities of the limbs. The invalidments due to tuberculosis, mental diseases, respiratory diseases, diseases of bones, joints and muscles, nervous diseases and ear and nose diseases stood out prominently in each year. V.C.Os. and I.O.Rs. were invalided at an increasing rate, from 33·61 in 1939 to 181·84 per 10,000 in 1944. This rate fell slightly to 165·33 per 10,000 in 1945. Until 1943 injuries in action caused invalidments at a rate lower than 1 per 10,000 but after 1943, their rates were 1·50 in 1944 and 4·04 in 1945. The last mentioned figure seems particularly high in this context, though it is a very low rate on the whole, in that year.

AVERAGE CONSTANTLY SICK

The daily average number of constantly sick in Burma and S.E.A.C., Ceylon, Sudan and Eritrea, Egypt and Western Desert and North Africa, Persia and Iraq were 28, 4, 14, 6 and 26 per 1,000 respectively.

On an average about 12,488 beds in the hospitals were occupied daily by V.C.Os. and I.O.Rs. in Burma and S.E.A.C. (excluding Ceylon) in 1943. In other words, 47 soldiers out of every 1,000 were in the hospitals during the year. The highest rate of beds occupied in Ceylon was 5·5 per 1,000 in 1944, in the Sudan and Eritrea 22 per 1,000 in 1941, in Egypt, the Western Desert and North Africa 8·2 per 1,000 in 1945, and in Persia and Iraq 30·6 per 1,000 during 1942. These rates are for active operational years on various fronts.

WAR WOUNDS AND SICKNESS

A study of morbidity and mortality figures of the Second World War shows that many more men were disabled by sickness than by enemy action. The striking wastage of man-power by disease is illustrated by the high ratio of sickness to war wounds, especially on the Indo–Burma front. The average ratio of war wounds to sickness (taking into consideration years of active operations only) was about 1 : 67. The ratio of mortality due to war wounds and to that due to sickness in different theatres was on an average 1 : 18, the highest being 1 : 36 in Persia and Iraq during 1941. The case mortality among the war wounded (deaths among those admitted for war wounds) on the Burma front during 1942–45 varied from 4·0 to 4·7 per cent. The case mortality among the war wounded in Egypt, Western Desert and North Africa, Sudan and Eritrea and Persia and Iraq was 0·3–13·0 per cent. 0·9–8·3 per cent. and 1·6 per cent. respectively.

For every soldier wounded on the Indo–Burma front 204 were sick in 1942 and 142 in 1943. The results of preventive measures, especially against malaria, are reflected in the ratio of battle and non-battle casualties in 1944 and 1945 when the ratios came down to 1 : 22 and 1 : 13 respectively. The ratio of casualties due to enemy action and non-enemy action in Ceylon was 1 : 7,264 for the obvious reason that it was not a theatre of active operations. The average ratio in Ceylon during 1942–45 was 1 : 2,872. It is interesting to observe that in 1943 and 1944, on the Indo–Burma front statistically every soldier was more than once in hospital, admission rates being 1,196·10 and 1,040·91 per 1,000 respectively. The figures also reveal that in 1944 (the year of highest admission rate due to war wounds) in the Indo–Burma theatre of operation, out of each group of 1,000 soldiers about 48 were wounded, and of these 48 less than 3 died of war wounds. In 1943 (the year of low war wound admission rate) about 9 of every 1,000 soldiers were admitted with war wounds and of these less than one died of injuries due to enemy action. The relationship of casualties due to enemy and non-enemy action in Egypt, the Western Desert and North Africa (except for 1945) varied from 1 : 11 to 1 : 42. During 1945, the ratio was 1 : 479. This relatively high rate of sickness as compared with war wounds during 1945 was due to the fact that operational activities had practically ceased. It may be added that the ratio would have been more or less similar to that of Ceylon, but owing to the decreased rate of general morbidity the figure for sickness was only 479 times that of war wounds. In the Sudan and Eritrea the ratio of war wounds to sickness was 1 : 68 in 1940, 1 : 3 in 1941 and 1 : 364 in 1942. The ratio of war wounds to sickness in Persia and Iraq was: 1 : 176 in 1941, 1 : 929 in 1942, 1 : 612 in 1943, 1 : 594 in 1944 and 1 : 446 in 1945. The average ratio of war wounds to sickness in Aden and Scotra was 1 : 1,396 (the highest figure being 1 : 1,769 in 1942). This was due to the area being a non-operational one, as in the case of Ceylon.

VOLUNTARY ORGANISATIONS

The Second World War once again demonstrated the valuable rôle of voluntary organisations. Reference may be made to the International Red Cross, the Joint War Organisation of the Indian Red Cross Society and St. John Ambulance Association, St. Dunstan's for the War Blinded, the Queen Mary's Technical School for Disabled Indian Soldiers, the Friends Ambulance Unit in Burma, China and India, the American Field Service, the Seagrave Hospital, the Indian Tea Association, Eastern Frontier Projects and many other organisations and individuals who provided much needed assistance to the soldiers, sailors and airmen.

EPILOGUE

Medicine in peace and war is basically similar. Military medicine increases in complexity with the rapidly changing character of environments peculiar to the war situation, the weapons with which it is conducted and the urgency of action. New medical problems are created not only by the congregation of large numbers of people, by terrain and by climate, but also by the conduct of war. For example, the emergence of air power led to the development of aviation medicine, while nuclear weapons lead to radiation medicine. Military medicine becomes a highly specialised service, mobile, flexible and demanding skills in improvisation, technical knowledge and complex logistics. Logistics concern not only the number of trained man-power, transport, tonnage of stores and equipment but also factors such as the number of casualties requiring collection under hazardous circumstances, treatment under difficult conditions, evacuation by various methods, often over difficult country and the conservation of man-power. Consideration of physical, social and epidemiological factors, history, especially medical, and medical geography assume importance, and catastrophies can be avoided if the medical services are consulted at all stages of planning and operations. The skill of the medical leader lies in his explaining to the military commander the impact of medicine on the course of battle and in exploiting all available medical skill and resources, civil and military, to the maximum.

The medical man in war-time is faced with a paradoxical situation. His professional aim is to ameliorate suffering, to prevent sickness and death. At the same time he is linked to the forces of destruction of which he becomes an integral part for the defence of his country. His is an outstanding example of sacrifice and service for his fellow men. There is no doubt that the medical services, despite the unpreparedness, administrative and organisational difficulties, the almost insurmountable difficulties imposed by shortage of medical man-power and material and the lack of adequate executive authority vested in the Medical Services in the early stages of the war, made a major contribution to victory.

The manner and circumstances in which the medical services tackled the problems that war presented hold valuable lessons for those who may be called upon to assume similar responsibilities in the future.

The late Prime Minister Nehru, when addressing the Official Medical Historians Liaison Committee on March 5, 1952 in New Delhi, stressed the wide repercussions of these lessons in peace as well as in war. The benevolent effects of medicine, both in war and peace, have profound social consequences. The application of the art of healing can reach the minds and hearts of men and do much to prevent those conflicts which set us back on the path of progress.

PART VI

The Geneva Conventions

THE GENEVA CONVENTIONS*

Some suggested amendments to meet the conditions of modern warfare.

W. Franklin Mellor

Secretary, Commonwealth Official Medical Historians Liaison Committee.

THE emblem of the Red Cross on a white background, the reversed colours of the Swiss national flag, was adopted as a compliment to the founder of the Red Cross, Monsieur Henri Dunant and, under the Geneva Conventions, it is a sign which confers immunity from attack on its wearer and the occupants of buildings or vehicles exhibiting it. To this end International Conventions designed to protect specified individuals from the grosser hardships of war have been evolved. These Conventions have been successively elaborated and adapted to meet new conditions.

At the end of the Second World War the Conventions were revised by a Diplomatic Conference and their provisions conferring immunity on those engaged in the treatment of the wounded and sick, on land or sea and those relating to the treatment of prisoners-of-war and to the protection of civilian persons in time of war are set out in the Geneva Conventions of 12th August, 1949.†

With one important exception the Conventions were for the most part observed by the belligerents during the Second World War. Inevitably there were times when the Red Cross was not respected and so failed to offer cover for 'protected personnel' but such incidents were few and for some of them acceptable explanations can be found.

The exception concerned the Japanese, whose attitude to the Conventions, to which their Government had not subscribed, was entirely different from that of the other belligerents. Against the Japanese the Red Cross afforded little or no protection. This has been fully recorded and is now well known. Here one is confronted with a different conception of man's obligations to his fellow man, of the sanctity of human life and of the attitude to suffering. In such circumstances it is questionable whether any value can be attached to a signature on behalf of any nation whose philosophy and culture include no real belief in the principles to which it may have subscribed its name. As long as this

---

* This Note embodies suggestions made by the Commonwealth Official Medical Historians in the light of their researches into the events and medical problems of the Second World War.

† Cmd. 8033. H.M.S.O., London. 1950.

cleavage of spirit remains the full application of the humanitarian
Conventions can never be universally effective.

To aid in their remaining effective as fully as possible in those areas
of the world where the symbol of the Red Cross is respected, the
Commonwealth Official Medical Historians of the Second World War
offer a few suggestions which might be taken into consideration when
the Geneva Conventions are being redrafted.

I. PROTECTION AFFORDED BY THE RED CROSS EMBLEM FROM AERIAL ATTACK

During the Second World War some attacks from the air were made
on persons, buildings, vehicles, ships and aircraft bearing the Red
Cross. The circumstances in which these attacks occurred need to be
examined carefully for they have rendered the Geneva Cross largely
ineffectual as a means of protection.

All kinds of aircraft were used on a large scale—fighters, fighter-
bombers, torpedo aircraft, rocket-firing aircraft, light, medium and
heavy day and night bombers. Their performance was continually
being improved. They flew much faster and climbed much higher than did
those of the First World War. In that war pilots flew low enough and
slowly enough to see Red Cross markings on the ground and had ample
time to note them on other aircraft. That was no longer possible during
the Second World War and is even less so today.

Other factors which operate in modern warfare and which add to the
physical difficulties of identifying the Red Cross Emblem from the air
include:

(*a*) Attacking aircraft always make use of sun or cloud cover. This
shortens the time available for accurate identification.

(*b*) With the increasing use of radar the pilot of an attacking aircraft
may never see the target, all control being automatic or from the
ground.

(*c*) At night identification by visual methods is impossible.

(*d*) To avoid countermeasures by ground defences, pilots either
attack from a very great height or carry out dive-bombing, using
cloud cover until the last moment or approaching at great speed
and at zero feet.

(*e*) Even in perfect weather colour on the ground is difficult to
distinguish at heights over 5,000 feet, when the entire ground
surface looks a homogeneous shade of blue—rather as moorland
appears in the distance on a sunny day; even with close observation,
therefore, it would be very difficult to pick out the standard
Red Cross* as displayed by, for example, a field hospital.

---

* 40 ft. by 40 ft. in size.

(f) In low level attacks the pilot is too intent on the work in hand and the avoidance of low hazards, such as electric pylons and cables, to notice details such as identification marks on buildings.

(g) Attack by ground defences will cause the pilot to take evasive action which will interfere with meticulous viewing of the ground.

(h) High level bombing attacks are often delivered above cloud by the use of radar without the pilot ever seeing the ground.

(i) Bombing error from either high or low level can be very considerable in certain circumstances and buildings out of the target area may be affected.

(j) The position of the sun can sometimes cause dazzle, which completely obscures detail in a target.

Thus the Geneva Cross is no longer a shield against attack from the air and the time seems to have come when a more effective substitute must be found.

It is suggested that a possible alternative would be to match the new method of attack with new means of identification, as, for example, the use of an international radio beacon call sign, emitting impulses on a frequency agreed by the Signatories to the Conventions and known as the Red Cross Frequency. Such a beacon could be adopted by all ground medical installations, hospital trains and ships and by aircraft being used as air-ambulances. There is a risk that such beacons would provide navigation marks for enemy attack—a risk that might well have to be taken.

In cases where medical installations, such as Casualty Air Evacuation Units, must be in very close proximity to legitimate military targets, or when, in large scale advances and retreats ambulances are mixed indiscriminately with fighting vehicles on congested roads, the use of camouflage would appear to offer the safest course to adopt.

2. 'FLYING DOCTORS'

During the Second World War many medical officers accompanied war planes on operational sorties. A medical officer, concerned with the needs of flying personnel, must know the conditions under which crews operate. To do this he must fly with them. It is only in this way that the reactions of aircrew can be seen and assessed and advances made in such fields as the prevention of fatigue and eyestrain and the most effective use of oxygen.

It is suggested that provision should be made in the Conventions that any medical officer who falls into enemy hands while engaged in this work on an operational sortie shall not lose the full protection to which he is entitled under the Conventions.

3. USE OF AIRCRAFT TO REMOVE CASUALTIES FROM LARGE
   ISOLATED UNITS IN ENEMY TERRITORY.

On several occasions during the Second World War, particularly in
the Far East, considerable forces were cut off by the enemy (e.g., the
'Boxes' in Burma) or were introduced by design many miles behind
the enemy lines (the Chindits). In these circumstances supplies were
flown in by freighter aircraft, which were used on their return flight to
evacuate casualties. Similar situations arose on other fronts where the
battle was one of movement by fast mechanised and armoured forces.

It is suggested that in contingencies such as these freighter aircraft,
when used as air-ambulances or for ferrying medical supplies, should
receive protection, even though they are flying across enemy-held
territory or front lines.

4. INFRINGEMENTS OF THE CONVENTIONS THROUGH IGNORANCE
   OF THEIR PROVISIONS

Lack of knowledge of the Geneva Conventions among all ranks led
to some breaches during the Second World War. Redress usually
came when the matter was brought to the notice of higher authorities.

It is suggested that this difficulty might be obviated or, at least lessened
if, in future, every combatant, of every rank had pasted in, or sewn into,
his Pay Book a short, clear and concise summary of his rights and responsibilities under the Conventions. This easily understandable
summary should be identical in all the languages into which it is
translated and be carried by all combatants and 'Protected' persons at
all times.

5. PRISONER-OF-WAR CAMPS

It appears clear from the experience of the Second World War that a
representative of the International Red Cross should be authorised to
act as an independent Resident Observer and Liaison Officer in each
prisoner-of-war, concentration or labour camp. With such an arrangement the execution of the provisions of the Conventions would come
under constant international scrutiny and be better assured.

It is suggested that Signatory and non-Signatory Governments alike
should be invited to accede to this procedure in time of war.

6. POSITION OF MEDICALLY QUALIFIED SCIENTISTS ENGAGED
   IN WAR-TIME WORK UNRELATED TO THE TREATMENT OF THE
   SICK AND WOUNDED

Of increasing and far-reaching importance is the new rôle that the
medical services have come to assume in times of war as a consequence
of the recognised value of the contributions that biological science has
to make. In the early stages of a war the major problems are those

arising from the need to produce in ever-increasing quantity, machines and equipment of ever expanding ingenuity, precision and lethality. Later, the more pressing problems are those which relate to the numbers and quality of men, to their health, efficiency and morale. In the Second World War the Fighting Services leaned heavily upon the physical sciences for the production of weapons and equipment. Later, they were forced by shortage of man-power to turn to the biological and social sciences for the satisfaction of their most urgent requirement— the provision of personnel capable of making the fullest possible use of the tools with which physical science had so abundantly endowed them.

It became increasingly necessary to undertake investigations that were overtly concerned with matters relating to the human aspects of offensive training and tactics and with the design, development and employment of lethal weapons. Such information could only be supplied by the physiologist and psychologist. The great majority of these possessed medical qualifications and were therefore within the Army Medical Services. These activities and interests were such as could not be pursued by the doctor in uniform claiming the shelter of the Geneva Cross. For this reason, in the United Kingdom, they became the responsibility of the Scientific Adviser to the Army Council, to whose department they were transferred.

It is manifest that such as are engaged in work of this kind should not be enrolled in military medical services, wearing the badges that make the wearer a 'protected' person; they should belong to a combatant branch and make no claim to protection. Their presence within the Medical Services would render uncertain the protection afforded by the Conventions to personnel concerned exclusively with the care of the wounded and sick in war-time, as at present defined by the Conventions.

It is suggested that a new Article should be added to the Conventions stating that medically qualified scientists engaged in activities unrelated to the treatment of the sick or wounded, or to the prevention of disease, shall not be regarded as 'protected personnel'.

The Red Cross is a symbol of man's compassion and those whose task it is to work under its protection take on a truly positive and beneficent rôle in warfare. The cynic might suggest that the increasing power and speed of engines of war will nullify all their endeavours. That is not so. In war there has grown up a strong adherence of participants to a pattern of conduct. International Law, even if not always codified, has great force and weight and goes much of the way in setting moral as well as legal standards. Despite time and change the Geneva Cross and all it stands for will always be a powerful help to man in time of war.

(95349) Dd.'132727 K 10 9/68 Hw.